*Levick's*

# Introduction to Cardiovascular Physiology

## Sixth Edition

Levick's

# Introduction to Cardiovascular Physiology

## Sixth Edition

**Neil Herring** BM BCh MA DPhil (Oxon) MRCP FHRS
Associate Professor and BHF Intermediate Fellow, University of Oxford, UK
Tutor and Fellow, Keble College, Oxford, UK
Consultant Cardiologist, Oxford University Hospital NHS Foundation Trust, UK

**David J. Paterson** MSc (WAust) MA DPhil (Oxon) DSc (WAust) FRSB FPhysiol Hon FRSNZ
Professor of Cardiovascular Physiology & Hon. Director, Burdon Sanderson Cardiac Science Centre, Oxford, UK
Head of Department of Physiology, Anatomy & Genetics, University of Oxford, UK
Tutor and Fellow, Merton College, Oxford, UK

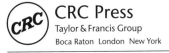

CRC Press
Taylor & Francis Group
Boca Raton London New York

CRC Press is an imprint of the
Taylor & Francis Group, an **informa** business

CRC Press
Taylor & Francis Group
6000 Broken Sound Parkway NW, Suite 300
Boca Raton, FL 33487-2742

© 2018 by Taylor & Francis Group, LLC
CRC Press is an imprint of Taylor & Francis Group, an Informa business

No claim to original U.S. Government works

Printed on acid-free paper

International Standard Book Number-13: 978-1-4987-3984-9 (Paperback)

**Visit the Taylor & Francis Web site at**
**http://www.taylorandfrancis.com**

**and the CRC Press Web site at**
**http://www.crcpress.com**

**Printed and bound in Great Britain by Bell and Bain Ltd, Glasgow**

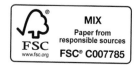

We dedicate this book to our pupils and teachers and the British Heart Foundation
who have supported our research

We shall not cease from exploration, and the end of all our exploring will be to arrive where we started and know the place for the first time.

*T. S. Eliot*

# Contents

Contents

Contents

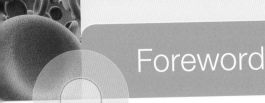

# Foreword

The seventeenth century physician William Harvey is known for his treatise on the motion of the heart and blood which was published in *De Motu Cordis et Sanguinis* in 1628. Harvey's description of experiments on many species unequivocally dispelled the long-held Galenic dogma that blood passed from the right side of the heart to the left through invisible pores in the ventricular septum. Harvey, using the scientific method, proved there were no such pores and that blood had to move in a circular fashion. He showed that the amount of blood pumped by the heart per minute was many times the volume of blood. Harvey wrote

*...I found the task so truly arduous... that I was almost tempted to think... that the movement of the heart was only to be comprehended by God. For I could neither rightly perceive at first when the systole and when the diastole took place by reason of the rapidity of the movement...*

Anyone who has watched the heart beat, has placed a catheter in an artery or has recorded electrical activity of the heart cannot be anything other than awestruck by the power and complexity of the heart and circulation. It is, indeed, as Harvey wrote an almost spiritual experience. Interestingly, William Harvey was Warden of Merton College at Oxford University in 1645; the same institution where Professors Paterson and Herring now reside.

The publication of the sixth edition of *Introduction to Cardiovascular Physiology* continues a rich tradition of education in cardiovascular science at Oxford. This edition is more than just an introductory textbook. It is, in our opinion, one of the most well-written and well-organized cardiovascular textbooks ever published. It is comprehensive in its scope and at the same time elegant in its simplicity.

This book covers every aspect of the heart and circulatory system. Chapters build on the anatomical, biophysical, molecular and cellular underpinning of function, to the integrative nature of each component of cardiovascular regulation. Objectives are clearly laid out, experimental evidence is highlighted, technical advances are discussed and the clinical relevancy of each component is nicely woven into the fabric of the book. One of most outstanding aspects of this text are the figures, which are both drawn *de novo* and are modified from existing research and review publications. Figures are vibrant and well described. They help to bring the reader along a logical sequence in understanding the progression and complexity of each component.

Clearly, the book is not a novel by any means, but in reading this text, one wonders how it will end. The authors pull the physiological concepts presented in chapters 1–16 together with two additional chapters devoted to adaptive responses of the cardiovascular system to environmental stimuli, exercise, aging and pathological situations. Chapter 19 and 20 focus on the experimental approach and modern techniques in cardiovascular research. Importantly, the denouement of the scientific discussions is the section on clinical case scenarios and problem-based learning, an excellent way for medical students to utilize prior information to understand the scientific rationale underpinning diagnosis and therapeutics.

This book should be part of the library of every medical student and physiology graduate student, even if their major interest is not cardiovascular science. In our opinion, there is no better compendium of basic cardiovascular function than Levick's sixth edition. We are certain that this book will surely entice young readers and new entrants in the field to seriously consider a career in cardiovascular medicine and science!

**Irving H. Zucker, PhD**
*Department of Cellular and Integrative Physiology*
*University of Nebraska Medical Center*
*Omaha, NE, USA*

**Kalyanam Shivkumar, MD, PhD**
*UCLA Cardiac Arrhythmia Center &*
*Neurocardiolgy Research Program of Excellence*
*Division of Cardiology*
*Department of Medicine*
*University of California Los Angeles*
*Los Angeles, CA, USA*

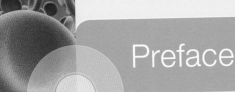

# Preface

The first edition of *An Introduction to Cardiovascular Physiology* by Rodney Levick was published in 1990 and has been an invaluable textbook for generations of medical and biomedical science students. Over the years, we have used its many editions extensively and with great fondness as both students and teachers. We were therefore honoured to be asked to take this textbook forward into its sixth edition. Given Professor Levick's huge contribution to this work, we have renamed the sixth edition as *Levick's Introduction to Cardiovascular Physiology*.

One of the first things we did when embarking on this task, was to consult a broad group of peers and students about what they thought of the previous edition. The striking and consistent finding was that the textbook was much loved and required 'evolution rather than revolution'. Nevertheless, we have introduced several key changes. The content has been widely updated given recent advancements, particularly in chapters 4, 5, 9, 12, 13, 15, 16, 17 and 18, and the clinical cases. Although this is a textbook of cardiovascular physiology rather than pathology, it is hard to ignore the significant progress in the areas of arrhythmias, hypertension and heart failure, and we have highlighted how this has improved our understanding of the underlying physiology. We are very grateful to Dr Julian Ormerod, and Associate Professors Ian Le Grice, Keith Dorrington, Pawel Swietach, Paolo Tammaro, and Professors Kim Dora, Chris Garland, Jeff Ardell, Bruce Smaill Peter Kohl and David Eisner for their help in this regard, although any inaccuracies remain our own. We are also grateful to Dr Nikant Sabharwal, Dr Jim Newton, and Associate Professors Oliver Rider and Rajesh Kharbanda for providing clinical images from the Oxford Heart Centre. We have updated the references for every chapter, and while the focus is on reviews from leading experts in the field, we have included classical original research papers throughout. References are now ordered with the most contemporary reviews and studies cited first. By popular demand, the figures and illustrations are now in full colour throughout the book.

The biggest change we have made is the addition of two substantial new chapters (19 and 20). There is a vast gulf to be bridged between reading a traditional textbook and reading original research papers, as required when undertaking a bachelor's degree in medical science, research dissertation or a higher research degree. It is overcoming this hurdle that students consistently find the most difficult aspect of their education. The aim of chapters 19 and 20 is to introduce students to the experimental approach and design, and simply describe the increasingly complex techniques that are used in cardiovascular research as well as their advantages and limitations. We hope that this will widen the book's use and audience, and build on the outstanding foundations it has provided in teaching cardiovascular physiology over the last 28 years.

**Neil Herring and David J. Paterson**
*Burdon Sanderson Cardiac Science Centre*
*Department of Physiology, Anatomy and Genetics*
*University of Oxford*
*February 2018*

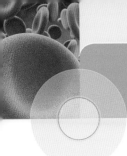

# A note on active and problem-based learning

One may read a textbook and gain a primary level of understanding of its subject; however, to master the subject thoroughly *active, 'hands-on' engagement with the subject matter is essential*. In other words, *self-expression* is vital. One may think one knows the subject, but there is nothing like verbalizing and answering questions to promote learning. To this end, learning objectives are given at the start of each chapter, and five clinical cases, with questions and answers, are included at the end of the book.

## USING THE LEARNING OBJECTIVES

Active learning is traditionally promoted by essay writing and question and answer tutorials. The *learning objectives* at the start of each chapter can be used as short-notes questions (e.g. 'draw and explain a delayed afterdepolarization', Chapter 3). The sections containing the answers are cited after each learning objective. Another excellent way to learn actively is to write brief notes on each learning objective. The notes will prove invaluable when revising for examinations.

## PROBLEM-BASED LEARNING

To encourage active learning and clinical relevance, medical schools increasingly base teaching on clinical cases, although this has serious drawbacks, as well as advantages, in the early years. Clinical cases are challenging, because they bring together many different topics and cut across many different chapters of the book. For example, heart failure (Case 1) involves altered cardiac excitation–contraction coupling (Chapters 3 and 18), the Frank–Starling law of the heart (Chapter 6), haemodynamics (Chapter 8), microvascular fluid exchange (Chapter 11) and extrinsic control of the circulation (Chapter 14). Clinical cases are therefore presented at the end of the book, with questions and answers linked to the main text.

# List of abbreviations

| | |
|---|---|
| 20-HETE | 20-hydroxyeicosatetraenoic acid |
| 5HT | 5-hydroxytryptamine |
| AAV | adeno-associated virus |
| ABP | arterial blood pressure |
| ABPI | ankle–brachial pressure index |
| ACE | angiotensin-converting enzyme |
| ACh | acetylcholine |
| ADH | antidiuretic hormone |
| ADP | adenosine diphosphate |
| AF | atrial fibrillation |
| AHN | anterior hypothalamic nucleus |
| Ang II | angiotensin II |
| ANP | atrial natriuretic peptide |
| ANS | autonomic nervous system |
| AP | arterial pressure |
| ARB | angiotensin receptor blocker |
| AT | atrial tachycardia |
| AT1R | angiotensin II receptor type 1 |
| ATP | adenosine triphosphate |
| AV | atrioventricular |
| AVA | arteriovenous anastomosis |
| aVF | augmented Vector Foot |
| aVL | augmented Vector Left |
| AVNRT | atrioventricular nodal re-entry tachycardia |
| aVR | augmented Vector Right |
| AVRT | atrioventricular re-entry tachycardia |
| $BK_{Ca}$ | large or big conductance $Ca^{2+}$-dependent $K^+$ channel |
| BNP | brain natriuretic peptide |
| BP | blood pressure |
| CaMKII | $Ca^{2+}$-calmodulin-dependent protein kinase II |
| cAMP | cyclic adenosine monophosphate |
| Cas | CRISPR-associated system |
| CCP | critical closing pressure |
| CeBF | cerebellar blood flow |
| CFP | cyan fluorescent protein |
| cGMP | cyclic guanosine monophosphate |
| CGRP | calcitonin gene-related peptide |
| CICR | $Ca^{2+}$-induced calcium release |
| CNP | C-type natriuretic peptide |
| CO | cardiac output |
| COP | colloid osmotic pressure |
| COX | cyclooxygenase |
| CRAC | $Ca^{2+}$-release activated channel |
| CRISPR | clustered regularly interspaced short palindromic repeats |
| crRNA | CRISPR RNA |

| | |
|---|---|
| CRTD | cardiac resynchronization defibrillator |
| CRTP | cardiac resynchronization therapy pacemaker |
| CSF | cerebrospinal fluid |
| CT | computed tomography |
| CVLM | caudal ventrolateral medulla |
| CVP | central venous pressure |
| CVS | cardiovascular system |
| DAD | delayed afterdepolarization |
| DAG | diacylglycerol |
| DAPI | 4',6-diamidino-2-phenylindole |
| DD | diastolic depolarization |
| DIC | differential interference contrast |
| DMNV | dorsal motor nucleus of the vagus |
| DRG | dorsal root ganglion |
| dsRNA | double-stranded RNA |
| EAD | early afterdepolarization |
| ECG | electrocardiogram |
| EDD | end-diastolic dimension |
| EDH | endothelium-dependent hyperpolarization |
| EDHF | endothelium-derived hyperpolarizing factor |
| EDP | end-diastolic pressure |
| EDV | end-diastolic volume |
| EET | epoxyeicosatrienoic acid |
| EJP | excitatory junction potential |
| ELISA | enzyme-linked immunosorbent assay |
| EMG | electromyogram |
| ENaC | epithelial $Na^+$ channel |
| eNOS | endothelial nitric oxide synthase |
| EPAC1 | exchange protein directly activated by cAMP 1 |
| ESC | embryonic stem cell |
| ESD | end-systolic dimension |
| ESV | end-systolic volume |
| ET | endothelin |
| FOXC2 | forkhead box protein C2 |
| FRET | Förster resonance energy transfer |
| GA | general anaesthetic |
| GAG | glycosaminoglycan |
| GDP | guanosine diphosphate |
| GFP | green fluorescent protein |
| GI | gastrointestinal |
| $G_i$ | inhibitory GTP-binding protein |
| GP | glycoprotein |
| GPCR | G protein-coupled receptor |
| gRNA | guide RNA |
| $G_s$ | stimulatory guanosine triphosphate-binding protein |
| GTN | glyceryl trinitrate |

| | | | |
|---|---|---|---|
| GTP | guanosine triphosphate | NAd | noradrenaline |
| HCN | hyperpolarization-activated cyclic nucleotide-gated | NAME | nitroarginine methyl ester |
| | | NANC | non-adrenergic, non-cholinergic |
| HCN4 | hyperpolarization-activated cyclic nucleotide-gated 4 | NET1 | norepinephrine transporter 1 |
| | | NET2 | norepinephrine transporter 2 |
| HDL | high-density lipoprotein | NF | natriuretic factor |
| HEK 293 | human embryonic kidney cells 293 | NO | nitric oxide |
| HF-PEF | heart failure with preserved ejection fraction | NOAC | novel oral anticoagulant |
| HIF-1 | hypoxia inducible factor 1 | NOS | nitric oxide synthase |
| HIP | hydrostatic indifferent point | NOS1-AP | nitric oxide synthase adaptor protein |
| HIT | high-intensity training | NP | natriuretic peptide |
| HPV | hypoxic pulmonary vasoconstriction | NPY | neuropeptide Y |
| HR | heart rate | NTS | nucleus tractus solitarius |
| HRE | HIF responsive element | NZGH | New Zealand genetically hypertensive (rat) |
| IAP | intra-abdominal pressure | OVLT | organum vasculosum lamina terminalis |
| ICA | internal carotid artery | $P_A$ | arterial pressure |
| ICC | intercellular cleft | $PaCO_2$ | partial pressure of $CO_2$ |
| ICD | implantable cardioverter defibrillator | PAF | platelet-activating factor |
| ICP | intracranial pressure | PAG | periaqueductal grey |
| ICS | intercostal space | PAH | para-aminohippuric acid |
| $IK_{Ca}$ | intermediate-conductance $K_{Ca}$ | $PaO_2$ | partial pressure of $O_2$ |
| IL-1β | interleukin-1β | $PAO_2$ | arterial $PaO_2$ |
| IML | intermediolateral nucleus | $P_C$ | capillary pressure |
| IOI | integrated optical intensity | PCI | percutaneous coronary intervention |
| $IP_3$ | inositol 1,4,5 trisphosphate | PCR | polymerase chain reaction |
| iPSC | induced pluripotent stem cell | $P_d$ | diastolic artery pressure |
| ITP | intrathoracic pressure | PDE2 | phosphodiesterase 2 |
| JAM | junctional adhesion molecule | PDE5 | phosphodiesterase 5 |
| JGA | juxtaglomerular apparatus | PDGF | platelet-derived growth factor |
| $K_{ATP}$ | ATP-dependent $K^+$ channel | PDGF-β | platelet-derived growth factor subunit B |
| $K_{Ca}$ | $Ca^{2+}$-activated $K^+$ channel | PE | phycoerythrin |
| $K_{ir}$ | inwardly rectifying $K^+$ channel | PECAM | platelet endothelial cell adhesion molecule |
| $K_v$ | voltage-dependent $K^+$ channel | PG | prostaglandin |
| LA | left atrium | $PGI_2$ | prostacyclin |
| LCN | local circuit neuron | $P_i$ | internal pressure |
| LD | lamina densa | $PI_3$ | phosphatidyl inositol-3 |
| LDH | lactic dehydrogenase | $P_iO_2$ | inspired partial pressure of $O_2$ |
| LHA | lateral hypothalamic nucleus | $PIP_2$ | phosphatidyl inositol bisphosphate |
| L-NMMA | L-N$^G$-monomethylarginine | PKA | protein kinase A |
| loxP | locus of X-over P1 | PKB | protein kinase B |
| LPBN | lateral parabrachial nucleus | PKC | protein kinase C |
| LQTS | long- QT syndrome | $PLA_2$ | phospholipase $A_2$ |
| LR | lamina rara | PLB | phospholamban |
| LV | left ventricle | PLC | phospholipase C |
| LVEDP | left ventricular end-diastolic pressure | $P_o$ | external pressure |
| MAP | mean arterial pressure | PP1 | protein phosphatase 1 |
| MCA | middle cerebral artery | PP2 | protein phosphatase 2 |
| MCP | mean circulatory pressure | PROX1 | prospero homeobox protein 1 |
| MHC | myosin heavy chain | PRU | peripheral resistance unit |
| MLC | myosin light chain | $P_v$ | venous pressure |
| MLCK | myosin light chain kinase | pVHL | von Hippel–Lindau tumour suppressor |
| MPI | myocardial perfusion imaging | PVN | paraventricular nucleus |
| MRI | magnetic resonance imaging | RA | right atrium |
| MSA | muscle sympathetic activity | Rac1 | Ras-related C3 botulinum toxin substrate 1 |
| MVC | maximal voluntary contraction | Rap1 | Ras-related protein Rap-1A |
| NA | nucleus ambiguus | RCT | randomized controlled trial |

| | | | | |
|---|---|---|---|---|
| REM | rapid eye movement | | TGF-$\beta$ | transforming growth factor $\beta$ |
| RhoA | Ras homolog gene family, member | | TNF$\alpha$ | tumour necrosis factor $\alpha$ |
| RNAi | interference RNA | | tPA | tissue plasminogen activator |
| ROC | receptor-operated channel | | TPR | total peripheral resistance |
| ROCK | Rho-associated protein kinase | | TRE | Tet response element |
| RV | right ventricle | | TRP | transient receptor potential |
| RVEDP | right ventricular end-diastolic pressure | | TRPC | transient receptor potential channel |
| RVLM | rostral ventrolateral medulla | | tTA | tetracycline transactivator |
| RVMM | rostroventral medial medulla | | TTX | tetrodotoxin |
| RyR | ryanodine receptor | | TXA$_2$ | thromboxane A$_2$ |
| SA | sino-atrial | | US | ultrasound |
| SAC | stretch-activated channel | | VCAM-1 | vascular cell adhesion molecule 1 |
| SERCA2a | sarcoplasmic/endoplasmic reticulum Ca$^{2+}$ ATPase 2a | | VDCC | voltage-dependent Ca$^{2+}$ channels |
| | | | VE-cadherin | vascular endothelial cadherin |
| SFO | subfornical organ | | VEGF | vascular endothelial growth factor |
| SGP | sialoglycoprotein | | VEGFA | vascular endothelial growth factor A |
| SHR | spontaneously hypertensive rat | | VEGFR-2 | vascular endothelial growth factor receptor 2 |
| siRNA | small interfering RNA | | VEGFR-3 | vascular endothelial growth factor receptor 3 |
| SK$_{Ca}$ | small-conductance K$_{Ca}$ | | VF | ventricular fibrillation |
| SNP | single nucleotide polymorphism | | VIP | vasoactive intestinal polypeptide |
| SOC | store-operated channel | | VSCC | voltage-sensitive Ca$^{2+}$ channel |
| SON | supraoptic nucleus | | VSM | vascular smooth muscle |
| SP | substance P | | VT | ventricular tachycardia |
| SPECT | single-photon emission computerized tomography | | vWF | von Willebrand factor |
| | | | WCT | wide complex tachycardia |
| SR | sarcoplasmic reticulum | | XDH | xanthine dehydrogenase |
| SSA | skin sympathetic activity | | XO | xanthine oxidase |
| SV | stroke volume | | YFP | yellow fluorescent protein |
| SV40 | simian vacuolating virus 40 | | ZO-1 | zonula occludens-1 |
| Tet | tetracycline | | | |

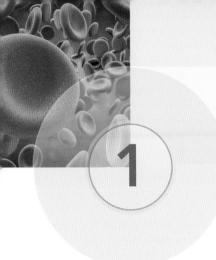

# Overview of the cardiovascular system

## LEARNING OBJECTIVES

*After reading this chapter you should be able to:*

- outline the distance limitation of diffusive transport and the roles of diffusion versus convection in oxygen transport (1.1);
- list the differences between the pulmonary and systemic circulations (1.3);
- sketch out how blood pressure (BP), velocity and total cross-sectional area change from the aorta to the microcirculation and to the vena cava (Figure 1.10);

- write down the basic law of flow (1.5) and apply it to work out the main source of vascular resistance;
- sketch the structure of the blood vessel wall (Figure 1.11) and state the roles of the endothelium, elastin, collagen and vascular smooth muscle;
- name five main functional categories of blood vessel and state their roles (1.7);
- define a 'portal circulation' and explain its functional value (1.8).

The heart and blood vessels evolved to transport $O_2$, nutrients, waste products and heat around the body rapidly. This is crucial for tissue viability, so the cardiovascular system (CVS) develops at an early stage in the embryo. However, very tiny organisms lack a circulatory system – their $O_2$ needs are satisfied by diffusion from the environment. Even large animals, such as humans, rely on diffusion for the transport of materials between the bloodstream and cells. Why, then, do we also need a CVS? The answer lies in the distance limitation of diffusive transport.

## 1.1 DIFFUSION: ITS VIRTUES AND LIMITATIONS

### Diffusion is brought about by a molecular 'drunkard's walk'

Diffusion is a 'passive' transport process, in the sense that it is driven by the rapid, random thermal motion of molecules, not by metabolic pumps. When a concentration gradient is present, the randomly directed step movements of individual solute molecules result in a net movement down the concentration gradient, i.e. a net diffusive transport (Figure 1.1).

### Distance dramatically slows diffusion

The rate of diffusive transport is important because nutrient delivery must keep up with cellular demand. Fortunately, diffusive transport is very fast over short distances; for example, diffusion from a capillary to tissue cell, a distance of ~10 μm, takes only ~50 ms. Unfortunately, as Einstein showed, the time $t$ that randomly jumping particles take to move a distance $x$, in one specific direction, increases as the square of the distance:

$$t \propto x^2 \qquad (1.1)$$

Thus, diffusion is incredibly slow over long distances (Table 1.1). Over 1 cm, which is the thickness of the human left ventricle wall, diffusion would take more than half a

**Compartment A     Compartment B**

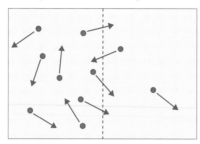

Time 1 (before random jumps):
concentration A = 8, concentration B = 2,
concentration difference ΔC = 6

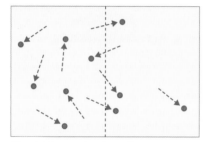

Time 2 (after random jumps):
concentration A = 6, concentration B = 4,
concentration difference ΔC = 2

**Figure 1.1** Spontaneous molecular steps in a random direction lead to a net movement of solute molecules (dots) down a concentration gradient. The probability of a randomly directed step from compartment A to B is greater than from B to A because there are more solute molecules in A than B, per unit volume. Note that an individual molecule, such as the top one in B, may move 'uphill', that is, into the more concentrated solution. Net diffusion is thus the result of unequal 'uphill' and 'downhill' fluxes.

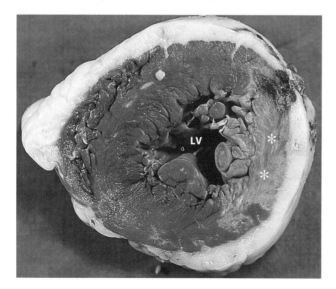

**Figure 1.2** Section of the human left ventricle after a coronary thrombosis; the myocardium has been stained for a muscle enzyme. The pale area (marked with two *) is an 'infarct', an area of muscle damaged or killed by lack of $O_2$. The pallor is due to the escape of enzymes from the dying muscle. The infarct was caused by a coronary artery obstruction, which halted the convective delivery of $O_2$. $O_2$ diffusion from blood in the main chamber (LV) is unaffected, yet only a thin rim of adjacent tissue (~1 mm) survived. (Courtesy of the late Professor M Davies, St George's Hospital Medical School, London.)

**Table 1.1** Time taken for a glucose molecule to diffuse specified distance in one direction

| Distance (x) | Time (t)[a] | Example *in vivo* |
|---|---|---|
| 0.1 μm | 0.000005 s | Neuromuscular gap |
| 1.0 μm | 0.0005 s | Capillary wall |
| 10.0 μm | 0.05 s | Capillary to cell |
| 1 mm | 9.26 min | Skin, artery wall |
| 1 cm | 15.4 h | Left ventricle wall |

*Source:* Einstein A. *Investigations on the Theory of the Brownian Movement* (trans. by Fürth R, Cowper AD, 1956). New York: Dover Publications; 1905.
[a] Einstein's equation states $t = x^2/2D$, where D is solute diffusion coefficient (glucose, $0.9 \times 10^{-5}$ cm$^2$ s$^{-1}$ at 37° C; oxygen in water, $3 \times 10^{-5}$ cm$^2$ s$^{-1}$, 37° C).

day. Sadly, nature often reminds us that Einstein's equation is correct. Figure 1.2 shows a section through a human heart after a coronary artery thrombus (clot) had blocked off the blood supply to the left ventricle wall. The pale area is cardiac muscle that died from lack of $O_2$, even though the adjacent chamber is full of oxygenated blood. The patient died because just a few millimetres reduced the rate of diffusive $O_2$ transport to a level that was too low to support life.

## Convection provides fast transport over long distances

For distances of >0.1 mm, a faster transport system is clearly needed. The CVS provides this (Figure 1.3). The CVS still relies on **diffusion** to transport $O_2$ across the short distance between gas and blood in the lungs; however, the absorbed $O_2$ is then washed rapidly along in a stream of pumped fluid, covering a large distance in seconds (~3 cm s$^{-1}$). This form of transport is called bulk flow or **convective transport**, and its energy source is the contraction of the heart. Convective transport carries $O_2$ a metre or more from the lungs to the smallest blood vessels of the human extremities in ~30 s, whereas diffusion would take more than 5 years! Nevertheless, diffusion takes over as the dominant transport process for the final 10–20 μm from blood to cell.

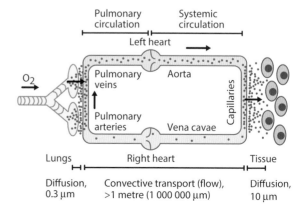

**Figure 1.3** Overview of the human circulation, highlighting the relative roles of diffusion and convection in $O_2$ transport.

## 1.2 FUNCTIONS OF THE CARDIOVASCULAR SYSTEM

There are four main functions of the cardiovascular system, as detailed below:

- The primary function of the CVS is the **rapid convective transport** of $O_2$, glucose, amino acids, fatty acids, vitamins, drugs and water to the tissues, and the rapid washout of metabolic waste products from the tissues (e.g. carbon dioxide ($CO_2$), urea, creatinine).
- The CVS is also a **control system**. It distributes hormones to the tissues and secretes bioactive agents itself (natriuretic peptides, renin, nitric oxide, endothelin, prostaglandins).
- The CVS is crucial for **body temperature regulation** because it transports heat from deep organs to the skin surface and regulates heat loss from the skin.
- In **reproduction**, the CVS provides the hydraulic mechanism for genital erection.

## 1.3 THE CIRCULATION OF BLOOD

The heart consists of two synchronous, muscular pumps, the right and left ventricles (Figure 1.4). Each pump is filled from a contractile reservoir, the right or left atrium. The right ventricle pumps deoxygenated blood through the pulmonary trunk to the lungs (Figure 1.5). Four pulmonary veins return oxygenated blood from the lungs to the left side of the heart, completing the short, low-pressure **pulmonary circulation**. The left ventricle pumps an equal volume of oxygenated blood to the tissues of the body. The tissues extract some of the $O_2$, and the partly deoxygenated blood returns via two great veins, the superior and inferior vena cava, to the right atrium. This completes the long, high-pressure **systemic circulation**. One-way valves in the heart and veins ensure that blood follows the circular pathway described earlier, as first demonstrated by the physician **William Harvey**. Harvey's originality and groundbreaking introduction of experimentation into physiology and medicine disproved the earlier ebb-and-flow dogma of the previous 1000 years. His elegant work is delightfully described in his book *De Motu Cordis* (trans. *Concerning the Motion of the Heart*, 1628).

### The right heart perfuses the pulmonary circulation

Venous blood enters the right atrium from the superior and inferior vena cava, and flows on through the tricuspid valve into the right ventricle. The ventricle is composed mainly of cardiac muscle and fills with blood while the muscle is relaxed. Cardiac relaxation is called **diastole** (pronounced dia-stol-i). Contraction, or **systole** (pronounced sis-tol-i), then follows. Systole pumps some of the ventricular blood into the pulmonary trunk at a low pressure. The trunk divides into the right and left pulmonary arteries, which supply each lung. Progressive branching leads to tiny blood vessels, called capillaries, in the walls of the minute air sacs of the lungs (alveoli). Here gases are exchanged by diffusion. Inhaled $O_2$ diffuses into the blood, raising its $O_2$ content from ~150 mL $L^{-1}$ (mixed venous blood, resting human) to ~195 mL $L^{-1}$. At the same time, $CO_2$ diffuses out of the blood into the alveolar gas and is exhaled. The oxygenated blood returns through the pulmonary veins and passes through the left atrium into the left ventricle.

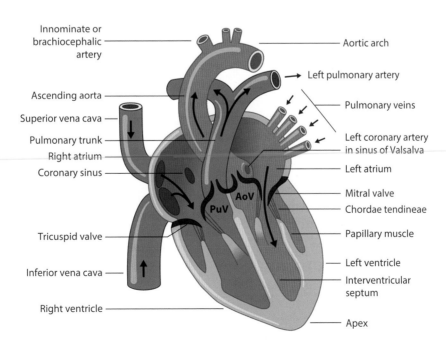

**Figure 1.4** Structure of the mammalian heart. Red indicates oxygenated blood; blue is deoxygenated blood. AoV, aortic valve; PuV, pulmonary valve.

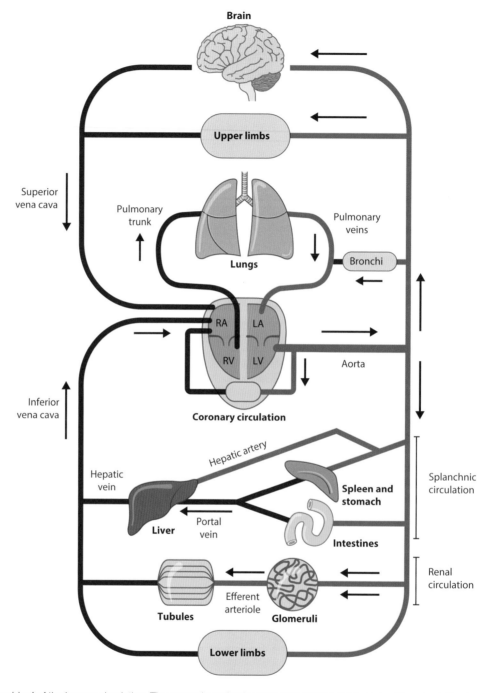

**Figure 1.5** 'Plumbing' of the human circulation. The systemic and pulmonary circulations are in series. The circulation to most systemic organs is in parallel (e.g. brain, myocardium, limbs), but the liver and renal tubules have an 'in-series' or portal blood supply. Bronchial venous blood drains anomalously into the left atrium, slightly desaturating it. Red, oxygenated blood; blue, deoxygenated blood; RA, right atrium; LA, left atrium; RV, right ventricle; LV, left ventricle.

## The left heart perfuses the systemic circulation

The left ventricle contracts at the same time as the right ventricle and ejects the same volume of blood, but at a much higher pressure. The blood flows through the aorta, which gives off the major named branches shown in Figure 1.6. Repeated arterial branching leads, ultimately, to millions of microscopic, thin-walled capillaries (Figure 1.7). Here the ultimate function of the CVS is fulfilled; dissolved gases, glucose and other metabolites diffuse between the capillary blood and the cells of the body. The deoxygenated blood returns through a convergent system of veins that, broadly speaking, accompany the named arteries and drain into the superior and inferior vena cava (Figure 1.8).

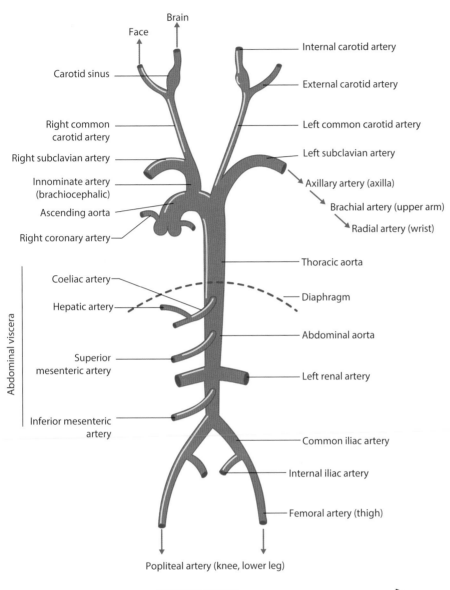

Brain

Face

Carotid sinus

Right common carotid artery

Right subclavian artery

Innominate artery (brachiocephalic)

Ascending aorta

Right coronary artery

Abdominal viscera

Coeliac artery

Hepatic artery

Superior mesenteric artery

Inferior mesenteric artery

Internal carotid artery

External carotid artery

Left common carotid artery

Left subclavian artery

Axillary artery (axilla)

Brachial artery (upper arm)

Radial artery (wrist)

Thoracic aorta

Diaphragm

Abdominal aorta

Left renal artery

Common iliac artery

Internal iliac artery

Femoral artery (thigh)

Popliteal artery (knee, lower leg)

**Figure 1.6** Simplified anatomy of the human arterial system. Paired thoracic intercostal arteries are not shown.

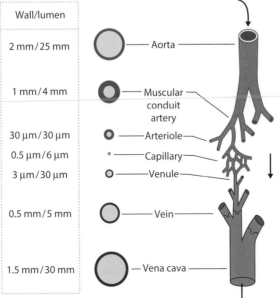

Wall/lumen

2 mm/25 mm — Aorta

1 mm/4 mm — Muscular conduit artery

30 µm/30 µm — Arteriole

0.5 µm/6 µm — Capillary

3 µm/30 µm — Venule

0.5 mm/5 mm — Vein

1.5 mm/30 mm — Vena cava

**Figure 1.7** Different types of blood vessel, seen in cross section and plan view. The thickness of the wall relative to the lumen is greatest in arterioles, though the ratio varies with vascular tone. The large vessel dimensions apply to humans. (After Caro CG, Pedley TJ, Schroter RC, et al. *The Mechanics of the Circulation*. Oxford: Oxford University Press; 1978; and Burton AC. *Physiology and Biophysics of the Circulation: an Introductory Text*. Chicago, IL: Year Book Medical Publishers; 1972.)

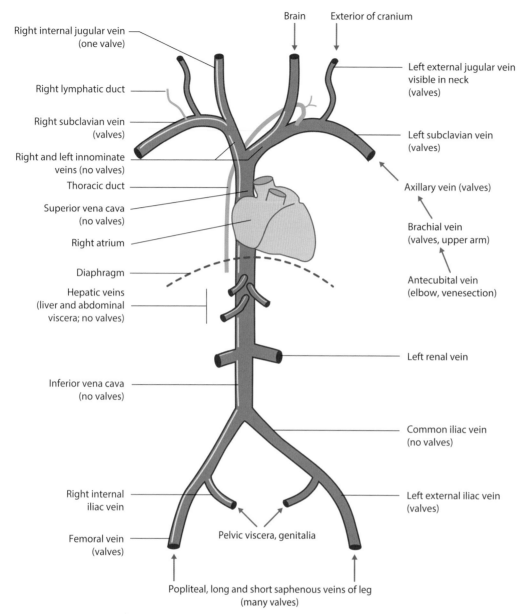

Right internal jugular vein (one valve)

Brain    Exterior of cranium

Left external jugular vein visible in neck (valves)

Right lymphatic duct

Right subclavian vein (valves)

Left subclavian vein (valves)

Right and left innominate veins (no valves)

Thoracic duct

Axillary vein (valves)

Superior vena cava (no valves)

Brachial vein (valves, upper arm)

Right atrium

Diaphragm

Antecubital vein (elbow, venesection)

Hepatic veins (liver and abdominal viscera; no valves)

Left renal vein

Inferior vena cava (no valves)

Common iliac vein (no valves)

Right internal iliac vein

Left external iliac vein (valves)

Femoral vein (valves)

Pelvic viscera, genitalia

Popliteal, long and short saphenous veins of leg (many valves)

**Figure 1.8** Simplified anatomy of the human venous system. Valves occur in limb veins but not central veins. The drainage of the main lymphatic vessels, the thoracic and right lymphatic ducts, into the neck veins, is shown. The lymphatic system develops as an outgrowth of the venous system during embryogenesis.

## 1.4 CARDIAC OUTPUT AND ITS DISTRIBUTION

Cardiac output is defined as the volume of blood ejected by one ventricle in 1 min. Cardiac output therefore equals **stroke volume** (the volume ejected per contraction) multiplied by **heart rate** (the number of contractions per minute). In a resting adult, the stroke volume is typically 70–80 mL and the heart rate is 60–75 bpm. Resting cardiac output is thus ~75 mL × 70 min$^{-1}$, or ~5 L min$^{-1}$. The output can increase greatly in response to increased peripheral $O_2$ demand, rising four- to fivefold during strenuous human exercise. How this increase is brought about, via autonomic nerves and physical distension, is described in Chapters 3–6.

### Cardiac output is distributed in proportion to metabolic and functional demand

As a rough rule, the left ventricular output is distributed to the tissues of the body in proportion to their metabolic rate. For example, skeletal muscle accounts for ~20% of human $O_2$ consumption at rest and receives ~20% of the cardiac output (Figure 1.9). However, this egalitarian principle is overridden in the kidneys because their excretory function requires a high blood flow. The kidneys account for only 6% of human $O_2$ consumption, yet they receive 20% of the cardiac output to generate an adequate excretion of water and urea. Since renal blood flow is so enormous, some other tissues must receive less than their 'fair' share of the cardiac output; surprisingly, cardiac muscle (myocardium) is one of them.

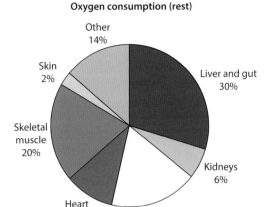

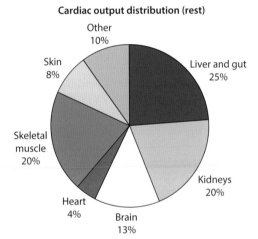

**Figure 1.9** Comparison of $O_2$ usage and cardiac output distribution in humans at rest. (Data from Wade OL, Bishop JM. *Cardiac Output and Regional Flow.* Oxford: Blackwell; 1962.)

To compensate for its relative underperfusion, the myocardium extracts an unusually high proportion of the $O_2$ in arterial coronary blood, namely 65%–75%. The norm for most tissues is only ~25%.

The distribution of cardiac output between tissues is actively adjusted to match changing demands. For example, during exercise the fraction of the output that goes to skeletal muscle can be increased to ~80%. This is brought about by the **vasodilatation** (reversible widening) of tiny arterial vessels in the exercising muscle, called arterioles (Figure 1.7). Vasodilatation allows blood to flow more easily into the active muscle.

## 1.5 INTRODUCING 'HYDRAULICS': FLOW, PRESSURE AND RESISTANCE

### Gradients of pressure drive the flow

What drives blood along a blood vessel? The chief factor is the gradient of blood pressure (BP). Ventricular ejection raises aortic BP to ~100 mmHg above atmospheric pressure. However, pressure in the great veins is close to atmospheric pressure. There is thus a large pressure difference driving blood from artery to vein. The usual cardiovascular units of pressure are 'mmHg above atmospheric pressure' because human BP was, until recently, measured using a mercury column, with atmospheric pressure as the reference or zero level.

Arterial pressure is **pulsatile** because the heart ejects blood intermittently (systole), with rests in-between (diastole). During diastole, the systemic arterial pressure decays from a peak of ~120 mmHg to a trough of ~80 mmHg; pulmonary artery pressure decays from 25 to 10 mmHg (Figure 1.10). This is conventionally written as 120/80 mmHg and 25/10 mmHg, respectively.

### A simple law links flow, pressure and conductance

Although arterial pressure and flow pulsate, many aspects of the circulation are best understood by using **average levels**. To get at the basic rule governing flow, let us consider a steady, non-pulsatile flow of water or plasma along a long rigid tube, driven by a constant pressure head. Under these conditions, flow $\dot{Q}$ is proportional to the pressure drop between the inlet (pressure $P_1$) and outlet (pressure $P_2$):

$$\dot{Q} \propto (P_1 - P_2) \qquad (1.2)$$

(Flow is often represented by a dotted $Q$ in physiology, because $Q$ stands for quantity of fluid and the dot denotes rate of passage in Newton's original calculus notation.) Flow is, by definition, the **volume transferred per unit time**. Flow is thus a rate of transport, and the common expression 'rate of flow' is both tautologous and dimensionally incorrect!

If we insert a proportionality factor, $K$, into equation 1.2, we obtain a basic **law of flow** that tells us how much flow is generated by a given pressure difference:

$$\dot{Q} = K(P_1 - P_2) \qquad (1.3)$$

The proportionality factor $K$ is called the **hydraulic conductance** of the tube. It is a measure of the ease of flow and depends on tube width. The wider the tube, the greater the conductance and the bigger the flow generated by a given pressure gradient. Thus, a large artery has a bigger conductance and carries a bigger flow than a narrow arteriole.

### Resistance is the opposition to flow

Instead of considering ease of flow (conductance), it is often more convenient to quantify the **difficulty** blood experiences in passing through a vessel, that is, the vessel's opposition to flow, or 'hydraulic resistance'. The hydraulic resistance of a tube is simply the inverse of its conductance (ease of flow);

current = voltage difference/electrical resistance.) Darcy's law tells us that $R = (P_1 - P_2)/\dot{Q}$, so **resistance is the difference in mean pressure needed to drive one unit of flow in the steady state**, and its units are mmHg mL min$^{-1}$. The bigger the resistance, the bigger the difference in pressure needed to drive a given flow.

Resistance is low in wide vessels, such as the named arteries and veins, and is high in narrow vessels, such as arterioles. Thus, arteries need only a small pressure drop to drive the cardiac output through them, whereas arterioles need a much bigger pressure drop (Figure 1.10). **The drop in pressure across a given class of vessel is thus an index of its resistance**. In this way we know that, in a resting human, the named large arteries account for only 2% of the total resistance of the systemic circulation; the smallest arteries and the arterioles ~60%; the capillaries ~20%; and the venous system ~15%.

## The resistances of tubes in series summate

When two tubes are joined in series (end-to-end), the resistances add up. Consequently, although the resistance of the aorta is low, the resistance of the systemic circulation is high, because of the additional high resistances of the narrow arterioles and capillaries. (Linkage in parallel is considered in Chapter 8.) The total resistance of the human systemic circulation is ~0.02 mmHg min mL$^{-1}$. The resistance of the pulmonary circulation is only one seventh as much, 0.003 mmHg min mL$^{-1}$, because pulmonary vessels are shorter and wider than their systemic counterparts. Consequently, a low pulmonary arterial pressure suffices to drive the cardiac output through the lungs.

## Active contraction/relaxation of arterioles adjusts peripheral resistance and local blood flow

Darcy's law of flow helps us to understand how the blood flow to a peripheral organ or tissue is regulated; for example, how it is increased to an exercising muscle or a secreting gland. Equation 1.4 shows that there are only two ways to raise blood flow – either the driving pressure must be raised or the vascular resistance reduced. Arterial BP is generally kept within a narrow range by nervous reflexes, so it is normally **changes in vascular resistance that regulate local blood flow**. For example, when we salivate, the blood flow to the salivary gland increases tenfold, because the vascular resistance of the gland is reduced to one tenth of its former value through arteriolar vasodilatation; the arterial pressure driving the flow is unchanged. Changes in vascular resistance are brought about by the contraction and relaxation of the narrow, terminal branches of the arterial system, so we must next consider the structure of blood vessels.

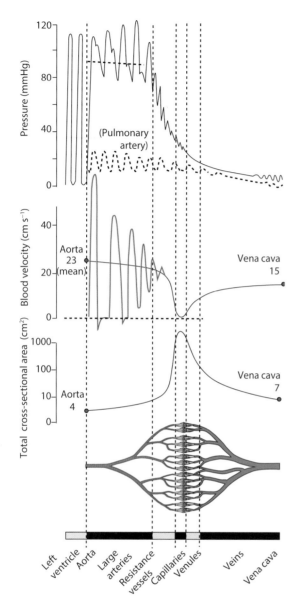

**Figure 1.10** Pressure and blood velocity in the systemic circulation of a resting human. (**Top trace**) The drop in mean pressure across the main arteries (dashed line) is only ~2 mmHg. The large pressure drop across the terminal arteries and arterioles (diameter 30–500 μm) shows that they are the main resistance vessels. The low pulmonary pressure profile is also shown. (**Middle trace**) Pulsation of blood velocity (red line) and change in mean velocity across the circulation (black line). The same blood flow passes each vertical dashed line per minute, namely the cardiac output. Mean velocity is blood flow divided by the cross-sectional area of the vascular bed (see text). (**Bottom trace**) Increase in total cross-sectional area of the circulation in microvessels.

resistance $R$ is $1/K$. Thus, we can rewrite the basic law of flow as:

$$\dot{Q} = \frac{(P_1 - P_2)}{R} \tag{1.4}$$

This is called **Darcy's law** of flow. (As an aide-memoire, note its similarity to **Ohm's law**, i.e. flow of electrical

## 1.6 BLOOD VESSEL STRUCTURE

The aorta gives rise to named conduit arteries (Figure 1.6). These branch repeatedly to form tiny arteries with a diameter of 0.1–0.5 mm, which branch into even narrower vessels of very high resistance, the arterioles (Figure 1.7). Arterioles branch into a vast number of fine, thin-walled capillaries. Capillaries converge to form venules, which converge into small veins, which converge into large, named veins (Figure 1.8).

### Branching slows down the blood

Capillary numbers are colossal; the capillaries of an adult human would girdle the earth if laid end-to-end (40 000 km). The total cross-sectional area of the vascular system at a given branch level is the number of vessels $n$ times the cross-sectional area of an individual vessel, $\pi r^2$. As blood traverses the arterial tree, the increase in $n$ through branching outweighs the reduction in vessel size, $\pi r^2$. Consequently, the **total cross-sectional area of the circulation increases from aorta to capillary bed** (Table 1.2 and Figure 1.10). It then falls as venous vessels converge.

The broadening of the circulation with branching is important, because it slows down the blood, just as the current in a river slows down when the river banks widen. The **blood velocity** (cm s⁻¹) at a branch level equals the total **flow** (cm³ s⁻¹), namely the cardiac output, divided by the total **cross-sectional area** of the branches (cm²): velocity = flow/area. Consequently, capillary blood velocity is ~1/200th of arterial blood velocity because of the vast increase in cross-sectional area (Figure 1.10). The slow blood velocity in systemic and pulmonary capillaries is important, because it gives the red cells **sufficient time to exchange O₂ and CO₂**.

### The vascular wall has three layers

The wall of all blood vessels, except capillaries, consists of three layers (Figure 1.11): the tunica intima (innermost coat); tunica media (middle coat); and tunica adventitia (outer coat).

The **intima** is a sheet of flattened endothelial cells resting on a thin layer of connective tissue. The endothelial layer is the main barrier to the escape of plasma. It also secretes many vasoactive chemicals, including the antithrombotic vasodilator, nitric oxide.

The **media** supplies mechanical strength and contractile power. It consists of spindle-shaped, smooth muscle cells, arranged helically and embedded in a matrix of elastin and collagen fibres. Two sheets of elastin, called the internal and external elastic laminae, mark the boundaries of the media. Intimal endothelial cells send processes through the internal elastic lamina in places, to make contact with smooth muscle cells. These myoendothelial junctions transmit signals from the intima to the media.

The **adventitia** is a connective tissue sheath with no distinct outer border. Its role is to tether the vessel loosely to the surrounding tissue. The adventitia of most vessels contains **sympathetic fibre terminals**. Each terminal has numerous bead-like swellings ('varicosities') that release a vasoconstrictor agent, noradrenaline, which regulates local resistance and blood flow. In large arteries and veins, the adventitia also contains small blood vessels, called **vasa vasorum** (literally 'vessels of vessels'), which nourish the thick media. In limb veins, the adventitia contains **nociceptive nerve fibres**, which mediate the pain of thrombophlebitis.

### Blood vessels develop from endothelium in the embryo

The CVS is the first organ system to form in the embryo, because it is needed to deliver O₂ and nutrients to the developing tissues. Embryonic blood vessel formation, or **vasculogenesis**, is controlled by signalling molecules. Vasculogenesis begins when mesodermal precursor cells express a receptor for **vascular endothelial growth factor A** (VEGF-A). Embryos lacking VEGF-A, or its receptor **vascular endothelial growth factor receptor 2** (VEGFR-2), fail to form blood vessels and die. Vasculogenesis starts at two sites, one in the yolk sac and one in the embryo proper. In the yolk sac, VEGFR-2-positive cells develop into islands of endothelium that enclose blood precursor cells (haemangioblasts). The islands then fuse to form a primary capillary plexus. In the embryo itself, VEGFR-2 cells form endothelial tubes that develop into the heart (see Section 2.1), the dorsal aorta and the primary (cardinal) vein. The primary vessels then develop connections with the capillary plexus. After this, the system remodels under genetic and

**Table 1.2** Comparison of number and size of different types of blood vessels in the dog mesentery[a]

| Vessel | Number | Length (mm) | Diameter (mm) | Total cross-sectional area (mm²) | Volume (% of total) |
|---|---|---|---|---|---|
| Main artery | 1 | 60 | 3 | 7 | 2.5 |
| Arterioles and smallest arteries | 1 380 000 | 1.5–2 | 0.024–0.031 | 739 | 8.1 |
| Capillaries | 47 300 000 | 0.4 | 0.008 | 2378[b] | 5.7 |
| Venules | 2 100 000 | 1.0 | 0.026 | 1151 | 6.9 |
| Small veins | 180 000 | 1–14 | 0.075–0.28 | 1019 | 21.3[c] |
| Large veins | 61 | 39–60 | 1.5–6 | 174 | 46.7[c] |

*Source:* After Schleier J. *Archiv Gesamte Physiologie*. 1918; 173: 172–204.
[a] In the mesentery, unlike most tissues, microvessels are easy to see and therefore quantify.
[b] Capillaries have the largest cross-sectional area and therefore slowest flow.
[c] Veins contain most of the circulating blood volume.

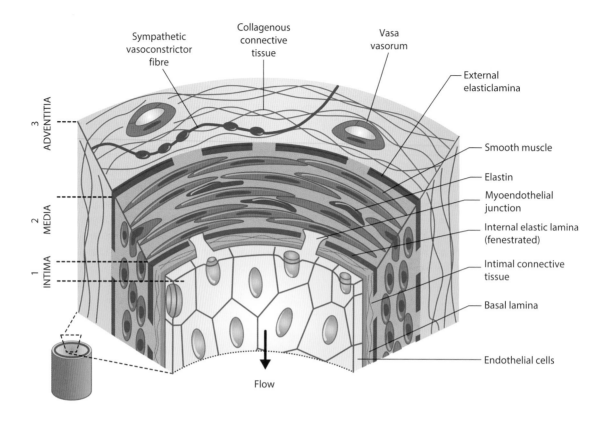

**Figure 1.11** Structure of the wall of a small artery.

haemodynamic influences to form arteries, capillaries and veins. Smooth muscle cells differentiate under the influence of transforming growth factor beta, and are recruited to blood vessels by an endothelial secretion, platelet-derived growth factor. Endothelial membrane proteins called **ephrins** determine which tubes become arteries, as opposed to veins.

Endothelial cell proliferation and VEGF-A also play a key role in the growth of new blood vessels in children and adults, for example, in wound healing and cancer. This is called **angiogenesis** (cf. vasculogenesis); see Chapter 9. The inhibition of angiogenesis in cancers is now a therapeutic target, because cancer cannot grow to a large size without a growing blood supply.

## 1.7 FUNCTIONAL CLASSES OF VESSEL

The mature circulation has evolved along sound economic principles, namely that each vessel must fulfil at least one extra role besides conducting blood. On this basis, the following major classes of vessel are recognized:

- elastic arteries;
- conduit and feed (muscular) arteries;
- resistance vessels;
- exchange vessels;
- capacitance vessels.

In each class of vessel, the structure of the wall is specially adapted to its role, as follows.

## Elastic arteries accommodate the stroke volume and smooth the flow

The heart ejects blood only during systole. Therefore, if arteries were completely rigid, there would be no peripheral blood flow during diastole. This potential problem is circumvented by the distensibility of the largest arteries, which is caused by an abundance of **elastin** (Table 1.3). The extracellular protein elastin is six times more extensible than rubber. The distensibility conferred by elastin enables the aorta, iliac arteries and pulmonary trunk (diameter 1–2 cm in humans) to act as temporary blood storage vessels; they expand by ~10% during each heartbeat to accommodate the ejected blood. The stretched elastin also stores mechanical energy. During diastole, the stored mechanical energy (tension) maintains the arterial BP, which drives the blood through the resistance vessels.

**Table 1.3** Composition of the blood vessel wall (%)

|  | Endothelium | Smooth muscle | Elastin tissue | Collagen |
|---|---|---|---|---|
| Elastic artery | 5 | 25 | 40 | 27 |
| Arteriole | 10 | 60 | 10 | 20 |
| Capillary | 95 | 0 | 0 | 5 (basal lamina) |
| Venule | 20 | 20 | 0 | 60 |

*Source:* After Caro CG, Pedley TJ, Schroter RC, et al. *The Mechanics of the Circulation*. Oxford: Oxford University Press; 1978; and Burton AC. *Physiology and Biophysics of the Circulation: an Introductory Text*. Chicago, IL: Year Book Medical Publishers; 1972.

Thus, even though the heart ejects blood only intermittently, arterial BP does not fall below ~80 mmHg, and blood flows continuously through the peripheral tissues (Figure 1.10).

**Collagen** is the other major extracellular protein of elastic arteries. Collagen fibrils are ~100 times less distensible than elastin. They form a partly slack network in the media and prevent overdistension if BP rises. The elastic artery wall is thus a composite material, similar in many respects to a car tyre; the rubber/elastin allows expansion up to a certain volume, beyond which increasing tension in inelastic fibres prevents overexpansion. As elastin fragments with age, the stiffer collagen increasingly dominates the properties of elastic vessels. This is a process called 'arteriosclerosis' (Chapter 18).

## Conduit and feed arteries deliver blood to the organs

Medium-size conduit arteries include the brachial, radial, femoral, cerebral and coronary arteries (diameter 0.1–1.0 cm in humans). Their tunica media contains more smooth muscle and is thicker, relative to the lumen, than in elastic arteries (Figure 1.7). The thick wall prevents collapse at sharp bends, such as the elbow and knee. The primary role of these **conduit** or **conducting arteries** is to conduct the flow from the elastic arteries to smaller arteries that feed the resistance vessels (**feed arteries**).

Conduit and feed arteries have a rich sympathetic innervation and can change their diameter actively. **Dilatation** facilitates the local increase in blood flow to skeletal muscle during exercise. **Contraction** reduces peripheral blood flow, spectacularly so in diving mammals. **Vasospasm** is an intense and sustained contraction of conduit arteries. This can be lifesaving in accidents, as demonstrated by a motorcycle crash victim brought into the Accident and Emergency department with one leg severed at the knee. Although the popliteal artery was torn in half, it was scarcely bleeding because shed blood platelets had triggered vasospasm. This prevented the patient from bleeding to death. Less beneficial is the cerebral artery vasospasm evoked by cerebral haemorrhage, which can cause a stroke, and the vasospasm of diseased coronary arteries, which can cause cardiac angina at rest (variant angina).

## Pressure falls sharply across resistance vessels (terminal arteries and arterioles)

From the small feed arteries, blood enters narrow terminal arteries (diameter 100–500 μm) and the final branches of the arterial tree, the arterioles (diameter 10–100 μm). These vessels dominate the resistance of the entire circulation, as shown by the **pressure profile of the circulation** (Figure 1.10). Mean BP falls very little along the elastic and conduit arteries (~2 mmHg from the aorta to the radial artery), because their wide diameter creates little resistance to flow. (The odd 'peaking' of the pressure wave in peripheral arteries is explained in Chapter 8.) **The major fall in BP occurs across the terminal arteries and arterioles**. From the law of flow (Equation 1.4), we see that there is only one possible explanation for a large pressure drop. These vessels must offer a large resistance to flow; resistance = pressure drop per unit flow. The terminal arteries and arterioles are therefore called **resistance vessels**.

The **proximal resistance vessels**, namely the terminal arteries, are richly innervated by sympathetic vasoconstrictor nerve fibres, and the muscular wall is thick relative to the lumen (Figure 1.7). The **distal resistance vessels**, namely the terminal arterioles, are poorly innervated, and the media comprises just one to three layers of smooth muscle cells. Some researchers define an arteriole as a vessel with just one layer of muscle, while others define it as an arterial vessel with a diameter of ~100 μm. The terminal arteries and arterioles have a high resistance because the lumen is narrow and the number of vessels is relatively low (Table 1.2).

## Resistance vessels act as 'taps' regulating local blood flow and capillary perfusion

Since the resistance vessels dominate the net resistance to blood flow, they act as the taps of the circulation; that is, they can turn local blood flow up or down to match local demand. When the resistance vessels dilate (**vasodilatation**), resistance to flow falls, so local blood flow increases. Conversely, **vasoconstriction** raises local resistance and reduces local blood flow. The terminal arterioles also adjust the number of capillaries perfused with blood. This task used to be attributed to imaginary 'precapillary sphincters', but it is now generally accepted that true sphincters rarely exist in blood vessels.

## Exchange vessels transfer $O_2$ and nutrients to the tissue

The exchange of $O_2$, $CO_2$, metabolites and fluid between blood and tissue occurs chiefly in the capillaries. **Capillaries** are tiny (diameter 4–7 μm) and very numerous, so most cells lie within 10–20 μm of the nearest capillary. The capillary wall comprises a single layer of endothelial cells 0.5-μm thick, with no media or adventitia. The extreme thinness facilitates the rapid passage of solutes. Some $O_2$ exchange also occurs through the walls of the arterioles, upstream of the capillaries, and some fluid exchange occurs downstream, in the **postcapillary or pericytic venule** (microscopic venule that lacks a complete smooth muscle coat; diameter 15–50 μm). Strictly speaking, therefore, the term **exchange vessel** includes capillaries and microvessels immediately upstream and downstream.

Although capillaries are very narrow, the capillary bed has a surprisingly low resistance to flow, and the pressure drop across it is only ~20 mmHg (Figure 1.10). The low resistance is due to multiple factors: the very large numbers of capillaries running in parallel (Table 1.2); their shortness (~1 mm); and a special kind of flow called bolus flow (Chapter 8). The large cross-sectional area of the capillary bed slows the blood velocity to 0.5–1 mm s$^{-1}$ (Figure 1.10). As a result, the '**transit time**' for a red cell to traverse a systemic capillary is ~0.5–2 s. This allows the red cell sufficient time to unload $O_2$ and take up $CO_2$ from the tissue.

## Arteriovenous anastomoses regulate heat exchange

A few tissues, notably the skin and nasal mucosa, possess wide shunt vessels with a diameter of 20–130 μm that connect arterioles directly to venules, bypassing the capillaries. These shunts are called **arteriovenous anastomoses** (singular, anastomosis). Their thick muscular walls are richly innervated by sympathetic vasoconstrictor fibres. In the skin, they are involved in the control of body temperature, and in the nasal mucosa they help to warm the inspired air. Arteriovenous anastomoses are not common in other tissues.

## Capacitance vessels are venous vessels that act as blood reservoirs

Venules (diameter 50–200 μm) and veins differ chiefly in size and number. The thin wall comprises the intima, a thin media of smooth muscle and collagen, and the adventitia. In limb veins, the intima has **semilunar valves** at intervals, as described by Harvey's teacher, the gloriously named Hieronymus Fabricius ab Aquapendente (Girolamo Fabrizio), at Padua University in 1603. The semilunar valves prevent the backflow of venous blood in the limbs under the drag of gravity (Figure 8.26). By contrast, the large central veins and the veins of the head and neck lack functional valves.

Venules and small veins are more numerous than the corresponding arterioles and arteries (Table 1.2), so their net resistance is low. Consequently, a pressure drop of only 10–15 mmHg is sufficient to drive the cardiac output from the venules to the right atrium.

Because of their large number and size, veins and venules contain about two thirds of the circulating blood at any one instant, and are therefore called '**capacitance vessels**' (Figure 1.12). The volume of blood in this venous reservoir is variable, partly because the thin venous wall is easily distended/collapsed, and partly because many veins are innervated by sympathetic vasoconstrictor fibres. At times of physiological stress, an increase in sympathetic fibre activity causes the capacitance vessels to contract, displacing blood into the heart and arteries to help maintain arterial pressure.

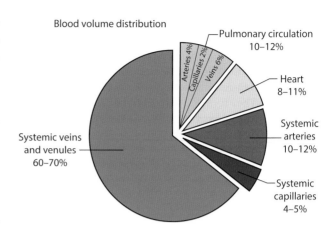

**Figure 1.12** Approximate distribution of 5.5 L of blood in a supine, resting man. On standing, the percentage of blood in the lungs falls by about one third, as does the volume in the heart, while the volume in the peripheral veins increases. (Adapted with permission from Folkow B, Neil E. *Circulation*. New York: Oxford University Press; 1971.)

## 1.8 THE PLUMBING OF THE CIRCULATION

### 'In-parallel' versus 'in-series' circulations

The systemic circulation is divided into specialized, individual circuits, each supplying a specialized tissue or organ (e.g. brain, heart wall, kidneys, intestine). The arterial supply to each organ usually comes from the aorta, so that each organ is supplied directly with arterialized blood. This form of plumbing is called an **in-parallel** arrangement (Figure 1.5). However, in a few organs the main blood supply is the venous outflow from another organ upstream. The two organs are thus connected **in-series**, not in-parallel. This type of arrangement is also called a **portal system**, and it has certain advantages and disadvantages, as follows.

### Portal circulations provide a direct delivery service

The **liver** has the largest portal system in the body. Around 72% of the liver's blood supply comes from the portal vein, which contains deoxygenated venous blood from the intestine and spleen (Figure 1.5). The portal vein enters the liver at the 'porta hepatis' (gateway of the liver), from which the term 'portal system' originates. In addition, the liver receives about a quarter of its blood flow via the hepatic artery; so, its circuitry is partly in-parallel, as well as in-series. Portal systems have the advantage that they transport valuable substances directly from one site to another. For example, the portal vein transports the products of digestion directly from the intestine to the liver, for immediate metabolic processing or storage.

Portal systems also exist in the **kidney**, where effluent blood from the glomerulus supplies the tubules, and in the **brain**, where a portal vein carries releasing hormones from the hypothalamus to the anterior pituitary gland.

However, a portal system has one obvious drawback. The downstream tissue receives partially deoxygenated blood under a reduced pressure head. As a result, the downstream tissue is vulnerable to damage during episodes of hypotension (low arterial pressure). For example, renal tubular damage is a relatively common complication of severe hypotension.

## 1.9 CONTROL SYSTEMS

The heart and blood vessels continually adjust their contractile state to meet the varying demands of daily life, such as standing, exercise, salivation, stress and so on. Such changes are brought about by nervous and endocrine reflexes, and are co-ordinated by the brain. One of the most important cardiovascular reflexes is the **arterial baroreceptor reflex**, which stabilizes arterial BP and thus maintains the pressure driving blood to the brain. The reflex is initiated by stretch receptors, called baroreceptors, in the walls of major arteries. The baroreceptors sense changes in BP and relay the information to the brainstem. This elicits reflex changes in the activity of autonomic nerves controlling the heart and blood vessels.

The resulting changes in cardiac output, peripheral resistance and venous capacitance help restore arterial BP to normal.

Where should we go from here? In a system as complex as the CVS, there is a danger of not seeing the wood for the trees, but the outline provided in this chapter should help avoid this. In Chapters 2–14 (cardiac electricity, haemodynamics and so on), we bump into the trees and even peep under the bark. In Chapters 15–18, we stand back again, to gain a broader perspective of how the system as a whole responds to physiological and medical challenges.

---

**CONCEPT BOX 1.1**

### VASCULAR RESISTANCE AND CONDUCTANCE

- Resistance to flow is defined as the pressure difference needed to drive unit flow through a vessel or set of vessels. This stems from the basic law of flow, Darcy's law: flow = pressure drop/resistance.
- Since the biggest pressure drop occurs across the terminal arteries and arterioles, these vessels are the main site of resistance to blood flow (resistance vessels).
- The resistance vessels regulate local blood flow (their 'tap' function). If they dilate, resistance falls and blood flow to the downstream tissue increases, e.g. in exercising muscle.
- Conductance is the inverse of resistance. If resistance halves, conductance doubles, raising the blood flow.

---

## SUMMARY

- The beating of the heart generates a rapid, convective transport of $O_2$, nutrients, waste products, hormones and heat around the body. The branching vascular tree conveys $O_2$ to within 10–20 μm of most cells; the short final distance is covered by diffusion. Since diffusive transport time increases as the square of distance, tissues die in the absence of convective transport (e.g. myocardial infarction).

- The right ventricle is filled via the right atrium and pumps deoxygenated blood at low pressure (mean ~15 mmHg) through the low-resistance pulmonary circulation for oxygenation. The left ventricle is filled via the left atrium and pumps oxygenated blood at high pressure (mean ~90 mmHg) through the high-resistance systemic circulation.

- Human resting cardiac output is ~5 L min⁻¹. Output equals heart rate (60–70 beats min⁻¹) times stroke volume (70–80 mL). The distribution to individual tissues is controlled by the local resistance vessels. Blood flow is generally allocated to a tissue in proportion to its metabolic activity, but the kidneys receive a disproportionate 20% of the cardiac output to satisfy their excretory role.

- Blood flow $\dot{Q}$ is driven by the pressure drop from artery to vein, $P_A - P_V$. Darcy's law of flow states that $\dot{Q} = (P_A - P_V)/R$, where $R$ is resistance to flow. Resistance is located chiefly in the tiny terminal arteries and arterioles, as shown by the large pressure drop across them. These 'resistance vessels' can actively constrict or dilate to match local blood flow to local demand.

- Other functional categories of vessel are as follows. Elastic arteries (e.g. aorta) receive the intermittently ejected stroke volume and convert it into a continuous, albeit pulsatile peripheral flow. Exchange vessels (capillaries, postcapillary venules) allow solute and water to exchange with the tissue. Capacitance vessels (venules, veins) contain about two thirds of the circulating blood volume and act as a controlled, variable reservoir of blood.

- Except in capillaries, the vascular wall comprises three layers: the tunica intima (endothelium); tunica media (vascular smooth muscle, collagen, elastin); and tunica adventitia (connective tissue, nerve fibres). The smooth muscle regulates the vessel diameter and thereby regulates local blood flow and the distribution of blood volume.

- Vascular smooth muscle is controlled by autonomic nerves, circulating hormones and local factors. Autonomic nerves and circulating hormones also regulate the rate and force of the heartbeat. In this way, the brain and reflexes can control the CVS. For example, the baroreflex stabilizes arterial BP.

- Most specialized circulations (e.g. coronary, cerebral) are plumbed in parallel to each other, so that each organ receives fully oxygenated blood. Portal circulations are in series with an upstream tissue and thus receive venous blood. For example, the portal vein supplies the liver with venous blood from the intestine.

## FURTHER READING

Loukas M, Youssef P, Gielecki J, et al. History of cardiac anatomy: a comprehensive review from the Egyptians to today. *Clinical Anatomy* 2016; **29**(3): 270–84.

Herring N, Paterson DJ. Part II. Section B: Adaptation and response. Adaption and responses: myocardial innervations and neural control. In: Hill J, Olson EN, eds. *Muscle: Fundamental Biology and Mechanisms of Disease*. London: Elsevier; 2012. pp. 275–84.

Aird WC. Discovery of the cardiovascular system: from Galen to William Harvey. *Journal of Thrombosis and Haemostasis* 2011; **9**(Suppl 1): 118–29.

Ritman EL, Lerman A. The dynamic vasa vasorum. *Cardiovascular Research* 2007; **75**(4): 649–58.

Jones EA, le Noble F, Eichmann A. What determines blood vessel structure? Genetic prespecification vs. hemodynamics. *Physiology (Bethesda)* 2006; **21**: 388–95.

Coultas L, Chawengsaksophak K, Rossant J. Endothelial cells and VEGF in vascular development. *Nature* 2005; **438**(7070): 937–45.

Paterson DJ, Coote JH. Neural control of cardiac function. In: Dyck PJ, Thomas PK, eds. *Peripheral Neuropathy*, 4th edn. London: Elsevier; 2005. pp. 217–232.

Fenger-Gron J, Mulvany MJ, Christensen KL. Mesenteric blood pressure profile of conscious, freely moving rats. *The Journal of Physiology* 1995; **488**(Pt 3): 753–60.

Harvey W. *On the Motion of the Heart and Blood in Animals* ('*De Motu Cordis*', trans. by Willis R). London: Prometheus Books, 1993.

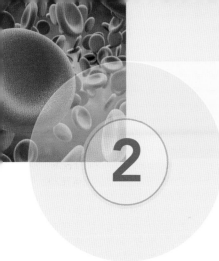

# The cardiac cycle

## 2

### LEARNING OBJECTIVES

*After reading this chapter you should be able to:*
- state the significance of the fibrotendinous ring, the four valves, papillary muscle, ventricle wall thickness and the pacemaker (2.1);
- list the four phases of the ventricular cycle and related valve positions (2.2);
- sketch the changes in atrial and ventricular pressures over the cardiac cycle (Figure 2.5);
- draw a ventricular pressure-volume loop, labelling each side and corner (Figure 2.6);
- define ejection fraction and give typical values (2.2);
- give the relative timings of diastole and systole at rest and during maximal exercise (2.2 and 2.4);
- state the origins of (1) the apex beat (2.1); (2) the heart sounds (2.5); (3) cardiac murmurs (2.5);
- outline briefly the nature and use of echocardiography, cardiac magnetic resonance imaging, nuclear cardiology, cardiac computer tomography and cardiac catheterization (2.6).

An adult human heart weighs only 250–350 g, yet it pumps out ~200 million litres of blood, via ~3 billion ($3 \times 10^9$) contractions over our allotted lifespan, making the heart one of the most heavily used muscles in the body. This chapter describes the mechanical events that generate the heart's truly remarkable output.

## 2.1 THE GROSS STRUCTURE OF THE HEART

The human heart is a four-chambered, hollow muscle, roughly conical in shape, ~12-cm long × 9-cm wide. It lies obliquely across the midline of the chest with the tip of the cone (the **cardiac apex**) behind the fifth left intercostal space (ICS) (Figures 2.1 and 2.2). The heart is rotated around its long axis so that the right atrium and right ventricle form the anterior surface.

The four cardiac chambers are built on a ring of fibrous fatty tissue called the **annulus fibrosus**, located at the atrioventricular junction. The atrioventricular plane is called the **base of the heart**, and it moves towards the apex during systole. The annulus fibrosus has three roles. First, it acts as a mechanical base for the atria and ventricles, which are attached to its upper and lower sides, respectively. Second, it defines four apertures, each containing a valve. Third, it insulates the ventricles electrically from the atria.

The cardiac chambers are lined internally by the **endocardium** (endo = inside), comprising a thin sheet of flattened endothelial cells over connective tissue and, in places, scanty smooth muscle cells. The endothelium also lines the valve surfaces and all blood vessels. The outer surface of the heart is covered by **epicardium** (epi = outside), a thin layer of flattened mesothelial cells over connective tissue. The entire heart is enclosed in a fibrous sac or **pericardium** (peri = around). The narrow, mesothelium-lined space between the epicardium and pericardium contains **pericardial fluid**, which lubricates the cardiac surfaces. The lower surface of the pericardium is fused to the diaphragm. Consequently, each time the diaphragm descends during inspiration, the heart is dragged into a more vertical orientation.

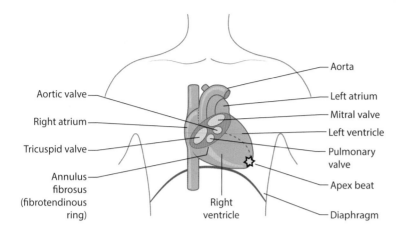

**Figure 2.1** Orientation of the heart and valves in the human thorax. The heart lies obliquely and is rotated so that the right atrium and right ventricle form most of the anterior surface. A fibrotendinous ring forms the 'base' of the heart. The tip of the ventricle forms the 'apex'. The inferior surface and the pericardium (not shown) rest on the central tendon of the diaphragm. The four valves are grouped closely in an oblique plane behind the sternum.

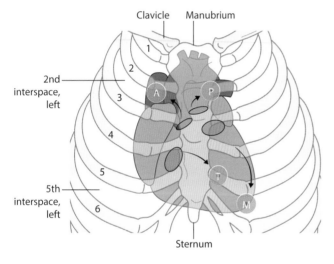

**Figure 2.2** Location of the cardiac valves and auscultation areas. A, aortic valve area; P, pulmonary valve area; T, tricuspid area; M, mitral area.

## Right atrium and tricuspid valve

The right atrium is the thin-walled, muscular chamber that receives the venous return from the two venae cavae and the coronary sinus. The coronary sinus is the main vein draining the heart muscle (Figure 1.4). The **pacemaker**, which is the 'sparking plug' that initiates each heartbeat, is found in the wall of the right atrium, close to the entrance of the superior vena cava.

A valve with three cusps, the tricuspid valve, connects the right atrium to the right ventricle. Each cusp is a thin, baggy flap, ~0.1-mm thick, composed of connective tissue and covered by endothelium. The free margin of each cusp is tethered by tendinous strings, the **chordae tendineae**, to an inward projection of the ventricle wall called the **papillary muscle** (Figure 1.4). The papillary muscles contract and tense the chordae tendineae during systole. This prevents the valve from inverting into the atrium as pressure builds up in the ventricle.

## Right ventricle and pulmonary valve

The free wall of the human right ventricle is ~0.5-cm thick and resembles a pocket tacked around the interventricular septum (Figure 2.3). The expulsion of blood is produced partly by the free anterior wall approaching the septum, as in old-fashioned bellows, and partly by movement of the base (tricuspid valve) towards the apex. The outlet from the ventricle into the pulmonary artery is guarded by the pulmonary valve, which has three equally sized, baggy cusps.

## Left atrium and mitral valve

The left atrium receives blood from the four pulmonary veins and transmits it into the left ventricle through a bicuspid valve. The large anterior and small posterior cusps were thought to look like a bishop's mitre, hence the name mitral valve. The cusp margins are tethered by chordae tendineae to two papillary muscles in the left ventricle, which prevents eversion (Figure 1.4).

## Left ventricle, apex beat and aortic valve

The left ventricle wall is about three times thicker than that of the right ventricle, because the left side must generate higher arterial pressures. Blood is ejected by a reduction in diameter (~40% of stroke volume) and length (~60% of stroke volume). The latter is due chiefly to the contracting muscle dragging the base (mitral plane) towards the apex, rather than the apex towards the base. The muscle fibres are wrapped around the chamber somewhat like a turban, that is, their orientation changes progressively. The innermost or **subendocardial muscle fibres** are orientated longitudinally, running from the base (fibrotendinous ring) to the apex (tip of the left ventricle). The central fibres run circumferentially, the outermost or **subepicardial fibres** again run longitudinally and the intermediate fibres run obliquely (Figure 2.3). When the chamber contracts, it twists forwards and the apex taps against the chest wall, producing a palpable **apex beat**.

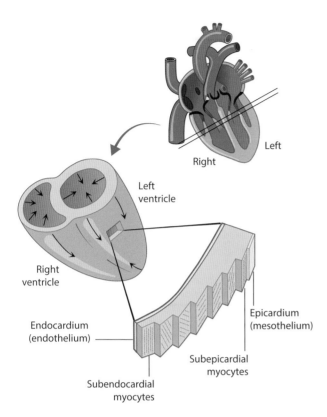

**Figure 2.3** Direction of ventricle wall motion during contraction (middle) and orientation of muscle fibres in the ventricle wall (bottom). The longitudinal shortening of the left ventricle length during systole accounts for ~60% of the stroke volume and is due chiefly to the base (atrioventricular plane) descending towards the apex, rather than the apex moving towards the base.

This is normally felt in the fifth, left ICS, about 10 cm from the midline (the mid-clavicular line). Cardiac enlargement can be detected by the deviation of the apex beat from its normal location.

The root of the aorta contains a three-cusp valve. Occasionally it has only two cusps, and such valves are prone to narrowing (**stenosis**) in later life. Next to each cusp, the root of the aorta bulges out into the **sinuses of Valsalva**. The two coronary arteries originate in the sinuses, just behind the valve leaflets (Figure 1.4).

## Cardiac embryogenesis and congenital cardiac abnormalities

The heart starts out as a simple endothelial tube located between the main embryonic vein and dorsal aorta. A coat of mesodermal cells differentiates into myocardial cells, which begin to contract rhythmically by day 19–20 in humans. The tube folds into an S-shape as it grows, and develops constrictions that delineate a primitive single atrium and ventricle. Each chamber is then subdivided into two. However, the two atria remain connected via an opening, the **foramen ovale** (see Figure 4.1). This shunts most blood from the right

atrium directly into the left atrium, since there is no need to perfuse the lungs for $O_2$ uptake in utero. Right atrial and ventricular blood is well oxygenated because it comes partly from the placental vein. Residual right-side blood that has not been diverted through the foramen ovale passes into the pulmonary trunk, from where much of it flows directly into the aorta through a connection called the **ductus arteriosus**. Thus, most blood bypasses the lungs. The ductus arteriosus and foramen ovale normally close soon after birth, redirecting the entire blood flow from the right side into the lungs for oxygenation.

Because of the intricacy of cardiac development, congenital cardiac abnormalities are relatively common (~1 per 100 live births). They fall into four categories:

- defects in the ventricular septum or atrial septum;
- persistent patent ductus arteriosus;
- aortic coarctation (narrowing of the aorta near the ductus arteriosus insertion);
- transposition of the major vessels. In Fallot's tetralogy, for example, the aortic orifice overlies the ventricular septum, and there is a ventricular septal defect, narrow pulmonary trunk and hypertrophied right ventricle.

Most of these conditions require surgical correction.

## 2.2 THE VENTRICULAR CYCLE

The cycle of atrial and ventricular contraction is called the cardiac cycle (Figure 2.4). The ventricular cycle is divided into four phases, based on the positions of the inlet and outlet valves. Let us begin with the moment when both the atria and ventricles are relaxed (diastole). The timings shown refer to a human cycle lasting 0.9 s, which corresponds to 67 bpm. The information has been acquired by echocardiography (see Section 2.6), cardiac catheterization (see Section 2.6) and electrocardiography (Chapter 5).

### Ventricular filling

| | |
|---|---|
| Duration: | 0.5 s (resting human) |
| Inlet valves (tricuspid, mitral): | Open |
| Outlet valves (pulmonary, aortic): | Closed |

Ventricular diastole occupies nearly two thirds of the cardiac cycle in a resting human, providing ample time to fill the ventricles. Initially, the atria are likewise in diastole, so blood flows passively from the superior and inferior vena cava through the relaxed atria and the open atrioventricular valves into the ventricles. Filling is very fast over the initial 0.15 s (Figure 2.5, ventricle blood volume plot). This **initial rapid-filling phase** displays a curious feature, namely ventricular pressure falls initially, despite blood volume increasing. The explanation is that the relaxing ventricle is recoiling elastically

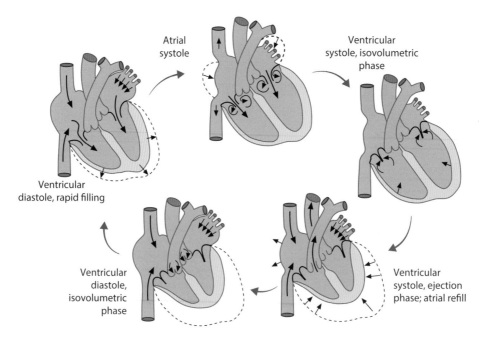

**Figure 2.4** Changes in valves, atrial and ventricular volumes during the cardiac cycle. For clarity, the apex is drawn here as if shifted towards the atrioventricular plane (base) during systole, but imaging shows that much of the longitudinal shortening is due to the base being pulled down towards the apex.

from its deformed end-systolic shape and is thus sucking blood into its chamber in early diastole.

As the ventricle reaches its inherent, relaxed volume, the rate of filling slows down (**diastasis**). Further filling is driven by the venous pressure, which distends the ventricle and causes ventricular pressure to rise gradually.

In the final third of the filling phase, **atrial contraction** pumps extra blood into the ventricle. In young adults, atrial systole boosts the ventricular filling by 10%–20% at rest, but the proportion increases with age, reaching 46% by 80 years. The atrial boost becomes more important during exercise, especially in the young, because the raised heart rate leaves less time for passive ventricular filling.

The volume of blood in a ventricle at the end of its filling phase is called the **end-diastolic volume** (EDV). The EDV is typically ~120 mL in a standing man (Figure 2.5), and ~150 mL supine. The corresponding **end-diastolic pressure** (EDP) is just a few mmHg. EDP is a little higher on the left side than on the right (Table 2.1), because the thicker left ventricle wall requires a higher pressure to distend it. Since pressures are higher in the left atrium than right atrium, congenital defects in the atrial septum in neonates usually result in a left-to-right

flow of blood. Such defects do not, therefore, deoxygenate the arterial blood or cause 'blue baby syndrome'.

## Isovolumetric contraction

| | |
|---|---|
| Duration: | 0.05 s |
| Inlet valves: | Closed |
| Outlet valves: | Closed |

Atrial systole is followed by ventricular systole. This lasts 0.35 s and is divided into a brief isovolumetric phase and a longer ejection phase. As soon as ventricular pressure rises just above atrial pressure, the atrioventricular valves are closed by the reversed pressure gradient. Backflow during closure is minimal because vortices approximate the valve cusps during the late filling phase (Figure 2.4, top). Since the ventricle has temporarily become a closed chamber, the tension of its contracting wall causes the pressure of the trapped blood to rise rapidly. The maximum rate of rise of pressure, $dP/dt_{max}$, is often used as an index of cardiac contractility (Figure 2.5).

## Ejection

| | |
|---|---|
| Duration: | 0.3 s |
| Inlet valves: | Closed |
| Outlet valves: | Open |

When ventricular pressure exceeds arterial pressure, the outflow valves are pushed open and ejection begins. Three quarters of the stroke volume is ejected in the first half of the

**Table 2.1** Mean pressures during the human cardiac cycle (mmHg)[a]

| | Right | Left |
|---|---|---|
| Atrium | 3 | 8 |
| Ventricle | | |
| End of diastole | 4 | 9 |
| Peak of systole | 25 | 120 |

[a] Adult, at rest and supine.

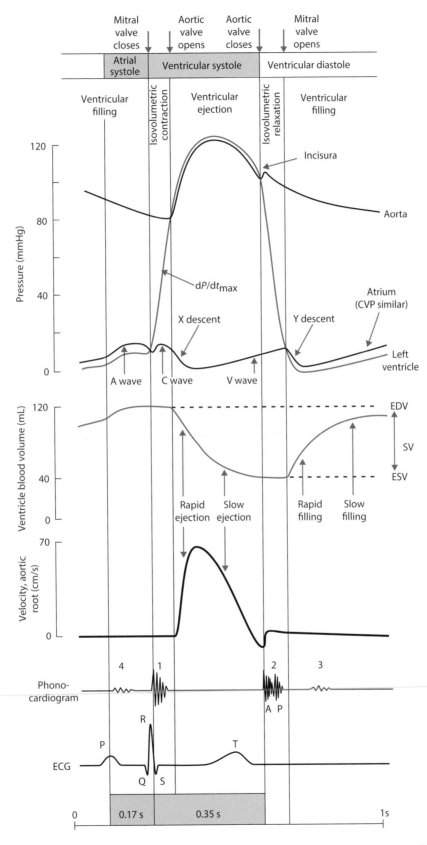

**Figure 2.5** Changes in pressure, volume and flow in the aorta, left ventricle and left atrium during the human cardiac cycle (subject is upright). The right side (not shown) has similar patterns but lower pressures. The jugular venous pulse in the neck and the right atrial wave are like the left atrial wave shown here. The second heart sound splits into aortic (A) and pulmonary (P) components. EDV, end-diastolic volume; ESV, end-systolic volume; SV, stroke volume. (After Noble MI. The contribution of blood momentum to left ventricular ejection in the dog. *Circulation Research* 1968; 23(5): 663–70.)

ejection phase – the **rapid ejection phase** (~0.15 s). Since the blood is ejected faster than it can drain away through the peripheral vessels, most of the stroke volume is accommodated temporarily in the distended elastic arteries. This drives the arterial pressure up to its maximum or 'systolic' level. During ejection, the cusps of the open aortic valve lie close to the entrances to the coronary arteries but do not block them because vortices behind the cusps cause them to 'float' between midstream and the aorta wall. The vortices are due to outpouchings of the root of the aorta, the sinuses of Valsalva (Figure 1.4).

Later in systole, the ejection rate slows down (Figure 2.5, aortic velocity trace). Because the rate at which aortic blood is draining away into the peripheral circulation now exceeds ventricular ejection, pressure begins to fall. Although ventricular pressure soon falls 2–3 mmHg below arterial pressure (Figure 2.5, top trace), the outward momentum of the blood prevents immediate closure of the aortic valve. However, the reversed pressure gradient gradually decelerates the outflow (Figure 2.5, velocity curve), until finally a brief backflow closes the outflow valve. Backflow is normally <5% of the stroke volume, though this figure increases greatly if the aortic valve is leaky (aortic incompetence). Valve closure creates a notch in the arterial pressure trace called the **incisura**. For the rest of the cycle, the arterial pressure declines gradually as blood drains away into the periphery.

Only two thirds of the end-diastolic blood volume is ejected in a resting human. The ejected volume, or **stroke volume**, is 70–80 mL and the residual or **end-systolic volume** is ~50 mL. The proportion ejected, or **ejection fraction**, is the stroke volume divided by EDV, and averages 50%–70% at rest. The end-systolic volume serves as a reserve that can be drawn on to raise the stroke volume and ejection fraction during exercise.

## Isovolumetric relaxation

| | |
|---|---|
| Duration: | 0.08 s |
| Inlet valves: | Closed |
| Outlet valves: | Closed |

When the aortic and pulmonary valves close, each ventricle becomes, briefly, a closed chamber, and the elastic recoil of the deformed, relaxing myocardium causes the ventricular blood pressure (BP) to fall rapidly. When ventricular BP falls just below atrial pressure, the pressure difference pushes open the atrioventricular valves, which terminates the isovolumetric relaxation phase. Blood floods in from the atria (which have themselves been filling up during ventricular systole), and the next cycle begins.

## The ventricular pressure-volume loop

A plot of ventricular BP against ventricular blood volume creates a roughly rectangular, closed loop (Figure 2.6),

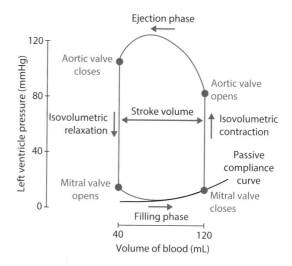

**Figure 2.6** Ventricular pressure-volume loop of the human left ventricle (subject resting, upright).

which proves very useful when discussing left ventricular performance (Chapter 5). The bottom left corner of the loop represents the opening of the mitral valve. Moving anti-clockwise with time, the bottom line shows the progressive filling of the ventricle in diastole. In the initial, rapid-filling phase, the pressure is falling because of the suction exerted by the elastic recoil of the ventricle. In the later, slow-filling phase (diastasis), the line coincides with the passive pressure-volume relation of the relaxed ventricle, or **compliance curve**.

At the onset of systole, the mitral valve closes (bottom right corner) and isovolumetric contraction raises the ventricular pressure (vertical, right side of the loop). When ventricular pressure reaches arterial BP, the aortic valve opens (top right corner). Volume then decreases as ejection occurs (top line, direction right to left). At the end of systole, the aortic valve closes (top left corner) and the ensuing isovolumetric relaxation (vertical left side) leads to mitral opening and repetition of the cycle. Note that each corner of the loop represents a valve opening or closing, and each side represents one phase of the ventricular cycle. The width of the loop is the stroke volume and its area represents the work done per beat.

The atria refill with blood during ventricular systole, so we must consider next the atrial cycle.

## 2.3 THE ATRIAL CYCLE AND JUGULAR VENOUS PRESSURE WAVES

The jugular veins in the neck are in open communication with the right atrium. Consequently, the atrial pressure cycle creates a visible jugular venous pulse, which is readily seen in a slim, recumbent human (Figure 8.27). Inspection of the jugular pulse is part of the standard clinical examination of the cardiovascular system. Pressure recordings in the jugular vein or atrium reveal two main pressure waves per cardiac cycle, the A and V waves, and a third, smaller wave, the C wave (Figures 2.5 and 8.27). There are also two sharp falls in pressure, called the X and Y descents.

The **A wave** is the increase in pressure caused by atrial systole, the 'A' referring to atrial. Atrial systole produces a slight reflux of blood through the valveless venous entrance. This reverses the flow in the venae cavae briefly, and raises central venous pressure (CVP) to its maximum point in the cardiac cycle, typically 3–5 mmHg. Backflow is small, even though there are no venoatrial valves, because the incoming venous blood has considerable inertia.

The next event, the atrial **C wave**, is caused by the bulging of the cusps of the tricuspid or mitral valve into the atrium as the valves close. Since the jugular veins are some distance from the atria, the venous C wave occurs slightly later. The jugular C wave is also caused partly by the systolic expansion of the adjacent carotid artery, hence the nomenclature 'C' for carotid.

After the C wave, the pressure falls sharply – the **X descent**. The X descent is caused by atrial relaxation and by the downwards movement of the base of the ventricle (annulus fibrosus) as the ventricle contracts (Figure 2.3). The downward movement of the base stretches the atria, sucking blood into them, so venous inflow reaches its peak velocity at this point (Figure 8.27).

As the atria fill, atrial pressure rises, creating the **V wave**; 'V' refers to the concomitant ventricular systole. Finally, the atrioventricular valves open and the atrial blood drains rapidly into the ventricles, producing a sharp drop in pressure, the **Y descent**.

Because the right atrial pressure cycle is mirrored in the internal and external jugular veins of the neck, a physician can assess the CVP cycle simply by inspecting the neck of a recumbent subject. What the eye particularly notices are two sudden venous collapses, corresponding to the X and Y descents. Certain cardiac diseases produce characteristic abnormalities of the jugular venous pulse. **Tricuspid incompetence**, for

example, produces exaggerated V waves in the neck, because ventricular systole forces blood back through the leaky valve into the right atrium and neck veins.

## 2.4 ALTERED PHASE DURATIONS WHEN HEART RATE INCREASES

The timings given earlier refer to a resting human. During strenuous exercise, the heart rate can reach 180–200 bpm, and the entire cardiac cycle lasts only about one third of a second (180 bpm). Consequently, each phase of the cycle must be shortened. However, the different phases do not shorten to an equal degree (Figure 2.7). Ventricular systole shortens moderately, to ~0.2 s, leaving a mere 0.13 s for diastole and ventricular refilling. The early rapid-filling phase remains important; diastasis is greatly curtailed, and atrial systole contributes more than at rest. Even so, 0.13 s is close to the minimum time for adequate refilling of the human ventricle. Further increases in heart rate, such as **pathological ventricular tachycardia**, cause cardiac output to decline because the diastolic interval is too brief to refill the ventricle adequately. **Diastolic refilling time thus sets a limit to the maximum useful heart rate**.

## 2.5 HEART SOUNDS AND VALVE ABNORMALITIES

Heart sounds are of great value to clinicians in assessing valve function.

### Normal heart sounds

When a cardiac valve closes, the cusps balloon back as they check the momentum of the refluxing blood. The sudden tensing of the cusps sets up a brief vibration, rather as a sail slaps audibly when filled by a sudden gust of wind. The vibration of the valve is transmitted through the tissues to the chest wall and can be heard through a stethoscope. With healthy valves, only closure is audible; opening is silent, as with a well-oiled door.

Two heart sounds are easily heard per beat – the first and second heart sounds. Heart sounds can be recorded through a microphone placed on the precordium (skin over the heart) and printed out as a **phonocardiogram** (Figure 2.5). The **first heart sound** is a vibration of ~100 cycles/s (100 Hz), caused by the near-simultaneous closure of the tricuspid and mitral valves. The **second heart sound**, of similar frequency, is caused by the closure of the aortic and pulmonary valves.

The second sound is sometimes audibly split into an initial aortic component and a fractionally delayed pulmonary component (**split second sound**). A first sound followed by a split second sound can be imitated as 'lubb-terrupp'. Splitting is most pronounced during inspiration for two reasons:

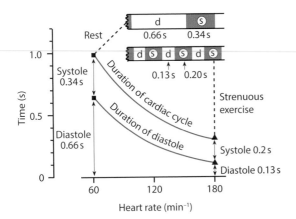

**Figure 2.7** The effect of heart rate on the diastolic period available for filling. Diastole is curtailed more than systole as heart rate increases. d, diastole; Ⓢ, systole. (Courtesy of Professor Horst Seller, University of Heidelberg.)

(1) inspiration lowers intrathoracic pressure, which increases right ventricular filling, which prolongs the right ventricular ejection time and delays pulmonary valve closure; (2) inspiration also expands the lung blood vessels, which transiently reduces the return of pulmonary blood to the left ventricle. This reduces the left ventricular stroke volume, shortens left ventricular ejection time and thus hastens aortic valve closure. Splitting of the second sound is caused, therefore, by equal and opposite movements of the aortic and pulmonary components.

Two further faint rumbles can be detected by phonocardiography, but they are of low frequency and difficult for the untrained ear to detect. The **third heart sound**, common in young people, is caused by the rush of blood into the relaxing ventricles during early diastole. The **fourth heart sound** occurs just before the first sound and is caused by atrial systole.

## Each valve has a separate auscultation (listening) area

All four heart valves lie close together under the sternum (Figure 2.2). Fortunately, each valve is best heard over a distinct, well-separated auscultation area, which is located over the chamber fed by the valve. The **mitral valve** is best heard in the mid-clavicular line of the fourth/fifth left ICS; the **tricuspid valve** in the fifth ICS at the left sternal edge; the **aortic valve** in the second ICS at the right sternal edge; and the **pulmonary valve** in the second ICS at the left sternal edge.

## Valve abnormalities cause cardiac murmurs

Valve abnormalities fall into two classes: incompetence and stenosis. **Valvular incompetence** is a failure of the valve to seal properly. This allows blood to regurgitate through the valve. **Valvular stenosis** is a narrowing of the open valve. As a result, an abnormally high pressure gradient is needed to drive blood through the open valve.

In **aortic valve stenosis**, systolic pressure in the left ventricle is raised, because a large pressure gradient is required to force blood through the narrowed valve (Figure 2.8, top). Also, the aortic pressure, which feeds the coronary arteries, is reduced. The combination of increased ventricular work and reduced coronary $O_2$ supply can cause angina during exercise. (Angina is reversible cardiac pain that arises when the myocardial $O_2$ demand exceeds coronary $O_2$ supply.) Clinical case 5 at the end of this book describes a patient with this condition.

Blood flows through a stenosed or incompetent valve as a turbulent jet, which creates a high-frequency vibration. The vibration can be heard through the stethoscope and is called a **murmur**. Since there are four valves and two pathologies, there are eight basic valve murmurs. Three common examples

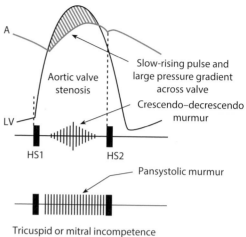
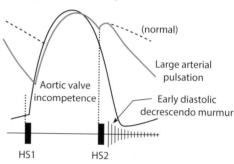

**Figure 2.8** Three cardiac murmurs caused by valve pathology. (Top) Aortic valve stenosis creates a large pressure gradient between the aorta (A) and left ventricle (LV) during ejection (hatched zone). The slow-rising arterial pulse is associated with a crescendo–decrescendo ejection murmur. (Middle) In tricuspid or mitral incompetence, regurgitation from the ventricle to the atrium during systole creates a pansystolic murmur. (Bottom) In aortic valve incompetence, diastolic leakage from the aorta to the LV causes a characteristic wide pulse pressure (systolic minus diastolic) and an early diastolic decrescendo murmur as the pressure head decays. Pressure and time axes as in Figure 2.5.

are illustrated in Figure 2.8. **Aortic valve stenosis** is characterized by a systolic **crescendo–decrescendo murmur** (one that rises and falls as ejection waxes and wanes), loudest over the aortic area (Figure 2.8, top). In **mitral incompetence**, blood regurgitates into the left atrium during ventricular systole. This creates a **pansystolic murmur** (one that extends throughout systole), loudest over the mitral area (Figure 2.8, middle). The sound may be represented roughly as 'lu-shsh-shsh-tupp'. By contrast, **aortic valve incompetence** produces an early **diastolic decrescendo murmur** (one that dies away), sounding roughly like 'lubb-dubbshsh' (Figure 2.8, bottom). Additional noises (clicks and snaps) can also occur.

Murmurs can arise from other causes besides valve disease. A **benign systolic murmur** is common in young people; it is caused by turbulence in the ventricular outflow tract. Benign systolic murmurs are common during pregnancy, strenuous exercise and anaemia (Section 8.2). Ventricular septal defects can also cause murmurs.

## 2.6 CLINICAL ASSESSMENT OF THE CARDIAC CYCLE

The human cardiac cycle is assessed at the bedside by examining five physical signs, namely:

- the arterial pulse (to assess heart rate and force);
- systolic and diastolic arterial BP;
- the jugular venous pulse;
- the apex beat;
- the heart sounds.

If pathology is suspected, more specialized investigations may be undertaken, as follows.

### Electrocardiography

The electrocardiogram (ECG) is a cutaneous recording of cardiac electrical events, which is described fully in Chapter 5. Here, we simply note the relation of the ECG waves to the cardiac cycle (Figure 2.5). The ECG **P wave** is produced by electrical activation of the atria, so it marks the onset of atrial contraction. The **QRS complex** is produced by electrical activation of the ventricles, so it is followed almost immediately by the onset of ventricular contraction and the first heart sound. The **T wave** is produced by the electrical recharging of the ventricles. Since this marks the onset of diastole, the T wave is closely followed by the second heart sound.

### Non-invasive imaging: echocardiography, magnetic resonance imaging, nuclear cardiology and computed tomography

#### Echocardiography

**Echocardiography** is a non-invasive tool that records the motion of the heart walls and valves. A beam of ultra-high-frequency sound is directed across the heart from a precordial emitter, namely a piezoelectric crystal emitting 1000 brief pulses of ultrasound per second (Figure 2.9). Between each microsecond pulse, there is a millisecond 'listening' interval, during which sound reflected by the chamber walls and valve cusps is collected. The reflected sound is computer-processed to build up a picture of cardiac structure and motion as follows.

In **two-dimensional (2-D) mode**, an anatomical image of a slice through the heart is displayed at successive instants

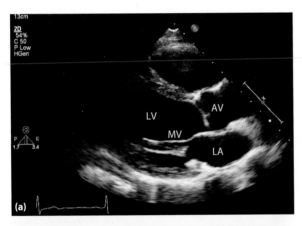

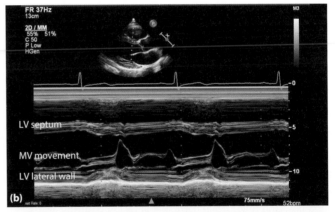

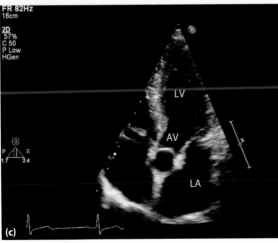

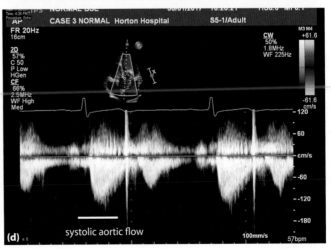

**Figure 2.9** Transthoracic echocardiography images. **(a)** A two-dimensional (2-D) image in the parasternal long axis view shows the left atrium, left ventricle (LV), and aortic (AV) and mitral valves (MV). **(b)** M-mode shows the motion of the mitral cusps and walls of the left ventricle over time along the dotted line in the 2-D figure image at the top. **(c)** An apical five-chamber view shows the LV and AV and **(d)** allows a Doppler flow measurement to be taken through the AV during systole. The electrocardiogram is shown as a green trace in panels **(a)**, **(c)** and **(d)**.

Table 2.2 Echocardiography results for a normal human left
ventricle (LV)[a]

| LV interventricular septal thickness | 0.6–1.2 cm |
| End-diastolic internal diameter | 3.9–5.3 cm (female) |
| | 4.2–5.9 cm (male) |
| Ejection fraction | >55% |
| Aortic valve area | >2.0 cm² |

[a] Values from the British Society of Echocardiography guidelines for valve and chamber quantification.

in time. This produces a moving image of the valve leaflets and heart wall, and reveals pathologies such as valve lesions, abnormal wall motions (e.g. infarcts) and left ventricular hypertrophy (wall thickening). Also, ejection fraction and cardiac contractility can be estimated from the change in left ventricular dimensions over the cycle (Table 2.2). Figure 2.9 shows still 2-D images.

In **M-mode** the positions of the anatomical features are plotted against time. This gives a linear display of the motion of the heart walls and valve leaflets, as shown in Figures 2.9b and 6.24.

Additional information is extracted from the frequency of the reflected ultrasound, which is altered by the moving blood cells (**Doppler shift**). From the Doppler shift, a colour-coded map of blood flow through a valve and chamber can be constructed and the velocity measured over time as shown in Figure 2.9d. This provides a non-invasive measure of the degree of stenosis or regurgitation across valves.

## Magnetic resonance imaging

**Magnetic resonance imaging** (MRI) is a further, non-invasive technique used to image the cardiac chambers and walls using rapid imaging acquisition timed with the ECG, so that acquisition can be taken at different points in the cardiac cycle (ECG gating). As well as producing highly accurate images of cardiac structure, the technique can be used to measure blood flow and myocardial perfusion at rest and during stress

with contrast agents such as those based on gadolinium (see Figure 2.10a–c).

## Nuclear cardiology

**Myocardial perfusion imaging (MPI)**, a nuclear cardiology technique, uses a γ-ray-emitting isotope, such as technetium, which is injected into a peripheral vein. The ensuing γ-ray emission from the heart is recorded by a gamma camera over the precordium. Images of the heart are computed in diastole and systole, and the ejection fraction is calculated from the change in counts per ejection. Alternatively, the uptake of the isotope from circulating blood into the myocardium itself via the coronary arteries can be compared at rest and during stress to assess coronary perfusion (see Figure 2.11a–c).

## Computed tomography

**Cardiac computed tomography** (CT) uses X-rays and the injection of an iodine-based contrast. Acquisition must be gated from the ECG and the heart rate slow enough (ideally <60 bpm, with the aid of β-blockers if necessary), so that good-quality images can be acquired using multi-detectors. These image slices can be combined to create a three-dimensional model of the heart (see Figure 2.12a,b). This provides a useful way of detecting stenosis and calcification in the coronary arteries (a CT coronary angiogram), as well as structural problems with the aorta, heart and pericardium. Cardiac CT exposes the patient to radiation (1–5 mSv with modern scanners), although this is generally at a lower dose than MPI (6–10 mSv using technetium).

## Cardiac catheterization

This is a powerful but invasive investigative technique. Under local anaesthesia, a catheter is introduced through the radial or femoral artery and advanced, under X-ray guidance, to access the aorta, coronary arteries and left ventricle. Similarly, a fine

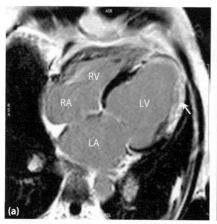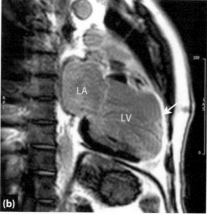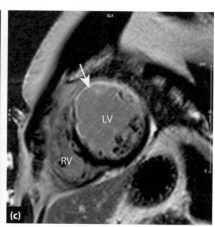

**Figure 2.10** Cardiac magnetic resonance images of the heart in **(a)** the horizontal long axis, **(b)** vertical long axis and **(c)** short axis views of the heart. After the injection of a gadolinium-based contrast agent via a peripheral vein, the gadolinium enters the coronary circulation. Most contrast agent leaves via the coronary veins, but in an area of scarring, gadolinium can accumulate in the extracellular space and remain. In the images above, there is late enhancement (bright white colour labelled with arrows) in the anterior wall, apex and distal septum consistent with a myocardial infarction in the territory of the left anterior descending coronary artery.

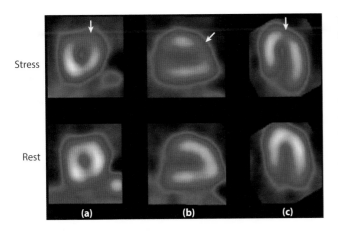

**Figure 2.11** Myocardial perfusion imaging with technetium from a patient with chest pain during exercise (stable angina). Images of the heart are taken with a gamma camera at rest and during increased cardiac work (e.g. exercise or dobutamine infusion) and images are displayed in **(a)** the left ventricular short axis, **(b)** antero-posterior and **(c)** septal-lateral axis views. The white arrows indicate areas of restricted tracer uptake during stress in the anterior wall and apex consistent with a left anterior descending coronary artery flow-limiting lesion.

catheter can be threaded through the femoral or jugular vein to the right atrium, the right ventricle or pulmonary artery. The cardiac catheter can then be put to several uses, as follows.

## Contrast angiography

A radio-opaque contrast medium is injected through the catheter and its progress through the cardiac chambers or coronary arteries is recorded by X-ray cinematography. This displays the movement of the heart wall and any valvular regurgitation. It also reveals atheromatous obstructions in the coronary arteries (see Figure 2.13a–d). A diagnostic angiogram usually has a low radiation exposure for the patient (2–5 mSv), although longer cases where interventions to treat coronary

artery disease are undertaken with balloon angioplasty and stenting carry higher exposure doses (5–40 mSv).

## Intracardiac pressure measurement

Chamber pressures can be measured by an external pressure transducer connected to the cardiac catheter, or by a miniature transducer mounted in the catheter tip. A reduced pressure difference across a closed valve is the gold standard test for valvular incompetence. Conversely, an elevated pressure gradient across an open valve indicates stenosis (Figure 2.8, top). A pulmonary artery catheter can be wedged in the pulmonary arterioles to record 'pulmonary wedge pressure', which is used as an estimate of left-sided filling pressure.

## Intracardiac pacing

This is a therapeutic, rather than a diagnostic, application of cardiac catheterization. In conditions where there is complete atrioventricular node block or sinus node disease, which compromises a patient haemodynamically, a temporary pacing lead can be introduced via the jugular or femoral vein, through the right atrium and tricuspid valve into the right ventricle and used to stimulate each heartbeat from an external pacing device. If the cause of heart block is recurrent or irreversible, the temporary pacing system should be replaced with a permanent pacemaker where the pacing leads are attached to a subcutaneous pulse generator located either pre-pectorally or underneath the pectoral muscle.

## Measurement of cardiac output by thermal dilution

This application of cardiac catheterization is described in Section 7.2.

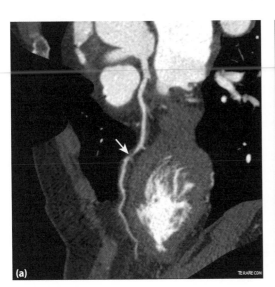

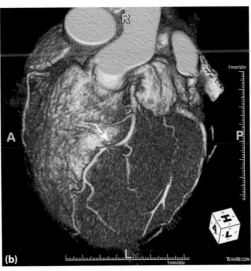

**Figure 2.12** Cardiac computed tomography showing **(a)** an image slice and **(b)** three-dimensional reconstruction from multiple slices. There is a tight narrowing in the mid-left anterior descending coronary artery highlighted by the white arrow in both images.

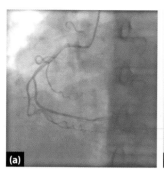 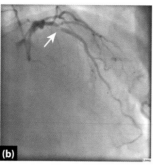 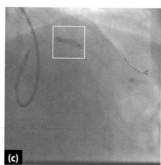 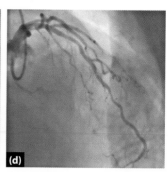

**Figure 2.13** Coronary angiogram showing **(a)** a normal right coronary artery and **(b)** the left coronary system with a tight stenosis (white arrow) in the proximal left anterior descending artery. **(c)** The lesion was treated by inflating a balloon in the coronary artery (angioplasty), surrounding which is a metal expandable frame called a stent. The two markers in the image demonstrate the beginning and end of the balloon and stent, as highlighted by the white box. Overall blood flow is restored with a good result **(d)**.

## SUMMARY

- The four muscular chambers of the mammalian heart are based on a fibrotendinous ring (*annulus fibrosus*) with four apertures, each occupied by a valve. The ring isolates the atria electrically from the ventricles.

- The ventricular cycle comprises *four phases* of unequal duration, with the right and left sides essentially in synchrony.

- During the *filling phase*, the ventricle is in diastole. The arterial outlet valves (aortic and pulmonary) are closed. The atrioventricular inlet valves (tricuspid and mitral) are open. Initial rapid, passive filling is aided by the elastic recoil of the ventricles. Filling then slows (diastasis). Late filling is boosted by *atrial systole*, especially in exercise and older patients.

- During the *isovolumetric contraction phase*, the onset of ventricular systole raises ventricular pressure, which closes the atrioventricular valves and creates the *first heart sound*. Pressure in the closed chamber rises rapidly, and this short phase is quickly terminated by the opening of the arterial outlet valves.

- During the ensuing *ejection phase*, two thirds of the ventricular blood (the *ejection fraction*) is expelled in resting subjects, and more during exercise.

- As the ejection wanes and pressures fall, a slight backflow closes the aortic and pulmonary valves. The resulting *second heart sound* is split during inspiration. During the ensuing

- *isovolumetric relaxation phase*, ventricular pressure falls rapidly until below atrial pressure. The atrioventricular valves then open and the cycle repeats.

- The *ventricular pressure-volume loop* is roughly rectangular. Each corner represents a valve action, each side a phase. The width equals stroke volume. The area equals stroke work.

- The right atrial cycle is reflected in the jugular veins, visible in the neck during recumbence. The *A wave* (atrial systole) and *C wave* (closure of the tricuspid valve) are followed by the *X descent* (atrial diastole). Pressure rises again as venous return continues (*V wave*), then falls as the opening of the tricuspid valve dumps the atrial contents into the ventricle (*Y descent*).

- *Phase duration* depends on heart rate. Ventricular diastole occupies two thirds of the cycle at rest but only one third at high heart rates. The fall in filling interval limits the maximum useful human heart rate to $180-200$ min$^{-1}$.

- *Abnormalities of the human cardiac cycle* may be detected at the bedside by inspecting the jugular venous pulse, measuring arterial BP and pulse rate, palpating the apex beat and auscultating the heart sounds. Characteristic *murmurs* are caused by valve stenosis or incompetence.

- *Further investigations* include electrocardiography, echocardiography, cardiac MRI, MPI, cardiac CT and diagnostic cardiac catheterization.

## FURTHER READING

Fisher DB, Lilly LS. The cardiac cycle: mechanisms of heart sounds and murmurs. In: Lilly LS, ed. *Pathophysiology of Heart Disease*, 6th edn. Philadelphia, PA: Lippincott Williams & Wilkins; 2015. pp. 26–42.

López DM, Come, PC. Cardiac imaging and catheterization. In: Lilly LS, ed. *Pathophysiology of Heart Disease*, 6th edn. Philadelphia, PA: Lippincott Williams & Wilkins; 2015. pp. 43–73.

Nishimura RA, Otto CM, Bonow RO, et al. 2014 AHA/ACC guideline for the management of patients with valvular heart disease: a report of the American College of Cardiology/American Heart Association Task Force on Practice Guidelines. *Journal of the American College of Cardiology* 2014; **63**(22): e57–185.

Otto CM. *Textbook of Clinical Echocardiography*, 5th edn. Philadelphia, PA: Elsevier/Saunders; 2013.

Vahanian A, Alfieri O, Andreotti F, et al. ESC Guidelines on the management of valvular heart disease. *European Heart Journal* 2012; **33**(19): 2451–96.

Carlsson M, Ugander M, Mosén H, et al. Atrioventricular plane displacement is the major contributor to left ventricular pumping in healthy adults, athletes and patients with dilated cardiomyopathy. *American Journal of Physiology* 2007; **292**(3): H1452–9.

Bourassa MG. The history of cardiac catheterization. *Canadian Journal of Cardiology* 2005; **21**(12): 1011–14.

Burkhoff D, Mirsky I, Suga H. Assessment of systolic and diastolic ventricular properties via pressure-volume analysis: a guide for clinical, translational and basic researchers. *American Journal of Physiology* 2005; **289**(2): H501–12.

Chung CS, Karamanoglu M, Kovács SJ. Duration of diastole and its phases as a function of heart rate during supine bicycle exercise. *American Journal of Physiology* 2004; **287**(5): H2003–8.

Udelson JE, Bacharach SL, Cannon RO, et al. Minimum left ventricular pressure during beta-adrenergic stimulation in human subjects: evidence of elastic recoil and diastolic 'suction' in the normal heart. *Circulation* 1990; **82**: 1174–82.

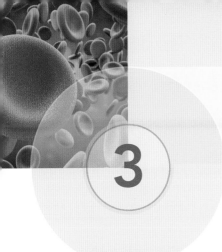

# The cardiac myocyte: excitation and contraction

# 3

## LEARNING OBJECTIVES

*After reading this chapter you should be able to:*

- outline the ultrastructure and functions of the sarcomere, sarcoplasmic reticulum (SR), transverse tubules and gap junctions (3.2);
- explain how the interactions between calcium ($Ca^{2+}$), actin and myosin produce contraction (3.3);
- sketch a ventricular action potential, label the various phases and name the ion channels responsible for each (3.6; 3.7);

- explain the link between the action potential plateau and contractility (3.9);
- describe $Ca^{2+}$ cycling in cardiac myocytes and the factors affecting $Ca^{2+}$ store size (3.9);
- state the effect of diastolic length on contractile force (3.9; 3.10);
- outline the effect of the following agents on contractile force: catecholamines; $Ca^{2+}$ channel blockers; phosphodiesterase inhibitors; digoxin (3.8; 3.9);
- draw and explain a delayed afterdepolarization (3.11).

Each heartbeat is triggered by an electrical system within the heart wall called the **pacemaker–conduction system**. This is composed of modified muscle fibres, not nerves. The pacemaker initiates an electrical discharge, which is conducted from one muscle fibre to the next by local electrical currents. When the electrical stimulus reaches the contractile muscle cells that make up the bulk of the heart (cardiac myocytes), they fire off an **action potential**, which raises the intracellular $Ca^{2+}$ ion concentration. The **$Ca^{2+}$ ions** then activate the myocyte's contractile machinery, which comprises **actin and myosin filaments**. The cardiac action potential lasts almost as long as the contraction, unlike the situation in skeletal muscle. Moreover, the cardiac myocytes are coupled together electrically, so every single one contracts during each heartbeat. This means that contractile force cannot be boosted by recruiting additional muscle fibres, as in skeletal muscle. Instead, contractile force is regulated by adjusting the intracellular $Ca^{2+}$ level and the stretch of the fibres in diastole.

## 3.1  THE IMPORTANCE OF CALCIUM

Both extracellular and intracellular $Ca^{2+}$ are essential for cardiac contraction. The need for extracellular $Ca^{2+}$ was demonstrated by the London physiologist **Sidney Ringer** between 1882 and 1885; as with many seminal discoveries, chance played a part. Ringer's assistant was tasked with preparing solutions of sodium chloride ($Na^+Cl^-$) and potassium chloride ($K^+Cl^-$), which maintained the beating of an isolated frog's heart for many hours. But when Ringer himself made up the 'same' solution, using distilled water, the heart quickly weakened and failed. Ringer discovered that his assistant had been using the 'hard' London tap water, and that the $Ca^{2+}$ in the water was essential to cardiac contraction. Indeed, if the extracellular $Ca^{2+}$ around an isolated myocyte is quickly washed away, the very next beat fails. This is because the entry of extracellular $Ca^{2+}$ into the space just beneath the cell membrane (the subsarcolemmal space), during the early phase of $i_{Ca}$ (an inward current of $Ca^{2+}$) is necessary to trigger the release of the $Ca^{2+}$ store in a compartment called the sarcoplasmic reticulum or SR ($Ca^{2+}$-induced $Ca^{2+}$ release), which then initiates crossbridge formation. The importance of this early observation by Ringer cannot be overplayed. Additionally, between 1880 and 1884, John Burdon Sanderson and FJM Page made the first recordings of electrical activity from the isolated frog's heart in a set of elegant experiments, noting that electrical activity always preceded contraction. This work set up the field of cardiac electrophysiology some 20 years before Willem Einthoven published his classical recordings of the human electrocardiogram (ECG) in 1902–3.

Although the heart wall comprises mainly muscle fibres, two other important cell types are present. Intermingled **fibroblasts** secrete collagen and other extracellular matrix polymers, which determine the stiffness of the wall and its elastic recoil from contraction during early diastole. **Endothelial cells** line the internal chambers to create a non-thrombogenic surface. The muscle fibres themselves fall into two categories, as indicated earlier. The great majority, the cardiac myocytes, do mechanical contractile work, and are quiescent until stimulated by the second type of muscle fibre, the pacemaker–conduction system. This chapter describes the electrical and contractile properties of the workhorse cardiac myocytes, while Chapter 4 describes the specialized pacemaker–conduction system.

## 3.2 ULTRASTRUCTURE OF A CARDIAC MYOCYTE

The human cardiac myocyte is a roughly cylindrical cell, 10–20 μm wide and 50–100 μm long. Some cardiac myocytes are branched; all possess a single central nucleus.

### Junctions provide mechanical and electrical connection

Adjacent myocytes are attached end-to-end at a stepped face, the **intercalated disc**. There are two distinct types of junction within the intercalated disc: the gap junction provides electrical conduction, and the desmosome provides mechanical strength (Figure 3.1).

The **gap junction**, or nexus, is oddly named, because the adjacent myocyte membranes approach each other extremely closely, to within 2–4 nm. Gap junctions transmit ionic currents, and hence electrical excitation, from one myocyte to the next, because the junction consists of hollow tubes. Six subunits of the protein connexin form a hollow tube, or **connexon**, spanning the cell membrane. Pairs of connexons from opposing myocytes unite end-to-end, so that the joined hemitubes create a continuous channel across the narrow intercellular gap. Ions can thus flow from the cytoplasm of one myocyte into the next. As a result, the entire muscle mass of the atria or ventricles behaves as an **electrically continuous sheet**, interrupted only by the annulus fibrosus. In myocardial

ischaemia, increases in intracellular acidity and $Ca^{2+}$ cause closure of some connexons, leading to poor electrical coupling, which facilitates arrhythmia.

**Desmosomes** provide mechanical strength by riveting the myocytes together. They are composed of cadherin, a transmembrane glycoprotein that spans the 25 nm-wide space between adjacent myocyte membranes. Cytoskeletal cables, called intermediate or desmin filaments, are anchored internally to the desmosomes. These cables run through the myocyte and give it tensile strength.

## The fundamental contractile unit is called a sarcomere

The myocyte is packed with long contractile bundles ~1-μm wide, called myofibrils. Each myofibril is composed of numerous basic contractile units called sarcomeres, joined end-to-end and aligned in register across the cell. The transverse alignment gives the cardiac myocyte its characteristic stripy appearance.

The resting length of a sarcomere is 1.8–2.0 μm. It comprises a set of filamentous proteins between two thin partitions, the **Z lines**, composed of the protein α-actinin (Figures 3.1 and 3.2); 'Z' is for 'zwischen', German for 'between'. Between the Z lines, there are two kinds of filament: thick filaments composed of the protein myosin; and thin filaments composed primarily of the protein actin. Cardiac myosin and actin are different isoforms to those found in skeletal muscle.

The **thick myosin filament** is 1.6 μm long × 11 nm wide. Multiple filaments are arranged in parallel in the central part of the sarcomere, which is called the A band because of its anisotropic appearance under polarized light. Each filament consists of ~400 myosin molecules. Each molecule resembles a golf club with a double head. The 'handle', 150 nm long, lies along the filament axis and the head protrudes from the side of the filament (Figure 3.3).

The **thin actin filament** is 1.05 μm long × 6 nm wide. Actin filaments are interposed between the myosin filaments, with one end free in the A band and the other rooted in the Z line. The actin filaments form the pale I (isotropic) band. The I band is only ~0.25 μm wide, because most of the actin filament is in the space between the myosin filaments, in the A band. In other words, the actin and myosin filaments interdigitate. The filamentous actin (F-actin) is a polymer of globular actin subunits (G-actin), which are bonded side-by-side. The thin filament consists of two such F-actin strings, arranged as a two-stranded helix (Figure 3.3). The groove of the double helix contains a regulatory protein, **tropomyosin**. Also, a regulatory complex composed of **troponins** is attached to the tropomyosin and actin at regular intervals. The tropomyosin–troponin complex plays a key role in initiating contraction.

Besides the contractile filaments, the sarcomere contains spring-like filaments of **titin**, which run from Z line to Z line. Their role is to align the myosin filaments and contribute elasticity to the heart wall, along with the extracellular collagen.

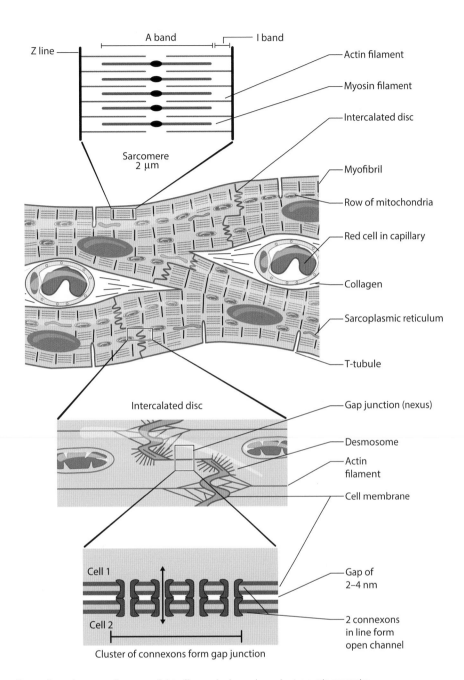

**Figure 3.1** Schematic section of myocardium parallel to fibre axis, based on electron micrographs.

## A transverse tubular system carries excitation into the interior

At each Z line, the surface membrane, or **sarcolemma**, is invaginated into a set of fine transverse tubules (**T-tubules**) that run into the cell interior (Figure 3.2). The T-tubules, like the surface membrane, possess $Na^+$ and $Ca^{2+}$ channels, so they transmit electrical excitation rapidly into the interior of the cell. This helps activate the numerous myofibrils virtually simultaneously. T-tubules are well developed in ventricular myocytes, but less so in atrial and Purkinje cells, and absent in the heart of birds and lower vertebrates.

## Sarcoplasmic reticulum contains a store of releasable calcium

Within the muscle cytoplasm (sarcoplasm) there is a second set of tubes, the SR, which is derived from the endoplasmic reticulum. The SR is a closed set of anastomosing tubes, 20–60 nm wide, that course over the myofibrils. The SR also passes very close to the T-tubules and sarcolemma in places, without opening into them. The SR is of major importance because it contains a store of $Ca^{2+}$ ions, which are partially released into the sarcoplasm when the cell is excited, leading to contraction.

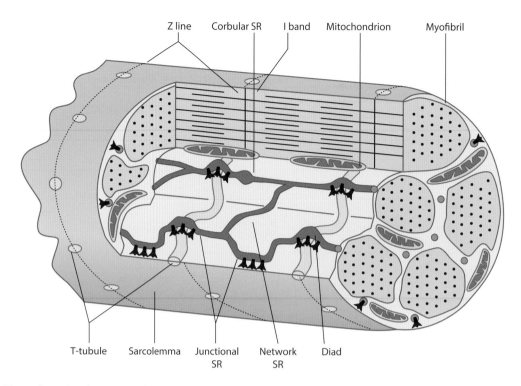

**Figure 3.2** Three-dimensional reconstruction of transverse tubular system (T-tubules) and sarcoplasmic reticulum (SR). The SR occupies ~5% of the cell volume. The black 'feet' are $Ca^{2+}$ release channels, also called ryanodine receptors.

The SR has two functionally distinct regions, with different roles in $Ca^{2+}$ handling, namely the junctional SR ($Ca^{2+}$ release) and network SR ($Ca^{2+}$ uptake) (Figure 3.2).

The **junctional SR** approaches to within 15 nm of the sarcolemmal surface or, more commonly, a T-tubule, forming a 'diad'. The lumen of the junctional SR contains a store of $Ca^{2+}$ ions loosely attached to a storage protein, calsequestrin. Tiny feet extend from the junctional SR towards the T-tubule or sarcolemma. Each foot is a gigantic protein, with a plethora of names: **$Ca^{2+}$ release channel** (describing its function); **ryanodine receptor (RyR)** (because it binds the drug ryanodine); or **calcium-induced calcium release (CICR)** channel (because it is activated by a rise in free $Ca^{2+}$).

The **network SR** comprises tubes that run over the myofibrils and actively take up sarcoplasmic $Ca^{2+}$ by means of abundant **$Ca^{2+}$-ATPase pumps**. Pump activity is regulated by an inhibitory protein, **phospholamban**.

As indicated earlier, when the myocyte is excited electrically, $Ca^{2+}$ is released from the junctional SR via the $Ca^{2+}$ release channels, and the released $Ca^{2+}$ activates the contractile machinery. This brings us to the question of how the contractile machinery works.

## 3.3 MECHANISM OF CONTRACTION

The contraction of the heart is brought about by the shortening of sarcomeres, as described here.

## Sarcomeres shorten by a sliding filament mechanism

Sarcomere contraction is brought about by the thin actin filaments sliding into the spaces between the thick myosin filaments, as described independently by Andrew Huxley and Rolf Niedergerke, and by Hugh Huxley and Jean Hanson, in 1954. Part of their evidence was that, during a contraction, both I bands shorten, but the A band does not. The filaments are propelled past each other by the repeated making, rotation and breaking of biochemical bonds, or **crossbridges**, between the thin and thick filaments. The crossbridges, noted by examining electron micrographs by Hugh Huxley in 1957, are the heads of myosin molecules protruding from the side of the thick filament. Each head acts as an **independent force generator**, and the swivelling action of hundreds of myosin heads per filament adds up to substantial force generation (Figure 3.3). The process can be likened to a rowing eight (the thick filament) moving up a river (the thin filaments) by repeatedly placing, moving and withdrawing their oar blades (myosin heads). The speed of crossbridge cycling, and hence filament sliding, is determined by the isoform of myosin; the adult human ventricle contains 97% slow-sliding β-myosin and 3% fast-sliding α-myosin.

## Calcium initiates shortening via the troponin–tropomyosin complex

Each actin subunit has a binding site for a myosin head, but the binding sites are blocked at rest by the ribbon-like tropomyosin molecule. Tropomyosin is a 42 nm-long protein that lies

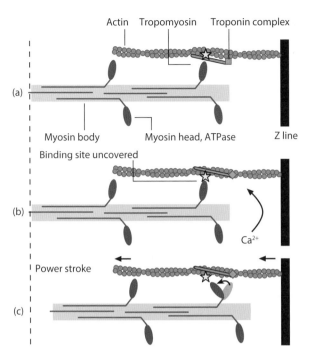

**Figure 3.3** Three stages of crossbridge cycling. (**a**) Rest. The actin binding sites (yellow stars) are blocked by tropomyosin. (**b**) Ca²⁺ displaces the troponin–tropomyosin complex, exposing actin binding sites. This allows the myosin head to form a crossbridge. (**c**) Flexion of the myosin head shifts the thin filament and Z line towards the sarcomere centre. The head then disengages and reattaches further along the actin filament. The figure shows only one of many actin binding sites, four of ~400 myosin heads and one of the two heads per myosin molecule.

in the groove of the F-actin double helix, and it overlies seven G-actin subunits. Each tropomyosin has a troponin complex attached to one end, composed of three units. Troponin C is a $Ca^{2+}$-binding protein; troponin I is inhibitory; and troponin T binds the complex to tropomyosin.

Exposure of the myosin-binding sites on actin is brought about by a sudden rise in the concentration of free $Ca^{2+}$ ions in the sarcoplasm, brought about mainly by $Ca^{2+}$ release from the SR store. Some of the $Ca^{2+}$ binds to troponin C. This causes a change in molecular configuration that shifts the tropomyosin–troponin complex deeper into the F-actin groove, thereby exposing the myosin-binding sites of the F-actin. The myosin head can now bind to the actin, forming a crossbridge, and contraction ensues.

Force and movement are generated by a change in the angle of the attached myosin head, which advances the filament by 5–10 nm. After this, the head disengages and the process repeats itself at a new actin site further along the thin filament. This process occurs in hundreds of myosin heads all along the filament, though not synchronously. Thus, to pursue the rowing analogy, the thick filament rows itself into the space between the thin filaments.

## The number of crossbridges determines the contractile force

In skeletal muscle, excitation raises the sarcoplasmic $Ca^{2+}$ concentration so high (10 µM) that troponin C is saturated and

crossbridge formation is maximal. Every twitch of an individual skeletal muscle fibre therefore occurs at full power. In the heart operating at resting outputs, this is not so. The $Ca^{2+}$ concentration during excitation reaches only 0.5–2 µM, which activates only a fraction of the potential crossbridge sites. Consequently, the contraction is **submaximal**, typically around 40% of maximal. Anything that increases the intracellular $Ca^{2+}$ level, such as adrenaline, therefore causes more crossbridges to form and increases the force of the heartbeat. In cardiac muscle, **the force of the contraction is proportional to the number of crossbridges formed**, and thus **depends on sarcoplasmic $Ca^{2+}$ concentration during excitation**.

## Adenosine triphosphate energizes the myosin head

Energy for the rowing movement of the myosin heads is supplied by adenosine triphosphate (ATP). ATP binds to an ATPase site on the myosin head. Flexion of the myosin head shifts the thin filament and Z line towards the centre of the sarcomere. The head then disengages and reattaches further along the actin filament (Figure 3.3c). Energy is released immediately from ATP by hydrolysis to adenosine diphosphate (ADP) and inorganic phosphate. The released energy activates the myosin head by cocking it back into a high-energy 'firing' angle (Figure 3.3a). 'Firing', that is, the power stroke in Figure 3.3b,c, is powered by the energy inherent in the cocked position.

## Contractile performance is tightly linked to oxygen supply

Each crossbridge cycle breaks down one ATP molecule, so a continuous supply of ATP is needed for contraction. Consequently, cardiac myocytes have an exceptionally high mitochondrial density. The mitochondria occupy 30%–35% of the cell volume, forming rows between the myofibrils. ATP is manufactured in the mitochondria by oxidative phosphorylation, for which $O_2$ is obligatory. Cardiac performance is therefore heavily dependent on the supply of $O_2$ by the **coronary arteries**. The partial pressure of $O_2$ in arterial blood ($P_{O_2}$; 100 mmHg) is much higher than in the myocyte (5–20 mmHg), so a large gradient drives the diffusion of $O_2$ into the myocyte. Moreover, myocyte sarcoplasm contains **myoglobin**, an $O_2$-binding protein, at ~3.4 g/L. Myoglobin is ~50% saturated at a $P_{O_2}$ of 5 mmHg, and therefore holds a small store of $O_2$. It also facilitates the rapid diffusion of $O_2$ through the sarcoplasm.

The release of the SR $Ca^{2+}$ store, which activates the contractile machinery, is itself triggered by an action potential. So, we must next consider the electrical properties of the cardiac myocyte.

## 3.4 RESTING MEMBRANE POTENTIAL

The potential difference between the interior and exterior of a myocyte can be measured by driving a fine, sharp-tipped microelectrode into the sarcoplasm (Figure 3.4).

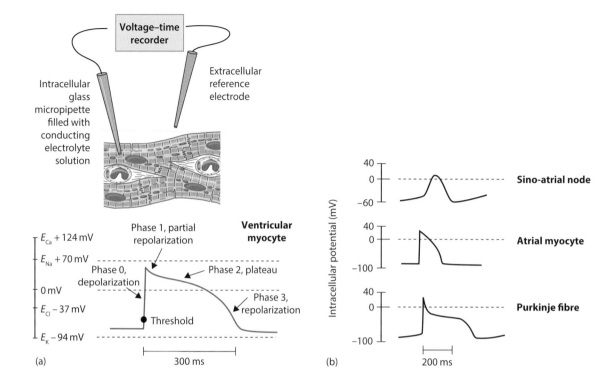

**Figure 3.4** (**a**) Intracellular potential of a ventricle subendocardial myocyte during an action potential. Resting potential –80 mV. Ion equilibrium potentials are marked for comparison. The top inset shows measurement of the potential. (**b**) Different forms of cardiac action potential. Sino-atrial node and some Purkinje fibres have unstable resting potentials. The atrial potential is triangular in many species, as shown here, but has a spike-and-plateau form in humans.

A **microelectrode** is a glass tube that has been heated, drawn out to a very fine point, filled with a conducting solution, and connected to an amplifier and voltmeter. The other lead of the voltmeter is connected to an extracellular electrode. The **intracellular potential** of the resting cardiac myocyte is –80 to –90 mV, that is, 80–90 mV lower than the extracellular fluid. In atrial and ventricular cells, the resting potential is stable (Figure 3.4), whereas in pacemaker cells and many conduction fibres (Purkinje fibres), it is unstable and drifts towards zero with time, a feature discussed in Chapter 4.

Membrane potentials are the result of differences in ion concentrations across the cell membrane and the presence of ion-conducting channels in the membrane. The ion channels have been characterized by **patch clamping**, in which a tiny patch of cell membrane is sucked onto the end of a micropipette and the electrical current through the channels in the patch is recorded (Figure 4.3). By applying different ions, potentials and blocking agents to the patch, specific ion channels can be identified. Cardiac myocytes express three classes of cation-conducting channel, namely $K^+$-, $Na^+$- and $Ca^{2+}$-selective channels, with many subtypes in each group. Channel selectivity is not absolute; for example, a 'potassium channel' has a $K^+/Na^+$ permeability ratio of ~100:1. Most of these channels can flip repeatedly between open and closed states, and the probability that one state predominates depends on the membrane potential and other factors.

## Potassium ions generate the resting membrane potential

The resting potential is the result of a high intracellular $K^+$ concentration (140 mM) relative to extracellular $K^+$ (4 mM), in combination with open $K^+$-permeable channels in the resting cell membrane. The membrane also has $Na^+$ and $Ca^{2+}$ channels, but these are mostly closed at negative potentials. By contrast, a specific type of $K^+$ channel, the inwardly rectifying channel ($K_{ir}$), is partly in the open state at negative potentials. (Mammals have a bewildering variety of $K^+$ channels, with at least 7 genes for inward rectifiers, 12 genes for voltage-activated $K^+$ channels and 5 genes for $Ca^{2+}$-activated $K^+$ channels.) Since intracellular $K^+$ concentration is ~35 times higher than extracellular $K^+$ concentration (Table 3.1), $K^+$ tends to diffuse

**Table 3.1** Concentration of ions in myocardial cells

|  | Intracellular (mM) | Extracellular (mM) | Nernst equilibrium potential (mV) |
|---|---|---|---|
| $K^+$ | 140 | 4 | –94 |
| $Na^+$ | 10 | 140 | +70 |
| $Ca^{2+}$ | 0.0001[a] | 1.2[b] | +124 |
| $Cl^-$ | 30 | 120 | –37[c] |
| pH | 7.0–7.1 | 7.4 | – |

[a] In a resting myocyte.

[b] The total $Ca^{2+}$ concentration in plasma is about double this, but only 1.2 mM is in ionic form.

[c] At –80 mV, the resting potential is the $Cl^-$ efflux through the $Cl^-$ channels. During an action potential, for example, +20 mV, there is $Cl^-$ influx through the $Cl^-$ channels.

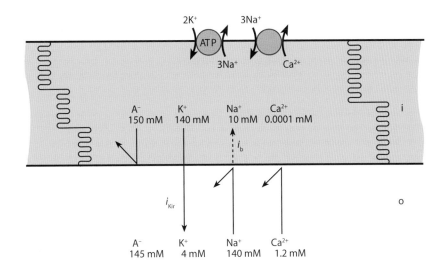

**Figure 3.5** Ion gradients and currents across the resting membrane (i, inside; o, outside). The 'A⁻' inside the cell refers to impermeant intracellular anions, mainly phosphate and charged amino acids. The straight arrows show concentration gradients for ions permeating the resting sarcolemma: $i_{Kir}$, outward background current of K⁺; $i_b$, inward background current (mainly Na⁺). Reflected arrows indicate ions unable to penetrate the resting membrane. Surface pump and Na⁺/Ca²⁺ exchanger shown at the top. ATP, adenosine triphosphate.

out of the cell through the $K_{ir}$ channels, creating a resting outward current of K⁺ ions, $i_{Kir}$ (or $i_{K^+}$). The negative intracellular ions, mainly organic phosphates and charged proteins, cannot accompany the K⁺ ions because the cell membrane is impermeable to them (Figure 3.5). Consequently, the outward leak of K⁺ ions quickly creates a tiny separation of charge, which leaves the cell interior negative with respect to the exterior. The electrical charge on a single ion is very large so just one excess negative intracellular ion per $10^{15}$ ion pairs is enough to generate a resting potential of −80 mV (see equation 3.1a). This minute imbalance is far too tiny to be detected by chemical analysis.

## The Nernst equation predicts the potassium equilibrium potential

If the intracellular potential were big enough (i.e. −94 mV), the negative intracellular potential attracting positive K⁺ ions

into the cell would exactly offset the tendency of K⁺ to diffuse out of the cell down the concentration gradient. There would then be no net movement of K⁺ out of the cell. The electrical potential at which this equilibrium would occur is called the K⁺ equilibrium potential ($E_K$). This **electrical potential** is, by definition, equal in magnitude to the outward-driving effect of the concentration gradient, or **chemical potential**. The chemical potential depends on the ion concentration outside ($C_o$) and inside the cell ($C_i$). The relationship between the electrical equilibrium potential of **any** ionic species X ($E_x$) and the concentration ratio is given by the **Nernst equation**:

$$E_x = (RT/zF) \log_e(C_o/C_i) \tag{3.1a}$$

where $R$ is the gas constant, $T$ is the absolute temperature, $z$ is the ion valency and $F$ is Faraday's constant. More simply, for a cation at the human body temperature (310 K or 37 °C), the equilibrium potential in mV works out to be:

$$E_x = (61.5/z) \log_{10}(C_o/C_i) \tag{3.1b}$$

Since the ratio $C_o/C_i$ for K⁺ is 1:35 and the valency is +1, the K⁺ equilibrium potential is −94 mV. Microelectrode measurements show that the resting membrane potential is close to $E_K$ but never quite equals it (Figure 3.6). This is explained in the next section.

The Nernst equation has important clinical implications, because the extracellular K⁺ concentration can rise excessively in some conditions, for example, renal failure, or locally in cardiac ischaemia. The Nernst equation tells us that this will reduce the resting membrane potential, that is, make it less negative (Figure 3.6). This can trigger a fatal cardiac arrhythmia.

## A sodium background leak creates non-equilibrium conditions

In reality, the resting membrane potential is never quite as big as the K⁺ equilibrium potential (Figure 3.6). This is due

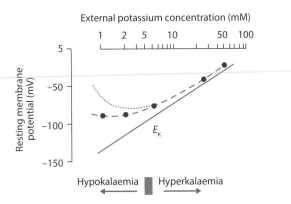

**Figure 3.6** Effect of extracellular K⁺ on the resting membrane potential of a myocyte (circles) or Purkinje fibre (dotted line). The solid line is the Nernst equilibrium potential $E_K$. Deviation from $E_K$ is due to the inward background Na⁺ current $i_b$. Increasing deviation in hypokalaemia is due to a fall in K⁺ conductance $g_K$. (Adapted from Noble D. *The Initiation of the Heart Beat*. Oxford: Clarendon Press; 1979.)

to a small, leak of Na⁺ ions, called the **inward background current** ($i_b$). Although the permeability of the resting membrane to Na⁺ is only 1/10th–1/100th of its permeability to K⁺, both the electrical and chemical gradient for Na⁺ are directed into the cell (Table 3.1). The sum of the two gradients, the **electrochemical gradient**, drives a small inward leak of Na⁺ into the cell (Figure 3.5). As a result, the resting potential is typically 10–20 mV more positive than the K⁺ equilibrium potential.

Since the resting potential is not quite negative enough to halt completely the outward diffusion of K⁺ ions, there is a continuous trickle of K⁺ out of the resting myocyte, creating an **outward background current** ($i_{Kir}$). The outward current $i_{Kir}$, along with another small outward current generated by the Na⁺/K⁺ pump, is equal and opposite to the inward current $i_b$. Thus, the resting membrane potential remains stable despite a continuous slow leak of K⁺ for Na⁺. This known as the 'pump-leak' model of the resting membrane potential.

## The membrane potential depends on the ratio of ionic permeabilities

A basic law of electricity, Ohm's law, can be used to understand how the relative permeability of the membrane to K⁺ and Na⁺ affects the membrane potential. **Ohm's law** states that current $i$ is proportional to the potential difference $\Delta V$ and the electrical conductance $g$ (1/resistance). In other words, $i = g.\Delta V$. The conductance of the cell membrane to an ion is proportional to its permeability to that ion. The potential difference $\Delta V$ that drives the outward background current of K⁺ ions ($i_{Kir}$) is the difference between the actual membrane potential $V_m$ and the K⁺ equilibrium potential $E_K$. Ohm's law thus tells us that the outward background current is:

$$i_{Kir} = g_K(V_m - E_K) \tag{3.2}$$

where $g_K$ is the membrane potassium conductance. By similar reasoning, the inward background current of sodium ions $i_b$ is:

$$i_b = g_{Na}(V_m - E_{Na}) \tag{3.3}$$

where $E_{Na}$ is the Na equilibrium potential (about +70 mV). As the Na⁺/K⁺ pump moves 3 Na⁺ ions out of the cell for every 2K⁺ ions it moves back in to the cell, the inward $i_{Kir}$ and outward $i_b$ must be in a 3:2 ratio to keep the resting potential stable. Combining the two expressions results in an equation describing the resting potential, called the **conductance equation**:

at rest $\quad i_{Kir} = -\dfrac{2}{3}i_b$

so $\quad g_K(V_m - E_k) = -\dfrac{2}{3}g_{Na}(V_m - E_{Na})$

$$V_m = \frac{E_K + E_{Na}(2g_{Na}/3g_K)}{1 + (2g_{Na}/3g_K)} \tag{3.4}$$

The conductance equation is a simple version of a more complex expression that also incorporates chloride currents (the Goldman–Hodgkin–Katz voltage equation); however, it is

ideal for our present purpose because it highlights the importance of the **Na⁺/K⁺ conductance ratio** $g_{Na}/g_K$ in setting the membrane potential. The conductance equation tells us that the resting potential is a K⁺ equilibrium potential ($E_K = -94$ mV) that has been reduced by a small fraction of the Na⁺ equilibrium potential ($E_{Na} = +70$ mV). The fraction is typically 1/10th because the $g_{Na}/g_K$ ratio is 1:10. Therefore, the conductance equation predicts that the resting potential should be $-94$ mV + 4.6 mV)/1.066, which is $-83.7$ mV. This is very close to the measured potential in resting cardiac myocytes. The conductance equation also tells us that if $g_{Na}$ becomes bigger than $g_K$, as happens during an action potential, the membrane potential will become positive – the characteristic feature of an action potential.

## Current–voltage relationships for ion channels are commonly non-linear

One problem in applying Ohm's law to ion channels is that the conductance $g$ of an ion channel, unlike that of a copper wire, often changes with the potential. Consequently, the current–voltage relationship is non-linear. An Ohmic equation such as (3.2) or (3.3) tells us the current at a given conductance and potential, but does not tell us the shape of the current–voltage

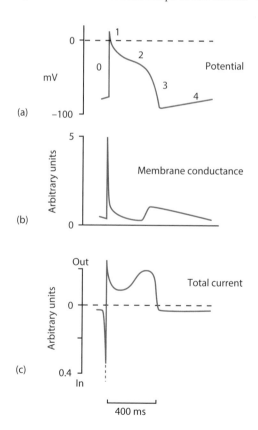

**Figure 3.7** Phases of cardiac action potential. (**a**) Changes in net electrical conductance of the membrane. (**b**) Net electrical current across the membrane. (**c**) Inward current downwards. The changes represent the sum of the individual K⁺, Na⁺ and Ca²⁺ changes shown in Figure 3.8. This myocyte is a Purkinje cell with an unstable resting potential and relatively negative plateau potential. (Weidmann's seminal observation of 1956, redrawn from Noble D. *The Initiation of the Heartbeat*. Oxford: Clarendon Press; 1979, by permission.)

relationship. The $K^+$ channel chiefly responsible for the resting potential, **the inwardly rectifying $K^+$ channel** $K_{ir}$, is a good example. Its conductance falls when the membrane is depolarized (loses charge), so less $K^+$ leaks out during the action potential (Figure 3.7). This is called inward rectification, and is important because it **conserves intracellular $K^+$ during the very long cardiac action potential**. The fall in channel permeability on depolarization is caused by positively charged magnesium ($Mg^{2+}$) ions and polyamines, which are drawn into the inner mouth of the channel and obstruct it.

## 3.5 ROLE OF PUMPS AND EXCHANGERS

### A sodium/potassium pump preserves the intracellular ion levels

The myocyte is a chemical battery, but the chemical that powers the battery, $K^+$, is slowly but continuously leaking out of the cell. Unchecked, the concentrations of $K^+$ and $Na^+$ would eventually equilibrate across the cell membrane, leaving the battery flat. This is prevented by active pumps in the sarcolemmal membrane, which preserve the chemical composition of the interior.

The **$Na^+/K^+$ pump** is an ATPase that uses metabolic energy to pump $Na^+$ ions out of the cell and, simultaneously, $K^+$ ions into the cell (Figure 3.5). Three $Na^+$ ions are expelled from the cell for every two $K^+$ ions pumped in. Therefore, the pump generates a net outflow of positive charge, and is said to be 'electrogenic'. However, the contribution of the pump current to the resting potential is a minor one because blocking the pump with ouabain, a cardiac glycoside, reduces the myocyte potential by only 2–4 mV. The pump rate is increased by a rise in intracellular $Na^+$ concentration or extracellular $K^+$.

The operation of several ion exchangers depends on the $Na^+$ gradient set up by the $Na^+/K^+$ pump. The **$Na^+/Ca^{2+}$ exchanger** is of major importance (see the next section). The **$Na^+/H^+$ exchanger** regulates intracellular pH by transporting protons out of the cell, in exchange for a flow of $Na^+$ into the cell down the gradient established by the $Na^+/K^+$ pump. The $Na^+/H^+$ exchanger is particularly important in myocardial ischaemia (see Section 3.11 and Figure 6.22).

### Calcium transporters regulate diastolic calcium and the calcium store

During diastole, myocytes expel the $Ca^{2+}$ ions that entered from the extracellular fluid during the preceding action potential (see the next section). The main $Ca^{2+}$ transporter in the surface membrane (sarcolemma) is the **$Na^+/Ca^{2+}$ exchanger**. This transmembrane protein is particularly abundant in sarcolemma close to the junctional SR. The exchanger operates in **'forward mode'** over most of the cardiac cycle, allowing three extracellular $Na^+$ ions into the cell in exchange for the expulsion of one intracellular $Ca^{2+}$ ion (Figure 3.5). The entry of the excess $Na^+$ ions creates a small inward current. The exchanger is not powered by ATP but is driven by the inwardly directed $Na^+$ concentration gradient, rather as a waterwheel is turned by a water gradient. Calcium expulsion thus depends, indirectly, on the active $Na^+/K^+$ pump, which creates the $Na^+$ gradient, a crucial point for understanding the cardiac drug digoxin (see Section 3.9).

Since the forward mode carries a net positive charge into the cell, it is also promoted by negative intracellular potentials. However, the exchanger is reversible and can be driven briefly into **reverse mode** ($Ca^{2+}$ entry, $Na^+$ expulsion) when the intracellular potential is positive (peak of the action potential), especially if intracellular $Na^+$ is high, as during treatment with the drug digoxin.

The $3Na^+/1Ca^{2+}$ exchanger accounts for around three quarters of $Ca^{2+}$ expulsion from cardiac myocytes. The other quarter is pumped out by a relatively small number of ATP-powered sarcolemmal **calcium pumps**. Calcium pumps are more abundant in the network SR, where they build up the $Ca^{2+}$ store. The active and passive $Ca^{2+}$ transporters together reduce the cytosolic $Ca^{2+}$ concentration to an extremely low level in resting myocytes, namely $10^{-7}$ M (0.1 µM).

## 3.6 CARDIAC ACTION POTENTIALS

### The cardiac action potential has five phases

An action potential is an abrupt reversal of the membrane potential to a positive value (Figures 3.4 and 3.7). The myocyte action potential is triggered by an action potential in the conduction system or an adjacent myocyte. The neighbouring action potential creates a current that reduces the negative resting potential (see Section 4.3). When the membrane potential reaches a **threshold** of −60 to −65 mV, the electrical conductance of the sarcolemma suddenly increases (Figure 3.8b), due to the opening of $Na^+$ channels (Figure 3.8). This allows a sudden, inward current of $Na^+$ ions (Figure 3.8). The resulting influx of positive charge causes the cell to **depolarize** extremely quickly and flip to a positive potential of +20 to +30 mV, called the **overshoot**. This is called phase 0 of the cardiac action potential (Figure 3.8).

In most myocytes, the membrane then begins to repolarize (phase 1). However, this early repolarization is only partial. When the membrane potential reaches 0 to −20 mV, it becomes relatively stable for a remarkably long period, 200–400 ms. This is called the **plateau**, or phase 2. Because of the plateau, myocardial action potentials last ~100 times longer than nerve or skeletal muscle action potentials (1–4 ms). The combination of a marked phase 1 and phase 2 gives the action potential a characteristic spike-and-plateau appearance in the human atrium, ventricular subepicardial (outer) muscle and Purkinje conduction fibres (Figure 3.4b). However, subendocardial myocytes lack a marked phase 1 (Figure 3.4a). Finally, the membrane **repolarizes** (phase 3), though at only 1/1000th of the rate of depolarization. Phase 4 is the resting potential.

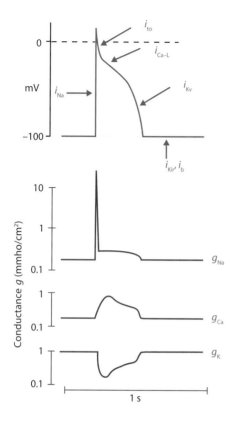

**Figure 3.8** Myocyte action potential, ionic currents responsible and changes in membrane conductance to individual ions, which together account for the net membrane conductance changes in Figure 3.7b. (Based on Noble D. *The Journal of Physiology* 1984; 353: 1–50, with permission from Wiley-Blackwell.)

The **shape of the cardiac action potential** differs between sites and between species (Figure 3.4a and Figures 3.8–311). Atrial potentials last only 150 ms and are triangular in many non-human species (Figure 3.4b). Ventricular potentials last longer (400 ms) and are more rectangular because of a distinct plateau at +30 to 0 mV (Figure 3.8). The phase 1 repolarization spike is well developed in subepicardial myocytes but not in subendocardial myocytes, so the subendocardial action potential lasts longer, a point that is important for understanding the ECG T wave (see Section 5.5). Purkinje cells have the longest action potentials of all (up to 450 ms), with a pronounced phase 1 spike and a low plateau potential, at around −20 mV (Figure 3.7a).

The myocardial action potential is generated by a sequence of changes in sarcolemmal permeability to Na⁺, Ca²⁺ and K⁺, which allows ionic currents to flow down their electrochemical gradients, as described next.

## Fast sodium channels cause rapid depolarization (phase 0)

Depolarization and overshoot are caused by an extremely rapid increase in sarcolemmal permeability to Na⁺ ions. **Fast sodium channels** open (activate) beyond their threshold of −60 to −65 mV, raising the net membrane conductance

abruptly by ~100-fold (Figure 3.8). This allows a rapid influx of Na⁺ ions, the **first inward current**, $i_{Na}$, down the electrochemical gradient (Figure 3.8). The inward current drives the potential towards the Nernst equilibrium potential for Na⁺, $E_{Na}$, which is +70 mV (Table 3.1). However, the potential never quite reaches $E_{Na}$ because there is still a small outward current of K⁺ ions. The situation at the **overshoot** is essentially a mirror image of that at rest, and the same equation (3.4) applies. Equation 3.4 predicts an overshoot membrane potential of +55 mV for a Na⁺:K⁺ conductance ratio of 10:1.

The fast Na⁺ channel is said to be **voltage-dependent** because it opens at a critical threshold potential; and **time-dependent** because its open state is of short duration. Because of the time dependency, Na⁺ channels **inactivate** automatically, and the overshoot is very brief. The molecular basis of these properties is explained in Section 3.7.

## Transiently open Potassium channels cause early repolarization (phase 1)

In myocytes with a marked phase 1, such as subepicardial myocytes and Purkinje fibres, the membrane next undergoes a rapid but incomplete repolarization because of a **transient outward current**, $i_{to}$ (Figure 3.8). The current is carried mainly by voltage-gated K⁺ channels, which open transiently in response to depolarization, then quickly inactivate (Figure 3.10). Also, an influx of Cl⁻ ions through chloride channels contributes to $i_{to}$.

Partial repolarization by $i_{to}$ has two roles: it enhances the electrochemical gradient for Ca²⁺ entry in the next phase and it **influences action potential duration**. For example, subepicardial myocytes express more transient outward K⁺ channels than subendocardial myocytes, so the subepicardial action potential is shorter. Conversely, in failing hearts, the K⁺ channel expression is reduced, so the action potential is prolonged.

## Long-lasting-type calcium channels cause the early plateau (phase 2)

The cardiac action potential next displays its unique feature, a plateau lasting 200–400 ms. The first part of the plateau is generated by a small but long-lasting inward current of Ca²⁺ ions, $i_{Ca}$. The Ca²⁺ current is the second inward current of the action potential ($i_{Na}$ being the first), and it prevents the myocyte from repolarizing rapidly, as would a nerve axon or skeletal muscle fibre. The existence of two different inward currents, $i_{Na}$ and $i_{Ca}$, can be demonstrated using tetrodotoxin, a dangerous poison from the Japanese pufferfish; this blocks fast Na⁺ channels and abolishes the initial spike of the action potential, but not the plateau phase (Figure 3.9). Figure 3.9 also shows that the plateau current $i_{Ca}$ is increased by adrenaline, a point we will return to later.

The inward Ca²⁺ current is driven by the electrochemical gradient, and is carried by channels called long-lasting-type or **L-type Ca²⁺ channels**. These are particularly abundant in

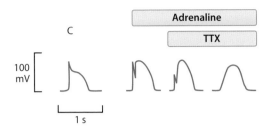

**Figure 3.9** Effect of adrenaline and tetrodotoxin (TTX) on the action potential of calf Purkinje fibre. The control recording (C) shows a normal Purkinje action potential. Adrenaline enhanced the plateau calcium current. TTX abolished the initial spike depolarization, because it blocked the fast Na$^+$ channels. The residual action potential resembles that of the sino-atrial node (see Figure 3.4). (Adapted from Carmeliet E, Vereeke J. *Pflüger's Archiv: European Journal of Physiology* 1969; 313: 303–15, with kind permission from Springer Science and Business Media.)

the T-tubules. L-type Ca$^{2+}$ channels are voltage-gated channels that are rapidly activated by depolarization (though not as rapidly as fast Na$^+$ channels); therefore, the $i_{Ca}$ current has already reached 40% of its peak during phase 1. The current peaks at 2–7 ms, then continues to flow at a declining rate for a long time, because L-type Ca$^{2+}$ channels inactivate slowly. Figure 3.8 shows the increase in Ca$^{2+}$ conductance and its prolonged, slow decay. The latter explains the decaying net membrane conductance during the plateau in Figure 3.7b. The L-type Ca$^{2+}$ channels can be partially inhibited by Ca$^{2+}$ channel blockers, such as verapamil and diltiazem.

The total conductance of the activated Ca$^{2+}$ channels is much lower than that of the fast Na$^+$ channels, so $i_{Ca}$ is a much smaller current. However, it is just the right size to counterbalance, very nearly, the repolarizing effect of the small outward K$^+$ current that flows throughout the action potential. In this way, the membrane potential is held close to 0 mV for hundreds of milliseconds.

The **outward K$^+$ current $i_{Kir}$ is reduced during the plateau**, because the membrane K$^+$ conductance falls on depolarization (Figures 3.8 and 3.10). This is the phenomenon of **inward rectification**, described earlier. Inward rectification is caused by the obstruction of the inner mouth of the K$_{ir}$ channels by intracellular Mg$^{2+}$ ions and polyamines during depolarization. Inward rectification is a helpful economy measure, because it minimizes the number of K$^+$ and Ca$^{2+}$ ions that are exchanged during the exceptionally long cardiac action potential, and thus reduces the energy cost incurred by an action potential.

## Sodium–calcium exchange maintains the late plateau

If Na$^+$ ions are removed from the fluid bathing an isolated myocyte, the plateau becomes shorter. This shows that the late part of the plateau, when more and more L-type Ca$^{2+}$ channels are closing, is maintained by an inward current of Na$^+$ ions. The plateau Na$^+$ current is carried by the Na$^+$/Ca$^{2+}$ exchanger (Figure 3.5), not the Na$^+$ channels. The exchanger

creates a net inward current because it lets three Na$^+$ ions into the cell for every Ca$^{2+}$ expelled. Moreover, the exchanger current increases during the plateau phase because of the rise in Ca$^{2+}$ concentration in the sarcoplasm. The exchanger current is most marked when the plateau is at a relatively negative potential (e.g. Purkinje fibres; Figures 3.4b bottom and 3.7a; cf. ventricular myocyte in Figure 3.4a) because the exchanger, being electrogenic, is affected by the membrane potential as well as ion concentrations. Indeed, during the positive overshoot phase of the action potential, the exchanger may even briefly go into reverse mode, helping to move Ca$^{2+}$ into the cell.

## Slow potassium channel opening causes repolarization (phase 3)

As the plateau progresses, the depressed net K$^+$ conductance begins to rise (Figure 3.8). This is due to the gradual opening of voltage-activated K$^+$ channels, called **delayed rectifier or slow K$^+$ channels** (K$_V$, K$_S$). Unlike the voltage-activated Na$^+$ and Ca$^{2+}$ channels, delayed rectifier channels activate very slowly (Figure 3.10). As they do so, the outward K$^+$ current $i_{Kv}$ gradually increases, until it outweighs the small, late-plateau inward current, and thereby initiates repolarization. As repolarization proceeds, the **inward rectifier** conductance is restored and contributes to the final stage of repolarization (Figure 3.10).

The magnitude of the inward K$^+$ current affects the **duration of the plateau**. When the heart rate is increased by sympathetic stimulation, channel phosphorylation increases the repolarizing K$^+$ current $i_{Kv}$, which induces early repolarization and thus shortens the plateau. This is a necessary step to allow more action potentials per minute (see Section 4.5). Action potential duration also alters in pathological conditions, shortening in hypoxia (Figure 3.10, top trace) and lengthening in

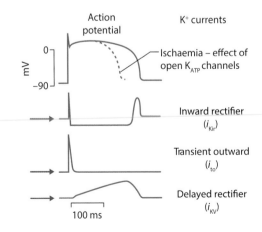

**Figure 3.10** Three K$^+$ currents contributing to the cardiac action potential. The arrows mark the zero current. The dashed line shows the effect of acute ischaemia; increased open probability of the K$_{ATP}$ channels shortens the action potential. Hypoxic shortening is abolished by the K$_{ATP}$ blocker glibenclamide, and by knockout of the pore-forming Kir6.2 protein in mice. (Adapted from Sanguinetti MC, Keating MT. *News in Physiological Sciences*, 1997; 12: 152–7, with permission from the American Physiological Society.)

chronic heart disease. A variant of the delayed rectifier protein gene *KCNQ1* (*potassium voltage-gated channel subfamily Q member 1*) impairs channel function, prolongs the plateau and causes a long QT interval in the ECG. This form of **long QT syndrome** (LQTS type 1) underlies some cases of sudden cardiac death in apparently healthy, young individuals. Long QT syndromes can also result from mutations of other channel proteins, such as the rapid delayed rectified K$^+$ channel *HERG+MiRP1* (LQTS type 2) and the Na$^+$ channel *SCN5A* (LQTS type 3).

## The refractory period and its relation to the contraction period

The myocyte is electrically inexcitable (refractory) throughout its prolonged depolarization. This is called the **absolute refractory period** (Figure 3.11). By the time repolarization reaches −50 mV, many but not all the fast Na$^+$ channels have reset from the inactivated state to a closed-but-activatable state. (The difference between 'inactivated' and 'closed' is explained in Section 3.7.) Consequently, the cell begins to regain some degree of electrical excitability at this point. However, a larger-than-normal excitatory stimulus is necessary because of the substantial number of Na$^+$ channels still inactivated. The period between −50 mV and full repolarization is therefore

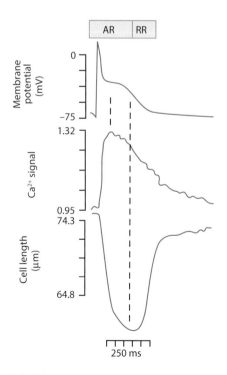

**Figure 3.11** Relationship between electrical, chemical and mechanical events in a single myocyte (rat). The myocyte was loaded with a fluorescent dye to measure free sarcoplasmic Ca$^{2+}$ concentration. Note the sequence of the peaks, first electrical, then chemical, then mechanical. Rat myocytes have an unusually negative plateau potential. AR, absolute refractory period to −50 mV repolarization; RR, relative refractory period from −50 mV to full repolarization. (Adapted from Spurgeon et al. *American Journal of Physiology* 1990; 258: H574−86.)

called the **relative refractory period**. After this, the myocyte regains its normal ease of electrical excitation.

**Myocyte contraction** starts about 10 ms or so after phase 0 and lasts 200–250 ms overall (Figure 3.11). Contraction therefore peaks near the end of the absolute refractory period, and the myocyte is into the relaxation phase by the end of the relative refractory period. Tension development is thus completed before the cardiac myocyte becomes re-excitable. This is important, because it limits the contractile behaviour of the heart to repeated **single twitches**. In skeletal muscle, by contrast, the very brief action potentials follow each other so quickly that one twitch fuses with the next one to generate a sustained contraction. This cannot happen in the heart, because the refractory period lasts as long as tension development. This seems an excellent arrangement, because a sustained myocardial contraction would quickly prove fatal!

## A relatively small quantity of ions is exchanged per action potential

The numerous ionic currents described in this chapter are all small, even the Na$^+$ current. Consequently, **the change in intracellular ion concentration caused by a single action potential is tiny**. Students often assume, wrongly, that the 'rush' of Na$^+$ ions into the cell must raise the intracellular Na$^+$ concentration substantially, but this is mistaking speed for quantity. Around 40 million Na$^+$ ions enter a myocyte during depolarization. Since a myocyte contains about 200 000 million Na$^+$ ions, Na$^+$ concentration rises by a mere 0.02%. The change is even smaller for K$^+$, a fall of 0.001%. The Na$^+$-K$^+$ and Na$^+$-Ca$^{2+}$ transporters can therefore restore the chemical composition of the sarcoplasm without excessive expenditure of metabolic energy.

The main ionic currents are summarized in Table 3.2. The numerous subtypes of channel are summarized in more detail, for reference purposes, in Table 4.2.

### 3.7 ADVANCED ASPECTS: STRUCTURE–FUNCTION RELATIONS OF ION CHANNELS

Although the molecular structure of ion channels is complex, a broad outline helps us to understand certain key properties, such as the time-dependent inactivation of Na$^+$ channels. Moreover, the genetic mutation of certain channel proteins underlies cardiac disorders, such as LQTS.

All ion channels are formed by transmembrane proteins arranged in a ring around a central, aqueous pore (Figure 3.12). In K$^+$ channels, four individual proteins, called α subunits, make up the ring; in Na$^+$ and Ca$^{2+}$ channels, four α-like domains of a single protein make up the ring. The simplest cardiac channel is the inwardly rectifying channel (K$_{ir}$), where each α subunit has two hydrophobic transmembrane helices. This probably evolved into the voltage-sensitive K$^+$ channels, with six transmembrane helices per α subunit. This, in turn,

**Table 3.2** Chief ionic currents in cardiac work cell (for a more detailed subdivision, see Table 4.2)

| Current | Ion | Direction[a] | Function | Blockers |
|---|---|---|---|---|
| $i_{K, total}$ | $K^+$ | Outward | 1. Generates resting membrane potential<br>2. Repolarization | $Ba^{2+}$<br>Tetraethylammonium hydroxide |
| $i_b$ | $Na^+$ (mostly) | Inward | Inward background current makes resting potential smaller than $E_K$ | – |
| $i_{Na}$ | $Na^+$ | Inward | Fast depolarization, to help propagate excitation | Tetrodotoxin, procainamide, lignocaine, flecainide |
| $i_{Ca}$ | $Ca^{2+}$ | Inward | 1. Excitation–contraction coupling<br>2. Plateau maintenance | $Mn^{2+}$, diltiazem, verapamil |
| $i_{Na^+/Ca^{2+}}$ | 3 $Na^+$ in<br>1 $Ca^{2+}$ out | Net inward current (forward mode of $Na^+/Ca^{2+}$ exchanger) | Sustains late plateau. Expels intracellular $Ca^{2+}$. Arrhythmogenic afterdepolarization in ischaemic $Ca^{2+}$ overload | – |

[a] 'Inward' means a flow of positive charge from the extracellular to the intracellular compartment.

---

**CONCEPT BOX 3.1**

**CARDIAC POTENTIALS ARE GENERATED BY IONIC GRADIENTS AND SEQUENTIAL ACTIVATION OF ION CHANNELS**

- The resting potential, –80 mV, is created by the tendency of intracellular $K^+$ to diffuse out of the myocyte through open, $K^+$-selective channels, leaving behind a slight excess of intracellular negative charge.

- The resting potential approaches the Nernst equilibrium potential for $K^+$, modified by a small, inward background leak of $Na^+$, because the membrane is far more permeable to $K^+$ than it is to $Na^+$ at rest. The $Na^+/K^+$ ATPase maintains the resting membrane potential by pumping $2K^+$ ions back into the cell and $3Na^+$ ions out of the cell. This is known as the 'pump-leak' model.

- Voltage-gated $Na^+$ channels admit a brief influx of positive ions into the cell at the start of an action potential, depolarizing the cell.

- The overshoot of the action potential (+30 mV) approaches a Nernst equilibrium potential for $Na^+$, modified by a small outward background current of $K^+$.

- The activation of long-lasting $Ca^{2+}$ channels then allows an influx of $Ca^{2+}$ ($i_{Ca}$). This nearly counterbalances the outward $K^+$ current and generates a long plateau at around 0 potential, lasting 200–400 ms.

- The plateau is terminated by an increasing efflux of $K^+$ ions through slowly activating, delayed rectifier $K^+$ channels. The $K^+$ efflux repolarizes the cell. Large $K^+$ currents shorten the plateau and small $K^+$ currents lengthen it.

probably evolved into $Na^+$ and $Ca^{2+}$ channels, where four α-like units are strung together as a single molecule.

## Inward rectifier potassium channel family

This family includes $K_{ir}$ and some related channels that we will meet later ($K_{ATP}$, $K_{ACh}$) (Figure 3.12, top). Mutation studies indicate that the $K^+$ selectivity of the central pore is conferred by a specific amino acid sequence motif, glycine-tyrosine-glycine, in an intramembrane loop lining the pore (P or H5 loop). There are no voltage-sensitive loops. However, depolarization reduces $K_{ir}$ conductance (inward rectification) because intracellular $Mg^{2+}$ ions and polyamines impede the inner mouth of the channel when current is flowing outwards.

## Voltage-gated potassium channel ($K_v$ family)

Two members of this family are particularly important for cardiac function.

### DELAYED RECTIFIER (SLOW) CHANNEL, $K_s$

Each α subunit is formed by protein KCNQ1 (potassium voltage-gated channel subfamily Q member 1), which has six hydrophobic transmembrane loops, S1–S6 (Figure 3.12, middle). Mutation studies show that positively charged arginine and lysine residues in the S4 loops act as a voltage sensor, making this a voltage-activated channel. Inactivation is brought about by a ball-on-chain (the last 20 amino acids of the intracellular N-terminal), which slowly blocks the intracellular opening following depolarization. Mutations of KCNQ1 impair channel function, leading to delayed repolarization and sudden death in young individuals (LQTS). The channel also has two regulatory β subunits-potassium voltage-gated channel subfamily E member 1 (KCNE1).

### TRANSIENT OUTWARD $K^+$ CHANNEL, $K_{to}$

This has a similar structure to $K_s$ but it is composed of different proteins, voltage-gated potassium channel subunit Kv4.3 (KCND3) and Kv channel-interacting protein 2 (KCIP2). It has a faster activation and inactivation than $K_s$. KCND3 expression is reduced in failing hearts, leading to prolonged action potentials.

**Inward rectifier channel K<sub>ir</sub>– two transmembrane helices per α subunit**

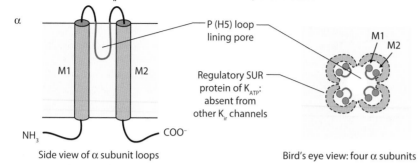

Side view of α subunit loops

Bird's eye view: four α subunits

**Voltage-gated K channel (K<sub>v</sub>, K<sub>to</sub>) – six transmembrane helices per α subunit**

**Na⁺ channel – four α-like domains in a single protein**

**Figure 3.12** Ion channel topography. The inward rectifier channel (Kir), with two transmembrane helices per α subunit, probably evolved into voltage-sensitive K⁺ channels, with six transmembrane helices, which evolved into Na⁺ and Ca²⁺ channels. In each case, a hollow channel is created by four proteins, called α subunits (K⁺ and transient receptor potential (TRP) channels), or by four α-like domains of a single protein (Na⁺ and Ca²⁺ channels). Each α subunit/domain has a P loop (red line) that dips into the lipid membrane to line the pore and determine its ion selectivity. The positively charged, arginine-rich S4 helix is the voltage sensor. S4 is uncharged in TRP channels (see Table 12.2). Phosphorylation of sites on intracellular loops by protein kinases can regulate channel activity, e.g. Ca²⁺ channel phosphorylation by cyclic adenosine monophosphate-activated protein kinase A promotes the open state, following adrenergic stimulation. The Ca²⁺ channel is broadly like the Na⁺ channel, but its slow inactivation gate may be the intracellular loop linking domains I and II.

## Voltage-gated sodium channel

The cardiac fast Na⁺ channel, Na$_V$1.5, is one of eight types of voltage-dependent Na⁺ channels in the genome. It is formed by a large single protein of ~2000 amino acids, which traverses back and forth across the cell membrane to form four near-identical groups called domains I–IV (Figure 3.12, bottom). Each domain has six hydrophobic transmembrane helices, S1–S6, as in K$_v$ channels. Positively charged arginine and lysine residues in S4 again act as the voltage sensor, and amino acids in the pore-lining P loop confer Na⁺ selectivity. The antiarrhythmic drugs lidocaine, procaine and quinidine inhibit Na⁺ channels by plugging the pore.

The excitation–inactivation cycle of the Na⁺ channel is due to the operation of two 'gates', which are parts of the polypeptide chain (Figure 3.13). The m or **activation gate** (probably the S6 helices) is closed at resting potentials, blocking the pore. A second intracellular gate, the h or **inactivation gate**, is open at a resting potential. The inactivation gate is a hinged lid over the channel entrance, formed by the positively charged intracellular loop linking domains III and IV. A channel in this configuration is closed but excitable ('deactivated'). When the membrane is depolarized to the threshold potential, an outward shift in the positively charged, voltage-sensitive S4 helices open the activation gate, allowing Na⁺ passage. However, at the same time, the inactivation gate begins to close. Because the inactivation gate moves more slowly than the activation gate, there is a millisecond or so when the channel is open, before the inactivation gate closes. This is the instant in which the brief first inward current $i_{Na}$ flows. Once the second gate has closed, the channel is inactivated. It cannot be re-excited until it has been reset to the closed-but-activatable starting configuration (Figure 3.13, bottom). This requires repolarization to beyond −70 mV.

## Voltage-gated, L-type calcium channel

The cardiac L-type Ca²⁺ channel comprises a single pore-forming protein, voltage-gated calcium channel subunit alpha Cav1.2 (CAC1C) (the α1 subunit), and several regulatory subunits. Like the Na⁺ channel, CAC1C has four

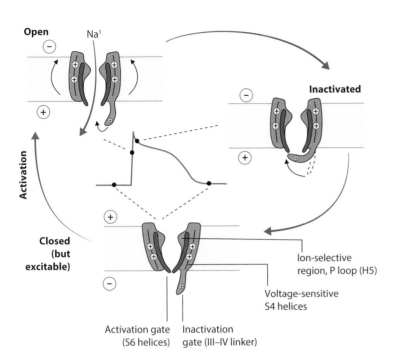

**Figure 3.13** Excitation–inactivation cycle of voltage-sensitive Na$^+$ channel. Outward displacement of the charged S4 helices of each domain by depolarization opens the activation gate (S6 helices). The slower inactivation gate is a hinged lid, formed by the intracellular loop linking molecular domains III and IV. Enzymatic cleavage of this loop abolishes inactivation. As long as the inactivation gate is closed, the myocyte is incapable of re-excitation (refractory).

domains, each with six transmembrane segments, including a charged S4 voltage sensor. Ca$^{2+}$ selectivity is attributed to glutamate residues in the pore-lining P loop. As with Na$^+$ channels, time-dependent inactivation is brought about by an intracellular lid docking process; however, the lid may be the intracellular loop linking domains I and II. Closure of the inactivation gate is enhanced by intracellular Ca$^{2+}$ via a binding protein, calmodulin (Ca$^{2+}$-dependent inactivation). Consequently, the rise in intracellular Ca$^{2+}$ during the action potential helps to terminate opening. Adrenergic stimulation leads to the phosphorylation of the C-terminus domain by protein kinase A, increasing the duration of the open state.

## 3.8 PHYSIOLOGICAL AND PATHOLOGICAL CHANGES IN ACTION POTENTIAL

As noted earlier, differences in transient outward K$^+$ channel expression result in a gradient of action potential duration across the ventricle wall. The action potential can also be regulated physiologically, and can be altered by disease, as described next.

### Catecholamines boost the plateau current and contractile force

The contractile force of a cardiac myocyte is proportional to the size of the plateau current $i_{Ca}$, which can be increased by circulating **adrenaline** and by **noradrenaline** from cardiac sympathetic fibres. The increased current creates a dome-shaped plateau (Figure 3.9) and leads to a bigger free Ca$^{2+}$ transient and contractile force. This is called the **inotropic** (strengthening) action of catecholamines. The biochemical steps that lead to the rise in $i_{Ca}$ are described in Section 4.5, and the way in which $i_{Ca}$ influences the size of the cytosolic Ca$^{2+}$ transient is described in Section 3.9. **L-type Ca$^{2+}$ channel blockers**, such as verapamil and nifedipine, have the opposite effect; they attenuate $i_{Ca}$ and thus weaken the heartbeat.

### Acute ischaemia shortens the action potential via the K$_{ATP}$ channels

During a coronary artery thrombosis, the acute myocardial hypoxia reduces plateau duration (Figure 3.10, top). This is due to the activation of a specialized form of K$_{ir}$ channel, the K$_{ATP}$ channel (Figure 3.12, top). At a normal intracellular ATP concentration of ~5 mM, the open probability of K$_{ATP}$ channels is low; however, the open probability increases as ATP concentration falls, and as ADP, adenosine and H$^+$ concentration rise in hypoxic cells. The increased K$^+$ conductance induces early repolarization. This shortens the plateau, which in turn truncates Ca$^{2+}$ entry. This may be helpful, in that it reduces the work of the Ca$^{2+}$ pumps/exchangers, and thus reduces O$_2$ demand during hypoxia.

### Chronic heart disease prolongs the action potential

Whereas acute hypoxia shortens the action potential, chronic cardiac failure, ventricular hypertrophy and chronic infarction lengthen it, by reducing K$^+$ channel expression, especially the transient outward K$^+$ channel. The reduced K$^+$ current leads to delayed repolarization, a prolonged plateau and a high frequency of arrhythmias. The importance of the timing of repolarization is vividly demonstrated by **LQTS**, which can be caused by genetic abnormalities in a range of ion channels including the delayed rectifier protein KCNQ1 (LQTS type 1). The prolonged plateau leads to Ca²⁺ overload and afterdepolarization (see Section 3.11), which in turn can trigger arrhythmias and sudden death in an otherwise healthy, young individual.

## 3.9 EXCITATION–CONTRACTION COUPLING AND THE CALCIUM CYCLE

### A sarcoplasmic calcium transient initiates contraction

The arrival of an action potential triggers a sharp rise in sarcoplasmic free Ca²⁺, from 0.1 to ~0.5–2 µM. Some of the Ca²⁺ binds to troponin C to activate contraction (Figure 3.3). To prove that sarcoplasmic Ca²⁺ causes contraction, Fabiato and Fabiato performed a classic experiment in 1975, in which the sarcolemma was stripped from the myocyte, so that intracellular Ca²⁺ could be equilibrated with a known Ca²⁺ concentration in the bathing fluid. These 'skinned' cells were found to relax at 0.1 µM Ca²⁺, contract moderately at 1 µM Ca²⁺ and contract maximally at >10 µM Ca²⁺. The correlation between contractile force and sarcoplasmic [Ca²⁺] was later confirmed in non-skinned myocytes, using intracellular Ca²⁺-sensitive fluorescent dyes; the fluorescent signal begins to rise immediately after depolarization and is quickly followed by contraction (Figure 3.11). Intact

myocytes are more sensitive to Ca²⁺ than skinned ones, and the free Ca²⁺ during a normal, submaximal twitch is probably ~0.55–0.75 µM.

How does the action potential induce an order of magnitude increase in sarcoplasmic Ca²⁺ concentration? As Figure 3.14 shows, Ca²⁺ comes from two sources: the main source is the SR store (~75%–90%) and the plateau current $i_{Ca}$ supplements it (~10%–25%).

### Calcium-induced calcium release from the sarcoplasmic reticulum is the main source of the calcium transient

The junctional SR contains a concentrated store of Ca²⁺ (~1 mM) and is studded with Ca²⁺ release channels (or RyRs). Each release channel is a giant protein with a molecular mass of 2.3 million Da. The protein forms a 'foot' with a T-shaped tube through its centre, through which Ca²⁺ is presumably released. The foot terminates only nanometres from the sarcolemma of a T-tubule or cell surface, and is thus extremely close to the L-type Ca²⁺ channels (Figure 3.14). In junctional regions, there is typically 1 L-type Ca²⁺ channel for every 10 Ca²⁺ release channels. The Ca²⁺ release channels are activated by a rise in free Ca²⁺ concentration in their local subsarcolemmal environment, brought about by the opening of the adjacent L-type Ca²⁺ channel. This is called Ca²⁺-induced Ca²⁺ release.

During diastole, the free intracellular Ca²⁺ concentration is so low that the release channels are closed, except for occasional random discharges, which can be seen as localized **Ca²⁺ 'sparks'** in myocytes loaded with Ca²⁺-sensitive fluorescent dye.

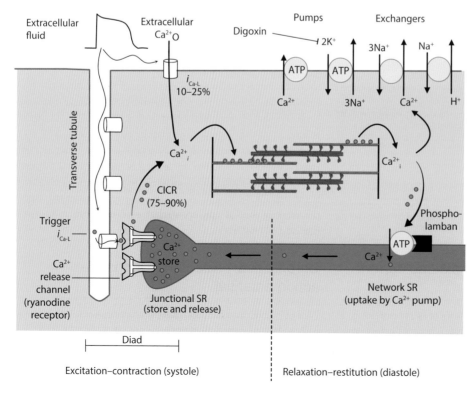

**Figure 3.14** The Ca²⁺ cycle during systole (left) and diastole (right). A T-tubule, L-type Ca²⁺ channel and adjacent cluster of ~10 Ca²⁺ release channels (only two are shown here) form a functional unit. CICR, calcium-induced calcium release; SR, sarcoplasmic reticulum.

Each spark represents a cluster of release channels, and most occur close to T-tubules, though some occur under the surface sarcolemma. When an action potential arrives, the sarcolemmal current $i_{Ca}$ quickly raises the $Ca^{2+}$ concentration in the subsarcolemmal space (Figure 3.14). This is called **trigger $Ca^{2+}$**. The trigger $Ca^{2+}$ from a single L-type channel probably activates a cluster of 6–20 release channels. Since this happens all over the cell, there is a near-synchronous firing of thousands of $Ca^{2+}$ sparks (~10 000 per cell), which releases a substantial fraction of the SR store, typically ~50%. This raises the sarcoplasmic $Ca^{2+}$ concentration roughly 10-fold over ~50 ms, from ~0.1 μM to a peak of ~1 μM. The released $Ca^{2+}$ diffuses rapidly into the sarcomere, and the cell begins to contract (Figure 3.11).

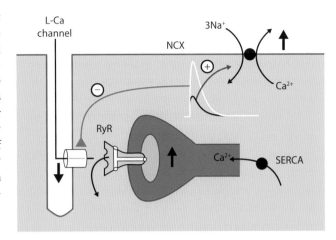

**Figure 3.15** The Eisner model of control of sarcoplasmic reticulum (SR) $Ca^{2+}$ content. An increase in SR content increases ryanodine receptor (RyR) $Ca^{2+}$ release and the whole cell $Ca^{2+}$ transient (represented by the white trace above). This increases (green arrow) $Ca^{2+}$ efflux via the $Na^+/Ca^{2+}$ exchanger (NCX) and decreases (red line) $Ca^{2+}$ entry via the L-type $Ca^{2+}$ channel. This leads to a decrease in cellular, and therefore SR, $Ca^{2+}$ content (through the sarco/endoplasmic reticulum $Ca^{2+}$-ATPase [SERCA]). Therefore, the 'set point' of SR $Ca^{2+}$ content depends on the activity of these key proteins (RyR, NCX, L-type $Ca^{2+}$ current and SERCA) and the negative feedback mechanism described.

## Sarcoplasmic reticulum calcium release is graded, not all-or-none

A potential problem with CICR is that positive feedback ($Ca^{2+}$ release causing more $Ca^{2+}$ release) could, in principle, cause an ungraded discharge of the entire SR store. This does not happen in practice; studies show unequivocally that a small $i_{Ca}$ causes a small $Ca^{2+}$ transient and weak contraction, while a large $i_{Ca}$ causes a large $Ca^{2+}$ transient and strong contraction. This is probably because the activation of release channels requires a **highly localized, very large rise** in subsarcolemmal $Ca^{2+}$ concentration, mediated by an immediately adjacent L-type $Ca^{2+}$ channel; a lesser, diffuse rise in cytosolic $Ca^{2+}$ is not sufficient to activate the release channels. Consequently, one cluster does not generally trigger others. Activation within a given cluster may possibly be all-or-none due to positive feedback (the cluster bomb model), but **the number of clusters activated is proportional to the size of $i_{Ca}$**. The greater the number and duration of L-type $Ca^{2+}$ channel opening events, the greater is the recruitment of subsarcolemmal release clusters and the greater the fraction of the SR store released.

The release channels activate rapidly, then inactivate slowly, over ~30–100 ms (mechanism unknown). Inactivation is followed by a slow recovery of the channel's resting ability to respond to $Ca^{2+}$. This is part of the process of restitution, the return of the system to its original resting state.

## Restitution: pumps in the network sarcoplasmic reticulum restock the store

The $Ca^{2+}$-ATPase pumps of the network SR are stimulated by the systolic rise in sarcoplasmic $Ca^{2+}$, and pump 75%–90% of the raised $Ca^{2+}$ back into the SR interior. The other 10%–25% is expelled by the sarcolemmal $Na^+/Ca^{2+}$ exchanger (Figure 3.14). Since sarcolemmal expulsion normally equals $Ca^{2+}$ entry during the action potential (as $i_{Ca}$), the cell $Ca^{2+}$ content is unchanged in diastole. As the sarcoplasm $Ca^{2+}$ concentration falls, $Ca^{2+}$ dissociates from the troponin–tropomyosin complex and the muscle relaxes. $Ca^{2+}$ uptake by the network SR is followed by restocking of the calsequestrin stores in the

junctional SR. The process of **restitution**, that is, the restocking of the store and restoration of release channel excitability, is normally completed well before the next excitation.

The SR $Ca^{2+}$ pumps are regulated by an inhibitory protein, **phospholamban**. The braking effect of phospholamban on the pump is reduced by adrenaline and noradrenaline. Consequently, adrenaline and noradrenaline increase the rate of myocardial relaxation (**lusitropic action**). The increased rate of SR $Ca^{2+}$ pumping also increases SR $Ca^{2+}$ content and hence the amount of $Ca^{2+}$ released to activate contraction. This, as well as an increase in $i_{Ca}$, results in an increase of force (**inotropic action**), as described in the next section.

Given the large contribution of the SR to the systolic rise of $Ca^{2+}$, it is important that SR $Ca^{2+}$ content is controlled. Emerging evidence from Eisner's group suggests that this is achieved by a simple negative feedback mechanism (Figure 3.15). An increase of SR $Ca^{2+}$ content increases the amplitude of the $Ca^{2+}$ transient. This increases $Ca^{2+}$ efflux on the $Na^+/Ca^{2+}$ exchanger and decreases $Ca^{2+}$ entry on the L-type $Ca^{2+}$ current. This imbalance of fluxes leads to a decrease of cell, and therefore SR $Ca^{2+}$ content. The 'set point' of SR $Ca^{2+}$ that is reached depends on the activity of the various $Ca^{2+}$ handling proteins: RyR, SERCA, $Na^+/Ca^{2+}$ exchanger and L-type $Ca^{2+}$ current.

## Beta-1 adrenergic stimulation increases the calcium transient and contractility

As well as providing the trigger $Ca^{2+}$, the current $i_{Ca}$ continues through the early plateau phase and accounts for ~10%–25% of the rise in sarcoplasmic $Ca^{2+}$ concentration. Consequently, the force of contraction correlates with the amplitude and duration of $i_{Ca}$. **Adrenaline** and **noradrenaline** increase $i_{Ca}$ via the signal transduction pathway shown in Figure 4.10. This increases the size of the free $Ca^{2+}$ transient, and hence contractile force, through two mechanisms. First, the increase in trigger $i_{Ca}$ in the subsarcolemmal space recruits more clusters of release channels, releasing a greater **fraction** of the $Ca^{2+}$ store. Second, the raised $i_{Ca}$ during the plateau increases the amount of $Ca^{2+}$ available for subsequent uptake into the SR store, leading to an increase in the **size** of the $Ca^{2+}$ store over several heartbeats. This focuses our attention on the important question, 'What governs the size of the $Ca^{2+}$ store?'

## Factors governing the size of the sarcoplasmic reticulum calcium store

The amount of $Ca^{2+}$ in the SR store depends on the balance between the influx of extracellular $Ca^{2+}$ during the plateau and its expulsion during diastole. Consequently, $Ca^{2+}$ store size depends on:

1. extracellular $Ca^{2+}$ concentration, which is normally very stable;
2. the size of the L-type $Ca^{2+}$ current, which is increased by the $\beta_1$-adrenoceptor ligands, noradrenaline and adrenaline, and reduced by $Ca^{2+}$ channel blockers;
3. heart rate, which affects the duration of systole (extracellular $Ca^{2+}$ influx) relative to diastole ($Ca^{2+}$ expulsion). Store size and contractile force generally increase with heart rate, as described under 'Bowditch effect' (see Section 6.11).

The size of the SR store can also be raised by pharmacological agents, such as **digoxin**, a drug used to treat chronic heart failure (next section). **Caffeine** at very high concentrations in vitro activates $Ca^{2+}$ release channels, leading to a sustained contraction called a contracture. However, at therapeutic lower levels, caffeine improves contractility by inhibiting phosphodiesterase, as does **milrinone**, a drug used to treat acute cardiac failure. The **phosphodiesterases** are a group of enzymes that degrade cyclic adenosine monophosphate (cAMP), which is the intracellular messenger mediating the effect of adrenaline and noradrenaline (Figure 4.10). Caffeine and milrinone elevate cAMP and thus mimic the contractility-enhancing action of adrenaline and noradrenaline. **Ischaemic heart disease**

can cause overloading of the SR store, leading to arrhythmias (Section 3.11).

## Digoxin increases the systolic calcium transient

Digoxin, a cardiac glycoside extracted mainly from foxglove, has been used for over two centuries to treat chronic cardiac failure. It enhances myocardial contractile force by increasing the size of the systolic $Ca^{2+}$ transient (Figure 3.16). Its pharmacological target is the sarcolemmal $Na^+/K^+$ pump, which it inhibits by ~25%. This raises the subsarcolemmal $Na^+$ concentration. Since the transmembrane $Na^+$ gradient drives the $Na^+/Ca^{2+}$ exchanger, $Ca^{2+}$ expulsion is slowed, the $Ca^{2+}$ store builds up and cardiac contractility improves. However, the toxic dose of digoxin is only a little higher than the therapeutic dose; at toxic doses, excessive accumulation of intracellular $Ca^{2+}$ causes store overload. This is a potent trigger for afterdepolarization and arrhythmias; so, a digoxin overdose can trigger arrhythmias (Section 3.9).

---

**CONCEPT BOX 3.2**

**CONTRACTILE FORCE IS PROPORTIONAL TO CROSSBRIDGE ACTIVATION**

- A crossbridge is a myosin head that extends from the thick myosin filament to a binding site on the thin actin filament. Flexion of the head generates contraction.
- Contractile force is increased by increasing the number of crossbridges.
- Crossbridge formation is induced by a rise in sarcoplasmic free $Ca^{2+}$ concentration.
- The free $Ca^{2+}$ transient is due chiefly to the partial discharge of the SR store of $Ca^{2+}$. Store discharge is triggered by the arrival of extracellular $Ca^{2+}$ as current $i_{Ca}$ at the start of an action potential ($Ca^{2+}$-induced $Ca^{2+}$ release).
- During a quiet heartbeat, the free $Ca^{2+}$ transient is only big enough to activate a fraction of the potential crossbridges.
- Sympathetic stimulation increases $i_{Ca}$ and stored $Ca^{2+}$, leading to bigger free $Ca^{2+}$ transients, increased crossbridge formation and increased contractile force.
- Stretching the cell increases its sensitivity to $Ca^{2+}$, and therefore increases crossbridge formation and contractile force.

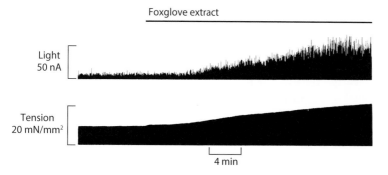

Foxglove extract

Light
50 nA

Tension
20 mN/mm²

4 min

**Figure 3.16** In 1785, William Withering reported that a folklore remedy based on an infusion of foxglove leaves (*Digitalis*) was beneficial for 'dropsy' (cardiac failure). The bicentennial experiment shown here confirms that foxglove extract increases contractile force and intracellular $Ca^{2+}$ concentration in ferret papillary muscle. Light emission from the aequorin-injected muscle (top trace) was used to measure systolic free $Ca^{2+}$ concentration; aequorin, a jellyfish protein, emits blue light in the presence of free $Ca^{2+}$. (From Allen DG, Eisner DA, Smith GL, et al. *The Journal of Physiology* 1985; 365: 55P, with permission from Wiley-Blackwell.)

## 3.10 REGULATION OF CONTRACTILE FORCE

The degree of activation of the contractile machinery is continually adjusted by physiological mechanisms during our daily lives (see Chapter 6). When we are at rest, only about 40% of the potential actin–myosin crossbridges are activated during systole, so the heartbeat is gentle. During exercise or stress, the number of crossbridges is increased, so the heart beats harder, that is, with increased force. There are two fundamentally different ways of increasing crossbridge formation:

1. The **systolic Ca$^{2+}$ transient** can be increased, as described earlier. This is normally brought about by noradrenaline released locally from cardiac sympathetic fibres, and circulating adrenaline from the adrenal gland.
2. **Stretching the myocyte** in diastole provides a second, fundamentally different way of increasing crossbridge formation. In normal life, the myocardium becomes more stretched whenever diastolic filling increases, for example, every time we lie down. Stretch increases the **sensitivity to Ca$^{2+}$**, rather than the size of the Ca$^{2+}$ transient. This is the basis of the fundamental **Starling law of the heart** or **length–tension relation** described in Chapter 6. An account of its underlying mechanism is deferred to that chapter.

## 3.11 STORE OVERLOAD, AFTERDEPOLARIZATION AND ARRHYTHMIA

Coronary artery disease can cause cardiac ischaemia, which often triggers an arrhythmia, such as fatal ventricular fibrillation (Chapter 5). The primary pro-arrhythmogenic change is often the **overloading of the SR calcium store**. The store becomes overloaded through two main mechanisms:

1. Ischaemia raises intracellular Na$^+$ concentration, partly because the energy supply for the Na$^+$/K$^+$ pump is reduced, and partly because intracellular acidosis stimulates the sarcolemmal Na$^+$/H$^+$ exchanger. A raised intracellular Na$^+$ concentration reduces the forward-mode turnover of the Na$^+$/Ca$^{2+}$ exchanger, leading to intracellular Ca$^{2+}$ accumulation (Figure 6.22).
2. Cardiac ischaemia reflexly increases cardiac sympathetic nerve activity, raising noradrenaline and adrenaline levels. This activates myocardial β-adrenoceptors, which, via intracellular cAMP (Figure 4.10), boost the plateau Ca$^{2+}$ current, $i_{Ca}$. High sympathetic activity in ischaemic

hearts thus promotes store overload and arrhythmias. Conversely, it is difficult to induce ventricular tachycardia or fibrillation by regional ischaemia in a chronically denervated heart. Phosphodiesterase inhibitors can have similar arrhythmogenic effects to high sympathetic activity because they too raise intracellular cAMP and hence $i_{Ca}$.

The overloaded Ca$^{2+}$ store is prone to spontaneous, **partial discharge during early diastole**, possibly exacerbated by increased leakiness of the Ca$^{2+}$ release channels (RyR2) due to β-adrenoceptor-driven phosphorylation. The diastolic rise in sarcoplasmic Ca$^{2+}$ stimulates Ca$^{2+}$ expulsion by the sarcolemmal 3Na$^+$/1Ca$^{2+}$ exchanger. Since this entails a net inward flow of positive charge, it causes a depolarization after the action potential (Figure 3.17). If the afterdepolarization reaches a threshold, a premature action potential follows and may trigger an arrhythmia. Afterdepolarization may occur after the cell has fully repolarized (**delayed afterdepolarization**) or during its repolarization phase (**early afterdepolarization**). Delayed afterdepolarizations probably trigger most of the arrhythmias associated with acute cardiac ischaemia, chronic cardiac failure, digoxin toxicity and phosphodiesterase inhibition.

Since an increased Ca$^{2+}$ current $i_{Ca}$, contributes to this chain of events, the risk of sudden death from arrhythmia after myocardial infarction can be reduced by β adrenergic receptor blockers (e.g. bisoprolol, metoprolol).

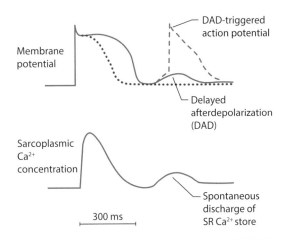

**Figure 3.17** Partial discharge of overloaded internal Ca$^{2+}$ store in diastole (lower trace) stimulates the electrogenic 3Na$^+$/1Ca$^{2+}$ exchanger, causing a net inflow of positive charge (Na$^+$) and a delayed afterdepolarization (DAD, upper trace). If DAD reaches a threshold, it triggers a premature action potential (dashed line). The dotted line shows the effect of replacing external Na$^+$ with Li$^+$, to inhibit the Na$^+$/Ca$^{2+}$ exchanger; the shortening of the plateau shows that the exchanger current normally contributes to the late plateau; also, the DAD is abolished. (Based on Benardeau et al. *American Journal of Physiology* 1996; 271: H1151–61, with permission from the American Physiological Society.)

## SUMMARY

- The myocyte **resting potential**, ~80 mV, approximates to a $K^+$ equilibrium potential, modified by a small inward background leak of $Na^+$ ions. The ATP-powered $3Na^+/2K^+$ pump maintains intracellular ion concentrations and contributes 2–4 mV to the potential.

- Contraction is initiated by an **action potential**. Voltage dependent $Na^+$ channels conduct a rapid inward current of $Na^+$, $i_{Na}$, which depolarizes the myocyte (spike of action potential, phase 0). The $Na^+$ channels rapidly inactivate, and a transient outward $K^+$ current, $i_{to}$, causes an early partial repolarization (phase 1). A second inward current, mainly of extracellular $Ca^{2+}$ ions, $i_{Ca}$, maintains a prolonged depolarization, the **plateau**, which lasts 200–400 ms (phase 2). An inward $Na^+$ current through the $3Na^+/1Ca^{2+}$ exchanger maintains the late plateau. Contraction begins during the plateau, and the cell is refractory to re-excitation.

- **Repolarization** by outward $K^+$ currents $i_{Kv}$ and $i_{Kir}$ terminates the plateau (phase 3). During tachycardia and hypoxia, increased $K^+$ currents shorten the plateau; in chronic heart disease, reduced $K^+$ currents lengthen it.

- Immediately after depolarization, extracellular 'trigger' $Ca^{2+}$ passes through L-type $Ca^{2+}$ channels into the subsarcolemmal space (early $i_{Ca}$). This activates clusters of $Ca^{2+}$ release channels (RyRs) in the junctional SR (**$Ca^{2+}$-induced calcium release**). The release of around half the SR $Ca^{2+}$ store transiently raises sarcoplasmic free $Ca^{2+}$ to ~1 μM.

- $Ca^{2+}$ binds to the troponin–tropomyosin complex on actin filaments, leading to the exposure of myosin-binding sites.

- Myosin heads then form **crossbridges**, extending from the thick myosin filaments to the thin actin filaments. The myosin heads swivel, rowing the thick myosin filaments into the spaces between the thin actin filaments. This generates tension and shortening. Recocking of the myosin heads consumes ATP, so mitochondrial density is high and normal contractility requires a high $O_2$ supply via the coronary arteries.

- **Contractile force**, typically ~40% maximal at rest, depends on the fraction of the potential crossbridges activated. This is regulated by two factors.

- Stretch of the sarcomere in diastole increases the *sensitivity* of the contractile machinery to $Ca^{2+}$, which leads to more crossbridge activation and contractile force (the length–tension relationship).

- The **size** of the systolic $Ca^{2+}$ transient determines the number of crossbridges activated at a given length. Adrenaline and noradrenaline increase $i_{Ca}$, which increases the store size and supplies more trigger $Ca^{2+}$, releasing a greater fraction of the store. This leads to bigger $Ca^{2+}$ transients and hence stronger contractions.

- In **ischaemia,** the SR $Ca^{2+}$ store becomes overloaded, especially when β-adrenoceptor stimulation by catecholamines is high. Spontaneous partial discharge of the overloaded store in diastole evokes afterdepolarization, due to the increased $3Na^+/1Ca^{2+}$ exchanger current. This can trigger premature action potentials and arrhythmia.

## FURTHER READING

Eisner, DA. Ups and downs of calcium in the heart. *The Journal of Physiology* 2018; **596**(1): 19–30.

Eisner DA, Caldwell JL, Kistamás K, et al. Calcium and excitation-contraction coupling in the heart. *Circulation Research* 2017; **121**(2): 181–95.

Vermij SH, Abriel H, van Veen TA. Refining the molecular organization of the cardiac intercalated disc. *Cardiovascular Research* 2017; **113**(3): 259–75.

Bers DM, Chen-Izu Y. Sodium and calcium regulation in cardiac myocytes: from molecules to heart failure and arrhythmia. *The Journal of Physiology* 2015; **593**(6): 1327–9.

Shattock MJ, Ottolia M, Bers DM, et al. $Na^+/Ca^{2+}$ exchange and $Na^+/K^+$-ATPase in the heart. *The Journal of Physiology* 2015; **593**(6): 1361–82.

Eisner D. Calcium in the heart: from physiology to disease. *Experimental Physiology* 2014; **99**(10): 1273–82.

Orchard CH, Bryant SM, James AF. Do t-tubules play a role in arrhythmogenesis in cardiac ventricular myocytes? *The Journal of Physiology* 2013; **591**(17): 4141–7.

Aidley DJ. The contractile mechanism of muscle. In: *The Physiology of Excitable Cells*, 4th edn. Cambridge: Cambridge University Press; 2008. pp. 336–71.

Bers DM. Calcium cycling and signaling in cardiac myocytes. *Annual Review of Physiology* 2008; **70**: 23–49.

Cheng H, Lederer WJ. Calcium sparks. *Physiology Reviews* 2008; **88**(4): 1491–545.

Sipido KR, Bito V, Antoons G, et al. Na/Ca exchange and cardiac ventricular arrhythmias. *Annals of the New York Academy of Sciences* 2007; **1099**: 339–48.

Jespersen T, Grunnet M, Olesen SP. The KCNQ1 potassium channel: from gene to physiological function. *Physiology (Bethesda)* 2005; **20**: 408–16.

Roden DM, Balser JR, George AL Jr, et al. Cardiac ion channels. *Annual Review of Physiology* 2002; **64**: 431–75.

Solaro RJ, Rarick HM. Troponin and tropomyosin: proteins that switch on and tune in the activity of the cardiac myofilaments. *Circulation Research* 1998; **83**(5): 471–80.

Fabiato A, Fabiato F. Contractions induced by a calcium-triggered release of calcium from the sarcoplasmic reticulum of single skinned cardiac cells. *The Journal of Physiology* 1975; **249**(3): 469–95.

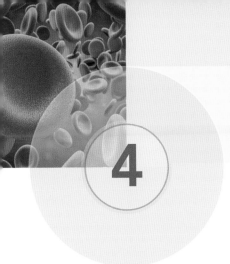

# Initiation and nervous control of heartbeat

# 4

## LEARNING OBJECTIVES

*After reading this chapter you should be able to:*

- sketch the anatomy of the cardiac excitation–conduction system and state the role of each component (4.1);
- explain 'dominance' (4.1) and the emergence of a slower pacemaker in heart block;
- draw the sino-atrial node potential over one cardiac cycle and state the ionic basis of each phase (4.2);
- explain how depolarization propagates through the myocardium (4.3);

- state the chronotropic actions of (1) sympathetic and (2) parasympathetic nerves, and the underlying mechanisms (4.5; 4.6);
- explain the inotropic and lusitropic effects of sympathetic stimulation (4.5);
- describe the deleterious effect of hyper- and hypokalaemia (4.8);
- state the actions of (1) β-blockers and (2) $Ca^{2+}$-channel blockers on the heart (4.9).

If the heart is excised from a cold-blooded animal and placed in a suitable solution of electrolytes, it will continue to beat for a long period. This simple experiment shows that the heartbeat is initiated from within the heart. Unlike skeletal muscle, extrinsic nerves are not necessary to initiate contraction. The heartbeat is initiated by an intrinsic electrical system composed of modified myocytes, not nerves. These specialized myocytes are organized into: (1) the sino-atrial (SA) node (pacemaker), a group of cells that discharge spontaneously at regular intervals to initiate the heartbeat; and (2) cells that conduct the electrical impulse across the annulus fibrosus into the ventricle wall, triggering ventricular systole. Although pacemaker activity does not depend on extrinsic nerves, the frequency of pacemaker firing can be modified by autonomic nerves; sympathetic activity increases it, parasympathetic activity decreases it. Sympathetic fibres also regulate the contractile force and therefore the stroke volume. Contrary to established dogma, the vagus nerve also innervates the ventricle and can depress contraction. Thus, both components

of the cardiac output, namely heart rate and stroke volume (SV), are under central nervous control and local circuit control within the heart itself (the heart's little brain), to regulate cardiac excitability and contractile strength. Importantly, the central nervous system also receives sensory afferent information from skeletal muscle, the heart, kidneys and arterial and cardiopulmonary receptors to help regulate cardiac function (see Figure 4.5).

## 4.1 ORGANIZATION OF THE PACEMAKER–CONDUCTION SYSTEM

### The sino-atrial node initiates the heartbeat

The SA node (pacemaker) is a strip of myocytes roughly 20mm long and 4mm wide in man, located on the posterior wall of the right atrium close to the superior vena cava (Figure 4.1). The mammalian SA node is so called because it evolved from

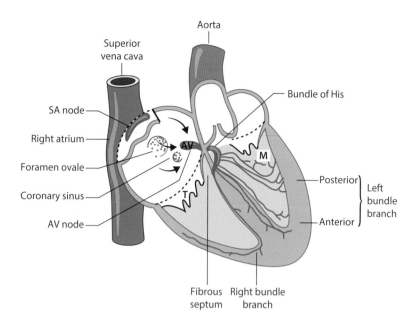

**Figure 4.1** The cardiac conduction system. The posterior fibres of the left bundle branch are seen facing forwards, running just inside the septum, then curling round in the left ventricular subendocardium. Black arrows show conduction through the atrial muscle. Note the proximity of the valves (T, tricuspid; M, mitral) to the bundle of His; valve lesions can affect the main bundle. The foramen ovale is the remnant of the fetal connection between right and left sides. The coronary sinus is the outlet of the main coronary vein. AV, atrioventricular; SA, sino-atrial.

the sinus venosus, an antechamber to the right atrium in lower vertebrates (relatively simple and primitive vertebrates). The SA node is made up of small myocytes that have scanty myofibrils and an unstable membrane potential capable of spontaneous depolarisation. Human nodal cells fire an action potential spontaneously about once every second at rest. This excites the adjacent atrial myocytes. The action potential is then conducted from myocyte to myocyte, creating a wave of depolarization that sweeps across both atria. The wave travels at ~1 m/s and initiates atrial systole.

## The atrioventricular node delays ventricular excitation

The electrical impulse quickly reaches the atrioventricular (AV) node, a small mass of cells and connective tissue in the lower, posterior region of the atrial septum. The AV node is the start of the only electrical connection across the annulus fibrosus, which otherwise insulates the atria from the ventricles (Section 2.1). The impulse is delayed in the node for ~0.1 s at resting heart rates. The delay is generated by the complex local circuitry and the small diameter of the nodal cells, 2–3 μm, which reduces the conduction velocity to ~0.05 m/s. The delaying role of the AV node is important, because it allows time for the atria to contract before the ventricles.

## The bundle of His and its branches excite the ventricles

The role of the ventricular conduction system is to excite the entire ventricular wall as near simultaneously as possible. A bundle of fast-conducting muscle fibres, the **bundle of His**, conveys the electrical impulse from the AV node through the annulus fibrosus into the fibrous upper part of the interventricular septum. Here the bundle turns and runs forwards along

the crest of the main muscular part of the septum (Figure 4.1). The bundle gives off a **left bundle branch**, which comprises two sets of fibres (or fascicles), one anterior and one posterior. These course down the left side of the muscular septum and supply the left ventricle. The remaining bundle, the **right bundle branch**, runs down the right side of the interventricular septum and supplies the right ventricle.

The bundle fibres are wide, fast-conducting myocytes arranged in a regular, end-to-end fashion. They terminate in an extensive network of large fibres in the subendocardium, described by the Czech histologist Johann Evangelist Purkinje in 1839. **Purkinje fibres** (correctly pronounced "P-oo-r-k-ih-n-y-eh" in Czech) are the widest cells in the heart (diameter 40–80 μm), and consequently have the highest conduction velocity (3–5 m/s). Their role is to distribute the electrical impulse rapidly to the subendocardial myocytes. From here, the impulse passes from myocyte to myocyte at ~0.5–1 m/s in a generally outward epicardial direction, until the whole wall has been excited. This takes ~90 ms.

## The fastest pacemaker dominates a hierarchy of slower, latent pacemakers

There are other potential pacemakers in the heart besides the SA node, but they have slower intrinsic frequencies of firing. The SA node normally determines the heart rate simply because its cells have the fastest frequency of firing, and therefore excite the heart before other slower pacemakers have reached their firing threshold. If the SA node is destroyed, myocytes in the atrium or AV node take over as the new pacemaker, because they have the next highest rate of firing. The bundle of His can also act as a pacemaker, but only at <40 bpm. Purkinje cells have an even slower pacemaking frequency, ~15 bpm, which is too slow to maintain an adequate cardiac output. There is thus a **gradient of intrinsic pacemaker frequencies along**

**the cardiac electrical system**. The slower lower centres are normally excited by the SA node before they have time to fire spontaneously. This is called **dominance**.

The emergence of a slow, distal pacemaker can be seen in the pathological condition of **heart block**. In complete heart block the AV node fails to transmit excitation through the annulus fibrosus, so the SA node can no longer dominate the ventricle. Pacemaker cells in the bundle of His then take over, driving the ventricles at <40 bpm (Figure 5.4). This is too slow for many daily activities, and such patients usually benefit from the insertion of an artificial, permanent pacemaker.

## 4.2 ELECTRICAL ACTIVITY OF THE PACEMAKER

### Pacemaker potential decay determines heart rate

The membrane potential of SA node cells is small and unstable. The initial potential is only −50 to −70 mV, because nodal cells express few inward rectifier K⁺ channels ($K_{ir}$), the channels responsible for the big, stable resting potential in atrial and ventricular myocytes. However, the pacemaker cell expresses voltage-dependent, delayed rectifier K⁺ channels, $K_v$ (Table 4.1), and K⁺ efflux through these channels generates the starting potential of around −60 mV.

The membrane potential then decays spontaneously with time (Figure 4.2). This slowly declining potential is called the **pacemaker potential**. When the pacemaker potential reaches a threshold of −40 to −55 mV, it triggers an action potential, which sparks off the next heartbeat. The rate of decay of the pacemaker potential, that is, its slope, is important, because it determines the time interval needed to reach the threshold, and thus the interval between heartbeats. The steeper the slope, the sooner the threshold is reached and the shorter the interval between the heartbeats. Thus, a steeply decaying pacemaker potential causes a high heart rate.

### Multiple ionic currents cause the potential to decay

The decay of the pacemaker potential is brought about by several different inward currents, and by a decay of the outward current, sometimes referred to as the sarcolemmal membrane "voltage clock".

The delayed rectifier, voltage-activated K⁺ channels, $K_v$, inactivate slowly with time at negative potentials, because of the ball-and-chain mechanism shown in Figure 3.12. This is why membrane electrical conductance declines during phase 4 in Figure 3.7. Consequently, the polarizing (negative-making) **outward current $i_K$ decays with time**. The decay in the outward K⁺ current allows inward, depolarizing currents to become increasingly dominant (Figure 4.2). The inward currents are as follows:

1. A small, inward current of Na⁺ ions slowly depolarizes the cell. The current may be partly the inward background current $i_b$, described in Chapter 3. In addition, many SA node cells possess a specialized pacemaker current called the **'funny' current**, $i_f$, which was discovered by Dario Francesco, Hilary Brown and Susan Noble in 1979; $i_f$ is only active at potentials positive to about −50 mV, and it is 'funny' in the sense that the channel is activated by hyperpolarization whereas most voltage-sensitive channels are activated by depolarization (e.g. $K_v$ and Ca²⁺ channels). Although the $i_f$ channel is non-selective between Na⁺ and K⁺, the $i_f$ current is carried chiefly by Na⁺ ions, because the electrochemical gradient favours Na⁺ influx at negative membrane potentials. Some believe this ion channel contributes little to pacemaking itself because it activates at membrane potentials more negative than seen in some isolated sinoatrial node cells and instead a 'Ca²⁺ clock' provides the main signal to generate spontaneous rhythm (see later in the chapter). However, circulating adrenaline ('epinephrine' in the American literature) shifts its potential more positively into the diastolic depolarization voltage range, because $i_f$ is a cyclic nucleotide-regulated ion channel (hyperpolarization-activated cyclic nucleotide-gated 4 [HCN4] protein) and is activated by second messengers, in particular **cyclic adenosine monophosphate (cAMP)**. Indeed, most single-cell experiments are done with Tyrode's solution where cAMP is not present, suggesting that the role of $i_f$ may be underestimated. Caesium ions block $i_f$ and slow the rate of pacemaker depolarization, as does a clinically used $i_f$ blocker, **ivabradine**. Inhibition of the current *in vivo* is estimated to reduce heart rate by approximately 15%–20%. These agents do not stop pacemaker decay completely, indicating the existence of additional pacemaking currents.

2. The **3Na⁺/Ca²⁺ exchanger** generates a net inward Na⁺ current, $i_{Na-Ca}$, that contributes substantially to pacemaker depolarization. Blocking this current can abolish the late part of the decay of the pacemaker potential.

3. As the membrane potential decays below approximately −55 mV, an **inward current of Ca²⁺ ions** begins to contribute to depolarization. The SA node expresses voltage-sensitive Ca²⁺ channels of a type called transient or **T-type**. T-type Ca²⁺ channels have an increased probability of being in the open state beyond −55 mV (Figure 4.3, left). As the potential declines further, voltage-sensitive **L-type** Ca²⁺ channels also begin to open. L-type channels activate at more depolarized (**Lower**) potentials than T-type Ca²⁺ channels (Figure 4.3, right). Thus, an increasing Ca²⁺ influx accelerates the depolarization rate in the late stages of the pacemaker potential, triggering the action potential and the next heartbeat.

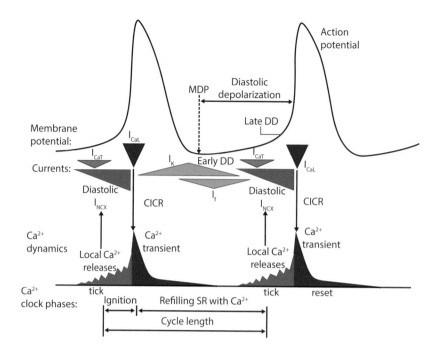

(a)

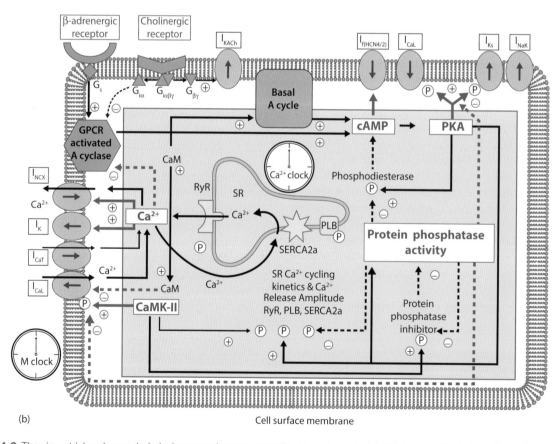

(b)

**Figure 4.2** The sino-atrial node coupled-clock pacemaker system and autonomic control. (**a**) Schematic illustration of key phases of the functional interactions between the membrane and Ca²⁺ clocks. (**b**) Schematic illustration of interactions of molecules comprising the full coupled-clock pacemaker. Note that the same regulatory factors (red) of the sarcoplasmic reticulum Ca²⁺ clock (grey intracellular area, black lettering) couple the Ca²⁺ clock to the membrane clock (blue membrane area, blue lettering). G protein-coupled receptors (green lettering) regulate both the Ca²⁺ clock and membrane clock via those same factors (red lettering) and other coupling factors (green shapes). CaMKII, Ca²⁺/calmodulin-dependent protein kinase II; cAMP, cyclic adenosine monophosphate; CICR, Ca²⁺-induced Ca²⁺ release; DD, diastolic depolarization; GPCR, G protein-coupled receptor; A cyclase, adenylyl cyclase; PKA, protein kinase A; PLB, phospholamban; SR, sarcoplasmic reticulum; RyR, ryanodine receptor; SERCA, sarco/endoplasmic reticulum Ca²⁺-ATPase. MDP, maximum diastolic potential; DD diastolic depolarization (pacemaker potential)

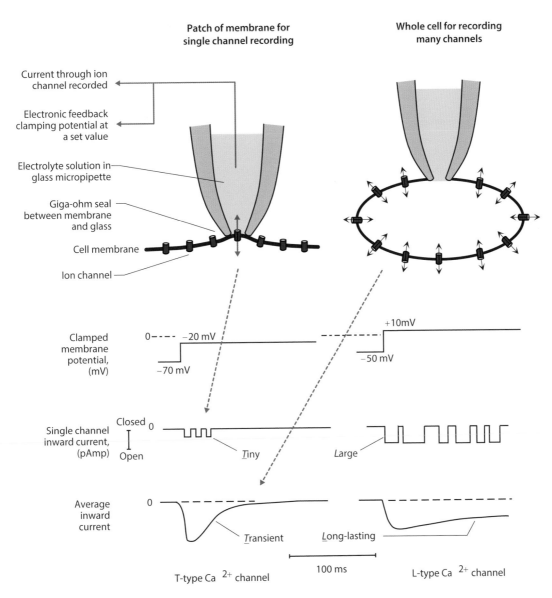

**Figure 4.3** Cardiac Ca²⁺ currents recorded by patch clamp. A tiny patch of membrane is sealed to the glass micropipette by suction to record single-channel activity (top left). The patch can be ruptured mechanically or chemically to record net current through all the ion channels in the cell ('perforated patch' or 'whole-cell' mode, top right). Depolarization beyond −55 mV (top left trace) caused a single T-type channel to flicker open sporadically (middle left), admitting tiny pulses of current. This soon ceases, so the average current passed by hundreds of T-type channels is transient (bottom left). When the membrane is depolarized further (top right trace), a single, higher-threshold L-type Ca²⁺ channel opens sporadically, admitting larger pulses of current, for longer (middle right). The average current passed by hundreds of such channels is thus long-lasting (bottom right) and inactivates only slowly. (Redrawn from Nilius B et al. *Nature* 1985; 316: 443–6, with permission from Macmillan Publishers Ltd.)

## Node action potentials are small, sluggish and calcium-based

Node action potentials are small in amplitude and slow-rising, like the tetrodotoxin-blocked myocyte of Figure 3.9. This is because the nodal cell has few functional fast Na⁺ channels. The action potential in both the SA and AV node is generated solely by an inward Ca²⁺ current (Table 4.1). Therefore, calcium channel inhibitors, such as verapamil, reduce the size of the nodal action potential and the pacemaker decay rate. Repolarization is brought about by an outward K⁺ current through delayed rectifier K⁺ channels, $K_V$ (Figure 3.10).

These voltage-gated channels activate very slowly during depolarization (time constant 300–400 ms), so they open gradually during the action potential. On repolarization, they begin to inactivate slowly, thus contributing to the next pacemaker cycle.

## Calcium clock hypothesis and calcium/calmodulin-dependent protein kinase II

With the advent of simultaneous submembrane Ca²⁺ imaging and ion current recordings with cell-attached patch electrodes, Ed Lakatta and colleagues have shown that

**Table 4.1** Main ionic currents in nodal pacemaker cells

| Current | Ion | Direction | Function | Channel inhibitor |
|---------|-----|-----------|----------|-------------------|
| $(i_{Na})$ | $(Na^+)$ | – | Voltage-operated $Na^+$ channels are largely absent/inactivated in nodal cells | – |
| $i_f$ and $i_b{}^a$ | $Na^+$ | Inward | Supply inward depolarizing current during initial part of pacemaker potential | $Cs^+$ and ivabradine block $i_f$ |
| $i_{Na-Ca}{}^b$ | $Na^+$ | Inward | Important contribution to later part of pacemaker depolarization | |
| $i_{Ca}$ | $Ca^{2+}$ | Inward | Contributes to last third of pacemaker potential Generates slow-rising action potential | $Mn^{2+}$, verapamil, diltiazem |
| $i_{Kv}$ | $K^+$ | Outward | Delayed rectifier, voltage-operated channel 1. Supplies decaying current during pacemaker potential 2. Supplies repolarization current | $Ba^{2+}$ |

$^a$ $i_f$ is funny current; $i_b$ is background current.
$^b$ Net inward current produced by the expulsion of one intracellular $Ca^{2+}$ in exchange for three extracellular $Na^+$ ions.

critically timed $Ca^{2+}$ release occurs during diastolic depolarization (DD) and activates the $Na^+/Ca^{2+}$ exchanger, contributing to the late DD, driving the membrane potential to the threshold for the rapid upstroke of the next action potential. These $Ca^{2+}$ release events are likely triggered by the T-type $Ca^{2+}$ current. Such rhythmic, spontaneous intracellular $Ca^{2+}$ cycling has been referred to as an 'intracellular $Ca^{2+}$ clock'. It has been proposed that this interacts with the classic sarcolemmal membrane voltage clock to form the overall pacemaker clock that is highly modulated by levels of high basal **$Ca^{2+}$/calmodulin-dependent kinase II (CaMKII)**. This protein modifies the phosphorylation state of the $Ca^{2+}$ cycling proteins **phospholamban** (PLB), RyR and L-type $Ca^{2+}$ channels by adjusting the local $Ca^{2+}$ release period to influence both normal and reserve cardiac pacemaker function (see Figure 4.2). It is most probable that a combination of both $i_f$ and the $Ca^{2+}$ clock hypothesis keeps us ticking. The dominance of each depends on the prevailing physiological state involving the autonomic nervous system (ANS), for example, during exercise.

## 4.3 TRANSMISSION OF EXCITATION

### Propagating currents spread the excitation

The spread of excitation through the atria, conduction system and ventricles is brought about by local electrical currents that act ahead of the action potential (Figure 4.4). In the active, depolarized region, the membrane interior is positively charged, while in the resting zone ahead, it is negative. The two regions are connected by an internal, electrically conductive pathway, namely the sarcoplasm and **gap junctions** (Figure 3.1). Positive charge therefore flows intracellularly into the resting membrane region, depolarizing it. Externally, the converse applies; the extracellular fluid is a conducting medium, so positive charge flows from the outside of the resting membrane to the active region, reducing the charge on the outside of the resting membrane. This process is in fact the **passive discharge of a capacitor**, namely the lipid

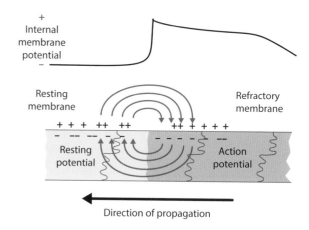

Direction of propagation

**Figure 4.4** Excitation is transmitted through the conduction system and myocardium by local currents acting ahead of the action potential. The internal current flows through the sarcoplasm and gap junctions of the intercalated disc. The external current flows through the extracellular fluid. The currents discharge the membrane ahead, triggering its action potential.

membrane. When the resting membrane potential reaches the threshold, an action potential is triggered, setting up fresh local currents to excite the next region and so on. Since the membrane to the rear is in its **refractory period**, excitation proceeds unidirectionally.

### The safety margin for propagation: conduction rate depends on fibre diameter and local current magnitude

The conduction of excitation is fastest in the widest cells, the Purkinje fibres. A **wide diameter** confers a low axial electrical resistance, which enables the local circuits in Figure 4.4 to reach out a greater distance ahead of the active region. Conduction rate also depends on the magnitude and rate of rise of the action potential. Conduction is fast in myocytes with large, rapid-rising action potentials, such as ventricular myocytes, because these potentials generate **big propagating currents**, and big currents can extend well ahead of the active region. The action potential depolarization rate, that is, the steepness of the phase 0, $Na^+$-mediated spike (500 V/s), is particularly important for the generation of big propagating currents and the reliable propagation of excitation. During ischaemia and hyperkalaemia, the deterioration in ventricular action potential size and phase 0 depolarization rate can impair conduction, contributing to ventricular arrhythmia (Section 5.10). Nodal cells, which have small, slow-rising action potentials, generate small propagating currents and have a **poor safety margin for conduction**; therefore, conduction is slow and easily blocked in nodal tissue.

## 4.4 REGULATION OF THE HEART RATE

The human heart beats 50–100 times per minute at rest and a little slower in endurance-trained athletes. In other mammals, the heart rate is proportional to $1/mass^{0.25}$: for example, the shrew's heart rate is 600 bpm and the elephant's is 25 bpm! The heart rate is modulated by sympathetic and parasympathetic autonomic nerves innervating the pacemaker and AV node. In the 17th century, Thomas Willis described the vagi nerves as the wandering nerves with cardiac projections. Weber and Weber made the first observation in the 1840s that right vagal stimulation slows the heart rate. The effects of vagal stimulation are abolished by atropine and mimicked by muscarine, strongly suggesting that the vagus nerve releases a chemical neurotransmitter. The work of Otto Loewi in 1921 (for which he was awarded the 1936 Nobel Prize jointly with Sir Henry Hallett Dale) proved this concept to be true. Stimulation of the right vagus nerve of an isolated frog heart decreased the heart rate, and the transfer of the perfusate to a second frog heart produced bradycardia in the donor. The chemical substance in the perfusate responsible for this action was named 'Vagusstoff' and was identified as acetylcholine (ACh) by Dale in the 1930s. The synthesis of ACh occurs in the cytosol via the transfer of an acetyl group from acetyl coenzyme-A to choline, which is catalysed by the enzyme choline acetyltransferase. Choline is taken up from the extracellular environment by the hemicholinium-sensitive transporter and this is thought to be the rate-limiting step in the synthesis.

Similar experiments showed that the sympathetic nervous system releases a chemical neurotransmitter 'Acceleranstoff', subsequently identified as noradrenaline by Ulf von Euler in 1946, leading to him sharing the Nobel Prize for Medicine or Physiology in 1970 with Sir Bernard Katz and Julius Axelrod. The arrival of an action potential in a sympathetic postganglionic terminal triggers the release of the neuroeffector **noradrenaline** ('norepinephrine' in the American literature); for details, see Section 14.1. This transmitter is synthesized via the hydroxylation of tyrosine to levodopa catalysed by tyrosine hydroxylase (the rate-limiting step) and then decarboxylation to dopamine by DOPA decarboxylase. Dopamine is then transported into vesicles via a reserpine-sensitive $H^+$/amine transporter

where the final hydroxylation to noradrenaline (catalysed by dopamine β-hydroxylase) occurs. As with vagal neurotransmission, depolarization of the nerve terminals causes $Ca^{2+}$ influx and the exocytotic release of neurotransmitter. Noradrenaline activates β1, β2 and α1 postsynaptic receptors in the heart (although >70% are β1 in higher-order mammals). It also binds to presynaptic autoinhibitory α2 receptors to modulate the release of transmitter. While ACh is rapidly metabolized by **cholinesterase**, noradrenaline has a longer half-life and is taken up into the nerve via norepinephrine transporter 1 (NET1) protein and to a far lesser extent postsynaptically via NET2. It is then metabolized by mitochondria-bound monoamine oxidase.

## Sympathetic fibres innervate the whole heart

The short preganglionic cardiac sympathetic fibres leave the spinal cord at segments T1-T4 and synapse in the paravertebral sympathetic ganglia. The much longer postganglionic fibres run along the surface of the great vessels to reach the heart. Unlike parasympathetic fibres, the sympathetic fibres richly innervate the ventricular muscle, the atria and the pacemaker–conduction system. The pacemaker is innervated chiefly by fibres from the right paravertebral ganglia, and the ventricles by fibres from the left paravertebral ganglia although there is a susbstnatial overlap (Figures 4.5 and 4.6).

## Parasympathetic fibres have a more restricted distribution

Cardiac parasympathetic fibres originate in the dorsal vagal motor nucleus and nucleus ambiguus of the brainstem, and the very long preganglionic fibres travel in the right and left vagus nerves (Figures 4.5 and 4.6). The right fibres generally innervate the pacemaker and the left the AV node, but there is considerable anatomical variation. The long preganglionic fibres synapse with the postganglionic **parasympathetic neurons** within the myocardium, mostly around the SA and AV nodes. Short postganglionic fibres innervate the nodes. The vagus nerve also innervates the ventricle, although the extent of this innervation is species-dependent. In the mouse and rat, this is sparse, but in the dog, it is extensive. In humans, the innervation is modest but functionally significant because the vagus nerve can depress ventricular contraction when heart rate is held constant.

## Autonomic fibres continuously modify the intrinsic pacemaker rate

Both the sympathetic and parasympathetic fibres are tonically (continuously) active, so the pacemaker firing rate is continuously influenced by them, even at rest. Increased sympathetic activity speeds up the heart rate (**tachycardia**) (Figure 4.7). Increased parasympathetic activity slows it down (**bradycardia**) (Figure 4.8). Although both autonomic systems are

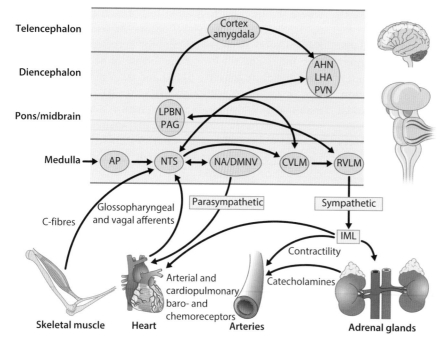

Telencephalon

Diencephalon

Pons/midbrain

Medulla

Cortex
amygdala

AHN
LHA
PVN

LPBN
PAG

AP → NTS ↔ NA/DMNV → CVLM → RVLM

C-fibres

Glossopharyngeal
and vagal afferents

Parasympathetic

Sympathetic

IML

Contractility

Catecholamines

Arterial and
cardiopulmonary
baro- and
chemoreceptors

Skeletal muscle    Heart    Arteries    Adrenal glands

**Figure 4.5** Neural control of the cardiovascular system. The medulla contains areas rich in cells that receive afferent feedback from the cardiopulmonary baroreceptors and arterial chemoreceptors, as well as sensory feedback from muscles and the heart itself. There is reflex efferent output to the heart, vasculature and the kidneys/adrenal glands via the autonomic nervous system. Subcortical areas are also able to drive autonomic outflow and are influenced by prefrontal structures involved in the fight or flight and exercise responses. AHN, anterior hypothalamic nucleus; AP, area postrema; CVLM, caudal ventrolateral medulla; DMNV, dorsal motor nucleus of the vagus; IML, intermediolateral nucleus; LHA, lateral hypothalamic nucleus; LPBN, lateral parabrachial nucleus; NA, nucleus ambiguus; NTS, nucleus tractus solitarius; PAG, periaqueductal gray; PVN, paraventricular nucleus; RVLM, rostral ventrolateral medulla. (Adapted from Herring N, Paterson DJ. Part II. Section B. Adaption and responses: myocardial innervations and neural control. In Hill J, Olson EN, eds. *Muscle: Fundamental Biology and Mechanisms of Disease.* London: Elsevier, 2012. pp. 275–84.)

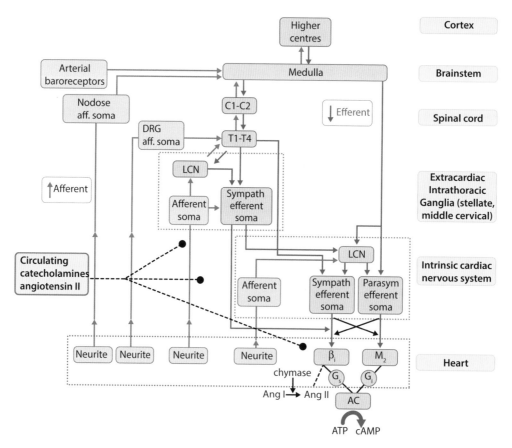

**Figure 4.6** Neurohumoral control and anatomical organization of cardiac innervation. The excitability of cardiac parasympathetic or sympathetic efferent pathways (labelled in red) depends on tonic inputs to synaptic junctions at different level in the brain, spinal cord and in the extrinsic and intrinsic cardiac ganglia. The highest level encompasses the spinal cord and brainstem with higher-centre modulation. Below that, are the extracardiac intrathoracic ganglia (such as the stellate ganglia) and the intrinsic cardiac nervous system. Cardiac afferent neurites (labelled in blue) and extra-cardiac circulatory receptors transmit beat-to-beat sensory information to the different levels producing feedback loops that maintain cardiac physiological stability. Aff, afferent; Ang, angiotensin; ATP, adenosine triphosphate; C, cervical; cAMP, cyclic adenosine monophosphate; DRG, dorsal root ganglion; LCN, local circuit neuron; T, thoracic. (Adapted from Fukuda et al. *Circ Res* 2015; 116(12): 2005–19.)

tonically active, the **parasympathetic, inhibitory effect predominates at rest**. This follows from the finding that the intrinsic heart rate is ~105 bpm in young humans after parasympathetic blockade by atropine and sympathetic blockade by propranolol. Physiological changes in heart rate are usually brought about by **reciprocal changes in sympathetic and parasympathetic activity**. For example, the tachycardia of exercise is brought about by reduced parasympathetic activity and increased sympathetic activity. This is also associated with increases in circulating catecholamines and angiotensin II (Ang II). These hormones act directly on cardiac receptors to increase cardiac rate and the force of contraction. Ang II can also facilitate the presynaptic release of noradrenaline.

## Parasympathetic regulation acts faster than sympathetic regulation

The tachycardia elicited by sympathetic stimulation is relatively sluggish in onset and decays relatively slowly when stimulation ceases (Figure 4.7). By contrast, the bradycardia elicited by parasympathetic stimulation has a very short latency and resolves more quickly when fibre activity ceases (Figure 4.8). Consequently, changes in parasympathetic activity account for rapid changes in heart rate, such as the slowing of the heart during each expiration (sinus arrhythmia) and fainting. The fast 'on' effect is brought about by a hyperpolarizing pathway activated by ACh (see later in the chapter). The fast 'off' effect is due to the rapid removal of ACh by the enzyme cholinesterase.

## The heart's little brain

The interconnected neural architecture of the heart's intrinsic nervous system has been elegantly explored and described by Armour (2008). This system is based on three levels of neural hierarchy and moves away from the historical notion of reciprocal cardiac control where the two arms of the ANS acted as 'accelerator and brake' on cardiac function. Instead, the excitability of cardiac parasympathetic pathways or sympathetic pathways depends on tonic inputs to synaptic junctions at several stages in the brain, spinal cord and extrinsic and intrinsic cardiac ganglia. Level 1 encompasses the spinal cord and medulla with higher-centre modulation. Level 2 incorporates extra-cardiac neurons, such as the stellate ganglia, and level 3 includes all the intrinsic cardiac ganglia and nerves. Cardiac afferents and extra-cardiac circulatory receptors serve to transmit beat-to-beat sensory information to levels 1, 2 and 3, and processing at these levels allows feedback loops that maintain physiological electrical and contractile stability in normal and stressed states (Figure 4.6).

Understanding this complex cardiac–neural axis has led to targeted autonomic modulation therapies for heart failure and arrhythmia aimed at the cervical cardiac vagus and sympathetic nervous system, respectively, because these diseases are also diseases of the ANS (see Chapters 5 and 18).

## Temperature also affects heart rate

The pacemaker rate is influenced by temperature. A **fever** causes the heart rate to increase by 10 bpm per degree

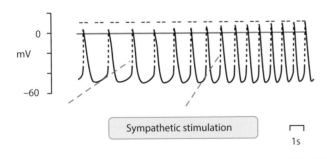

Sympathetic stimulation

1s

**Figure 4.7** Effect of continuous sympathetic stimulation (box) on pacemaker potential. Note the relatively sluggish onset of tachycardia. The dashed, red gradients highlight the increased slope of the pacemaker potential. The upper double-dashed line draws attention to the increase in action potential size, caused by the increased inward $Ca^{2+}$ current induced by noradrenaline-activated β adrenergic receptors. (From Hutter OF, Trautwein W. *Journal of General Physiology* 1956; 39: 715–33, with permission from Rockefeller University Press.)

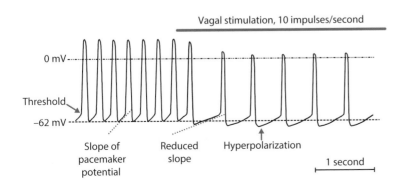

Vagal stimulation, 10 impulses/second

0 mV

Threshold

−62 mV

Slope of pacemaker potential    Reduced slope    Hyperpolarization    1 second

**Figure 4.8** Changes in the sino-atrial node pacemaker potential and attendant bradycardia caused by stimulation of vagal cardiac parasympathetic fibres in the guinea pig. Note the brisk hyperpolarization of the resting membrane and the sustained slope reduction (dashed red line), which increase the time needed to reach the threshold. (After Bolter CP, Wallace DJ, Hirst GDS. *Autonomic Neuroscience: Basic and Clinical* 2001; 94, 93–101, with permission from Elsevier.)

centigrade. Conversely, cooling can be used to slow the heart during open-heart surgery to preserve the metabolic integrity of cardiac cells.

## 4.5 EFFECTS OF SYMPATHETIC STIMULATION

### Sympathetic stimulation increases heart rate, contractility and relaxation rate

Noradrenaline binds to $\beta_1$ adrenergic receptors on the cardiac cell membrane. Cardiac myocytes also express $\alpha$ and $\beta_2$ adrenergic receptors, but $\beta_1$ receptors outnumber $\beta_2$ by around 4:1 in humans. The circulating hormone **adrenaline** (epinephrine), which is secreted by the adrenal medulla in response to sympathetic stimulation, likewise activates cardiac $\beta_1$ adrenergic receptors. Adrenaline and noradrenaline are known collectively as **catecholamines**. Activation of $\beta_1$ adrenergic receptors leads, over several beats, to:

- an increase in heart rate (the chronotropic effect; Figure 4.7);
- increased AV node conduction velocity (the dromotropic effect);
- shortening of the myocyte action potential (Figure 4.9);

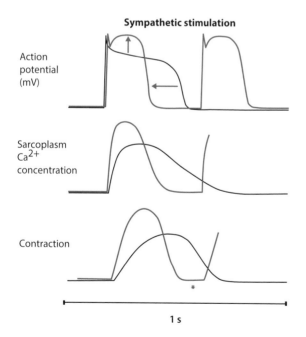

**Sympathetic stimulation**

Action potential (mV)

Sarcoplasm Ca²⁺ concentration

Contraction

1 s

**Figure 4.9** Effect of sympathetic stimulation on a ventricular myocyte. Heart rate approximately doubled in this illustration. (Top pair of traces) Membrane potential before (black) and after (red) sympathetic stimulation. Vertical arrow highlights increased inward Ca²⁺ current during the plateau, producing a domed appearance. Horizontal arrow highlights shortening of action potential by increased outward, repolarizing K⁺ current. (Middle traces) Increased sarcoplasmic Ca²⁺ transient and faster removal. (Bottom traces) The contraction is stronger and of shorter duration, and relaxation is more rapid. Despite this, the diastolic period for refilling is severely curtailed (asterisk).

- increased contractile force (the inotropic effect; Figures 4.9 and 6.18);
- increased rate of relaxation (the lusitropic effect; Figures 4.9 and 6.18).

The action of noradrenaline is terminated partly by diffusion into the bloodstream, which washes it away, and partly by reuptake into the sympathetic nerves. Because these processes are relatively slow, the recovery from sympathetic stimulation is also slow.

The intracellular pathways that lead to these dramatic changes in cardiac performance are discussed next.

### $\beta_1$-adrenergic receptors activate the cAMP–Protein Kinase A pathway

Activated $\beta_1$-receptors trigger a biochemical cascade that amplifies the signal and leads to multiple changes in ion channel and pump activity (Figure 4.10). Each receptor catalyses the dissociation of many molecules of an intramembrane G protein, $G_s$ ('s' for stimulatory). This trimeric (three-part) protein dissociates into $\alpha_s$ and $\beta\gamma$ subunits. The $\alpha_s$ subunit diffuses within the membrane and activates a membrane-bound enzyme, **adenylate (or adenylyl) cyclase**, which catalyses the conversion of numerous adenosine triphosphate (ATP) molecules into the intracellular messenger cAMP. Because of the substantial amplification along the pathway, the activation of a single adrenergic receptor generates many intracellular messenger molecules; cAMP has the following actions:

- cAMP interacts directly with **pacemaker $i_f$ channels** to increase their open-state probability. The rise in current $i_f$ accelerates the rate of pacemaker potential decay and contributes to the chronotropic effect.
- cAMP activates the intracellular enzyme **protein kinase A (PKA)**. PKA catalyses the phosphorylation of **L-type Ca²⁺ channels**, which increases their open-state probability and duration. In atrial and ventricular myocytes, the resulting increase in the plateau Ca²⁺ current creates a 'spike-and-dome' action potential, and contributes to the inotropic effect (Figure 4.9). In SA node myocytes, the increase in the Ca²⁺ current accelerates the pacemaker potential decay and thus contributes to the chronotropic effect.
- PKA phosphorylates the slow, **delayed rectifier K⁺ channels**. The resulting increase in the repolarizing outward current $i_{Kv}$ contributes to the shortening of the ventricular action potential (Figure 4.9). However, shortening also occurs during purely electrical pacing (cf. sympathetic stimulation), because the intracellular Na⁺ and Ca²⁺ concentrations rise when action potential frequency is increased. These ionic changes affect several currents influencing action potential duration. The reduction in action potential duration allows more excitations to fit into each minute, a necessary, permissive step when heart rate increases.

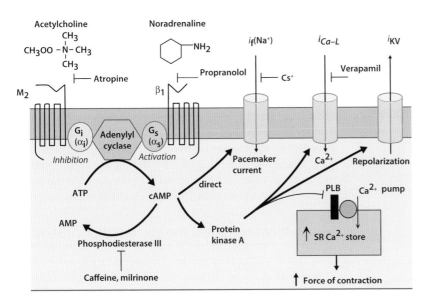

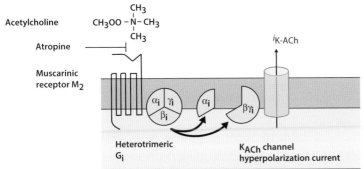

**Figure 4.10** Signal transduction pathways activated by the sympathetic transmitter nor-adrenaline and the parasympathetic transmitter acetylcholine, in a myocardial or pacemaker cell. Each G protein is a heterotrimer of α, β and γ sub-units. On activation, it dissociates into an α and a βγ subunit (lower panel). The $α_s$ subunit activates adenylate cyclase. The $α_i$ subunit inhibits adenylate cyclase. The $β_γ$ subunit activates the $K_{ACh}$ ($K_G$) channels. ATP, adenosine triphosphate; cAMP, cyclic adenosine monophosphate; Gi, inhibitory GTP-binding protein; Gs, stimulatory guanosine triphosphate (GTP)-binding protein; PLB, phospholamban; SR, sarcoplasmic reticulum.

- PKA phosphorylates **phospholamban**, reducing its inhibitory effect on the $Ca^{2+}$-ATPase pump of the network sarcoplasmic reticulum (SR). This 'disinhibition' increases the $Ca^{2+}$ affinity of the pump, and thus boosts $Ca^{2+}$ transfer from the sarcoplasm into the SR. This accounts for most of the lusitropic (relaxation-speeding) effect. β adrenergic stimulation may also phosphorylate the **$Ca^{2+}$ release channels** (ryanodine receptors RyRs), so that a bigger fraction of the raised $Ca^{2+}$ store is released per excitation.

This biochemical transduction pathway is relatively long and slow, so the 'on' response to sympathetic stimulation is slow (Figure 4.7). As well as the classic PKA pathway, long-term β adrenergic stimulation may activate another kinase, CaMKII. This phosphorylates phospholamban at a different site and maintains the inotropic effect of β adrenergic stimulation. To return the cell to its baseline state, the various phosphorylated proteins are dephosphorylated by the **phosphatase** proteins phosphatase 1 (PP1) and 2 (PP2A). Many of these regulatory enzymes – PKA, CaMKII, PP1 and PP2A – are organized into extremely large regulatory protein complexes around their sub-cellular targets (e.g. phospholamban, RyR).

The $β_1$ receptor itself is subject to continual turnover. While occupied by a catecholamine molecule, the receptor can be phosphorylated by a receptor kinase. This uncouples the receptor from the $G_s$-adenylate cyclase system and leads to its internalization (downregulation). Fresh $β_1$ receptors are normally inserted into the membrane to maintain the appropriate receptive level. However, the balance between removal and replacement goes awry in heart failure (Chapter 18).

## Chronotropic and dromotropic effects

The intracellular events discussed so far enhance cardiac performance as follows:

1. **The rate of decay of the pacemaker potential is increased**, so the threshold is reached sooner and the heart rate increases (Figure 4.7). The increased decay rate is caused by increases in the depolarizing currents $i_f$, $i_{Ca-L}$ and $i_{Na-Ca}$, aided by an increased rate of deactivation of the delayed rectifier $K^+$ channel, reducing $i_{Kv}$. For the heart to function effectively at a higher pacing rate, the cardiac cycle must also be shortened. Sympathetic stimulation brings this about as follows:

2. **Conduction through the AV node is speeded up** by the activated nodal $β_1$ receptors (dromotropic effect). This reduces the time lag between SA node firing and ventricular contraction and shortens the electrocardiogram (ECG) PR interval.

3. **The action potential of atrial and ventricular myocytes is shortened**, because of early repolarization (Figures 4.9 and 4.10). Without this change, the long plateau would limit the maximum possible heart rate. This change shortens the QT interval of the ECG.

## The inotropic effect is due to an increased calcium transient

Over the course of several beats, the raised plateau $Ca^{2+}$ current $i_{Ca-L}$ (Figures 3.9, 4.7 and 4.9), in conjunction with the increased $Ca^{2+}$ affinity of the SR pumps, increases the size of the SR store. The **enlarged $Ca^{2+}$ store** and **increased trigger $Ca^{2+}$** (increased $i_{Ca-L}$) generate a bigger, systolic-free $Ca^{2+}$ transient (Figure 4.9). This activates more crossbridges and thus increases the force of atrial and ventricular systole.

## The lusitropic effect is due mainly to faster calcium reuptake by the SARcoplasmic reticulum

The **duration of contraction falls** and the **relaxation rate increases** (Figure 4.9). This shortens the ejection and isovolumetric relaxation phases of the cardiac cycle, and thereby **minimizes the reduction in diastolic interval** (Figure 2.7). This is essential because the heart needs sufficient time to refill. The lusitropic effect is brought about chiefly by the accelerated removal of sarcoplasmic $Ca^{2+}$ by the network SR pumps. Studies of genetically engineered, phospholamban knockout mice show that 85% of the lusitropy is due to pump stimulation by phosphorylated phospholamban. The rest is due to the phosphorylation of thin filament troponin I, which speeds up crossbridge cycling and thus allows faster relaxation.

## cAMP-raising drugs mimic sympathetic stimulation

Intracellular cAMP concentration depends not only on the rate of production by adenylate cyclase but also on the rate of degradation by **phosphodiesterase**. Agents that inhibit phosphodiesterase, such as **caffeine**, **theophylline** and **milrinone**, raise intracellular cAMP. This is why your heart beats faster when you drink lots of strong coffee. Therefore, they mimic the effects of $\beta_1$-agonists, that is, they increase the heart rate and contractility. However, despite their beneficial cardiodynamic effects, these drugs increase the mortality rate in patients with heart failure.

## 4.6 EFFECTS OF PARASYMPATHETIC STIMULATION

## The main parasympathetic neurotransmitter is acetylcholine

The arrival of an action potential in a parasympathetic postganglionic terminal triggers the release of the ACh. ACh binds to and activates **muscarinic $M_2$ receptors** on the myocyte membrane. However, the ACh is quickly removed from the junctional region by the enzyme cholinesterase. Consequently, the heart rate picks up briskly when vagal activity is reduced.

Vagal parasympathetic fibres are tonically active, and the tonic activity is increased by endurance training, causing a fast heart rate recovery from exercise in athletes. The training bradycardia seen at rest in athletes is thought to be due predominantly to changes in intrinsic pacemaking. However, the amount of ACh released from the vagus nerve terminals can also be increased by a pathway involving neuronal nitric oxide (NO) synthase, which likewise is enhanced by training.

## Acetylcholine slows the pacemaker potential

Vagal stimulation produces bradycardia through two electrophysiological actions (Figure 4.8). The chief effect is to reduce the rate at which the pacemaker potential decays. In addition, the membrane is rapidly hyperpolarized, that is, made more negative. Because of these two effects, the potential takes longer to reach the threshold and the heart rate decreases. Of the two effects, the reduction in slope is the more important over long periods, because it can be elicited by a lower concentration of ACh and is better sustained. The chronic bradycardia of a trained athlete is an example of this effect.

## $M_2$ receptors inhibit adenylate cyclase and activate potassium channels

ACh reduces the pacemaker slope by reducing both the $Na^+$ current $i_f$ and the L-type $Ca^{2+}$ current $i_{Ca-L}$. The mechanism is the reverse of that triggered by $\beta_1$ adrenergic receptors. The $M_2$ receptor activates an inhibitory trimeric G protein, $G_i$, causing it to dissociate into $\alpha_i$ and $\beta\gamma_i$ subunits. The $\alpha_i$ subunit inhibits adenylate cyclase (Figure 4.10, top panel), leading to a fall in cAMP and reduced PKA activity. These changes in turn reduce the activity of $i_f$ and L-type $Ca^{2+}$ channels.

ACh-induced hyperpolarization is mediated by the $\beta\gamma_i$ subunit of the dissociated $G_i$ protein (Figure 4.10, bottom panel). The $\beta\gamma_i$ subunit rapidly activates a specialized form of inward rectifier $K^+$ channel, the $K_G$ or $K_{ACh}$ **channel**. The resulting increase in outward $K^+$ current shifts the membrane potential closer to the Nernst equilibrium potential for $K^+$, $-94$ mV (equation 3.1), causing hyperpolarization. The shortness of the $M_2$–$G\beta\gamma_i$–$K_G$ linkage accounts for the rapidity with which vagal stimulation slows the heart.

## Physiological roles

Examples of vagal bradycardia in man include:

- slowing of the heart during expiration;
- the low heart rate of a trained athlete;
- slowing of the heart during a dive (Chapter 17);
- transient arrest of the heart at the onset of fainting (vasovagal attack; Chapter 18).

An extreme example of vagal bradycardia has given rise to the everyday expression, 'playing possum'. To fool a predator, the possum feigns death by collapsing and developing a profound bradycardia:

*Quoth Fox to Brer Possum*
*'You're due in my antrum'.*
*Old possum smiled; he had a hunch*
*His flaccid apnoee-a*
*And bradycardee-a*
*Would leave Fox in no mood for lunch.*

## 4.7 LOCAL NEUROMODULATORS AND AUTONOMIC CO-TRANSMITTERS

Since the discovery of the classical neurotransmitters, several other transmitters have been discovered; this has given rise to co-transmission theory. To be a neurotransmitter, four broad criteria must be met: (1) the compound must be synthesized presynaptically; (2) the compound must be released on appropriate stimulation; (3) microapplication of the compound should mimic part of the effect of nerve stimulation; (4) the actions of the compound should be blocked pharmacologically. Co-transmitters are released during periods of high autonomic drive and are broadly viewed as neuromodulators because they can modulate the release of classical transmitters while at the same time binding to their own postsynaptic receptor.

Regarding the **sympathetic system**, Geoffrey Burnstock played a key role in the discovery of ATP, the first co-transmitter that binds to purinergic receptors. This is a widespread signalling system through the body; it is now known as the purinergic nervous system. Sympathetic neurons also contain neuropeptide Y (NPY) and galanin. Both noradrenaline and ATP have relatively short half-lives because noradrenaline is taken back into the nerve terminal via the noradrenaline transporter and ATP is rapidly metabolized. Conversely, while the half-lives of NPY and galanin are significantly longer, they are released in much smaller quantities. Therefore, the role of co-transmitters may be more important during conditions associated with high levels of adrenergic drive. For example, plasma NPY levels are elevated following myocardial infarction and during left ventricular failure in humans, where they correlate positively with 1-year mortality.

Many parasympathetic neurons within the heart also contain different co-transmitters including somatostatin and vasoactive intestinal polypeptide (VIP), and endogenous opioids, such as dynorphins. Whether these co-transmitters are released during physiological activation of the vagus nerve or change their expression profile in cardiovascular disease is not known.

Neuromodulators can act in an autocrine and paracrine fashion that is intrinsic to sympathetic ganglia or vagal neurons (such as the NO generated by neuronal NO synthase and its adaptor protein, CAPON). Here, the gaseous transmitter can influence the release of noradrenaline or ACh (autocrine action), diffuse to adjacent cells and change intracellular $Ca^{2+}$ handling (paracrine action). Neuromodulators may also act as either autoinhibitory or crosstalk communicating messengers between neuronal populations (e.g. the co-transmitters NPY, galanin and VIP). Substances released from cardiac myocytes and the coronary vasculature, including natriuretic peptides and Ang II, also influence neuronal function acting in a paracrine manner (see Figure 4.11). These signalling pathways converge on neuronal $Ca^{2+}$ handling, transmitter release

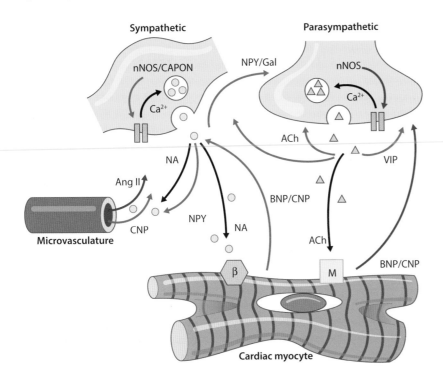

**Figure 4.11** Schematic representation of the neuromodulatory pathways influencing the release of noradrenaline(NA) and acetylcholine (ACh) from postganglionic sympathetic and parasympathetic neurons. NA and ACh release is triggered by the influx of calcium through neuronal voltage gated calcium channels (in grey) Neuromodulators can arise from the coronary microvasculature (e.g. angiotensin II [Ang II] and C-type natriuretic peptide [CNP]), myocytes (B-type natriuretic peptide [BNP]), as well as between neurons (neuropeptide Y [NPY], galanin [Gal], acetylcholine [ACh] and vasoactive intestinal peptide [VIP]) and within neurons (such as neuronal nitric oxide synthase [nNOS] and its activator protein, [CAPON]). Stimulatory pathways are represented by green arrows, and inhibitory pathways by red arrows. (Adapted from Habecker et al. *The Journal of Physiology* 2016; 594(14): 3853–75.)

and/or reuptake mechanisms. The plasma levels and protein expression of many of these neuromodulators are increased in both animal models and patients with cardiovascular disease. However, their functional significance and the potential to exploit these pathways pharmacologically in disease states are yet to be established.

## 4.8 DANGERS OF AN ALTERED IONIC ENVIRONMENT

Since cardiac function depends on ionic gradients, any severe disturbances of extracellular ion concentration is obviously bad for the heart. As Ringer showed, **hypocalcaemia** reduces myocardial contractility. Conversely, extreme **hypercalcaemia** arrests the heart in systole.

### Hyperkalaemia can cause arrhythmia

The plasma $K^+$ concentration in a resting human is normally maintained at 3.5–5 mM by means of renal excretion and cellular uptake by the $Na^+/K^+$ pump. Renal $K^+$ excretion is regulated by the renin–angiotensin–aldosterone system (Chapter 14), while the cellular pump is stimulated by a rise in extracellular $K^+$ concentration. Clinical hyperkalaemia can arise from reduced renal excretion (renal failure, angiotensin converting enzyme (ACE) inhibitors, spironolactone) or the escape of intracellular $K^+$ following acidosis (inorganic acid), tissue breakdown, crushing injury, transfusion of expired blood and haemolysis (e.g. freshwater drowning). Hyperkalaemia weakens the heartbeat and can lead to arrhythmia. A hyperkalaemia of 6–7 mM in a resting human can be a medical emergency, because a rapid increase can arrest the heart in diastole (**asystole**). Indeed, for cardiac transplant surgery, the donor heart is deliberately perfused with **cardioplegic solution** containing 20 mM $K^+$ to arrest the heart. An arrested heart needs less $O_2$, so it is better able to survive until transplantation.

Hyperkalaemia reduces the Nernst $K^+$ equilibrium potential and, therefore, the resting membrane potential (Figure 3.6). This in turn diminishes the action potential, because the low resting potential prevents many $Na^+$ channels from resetting from the inactivated state to the closed-but-activatable state (Figure 3.13, top right). At a resting potential of –70 mV about half the inactivation gates are closed, while at –50 mV most are closed. As a result, the action potential begins to lose its sharp phase 0, and it is eventually reduced to a sluggish rise of small amplitude dependent on $i_{Ca-L}$ (Figure 4.12). Since small, slow-rising action potentials generate less propagating current, electrical transmission is slower and less secure than normal. This can lead to heart block (Figure 5.4) or a pathological ventricular tachycardia/fibrillation. The raised extracellular $K^+$ also stimulates the electrogenic $3Na^+/2K^+$ pump and enhances the activity of the $K^+$ channels $K_{ir}$ and $K_{v(r)}$, causing early repolarization. This reduces the window for $Ca^{2+}$ entry resulting in a subsequent decrease in contractile function.

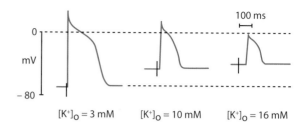

$[K^+]_O = 3$ mM    $[K^+]_O = 10$ mM    $[K^+]_O = 16$ mM

**Figure 4.12** Effect of hyperkalaemia on the membrane potential of a Purkinje fibre (see text). The spike to the left of each action potential marks stimulation by an external impulse some distance away. Note the increasing conduction time, reduced resting potential, reduced action potential size and slowed rate of rise. (Adapted from Myerburg RJ, Lazzara R. In: Fisch E, ed. *Complex Electrocardiography*. Philadelphia, PA: Davis, 1973.)

The attendant ECG changes include a wide QRS complex (because of slow electrical propagation in the ventricle) and a tall, peaked T wave (due presumably to the enhanced repolarizing $K^+$ current).

Some of these changes also occur in the ischaemic myocardium, because ischaemia causes a local increase in myocardial interstitial $K^+$ concentration (Figure 6.22). Treatment of the hyperkalaemia is by correction of the cause and, in an emergency, intravenous $Ca^{2+}$ gluconate to maintain inotropic support to the heart while $K^+$ is lowered with insulin and glucose, which causes a widespread cellular uptake of $K^+$.

Remarkably, and despite this catalogue of horrors, the plasma $K^+$ concentration in a normal human can double to 8 mM in severe exercise without evident harm. The $K^+$ is released following repolarization of the action potential during muscle contraction. Because there is an incomplete reuptake of $K^+$ by the $Na^+/K^+$ pump, hyperkalaemia occurs. It appears that the large increase in adrenaline and noradrenaline during exercise protects the myocardium against hyperkalaemia, probably by boosting the action potential current $i_{Ca-L}$.

### Hypokalaemia likewise can cause arrhythmia

Hypokalaemia occurs when extracellular $K^+$ concentration falls below 3.5 mM. Clinical hypokalaemia arises mainly from increased renal excretion (caused usually by $K^+$-losing thiazide diuretics), severe burns or severe diarrhoea and vomiting. The low extracellular $K^+$ reduces the activity of the electrogenic $3Na^+/2K^+$ pump and the $K^+$ channels $K_{ir}$ and $K_{v(r)}$, thereby reducing the repolarizing currents. This prolongs the plateau duration and phase 3 repolarization, particularly in the $K_v$-rich subepicardial myocytes. An upright T wave in the ECG depends on the fact that the subepicardial action potential is normally shorter than the subendocardial action potential (see Section 5.5). Prolongation of the subepicardial action potentials thus leads to flattened or inverted T waves, and sometimes a late wave called a **U wave**. Action potential prolongation can give rise to afterdepolarizations (arrhythmia) where another action potential is generated before the cell has had time to complete repolarization (see Chapter 5). This action potential is caused by the inability of the cardiac cell to deal with the load of intracellular $Ca^{2+}$ (during a long action potential duration), resulting in a net positive $Na^+$ influx as the cell attempts to extrude $Ca^{2+}$. So, the real villain is probably the rise in intracellular $Na^+$. If a run of extra depolarizations happens, then the heart prematurely contracts before it has had time to complete ventricular filling resulting in a reduced stroke volume (SV) and cardiac output. This in turn causes a collapse in arterial blood pressure and perfusion pressure to vital organs like the heart and brain, resulting in hypoxia and tissue death. High levels of catecholamines will further exacerbate the negative cardiac effects of hypokalaemia on the heart by causing increased intracellular $Ca^{2+}$ transients leading to more afterdepolarizations.

## Hydrogen ions and ischaemia weaken the heartbeat

Intracellular $H^+$ ions compete with $Ca^{2+}$ for the troponin C binding site. Consequently, intracellular acidosis weakens the contraction. Intracellular pH is normally held at 7.1–7.2 by membrane transporters, namely the $Na^+/H^+$ exchanger and $Na^+/HCO_3^-$ importer. However, these can be overwhelmed in ischaemia, leading to intracellular acidosis and weak contractions (Section 6.12).

## 4.9 PHARMACOLOGICAL MANIPULATION OF CARDIAC CURRENTS

Pharmacological manipulation consists of the following:

- **$Na^+$ channel blockers**. Procainamide, lidocaine, mexiletine and flecainide acetate are used as antiarrhythmic drugs.
- **β-blockers**. The tonic, stimulatory effect of sympathetic activity can be reduced by non-selective β adrenergic receptor blockers (e.g. propranolol) and specific $β_1$ adrenergic receptor blockers (short-acting metoprolol and long-acting bisoprolol). These agents attenuate the cardiac $Ca^{2+}$ currents and SR pump, leading to a fall in heart rate, contractile force and cardiac output. This is beneficial in the treatment of chronic stable heart failure (Section 18.4) and stable angina (ischaemic heart pain when cardiac work exceeds the capacity of diseased coronary arteries to deliver $O_2$ during exercise; see Section 15.1).
- **$K^+$ channel blockers**. Sotalol is a β adrenergic receptor blocker which, at higher concentrations, also blocks $K^+$ channels, making it a useful antiarrhythmic medication. Amiodarone also blocks $K^+$ channels (and $Na^+$ and $Ca^{2+}$ channels) and has some β adrenergic receptor blocking action. It is a potent antiarrhythmic medication, but unfortunately has many side effects including photosensitivity, thyroid disturbance, hepatitis and lung

scarring, if used long-term. Dronedarone is a similar medication that is less potent than amiodarone. While it is less likely to disturb thyroid function, monitoring of liver function is still required because rare but severe cases of hepatitis have been reported.
- **$Ca^{2+}$ channel blockers**. Verapamil and diltiazem partially inhibit L-type $Ca^{2+}$ channels, reducing the plateau current $i_{Ca-L}$. This shortens the action potential and has a negative inotropic (weakening) effect. Verapamil has a greater effect on the heart than nifedipine and is used to reduce cardiac work and hence $O_2$ demand in stable angina patients. Verapamil also slows AV node conduction, so it can suppress arrhythmias that depend on a 'circus' re-entry mechanism (see Section 5.8).
- **Adenosine**. Adenosine is sometimes given intravenously to slow or terminate **supraventricular tachycardia** (see Chapter 5), a pathologically high heart rate driven by an abnormal atrial or AV node-dependent rhythm. Adenosine acts on purinergic $A_1$ receptors to activate nodal $K^+$ channels, leading to hyperpolarization. This reduces the heart rate and slows AV node conduction.
- **'Funny' channel blocker**. Ivabradine blocks the pacemaker current $i_f$, thus reducing the rate of pacemaker depolarization. The attendant slowing of the heart rate reduces myocardial $O_2$ demand, so ivabradine is used to treat stable angina.
- **$K^+$ channel openers**. The metabolically sensitive $K_{ATP}$ channel, which we met in Section 3.7, can be activated by cromakalim, pinacidil, minoxidil and nicorandil. $K_{ATP}$ activation causes hyperpolarization. The main therapeutic effect is the relaxation of peripheral blood vessels, which helps to relieve stable angina.

## 4.10 MECHANO-ELECTRICAL FEEDBACK

A sharp thump on the chest can sometimes restart an arrested heart, or correct a pathological tachycardia. Therefore, mechanical stimuli can affect cardiac electrical activity. Mechanical stretch can activate stretch-activated channels (SACs), which transmit an inward, depolarizing cation current. The following effects are attributed to SACs (Table 4.2):

- **The Bainbridge 'reflex'**. Bainbridge discovered in 1915 that the rapid infusion of a large volume of saline into the venous system causes a transient tachycardia (Section 16.3). The tachycardia may be due in part to the activation of SACs in the pacemaker cells.
- **Mechanically-induced arrhythmia**. Mechanical stimulation of the wall of the atrium or ventricle during cardiac catheterization can trigger extra systoles and other arrhythmias. A mechanical impact on the chest wall, for example from an ice hockey puck, can also have the same effect. If the external impact coincides

**Table 4.2** Cardiac ion channels: advanced aspects. To paraphrase Denis Noble in *The Surprising Heart*, the description of ionic currents in the preceding text "may already have exhausted the reader, but it certainly does not exhaust the mechanisms that have been found". This table lists, for advanced students and reference purposes, the main ionic currents, component proteins and genes (in brackets) of the pore-forming α subunit. Regulatory β and other subunits are not listed. First-year students should not attempt to memorize these details!

| Channel and current | Properties and activators | Inhibitor | Roles |
|---|---|---|---|
| **Potassium-conducting channels based on Kir protein, non-voltage-gated** | | | |
| **Inward rectifier channel Kir** <br> – current $i_{K1}$ or $i_{Kir}$ <br> – heterotetramer[a] of Kir2.1 (*KCNJ2*) and Kir2.2 (*KCNJ12*) | Open at negative potentials. Little $K^+$ efflux at positive potentials because internal aperture blocked by $Mg^{2+}$ and polyamines | $Ba^{2+}$ | Supplies outward current for resting potential of myocytes and late phase of repolarization, from −20 mV to −80 mV. Few in the sino-atrial (SA) node, hence small resting potential |
| **Muscarinic G-protein activated $K_G$, $K_{Ach}$** <br> – current $i_{K-Ach}$ <br> – heterotetramer of Kir3.1 (*KCNJ3*) and Kir3.4 (*KCNJ5*) | Activated by acetylcholine (ACh) and adenosine receptors through release of $G_{\beta\gamma}$. Some spontaneous opening | $Ba^{2+}$ partially. Pertussis toxin blocks the $G_i$ protein | In the SA node, ACh and adenosine receptors slow heart rate via hyperpolarizing effect of $K_G$ channels. In SA node, $K_G$ contributes to background $K^+$ current |
| **ATP-sensitive K channel $K_{ATP}$, $K_{NDP}$** <br> – current $i_{K-ATP}$ <br> – octamer of 4 Kir6.2 surrounded by 4 SUR2 | Opened by low adenosine triphosphate (ATP) (<0.1 mM), raised nucleoside adenosine diphosphate (ADP), adenosine, $H^+$, nicorandil, cromakalim, pinacidil, diazoxide | Glibenclamide | Abundant. In ischaemia, opening terminates ventricle action potential early, reducing contractile force |
| **Potassium-conducting channels based on $K_v$ protein, voltage-gated** | | | |
| **Delayed rectifier, voltage-activated Kv: subtypes Ks, Kr** <br> – current $i_{Kv} = i_{Ks} + i_{Kr}$ <br> Ks gene *KvLQT1* (*KCNQ1*); Kr gene *HERG* (*KCNH2*) | Activates slowly on depolarization beyond −40 mV, then inactivates slowly ($i_{Ks}$) or rapidly ($i_{Kr}$). Shortens action potential. Ks is enhanced by β adrenergic stimulation | $Ba^{2+}$ TEA[b] 4AP[c] | Slow inactivation causes decaying $g_K$ of pacemaker potential. Terminates action potential by supplying initial repolarization current down to −20 mV. Increased by β adrenergic stimulation to shorten myocyte action potential. *KCNQ1* mutation causes ~50% cases of long QT syndrome; *HERG* less often |
| **Transient outward** <br> – current $i_{to}$ <br> – Kv4.3 (*KCND3*) | Activated by depolarization. More in subepicardial than subendocardial myocytes | 4AP | Causes phase 1 repolarization, shortening the subepicardial action potential. Shortens action potentials in rat and mouse to allow high heart rates. Downregulated in heart failure, causing prolonged action potentials |
| **Sodium-conducting channels** | | | |
| **Fast-inactivating Na channel, $Na_V$** <br> – current $i_{Na}$ <br> – cardiac isoform is $Na_V$1.5 (*SCN5A*) | Open state is voltage- and time-dependent | Tetrodotoxin, local anaesthetics | Depolarization spike of action potential in ventricles, atria. Scarce in the SA node, so no spike here. *SCN5A* mutations are a rare cause of long QT syndrome (<5% cases) |
| **Hyperpolarization-activated** <br> – 'funny' current $i_f$ <br> – tetramer of HCN1–4 | Opens slowly at potentials negative to −45, −60 mV. **H**yperpolarization-activated **c**yclic **n**ucleotide-gated, hence 'HCN' protein | $Cs^+$, ivabradine | Contributes to pacemaker depolarization; $Cs^+$ slows pacemaker depolarization by 10%–40%. Activity increased by cyclic adenosine monophosphate (cAMP) during β adrenergic stimulation; reduced by acetylcholine $M_2$ receptors |
| **Background** <br> – current $i_b$ | Passive background current | | Attenuates the resting membrane potential |

*(Continued)*

**Table 4.2 *(Continued)***

| Channel and current | Properties and activators | Inhibitor | Roles |
|---|---|---|---|
| **(Na–Ca exchanger, NCX)** <br> – current $i_{Na-Ca}$, $i_{NCX}$ | Not a channel but transfers 3 $Na^+$ into cell for each $Ca^{2+}$ expelled (forward mode). Activated by intracellular $Ca^{2+}$ | $Li^+$, $Cd^{2+}$, $La^{3+}$ | 1. Forward mode supplies net inward current in late plateau <br> 2. Brief reverse mode after $Na^+$ spike may contribute to early $Ca^{2+}$ influx <br> 3. Can generate DADs |
| **(Na–K pump)** <br> – current $i_{NaK}$ | Not a channel, but transfers 3 $Na^+$ out of cell for every 2 $K^+$ in, generating a small net outward current | Digoxin, ouabain | Minor outward current, contributing 2–4 mV to resting membrane potential |
| **Calcium-conducting channels** | | | |
| **L-type $Ca^{2+}$ channel** <br> – current $i_{Ca-L}$ <br> – protein $Ca_v1.2$, $\alpha1C$ (*CACN1AC*) | Voltage-operated; activated by depolarization. **L**ong-lasting activation. Inactivation is time-dependent and $Ca^{2+}$-dependent | Diltiazem, verapamil | 1. Supplies trigger $Ca^{2+}$ for CICR <br> 2. Carries most of the early plateau current <br> 3. Generates SA and atrioventricular node action potentials <br> 4. C-terminus phosphorylation following β adrenergic stimulation mediates increased $Ca^{2+}$ influx and contractility |
| **T-type $Ca^{2+}$ channel** <br> – current $i_{Ca-T}$ <br> – $Ca_v3.1-3.3$, $\alpha1H$ (*CACNA1H*) | Activates at more negative potentials than L-type, e.g. –55 mV. **T**ransient activation state | $Ni^{2+}$. Insensitive to verapamil or β agonists | Contributes to pacemaker depolarizing current |
| **Chloride-conducting channels** | | | |
| **cAMP-dependent** <br> – current $i_{Cl(AMP)}$ | Activated by cAMP and therefore $β_1$ agonists | | Contributes to phase 1 repolarization after $β_1$ activation, from positive potentials down to $E_{Cl}$ of –40 mV (Table 3.2) |
| **$Ca^{2+}$-dependent** <br> – current $i_{Cl(Ca)}$ | Activated by cytosol $Ca^{2+}$ | DIDS | $E_{Cl}$ is –40 mV, so contributes to phase 1 repolarization, pacemaker depolarization and DADs |
| **Swelling-activated** | Stretch-activated, opened by osmotic swelling of cell | | Regulates cell volume |
| **Stretch-activated channels (SACs)** | | | |
| **Non-specific cation conducting** <br> – TRP protein family | Activated by stretch | $Gd^{3+}$ | Mechano-electric feedback |
| **$K^+$-selective SAC** <br> – protein TREK-1 | Activated by stretch | | Mechano-electric feedback |
| **$Cl^-$-selective SAC** | See under **Chloride** | | See under **Chloride** |

*Note:* CICR, $Ca^{2+}$ induced $Ca^{2+}$ release; DAD, delayed afterdepolarization; DIDS, 4,4′-diisothiocyano-2,2′-stilbenedisulfonic acid; TRP, transient receptor potential.
[a] Composed of four subunits that are not all identical.
[b] TEA, tetraethylammonium.
[c] 4AP, 4-aminopyridine.

with a vulnerable window during the cardiac cycle (usually around the T wave), this can lead to ventricular arrhythmia and sudden cardiac death and is refered to as "commotio cordis". Gadolinium ions, $Gd^{3+}$, block SACs and prevent stretch-induced arrhythmias.

- Atrial myocytes secrete the polypeptide hormone **atrial natriuretic peptide** in response to stretch (Section 14.9). This response is presumably mediated by SACs.

## SUMMARY

- The SA node (pacemaker) initiates atrial contraction. The AV node delays the transmission of excitation to the ventricle, so that atrial contraction precedes ventricular contraction. The bundle of His and Purkinje system distribute the electrical impulse rapidly throughout the ventricular muscle mass.

- The membrane potential of a pacemaker cell decays with time (the pacemaker potential). The decay is caused by multiple inward currents ($Na^+$ currents $i_f$, $i_b$; exchanger current $i_{Na-Ca}$; $Ca^{2+}$ currents $i_{Ca-T}$, $i_{Ca-L}$), some driven by an internal '$Ca^{2+}$ clock', combined with a decaying $K^+$ permeability. The decay rate determines the time needed to reach threshold and fire an action potential that initiates the next heartbeat. Heart rate is thus controlled by the slope of the decaying pacemaker potential. The nodal action potential is small, sluggish and generated solely by L-type $Ca^{2+}$ channels.

- Sympathetic fibre terminals release noradrenaline, which activates cardiac $\beta_1$ adrenergic receptors. In the SA node, $\beta_1$ receptor activation accelerates the decay of the pacemaker potential and thus increases heart rate (chronotropic effect). The increased decay rate is due to increases in the depolarizing pacemaker currents $i_f$ and $i_{Ca-L}$, and an accelerated decay in $K^+$ permeability.

- Activation of $\beta_1$ adrenergic receptors on atrial and ventricular myocytes increases the open probability of L-type $Ca^{2+}$ channels, leading to a bigger plateau current, $Ca^{2+}$ store and trigger $Ca^{2+}$, and thus a bigger $Ca^{2+}$ transient and stronger contraction (inotropic effect). $Ca^{2+}$ reuptake by the SR pumps is enhanced, so systole is shortened and relaxation speeded up (lusitropic effect). The effects of $\beta_1$ receptor activation are mediated through the $G_s$-adenylate cyclase–cAMP–PKA cascade.

- Parasympathetic vagal fibres release ACh, which activates muscarinic $M_2$ receptors. This activates the $G_i$ protein, which inhibits the adenylate cyclase–cAMP–PKA pathway. The inhibition of PKA reduces the inward pacemaker currents $i_f$ and $i_{Ca-L}$, and thus slows pacemaker depolarization and heart rate. Muscarinic receptors also hyperpolarize pacemaker cells by activating $K_{ACh}$ channels. This produces an abrupt fall in heart rate, for example, on expiration or fainting.

- Electrical activity can be altered by ionic environment and drugs. Hyperkalaemia depolarizes the myocytes, leading to conduction impairment and arrhythmias. Hypokalaemia has the opposite electrophysiological effect but is also arrhythmogenic, especially in the presence of a high sympathetic drive. $\beta$-blockers such as metoprolol and bisoprolol, and $Ca^{2+}$ channel blockers such as diltiazem and verapamil, reduce the plateau current $i_{Ca}$, which reduces contractile force and heart rate. Since this reduces myocardial $O_2$ demand, these drugs are beneficial in stable angina.

## FURTHER READING

Weiss JN, Qu Z, Shivkumar K. Electrophysiology of hypokalemia and hyperkalemia. *Circulation: Arrhythmia and Electrophysiology* 2017; **10**(3): e004667.

Habecker BA, Anderson ME, Birren SJ, et al. Molecular and cellular neurocardiology: development, cellular and molecular adaptations to heart disease. *The Journal of Physiology* 2016; **594**(14): 3853–75.

Peyronnet R, Nerbonne JM, Kohl P. Cardiac mechano-gated ion channels and arrhythmias. *Circulation Research* 2016; **118**(2): 311–29.

Capel RA, Terrar DA. The importance of $Ca^{2+}$-dependent mechanisms for the initiation of the heartbeat. *Frontiers in Physiology* 2015; **6**: 80.

Coote JH, White MJ. CrossTalk proposal: bradycardia in the trained athlete is attributable to high vagal tone. *The Journal of Physiology* 2015; **593**(8): 1745–7.

D'Souza A, Sharma S, Boyett MR. CrossTalk opposing view: bradycardia in the trained athlete is attributable to a downregulation of a pacemaker channel in the sinus node. *The Journal of Physiology* 2015; **593**(8): 1749–51.

Herring N. Autonomic control of the heart: going beyond the classical neurotransmitters. *Experimental Physiology* 2015; **100**(4): 354–8.

Yaniv Y, Lakatta EG, Maltsev VA. From two competing oscillators to one coupled-clock pacemaker cell system. *Frontiers in Physiology* 2015; **6**: 28.

Coote JH. Myths and realities of the cardiac vagus. *The Journal of Physiology* 2013; **591**(17): 4073–85.

Zipes DP, Jalife J. *Cardiac Electrophysiology from Cell to Bedside*, 6th edn. Philadelphia, PA: WB Saunders, 2013.

El-Sherif N, Turitto G. Electrolyte disorders and arrhythmogenesis. *Cardiology Journal* 2011; **18**(3): 233–45.

DiFrancesco D. The role of the funny current in pacemaker activity. *Circulation Research* 2010; **106**(3): 434–46.

Eisner DA, Dibb KM, Trafford AW. The mechanism and significance of the slow changes of ventricular action potential duration following a change of heart rate. *Experimental Physiology* 2009; **94**: 520–8.

Lakatta EG, DiFrancesco D. What keeps us ticking: a funny current, a calcium clock, or both? *Journal of Molecular and Cellular Cardiology* 2009; **47**(2): 157–70.

Armour JA. Potential clinical relevance of the 'little brain' on the mammalian heart. *Experimental Physiology* 2008; **93**(2): 165–76.

Paterson DJ. Role of potassium in the regulation of systemic physiological function during exercise. *Acta Physiologica Scandinavica* 1996; **156**(3): 287–94.

Paterson DJ. Antiarrhythmic mechanisms during exercise. *Journal of Applied Physiology* 1996; **80**(6): 1853–62.

Noble D. The surprising heart: a review of recent progress in cardiac electrophysiology. *The Journal of Physiology* 1984; **353** (1), 1–50

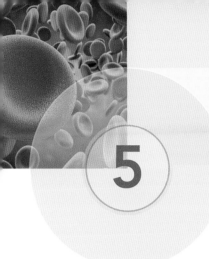

# Electrocardiography and arrhythmias

# 5

## LEARNING OBJECTIVES

*After reading this chapter you should be able to:*

- draw, label and scale a typical ECG trace, stating the chosen lead (5.1–5.3);
- state the origin of the P, QRS and T waves, and the PR and ST intervals (5.2);
- explain what a cardiac dipole is (5.4);
- sketch out how the cardiac dipole changes with time in the frontal plane during ventricular depolarization (5.5);
- explain why different leads record different QRS patterns during the same systole (5.6);
- outline the ECG changes caused by ischaemic heart disease (5.9);
- state the roles of triggers and substrate in initiating and maintaining arrhythmias (5.10, 3.11);

- give the meaning, mechanism and significance of:
  - heart block;
  - sinus arrhythmia;
  - ectopic beat;
  - atrial tachycardia;
  - atrioventricular nodal re-entrant tachycardia;
  - atrioventricular re-entrant tachycardia;
  - atrial flutter;
  - atrial fibrillation;
  - ventricular tachycardia;
  - ventricular fibrillation.

## 5.1 PRINCIPLES OF ELECTROCARDIOGRAPHY

The electrical activity of the heart was an incidental finding of two physiologists, Rudolf Albert von Kölliker and Heinrich Müller, working at the University of Würzburg in 1856. When a frog sciatic nerve/gastrocnemius muscle preparation accidentally fell onto an isolated frog heart such that the sciatic nerve touched the heart, both muscles contracted synchronously, suggesting that the heart generates electrical impulses. This electrical activity was directly recorded from the heart surface with Lippmann's capillary electrometer by the British physiologist John Burdon Sanderson. The electrocardiogram (ECG) is a recording of potential changes at the skin surface that result

from the depolarization and repolarization of the heart muscle. The method was developed in the early 20th century by Willem Einthoven in Leiden, who invented the string galvanometer, and Augustus Waller in London, whose demonstration involving his pet bulldog 'Jimmie' to the Royal Society in 1909 provoked protests in Parliament (Figure 5.1). The Nobel prize in Physiology or Medicine was awarded to Einthoven for the development of the ECG in 1924; if Waller had still been alive at the time, he would have undoubtedly shared the prize. As explained in Chapter 4 (Figure 4.4), the spread of cardiac excitation creates currents in the extracellular fluid. The currents generate small potential differences across the body surface, of around 1 mV, and these can be recorded by a sensitive voltmeter connected to metal electrodes placed on the skin surface. The potential difference is recorded on a strip of

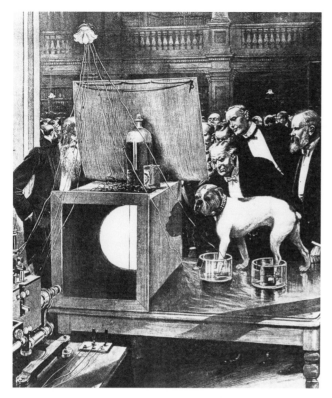

**Figure 5.1** Electrocardiogram demonstrated to the Royal Society by Waller's pet bulldog, Jimmie, in 1909; Waller is just behind Jimmie. Jimmie has his front and hind paws in pots of normal saline connected to a galvanometer (from the *Illustrated London News*, 22 May 1909).

*The Times* newspaper, July 9, 1909, reported that Mr Ellis Griffith (MP for Anglesey) questioned the Secretary of State in Parliament over Waller's 'public experiment' on a dog with 'a leather strap with sharp nails secured around the neck, his feet being immersed in glass jars containing salts connected by wires with galvanometers'. Had the Cruelty to Animals Act (1876) been contravened?

Mr Gladstone: "I understand the dog stood for some time in water to which sodium chloride had been added or in other words a little common salt. If my honourable friend has ever paddled in the sea he will understand the sensation. (Laughter) The dog – a finely developed bulldog – was neither tied nor muzzled. He wore a leather collar ornamented with brass studs. Had the experiment been painful the pain would no doubt have been immediately felt by those nearest the dog." (Laughter)

Mr MacNeill (Donegal South): "Will the right honourable gentleman inform the person who furnished him with his jokes that there are members in this House who regard these experiments on dogs with abhorrence?" (Hear)

Mr Gladstone: "I certainly shall not. The jokes, poor as they are, are mine own." (Laughter and cheers)

(From Waller AD. *Physiology; the Servant of Medicine: Chloroform in the Laboratory and in the Hospital*. London: Hodder and Stoughton; 1910.)

moving paper or computer screen to produce the familiar ECG trace. The paper speed is standardized at 0.2 s per large division (25 mm/s).

The magnitude of the skin potential difference depends on the size of the extracellular current, which in turn depends on the **mass of myocardium** that is activated. Consequently, the surface ECG detects the activity of atrial and ventricular muscle, but fails to detect the pacemaker. However, the activity of the latter can be recorded with a cardiac catheter.

## 5.2 RELATION OF ECG WAVES TO CARDIAC ACTION POTENTIALS

The human ECG shows three main deflections per cardiac cycle (Figure 5.2): the P wave is caused by atrial depolarization; the QRS complex by ventricular depolarization; and the T wave by ventricular repolarization. The trace returns to the baseline, or 'isoelectric state', during the PR interval and the ST segment. The lettering was allotted sequentially by Einthoven, reflecting a tradition in mathematics first used by Rene Descartes in the 17th century. The ECG waves are aligned with the underlying cardiac action potentials in Figure 5.3, and with the other events of the cardiac cycle in Figure 2.5.

### The P wave marks atrial excitation

The first ECG wave, the small, broad P wave, coincides with the upstrokes of thousands of right then left atrial action potentials, spread over ~0.08 s. The P wave thus marks atrial depolarization. Atrial contraction occurs during the PR interval.

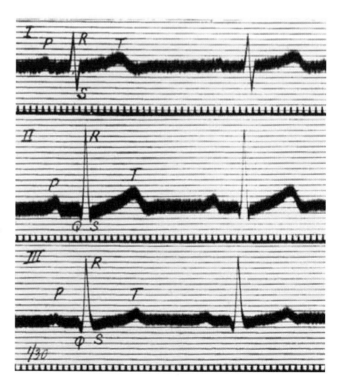

**Figure 5.2** Human ECG, Leads I–III. Lead II (60°) has the largest P, R and T waves. Lead I (0°) has a smaller R wave than Lead III, so this individual's electrical axis is between 60° and 90° (see Section 5.7). Ordinate divisions = 0.1 mV; time marks = 1/30th second. Thick baseline is an interference artefact of early string galvanometers, cf. Figure 5.4a. (From Sir Thomas Lewis's classic monograph, *The Mechanism and Graphic Registration of the Human Heart*. London: Shaw and Sons, 1920.)

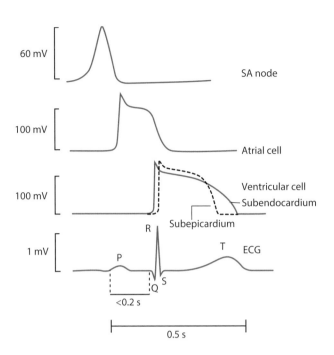

**Figure 5.3** Timing of ECG waves compared with intracellular recordings of cardiac action potentials. Subepicardial and apical myocytes (dashed trace) have shorter action potential durations than subendocardial and basal myocytes, so they repolarize first. This causes the T wave to be upright (Section 5.5). SA, sino-atrial.

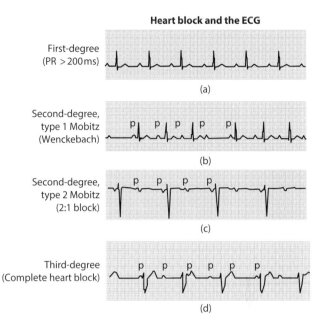

**Figure 5.4** Progressive stages of heart block and the ECG. **(a)** First-degree block; the PR interval is prolonged (>200 ms). **(b)** Second-degree block (Mobitz type 1 or Wenckebach); progressive prolongation of the PR interval until a P wave fails to conduct to the ventricle. **(c)** Second-degree block (Mobitz type 2); several P waves are present (in this case 2) for every QRS. **(d)** Third-degree block (complete heart block); QRS complexes are unrelated to P waves.

## The PR interval marks atrioventricular node delay

The interval between the start of the P wave and the start of the QRS complex is called the PR interval, even when it is strictly speaking a P–Q interval. The PR interval represents the time taken for excitation to spread across both atria, then through the atrioventricular (AV) node and the bundle of His–Purkinje system into the ventricle. Much of the PR interval represents the delay in transmission through the AV node, which allows atrial systole to precede ventricular systole. The PR interval should not exceed 0.2 s. Longer intervals indicate a defect in the conduction pathway called **heart block** (Figure 5.4a).

The ECG is isoelectric for much of the PR interval, despite the potential difference between the depolarized atria and polarized ventricles. This is because the insulating annulus fibrosus breaks the electrical circuit shown in Figure 4.4; consequently, no detectable extracellular current is flowing.

Atrial repolarization does not register on the ECG because it is coincident and slow (Figure 5.3); therefore, it does not generate sufficient extracellular current to be detected. It is often stated, incorrectly, that atrial repolarization is not seen because it is obscured by the QRS complex. The ECG of patients with third-degree heart block, where P waves are not followed by an 'obscuring' QRS wave, show clearly that atrial repolarization simply does not register on the ECG (Figure 5.4d).

## Atrioventricular node conduction block

The AV node, bundle of His or a bundle branch may begin to fail to transmit electrical excitation properly, because of tissue fibrosis or ischaemic heart disease. Three degrees of main AV nodal block are recognized. **First-degree heart block** is a lengthening of the PR interval to >0.2 s (e.g. 0.32 s in Figure 5.4a). This is caused by a slowing of conduction between the AV node and ventricle. **Second-degree heart block** is an intermittent failure of excitation to pass from the atria to the ventricles. In Figure 5.4b, for example, there are only three QRS complexes for four P waves; the PR interval lengthens with each beat, until a point is reached where transmission fails completely. This is known as **Type I Mobitz (Wenckebach) phenomenon**. If transmission from atria to ventricles fails so that there are two or more P waves with every QRS complex, then this is known as **Type II Mobitz** second-degree heart block (Figure 5.4c). In **third-degree or complete heart block**, the transmission fails completely, so the atria and ventricles beat independently, at different rates. In Figure 5.4d, the atria (P waves) are beating at 88 bpm, driven by the sino-atrial (SA) node. The ventricles are beating at 53 bpm, driven by a latent pacemaker in the bundle of His or Purkinje system that has escaped from dominance by the SA node. Type II Mobitz second-degree heart block and complete heart block often cause problems. The slow heart rate that results can cause breathlessness, particularly on exertion when heart rate should rise. If QRS complexes cease for more than 3 s (as can occur intermittently in the latter two conditions), this compromises cerebral perfusion causing **Stokes–Adams attacks** (sudden, temporary loss of consciousness). Such patients are treated with implantable cardiac pacemakers. Complete cessation of ventricular electrical activity is known as "asystole" and will cause a cardiac arrest and sudden cardiac death unless cardiopulmonary resuscitation is started promptly.

## The QRS complex marks ventricular excitation

The rapid depolarization of a large mass of ventricular muscle produces a large deflection, the QRS complex (Figure 5.3), which occurs just before the first heart sound. The Q wave is defined as the first downward spike (negative deflection), the R wave as the first upward spike (positive deflection) and the S wave as the second downward spike. All three components are not necessarily present in every record; the complex may be just RS (e.g. Figure 5.2, Lead I) or just QR. The complex normally lasts <0.12 s. Wider QRS complexes indicate slower activation of the ventricles, caused by either a ventricular ectopic beat or a block in one of the bundle branches. In bundle branch block, the R wave has a characteristic 'M or W'-shaped notch (depending on the lead and if it is the left or right bundle branch that is blocked), because of the staggered activation of the ventricles. The first heart sound follows just after the QRS complex (Figure 2.5). Hypertrophy of the ventricles can lead to particularly tall QRS complexes, although their size is also influenced by the amount of tissue between the heart and electrode.

## The ST segment is displaced in ischaemic heart disease

The ST segment extends from the end of the QRS wave to the start of the T wave. It coincides with the plateau of the ventricular action potential and rapid ventricular ejection. Since the ventricle is uniformly depolarized, no extracellular current is flowing and the ST segment is isoelectric. However, in ischaemic heart disease the ST segment can be depressed or elevated because of injury currents (Section 5.9).

## The T wave marks repolarization

Ventricular repolarization is slower and less synchronous than depolarization, so it generates a broad, but relatively low-magnitude wave, the T wave (Figure 5.3). The second heart sound follows closely after the T waves. Both the T and R waves are upright in most ECG recordings, even though repolarization is the electrical opposite of depolarization. The explanation of this oddity is deferred to Section 5.5, because it depends on the concept of 'cardiac dipole' (Section 5.4). Myocardial ischaemia can cause **T wave inversion** (see section 5.9 and Figure 5.10).

## 5.3 STANDARD ECG LEADS

To understand the waves of the ECG we must consider three factors: (1) the anatomical positioning of the recording electrodes relative to the heart; (2) the concept of an electrical dipole; and (3) the change in dipole orientation as depolarization spreads across the ventricles.

Let us deal first with the positioning of the recording electrodes. The most basic ECG is recorded using three **limb electrodes**, one on each arm and one on the left leg (Figure 5.5). Wrists and ankles/shins are usually used to minimize interference from contracting skeletal muscle electromyograms (EMGs). The exact position makes little difference to the recording; the limb simply serves as a tube of conducting electrolyte solution (the extracellular fluid) connected to the torso.

## There are three bipolar limb leads

Pairs of limb electrodes, called the bipolar limb leads, can be connected across a voltmeter in three different combinations. When the left arm is connected to the positive terminal of the voltmeter and right arm to the negative terminal, this is called a Lead I recording. If the potential on the left side of the body is more positive than on the right during cardiac excitation, Lead I records a positive potential. The three bipolar combinations (as shown in Figure 5.5) are as follows:

- left arm (+) to right arm (−) = lead I (angle of view 0°);
- left leg (+) to right arm (−) = lead II (angle of view +60°);
- left leg (+) to left arm (−) = lead III (angle of view +120°).

Because each limb serves as an electrical conductor connected to the trunk, the limb electrodes in effect record from each shoulder and the pelvis. They thus form a sensing triangle around the heart, called **Einthoven's triangle** (Figure 5.5). Each lead views the heart from a different angle in the frontal plane. Lead I, forming the top of Einthoven's triangle, is horizontal, and this angle is taken as zero. Lead II is at roughly 60° to Lead I and Lead III at roughly 120°.

## There are three unipolar limb leads

A cunning ruse provides three additional viewing angles from the same limb electrodes. The trick is to feed the signal from two arm electrodes simultaneously into the negative terminal of the voltmeter, thereby producing an averaged signal located roughly in mid-chest. When the signal from the foot is connected to the other terminal, the angle of view is from the pelvis to mid-chest, +90° to the horizontal (Figure 5.5). This is

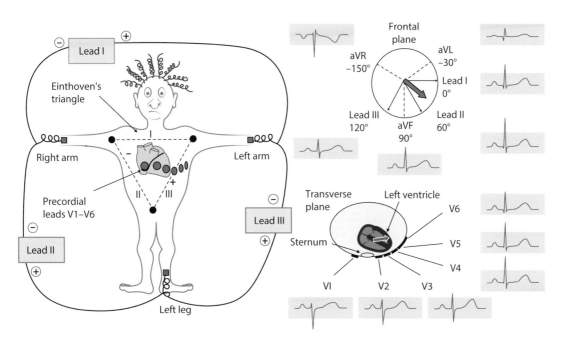

**Figure 5.5** Electrode positions to record a 12-lead ECG. The bipolar limb leads (I, II and III) and augmented limb leads (aVL, aVR and aVF) record in the frontal plane. Precordial chest leads V1–V6 record in the transverse plane. For explanation of augmented limb leads, see the text. Typical recordings on the right. Red arrows show direction of biggest potential difference during ventricular excitation (main dipole), in the frontal and transverse planes. aVF, augmented Vector Foot; aVL, augmented Vector Left; aVR, augmented Vector Right.

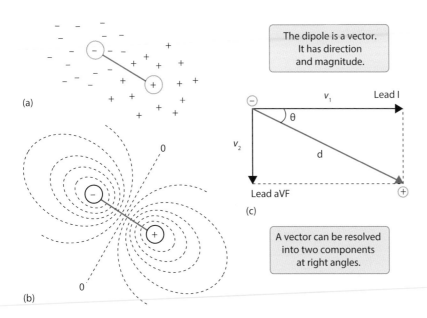

The dipole is a vector. It has direction and magnitude.

A vector can be resolved into two components at right angles.

**Figure 5.6** Properties of an electrical dipole. **(a)** Two diffuse groups of opposite charge can be represented by a dipole; that is, two points of opposite charge, like the terminals of a battery. **(b)** Equipotential lines around a dipole. The zero potential runs across the middle of the dipole. **(c)** Resolution of dipole vector (red arrow) into two components at right angles. The length of the red arrow represents vector magnitude d. The voltage difference $v_1$ detected by Lead I depends on angle $\theta$ ($v_1$ = d cosine $\theta$). If $v_1$ and $v_2$ are drawn the same lengths as the R waves in Leads I and aVF, respectively, the electrical axis of the heart equals $\theta$.

called a unipolar limb lead aVF (**a**ugmented **V**ector **F**oot). The three unipolar limb leads are:

- left arm to +terminal = aVL (angle of view −30°);
- right arm to +terminal = aVR (angle of view −150°);
- foot to +terminal = aVF (angle of view +90°).

Lead aVR (augmented Vector Right) looks into the inside of the ventricles, so it records negative rather than positive waves (Figure 5.5). Lead aVF records the inferior surface of the heart.

Since aVF is at a right angle to Lead I, it is useful for working out the cardiac electrical axis, as explained later in the chapter.

## There are six unipolar precordial leads

In clinical practice, an additional six electrodes, V1–V6, are placed across the chest for connection to the positive terminal of the voltmeter. All three limb leads are connected to the negative terminal to create a mid-chest reference point. The six precordial leads encircle the heart and 'look' transversely across the chest. This is useful, because the wave of excitation travels in three dimensions, not just the frontal plane recorded through the limb leads. Leads V1 and V2 lie over the fourth intercostal space (ICS), immediately right and left of the sternum, respectively; they record right ventricle activity best. V3 is between V2 and V4. V4 is placed over the fifth ICS in the mid-clavicular line. V3 and V4 record interventricular septal activity best. V5 and V6 are at the same level in the anterior axillary and mid-axillary line, respectively, and record the left ventricular activity best.

The ECG records an upward deflection when the positive pole of a potential difference is directed towards the left arm (Lead I) or left leg (Leads II and III), or a unipolar/precordial lead. We must therefore consider next the polarity of the heart during excitation.

## 5.4 THE CARDIAC DIPOLE

### Two clusters of charge can be represented by two poles

At any instant during the spread of excitation through the ventricle there is a resting zone, with a diffuse cloud of positive extracellular charges, and an excited zone, with a diffuse cloud of negative extracellular charges (Figure 5.6a). Just as a diffuse mass can be represented by a centre of gravity, so a diffuse charge can be represented as a single charge at its electrical centre, or pole. Thus, during the spread of excitation the ventricles can be represented by one negative pole and one positive pole, that is, by an electrical dipole. The size of the attendant ECG deflection depends not only on the **magnitude** of the dipole but also on its **orientation** relative to the recording lead, as follows.

### Detection depends on the angle of the recording leads

A dipole is surrounded by positive and negative potential fields, which grow weaker with increasing distance, like the fields around a magnet (Figure 5.6b). When the leads of a voltmeter are aligned with the two poles, the difference between the positive and negative potential fields is recorded optimally, whereas leads at right angles to the dipole detect no potential difference (Figure 5.6b). The potential difference recorded by the ECG voltmeter thus depends on the orientation of the recording electrodes relative to the dipole. You can get a sense of this effect by viewing a ruler face on, then slowly rotating it through 180°. The visible length changes from maximum to zero and back to maximum as the angle of view changes.

### The dipole can be resolved into vectorial components

The dipole is a **vector** quantity. That is, it possesses direction as well as magnitude, just like a mechanical force.

The symbol for a vector is an arrow whose length represents the size of the vector and whose direction represents the angle of the vector. Just as with a force vector, the electrical vector can be resolved into two components at right angles, and the ECG registers **the magnitude of the component aligned with the recording leads** (Figure 5.6c). But this raises another question: in which direction does the cardiac dipole point?

## 5.5 THE EXCITATION SEQUENCE

Both the magnitude and orientation of the cardiac dipole change continuously as excitation spreads through the ventricles. For simplicity, we will consider only changes in the frontal plane here; however, since the ventricles are three-dimensional bodies lying in an oblique, rotated position, the dipole size and direction change in the transverse plane too.

### The ventricular dipole swings anticlockwise in the frontal plane during depolarization

The first part of the ventricles to depolarize is the left side of the interventricular septum, which is activated by the left bundle branches (Figure 5.7). The dipole magnitude is small, because only a small mass of muscle has been activated; and the dipole angle is ~120° to the horizontal, that is, pointing down and rightwards. Next, the remaining septum and most of the subendocardium depolarize, while the subepicardium is still polarized. Since the bulky left ventricle predominates, the dipole magnitude is large and the dipole angle is ~60°, that is, pointing down and leftwards. The last region to be excited by the advancing wave of depolarization is the base of the ventricles, close to the annulus fibrosus. The bulky left ventricle again predominates, creating a small dipole pointing headward. The sequence of ventricular activation thus causes the cardiac vector to rotate anticlockwise in the frontal plane, and to wax and wane in size as it rotates. This entire sequence takes ~90 ms.

### Repolarization occurs in reverse, creating an upright T wave

We now have the information needed to answer a puzzle raised earlier – why is the T wave upright? This seems odd on first acquaintance, since repolarization is the electrical opposite of depolarization. The explanation is that the myocytes repolarize in reverse order to depolarization. In other words, the subepicardium repolarizes before the subendocardium (Figure 5.8). This is because the outer ventricular myocytes have shorter action potentials than the inner myocytes, perhaps due to a higher density of transient outward $K^+$ channels (Figure 5.3). Recent evidence also points to cellular coupling or 'electrotonic' influences, such that the action potential duration shortens the

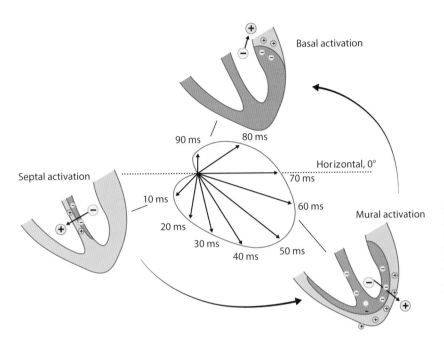

**Figure 5.7** Changes in size and angle of cardiac dipole (straight arrows) with time during ventricular excitation. Charges refer to extracellular, not intracellular, fluid. Pale pink areas are myocytes at resting potential, so they carry a positive extracellular charge. Red areas are depolarized myocytes with negative extracellular charge. The cardiac dipole rotates anticlockwise and waxes and wanes over ~90 ms. The electrical axis here is ~40° below the horizontal.

further away it is from a given stimulus. Therefore, repolarization begins in the subepicardium and spreads towards the subendocardium, whereas depolarization does the reverse. The same can be said regarding action potential duration between the base and apex of the heart, such that depolarization spreads from base to apex, and repolarization from apex to base. As a result, the same polarity develops transiently across the heart during repolarization as during depolarization (Figure 5.8). This is why the T wave is upright.

## 5.6 WHY THE QRS COMPLEX IS COMPLEX

Knowing the orientation of the ECG leads and dipole, we are now able to understand why the QRS complex has negative and positive waves, and why the same heartbeat generates differently shaped QRS complexes in different leads (Figure 5.5). To work through an example, let us consider the dipole at three instants, the beginning, middle and end of ventricular excitation, as detected by bipolar limb Leads I–III. In the individual shown in Figure 5.9, the small initial dipole at ~120° is directed obliquely away from Lead I. Resolving the vector, we find there is a small component directed at 180°. Since the positive pole points away from Lead I (0°), Lead I records a small, negative deflection, that is, a Q wave (point 'a' in Figure 5.9). However, at the same instant, Lead III (120°) detects the full dipole (120°), so it records a positive deflection, that is, the start of an R wave.

By 50 ms, the dipole has grown to its maximum size and swung anticlockwise to ~40°. The dipole now has a large vectorial component directed at Lead I (0°), which therefore records a substantial upward deflection – a large R wave (point 'b', Figure 5.9). Lead II (60°) is almost exactly aligned with the

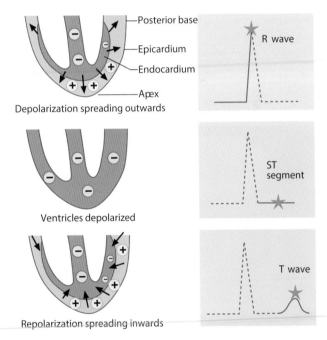

**Figure 5.8** Depolarization/repolarization state of ventricles at three points in time, namely partial depolarization (red zone; R wave, top), full depolarization (ST segment, middle) and partial repolarization (pale pink T wave, bottom). Signs refer to extracellular charge. Arrows show direction of advance of wavefront. Since myocytes repolarize in reverse order to depolarization, the dipoles are in the same direction. Consequently, the T wave is upright.

dipole, so **Lead II usually registers the biggest R wave**. Lead III (120°) is almost at right angles to the dipole, and so Lead III records little potential difference.

By 90 ms the dipole has dwindled in magnitude and, in the illustrated case, swung round to about –100°, creating a small, downward deflection in each limb lead, that is, an S wave. Thus,

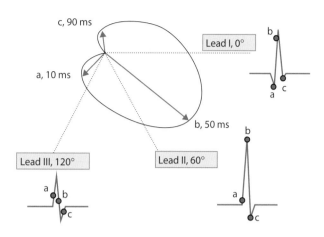

**Figure 5.9** Illustrationof how the changing magnitude and direction of the dipole (red arrows) creates different QRS complexes in different frontal leads. The dipole is shown at three instants in time: a; b; and c. The vectorial component recorded by Leads I, II and III at each instant is marked by a red dot on the corresponding ECG trace.

the same wave of ventricular excitation produced a QRS complex in Lead I, a very large RS complex in Lead II and a small RS complex in Lead III. Using similar reasoning, the reader should now be able to work out why the **P wave, QRS complex and T wave are all inverted in Lead aVR** (Figure 5.5), and why the Q wave generated by the initial depolarization of the interventricular septum is best seen in aVL.

The precordial (chest) leads record the dipole in the transverse plane. In this plane, the maximum dipole points towards the left axilla (Figure 5.5, bottom right, red arrow); so, the R wave increases in height from V2 to V3 and peaks in the axillary Leads V4 and V5. Since the maximum dipole points away from V1, the main wave of the QRS complex is downwards in V1.

Confusingly, not all ECG traces are identical to those in Figures 5.5 and 5.9. This is because the orientation of the cardiac dipole varies between individuals. For example, the subject of Figure 5.2 had the biggest R wave in Lead II, as expected, but Lead III showed a bigger R wave than Lead I. This indicates a more vertically orientated electrical axis, and brings us to the issue of the electrical axis of the heart.

## 5.7 THE ELECTRICAL AXIS OF THE HEART

The direction of the largest dipole in the frontal plane is called the electrical axis of the heart. In Figures 5.5 and 5.9, the electrical axis is ~40° below the horizontal. The electrical axis can be worked out numerically by comparing the height of the R wave in Leads I and aVF, using the method shown in Figure 5.6c. In a busy clinic, a quick estimate can be made as follows: (1) compare the size of the R wave in Leads I–III.

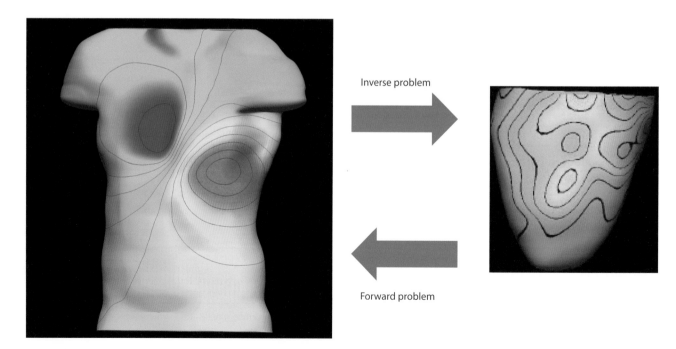

**Figure 5.10** Body surface electrical potential map (**left**) and epicardial ventricular electrical activation map (**right**). Predicting the temporal changes in body surface potentials based on the changes in electrical activity measured from the ventricles is known as the *forward problem* of electrocardiography (i.e. right to left arrow), while determining ventricular *activation from body surface recordings is known as the inverse problem* of electrocardiography (i.e. right to left arrow). The colours correspond to 'isochronal' lines. These are regions that are activated at the same point in time. (The dark blue represents regions activated first, through to red being the region activated last.) (Adapted from Paterson DJ. *The Journal of Physiology* 2013; 591(17): 4065–6 and Herring N, Paterson DJ. *Quarterly Journal of Medicine* 2006; 99(4): 219–30.)

**THE DEPOLARIZING VENTRICLE FORMS AN ELECTRICAL DIPOLE**

- During the 90 ms that it takes depolarization to spread through the ventricles, the excited region carries a cloud of negative extracellular charges (the negative pole) and the resting region a cloud of positive extracellular charges (the positive pole). A dipole thus forms across the heart.

- The dipole is biggest midway through excitation, because roughly half the wall is negative and half positive.

- The direction of the biggest dipole is called the electrical axis of the heart. It is typically −30° to +90° below the horizontal, in the frontal plane.

- An ECG lead detects the amount of the dipole that is parallel with the lead. Lead II, aligned at 60° to the horizontal, is roughly in line with the biggest dipole, so it usually has the biggest R wave.

- The dipole waxes and wanes, and swings anticlockwise, as excitation sweeps through the ventricles. The changes in dipole size and orientation generate the Q, R and S waves.

If the largest R wave is in Lead II, the electrical axis is closer to 60° than 0° or 120°; (2) look for the lead with the smallest QRS complex, with R and S waves of nearly equal height. This lead must be roughly at right angles to the electrical axis (e.g. Lead I in Figure 5.2).

The electrical axis has a very wide, normal range, from −30° to +90°. The axis depends partly on an individual's anatomy; the heart and electrical axis are more vertical in a tall, thin person than in a short, broad-chested individual. The axis also becomes more vertical during each inspiration because the descending diaphragm tugs on the pericardium and drags down the apex. The electrical axis depends also on the relative thickness of the right and left ventricle walls. Hypertrophy of the left ventricle (e.g. due to exercise training, hypertension or hypertrophic cardiomyopathy) shifts the electrical axis to the left (**left axis deviation**). Hypertrophy of the right ventricle (often due to pulmonary disease) produces **right axis deviation**.

## 5.8 THE INVERSE PROBLEM OF ELECTROCARDIOGRAPHY AND ECG IMAGING (ECG$_i$)

Biophysicists have attempted to calculate the temporal changes in body surface potentials based on the electrical activity measured from the ventricles in what is known as the *forward problem of electrocardiography*. However, the 'holy grail' of electrocardiology is to improve on the 12-lead ECG and solve the so-called '*inverse problem*', that is, to

determine ventricular activity from body surface recordings (see Figure 5.10). Determining the electrical axis of the heart as described previously is in fact a simple form of the 'inverse problem'. Several mathematical algorithms for this exist, although many more body surface electrodes are required to produce an accurate body surface map and knowing the position of the heart within the thorax is also crucial to their solutions. Electrocardiographic imaging uses a multi-electrode vest that records 256 body surface ECGs. Then, using geometrical information from a CT or MRI scan, it reconstructs electrograms, activation sequences (isochrones) and repolarization patterns on the heart's surface. While the epicardial activation and repolarization sequences can be reasonably well determined, the absolute magnitude of the potential changes on the heart cannot. This approach can detect electrophysiological changes and their location on the heart during left anterior descending artery occlusion before changes in the standard 12-lead ECG occur. It can also locate atrial pacing sites to within 6 mm, and has been used to map arrhythmias, including accessory pathways and electrical substrate within myocardial infarction scars in relation to the activation pattern of ventricular tachycardia (VT), before ablation procedures.

## 5.9 ECG IN ISCHAEMIC HEART DISEASE

Coronary artery disease is a common cause of local ventricular ischaemia, which can manifest itself as T wave inversion, new conduction defects (such as heart block or bundle branch block) or displacement of the ST segment above/below the isoelectric baseline. ST segment displacement is caused by a fall in resting potential and action potential magnitude in ischaemic myocytes. This creates a potential difference between the ischaemic myocytes and surrounding healthy ones, caused at least in part through opening of adenosine triphosphate-sensitive $K^+$ channels and accumulation of extracellular $K^+$. An **injury current** can then flow during normally isoelectric periods, which shifts the level of the ST segment.

Exercise-induced, or **stable angina** can cause ST segment depression, as explained in Figure 5.11a. The change is reversible with rest. This is usually caused by an atherosclerotic lesion producing a narrowing in a coronary artery that only limits oxygen delivery to the myocardium when demand is increased as heart rate rises during exercise.

By contrast, a large **ST-elevation myocardial infarction** is caused by acute atherosclerotic plaque rupture, thrombus formation and complete occlusion of one of the main epicardial coronary arteries (Figure 5.11b). This can be treated by emergency revascularization using a catheter and injection of dye (angiography) to identify the blockage, and passing a wire through the blockage and inflating a small balloon on the wire (angioplasty) surrounded by an expandable metal frame known as a stent. This is known as primary percutaneous coronary intervention and is indicated within 12 hours of the onset of pain if ST elevation occurs in 2 or

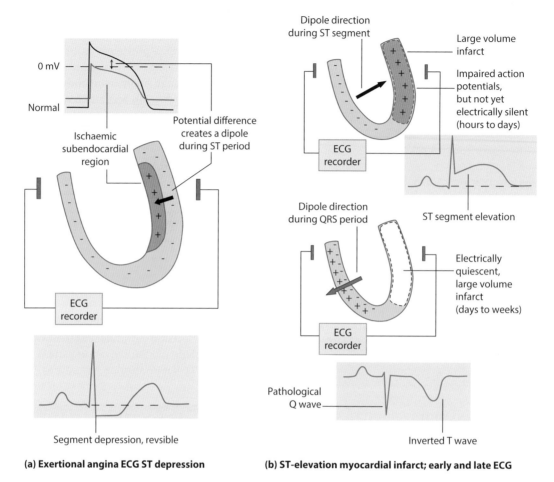

**(a) Exertional angina ECG ST depression**

**(b) ST-elevation myocardial infarct; early and late ECG**

**Figure 5.11** Effect of myocardial ischaemia on ventricle extracellular charge distribution and the ECG. **(a)** ST segment depression during exertional angina. The potential difference between normal myocytes and ischaemic myocytes (usually subendocardial) creates a dipole and injury current during the ST interval (cf. normally uniform depolarization; Figure 5.8, middle) and a reversed one during the T–P interval. This depresses the ST segment relative to the baseline. The ECG reverts to normal when the angina is relieved by rest. A partial-thickness, subendocardial infarct can likewise cause ST depression, but this is not relieved by rest. **(b)** An ST-elevation myocardial infarct, caused by occlusion of a main epicardial coronary artery. (Upper schematic) Ventricle during the ST interval, a few hours after infarction. The potential difference between the ischaemic and normal myocytes during ST creates a dipole and injury current, which causes ST elevation in the leads facing the infarct, for example, V1–4 for anterior infarcts, and aVF, II and III for an inferior infarct. (Lower schematic) Ventricle during spread of excitation, several days later. As ischaemic cells die (necrosis), they become electrically silent, so ST elevation dwindles and is replaced by pathological Q waves and T wave inversion. Pathological Q waves are deep Q waves (>2 mm, 0.2 mV) in leads not normally showing them, persisting for years. These features are caused by the altered dipole during excitation; cf. Figure 5.7. The infarcted myocardium acts as an 'electrical window' for leads facing it. A small-volume subendocardial infarct does not generate pathological Q waves.

more contiguous leads (>2 mm in the chest leads or >1 mm in the limb leads), or a new left bundle branch block develops, to minimize the amount of subsequent myocardial damage. This has been shown to improve morbidity and mortality in randomized clinical trials. If a large enough volume of ventricular tissue is infarcted, then broad, deep negative deflections in the ECG, known as Q waves, can develop over the subsequent days and remain permanently. These may represent endo-to-epicardial activation in the wall opposite to the scar 'window', becoming more prominent in some ECG leads.

It should be noted that during small ischaemic events (including **stable and unstable angina, and non-ST-elevation myocardial infarction**), there may be no detectable changes on a single 12-lead ECG and repeated ECGs are needed to look for subtle changes in the ST segments or T waves. Even then, the severity and location of ischaemia relative to the position of exploring electrodes limit the sensitivity of the ECG in detecting ischaemia. Measurements of plasma troponin levels released from damaged myocytes may be required to diagnose or exclude a myocardial infarction.

## 5.10 ARRHYTHMOGENIC MECHANISMS: A TRIGGER, VULNERABLE WINDOW AND SUBSTRATE

Given the millions of normal heartbeats we experience in a lifetime, why is it that on very rare occasions, abnormal rhythms are generated? The answer is complex, but a simple way of looking at it is that a pathological arrhythmia usually requires a **trigger** to generate an extra-stimulus within the heart. This extra-stimulus needs to have the right properties and be perfectly timed within a **vulnerable window**, and there needs to be a suitable **substrate** within the heart to maintain the propagation of the extra-stimulus. The substrate can be **structural and/or electrophysiological**, as well as **static and/or dynamic**.

## Triggers and a vulnerable window

Arrhythmic triggers include afterdepolarization and abnormal automaticity. With **abnormal automaticity**, there are repetitive, spontaneous phase 4 depolarizations in a group of cells outside the heart's usual primary (SA node) and secondary (AV node, bundle of His–Purkinje system) pacemakers. This can be driven by a $Ca^{2+}$ clock mechanism like that described in SA node cells in Chapter 4, and may sustain atrial tachycardias (ATs). They may also be driven by local injury currents from ischaemic regions depolarizing neighbouring border zones, which may account some ventricular tachycardia seen during ischaemia/reperfusion known as an accelerated idioventricular rhythm.

Triggered activity may result from afterdepolarizations as described in Section 3.11. Most pathological arrhythmias are triggered by a **delayed afterdepolarization (DAD)**, which results from the discharge of an overloaded sarcoplasmic reticulum (SR) $Ca^{2+}$ store (Figure 3.17). This is exacerbated by cardiac ischaemia and β adrenergic receptor stimulation by catecholamines. **Early afterdepolarizations (EADs)** are more common when the action potential is prolonged, such as during bradycardia, inherited long QT syndromes (LQTS) and hypokalaemia/hypocalcaemia, or in the presence of drugs that block $K^+$ channels. This is often characterized by the appearance of a U wave after the T wave. The mechanism for EADs during the plateau phase of the ventricular action potential is classically thought to be due to reactivation of L-type $Ca^{2+}$ channels. Like DADs, EADs are also more common during conditions of intracellular $Ca^{2+}$ overload (as occurs when action potential duration is prolonged) because the L-type $Ca^{2+}$ current can be enhanced by cytoplasmic calcium and phosphorylation by calcium/calmodulin-dependent protein kinase II. This is coupled to an increase in $Na^+$ conductance due to activation of the $Na^+/Ca^{2+}$ exchanger as the cell attempts to defend against the high levels of intracellular $Ca^{2+}$. Afterdepolarizations do not always result in the generation of an action potential and ectopic beat. They must be of sufficient magnitude to reach the threshold and follow the refractory period of the previous beat. Atrial or ventricular ectopic beats are common in completely normal, healthy hearts where they rarely lead to arrhythmias. They are therefore not the whole story. They must be perfectly timed during a **vulnerable window** (usually the latter half of the T wave, when some myocytes have repolarized, but some have not), and have a suitable substrate, so that the wave of excitation

they produce can form a self-sustaining arrhythmia. The shorter the duration of an ectopic beat action potential, and therefore refractory period, the more likely it is to be able to produce a re-entrant circuit (see the following section). The relationship between action potential duration and the preceding diastolic interval is known as **electrical restitution**.

## A sustaining substrate

Sometimes, an abnormal conduction pathway develops, so that the wave of excitation travels in a never-ending circle (**circus or spiral wave**, Figure 5.12). This concept was first demonstrated by George Ralph Mines, the pioneering English cardiac electrophysiologist. Myocytes emerging from their refractory period find themselves re-excited prematurely by the return of the local excitation wave (**re-entry**). A slow conduction velocity of wave propagation favours re-entry, as does a short refractory period, because it allows time for the myocytes to regain excitability. Re-entry also requires a central area of conduction block that may be anatomical (such as a myocardial infarction scar) or functional (such as a group of cells that are refractory and unable to be excited), and for one limb of the circuit to be refractory at initiation (known as unidirectional conduction block) as shown in Figure 5.12. That way, both waves of excitation

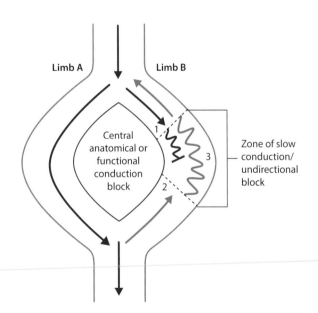

**Figure 5.12** The initiation of a re-entry arrhythmia. Limbs A and B represent two pathways with different electrophysiological properties surrounding an area of central anatomical or functional conduction block. Limb B has a region of slow conduction velocity and unidirectional conduction block (if the cells are refractory at that point in time at point 1 in limb B). Therefore, the initial impulse conducts anterogradely only through limb A and is blocked in limb B (labelled 1). The impulse then continues to conduct retrogradely into limb B (labelled 2) and through the zone of slow conduction velocity (labelled 3). As the wavefront returns, if limb A is no longer refractory, then the wavefront can propagate down limb A again and a re-entry circuit is formed. (Adapted from Bashir Y, Betts TR, Rajappan K. *Cardiac Electrophysiology and catheter ablation [Oxford Specialist Handbooks in Cardiology]*. Oxford: OUP; 2010.)

around the area of the central conduction block do not collide and extinguish each other. Re-entry therefore requires an appropriate **substrate**. This substrate may be anatomically fixed, such as with atrial flutter, the slow pathway of AV nodal re-entry tachycardia (AVNRT) or the bundle of Kent in AV re-entry tachycardia (AVRT; see the next sections). It may also develop because of genetic conditions, such as arrhythmogenic right ventricular cardiomyopathy, hypertrophic cardiomyopathy and inherited dilated cardiomyopathy (particularly *lamin A/C* [*LMNA*] gene mutations). It can be acquired because of local ischaemia that uncouples gap junctions, raises extracellular $K^+$, depolarizes the resting potential and thereby prevents some fast $Na^+$ channels from recovering from the inactivated state (Figure 3.13). The resulting impairment of the action potential upstroke reduces the propagating currents, which slows conduction (Figure 4.12). In ischaemic and dilated cardiomyopathy, there is scarring and fibrosis as well as remodelling of ion channels and sympathetic innervation, particularly in scar border zones. The substrate may also be dynamic because electrophysiological properties can be influenced by hypoxia, haemodynamics, metabolic/ionic changes, drugs and autonomic tone. Ventricular arrhythmias tend to occur during exercise or first thing in the morning when sympathetic drive is highest. One common feature that promotes re-entry is a substrate that is **heterogeneous** in terms of its conduction velocity, action potential duration and refractory period. Mines also described the vulnerable window during the cardiac cycle when a single stimulus can induce ventricular arrhythmias because all the conditions for initiating self-sustaining re-entry are met.

## Wave stability, wavebreak and fibrillation

A spiral wave that is fixed to a single anchoring source tends to produce a static regular ECG wave pattern (a monomorphic tachycardia). For example, in the ventricles this produces a regular, broad complex tachycardia on the ECG that is of a constant amplitude (see Section 5.11). However, if the spiral wave's position drifts backwards and forwards this can lead to variation in the amplitude of the tachycardia on the ECG. A good example of this in the ventricles is the polymorphic tachycardia seen in LQTS where the broad complex tachycardia fluctuates in amplitude. This was described in 1966 by Dessertenne as 'torsade de pointes'. This translates to 'turning of the points' which originates from a ballet sequence in which the dancer twists around their 'pointes' (or tips of their toes). If the wave of excitation splits up into more than one wavefront ('wavebreak'), then multiple wavelets can be formed, and this produces fibrillation. There is currently debate in the fields of both atrial and ventricular fibrillation (VF) research as to whether fibrillation is maintained via a single stationary 'mother' rotor from which wavelets emanate, or whether wavebreak itself plays a fundamental role in initiating and maintaining fibrillation, producing multiple ever-changing wavelets.

## General principles of treating arrhythmias

Pharmacological treatment of arrhythmias can be aimed at simply controlling their rate, if the patient is asymptomatic, or controlling the rhythm, that is, cardioverting back to sinus rhythm and preventing further episodes. **Rate control** is achieved for arrhythmias arising from the atria through drugs that block the AV node, such as $Ca^{2+}$ channel blockers, β-blockers and digoxin. If the AV node is a crucial part of the re-entrant circuit then transiently blocking the AV node with manoeuvres that activate the vagus nerve (such as carotid sinus massage, Valsalva manoeuvre or drinking ice-cold water to mimic the diving reflex) or drugs such as intravenous adenosine or verapamil can cardiovert back to sinus rhythm. **Rhythm control** is achieved for other arrhythmias with medications such as $Na^+$ channel blockers (e.g. class Ia: procainamide; class Ib: mexilitine or lidocaine; class Ic: flecainide acetate or propafenone) or $K^+$ channel blockers (e.g. sotalol or amiodarone), but care should be taken when there is impaired left ventricular function or underlying coronary artery disease because many antiarrhythmic drugs can be proarrhythmic in these conditions. The only antiarrhythmic medications to successfully prevent ventricular arrhythmias and improve mortality following a myocardial infarction or during congestive heart failure are β-blockers.

If medical therapy fails, or the patient is acutely haemodynamically compromised by their arrhythmia (i.e. has no pulse, low blood pressure, chest pain or cardiac failure), then **electrical direct current cardioversion** or defibrillation (under appropriate sedation if still conscious) is the treatment of choice. For those patients with recurrent symptomatic arrhythmias that are difficult to control pharmacologically, then a percutaneous electrophysiological study and ablation may be appropriate. This procedure involves cauterization of local regions of conduction using heat (radiofrequency ablation) or freezing (cryoablation), although the success of these procedures depends on the clinical arrhythmia.

## 5.11 ARRHYTHMIAS

## Sinus arrhythmia

Sinus arrhythmia is the normal, regular physiological slowing of the heart during expiration and speeding up during inspiration. Sinus arrhythmia is especially marked in children and young adults. The inspiratory tachycardia partially compensates for a fall in left ventricular stroke volume during inspiration. The latter is due to a fall in left ventricle filling as inspiration expands the pulmonary vascular bed.

Sinus arrhythmia is brought about by an increase in vagal activity during expiration, followed by a decrease during inspiration. This phasic change in vagal activity persists even when breathing is paralysed, suggesting that it originates primarily by a central (cf. reflex) mechanism, namely an input from the respiration centre to the vagal motor nuclei in the brainstem (Figure 16.17). Sinus arrhythmia can also be seen in some heart transplant patients and may result from direct stretch of the sino-atrial node (see the Bainbridge "effect", Chapter 4.10 and 16.3).

## Ectopic beats

Aberrant myocytes may occasionally fire before the SA node, triggering a premature beat, also known as an ectopic beat or extra systole (Figure 5.13). If the trigger site lies in the ventricle, the resulting QRS wave is broad and unsynchronized because excitation was not disseminated along the normal, rapid bundle of His–Purkinje pathway. The contraction is ill-co-ordinated and fails to eject blood normally. The subsequent, normal excitation wave from the SA node finds the ventricular myocytes still in their refractory period, so no contraction is elicited. This results in a long interval before the next normal beat, called a **compensatory pause**. The patient often notices this delay, commenting that "My heart keeps missing a beat".

Occasional ectopic beats are not uncommon in normal individuals, and are common after a heart attack. The ectopic beat is probably triggered by a DAD. The DAD is the result of a discharge of the SR $Ca^{2+}$ store in early diastole, which increases the net inward exchanger current, $i_{Na-Ca}$ (Figure 3.17). DADs are most likely to occur in ischaemic heart disease, or when the SR $Ca^{2+}$ store is overloaded due to the action of digoxin, catecholamines, caffeine and other phosphodiesterase inhibitors.

Ectopic beats can sometimes be suppressed with medication such as β-blockers and avoiding caffeinated drinks, although in the context of an otherwise structurally and electrophysiologically normal heart, they are benign and this is purely to help symptoms. If there is a very high frequency of unifocal (e.g. right ventricular outflow tract) ventricular ectopic beats (especially if >20% of all heartbeats), then there may be a risk of developing a tachycardia cardiomyopathy and treatment with percutaneous ablation could be considered.

## Atrial tachycardia

AT originates from a group of cells in the left or right atrium, other than the SA node, spontaneously generating a wave of excitation through abnormal automaticity or micro re-entry. The P waves that are generated are often of a different morphology to the patient's usual P waves (with left to right axis if arising from the left atria) and can continue through the QRS complexes and T waves, often being obscured if the rate is much faster than what the AV node can conduct. As the atria are depolarizing extremely rapidly with little time to relax and refill with blood, contraction is often ineffective, which can impair ventricular filling and cause breathlessness and light-headedness as well as palpitations. The lack of effective atrial contraction also predisposes to the development of a thrombus in the left atrium or left atrial appendage. There is therefore a **risk of thromboembolic stroke** with this arrhythmia, which is also seen with atrial flutter and atrial fibrillation (AF). This risk should be assessed for an individual patient with an appropriate risk calculator (e.g. the $CHA_2DS_2$-VASc score) and if high enough, the patient should be formally anticoagulated (with

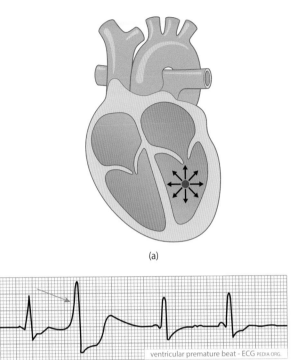

(a)

(b)

ventricular premature beat - ECG PEDIA.ORG.

**Figure 5.13** A ventricular ectopic beat is generated by the spontaneous excitation of a group of cells within the ventricle, as shown in **(a)**. **(b)** This is an early broad QRS duration (red arrow) on the ECG not triggered by a preceding P wave, and is usually followed by a short compensatory pause before the next sinus beat.

warfarin or a novel oral anticoagulant (NOAC), see Section 9.11 and Table 9.1). Otherwise treatment may be via rate control if the patient is asymptomatic (using AV blocking drugs such as $Ca^{2+}$ channel blockers, β-blockers or digoxin), or via rhythm control approach if symptomatic (e.g. using flecainide, sotalol, amiodarone, electrical cardioversion or percutaneous ablation).

## Atrioventricular nodal re-entry tachycardia

AVNRT is the most common pathological regular tachycardia with a narrow QRS complex (ie conducted via the AV node). It is a type of re-entry tachycardia that is dependent on the presence of both slow and fast conduction pathways within the AV node and the ability of the pathways to conduct retrogradely from ventricles to atria (Figure 5.14). In typical AVNRT, during the appropriate conditions (e.g. sympathetic stimulation), an ectopic beat may make the fast pathway refractory, so that conduction occurs anterogradely down the slow pathway and then, as the fast pathway has recovered, retrogradely up the fast pathway to complete a re-entry circuit that becomes self-sustaining. Occasionally in atypical AVNRT, re-entry can occur via fast–slow or even slow–slow pathway conduction. The patient usually experiences a rapid heart rate (palpitations). Cardioversion may be achieved through vagal manoeuvres or intravenous adenosine or verapamil to block the AV node. Preventative treatment can be through taking β-blockers or $Ca^{2+}$ channels blockers, or by performing a slow pathway modification

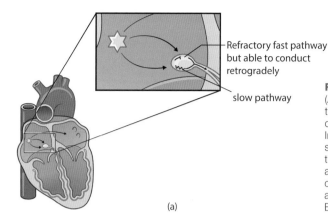

- Refractory fast pathway but able to conduct retrogradely
- slow pathway

(a)

**Figure 5.14** An atrioventricular (AV) nodal re-entry tachycardia (AVNRT) is dependent on the presence of both slow and fast conduction pathways within the AV node itself (see inset in **(a)**) and the ability of the pathways to conduct retrogradely from the ventricles to the atria. In typical AVNRT, during the appropriate conditions (e.g., sympathetic stimulation), an ectopic beat may make the fast pathway refractory so that conduction occurs anterogradely down the slow pathway and then, as the fast pathway has recovered, retrogradely up the fast pathway to complete a re-entry circuit that becomes self-sustaining. This produces a regular narrow complex tachycardia without clear P waves on the ECG **(b)**.

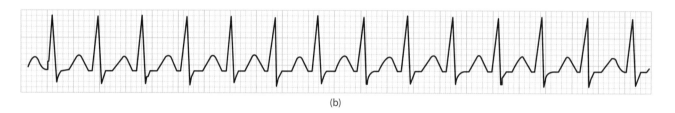

(b)

percutaneous ablation procedure. This has a 90%–95% success rate but comes with a risk of inducing complete heart block for which a permanent pacemaker would be required of <1%.

## Atrioventricular re-entry tachycardia

The unforgettably named **Wolff–Parkinson–White syndrome** comprises episodes of paroxysmal tachycardia, resulting from an anatomically definable re-entry pathway, the accessory bundle of Kent. This is an extra electrical connection across the annulus fibrosus, additional to the bundle of His. The re-entry circuit can form with anterograde conduction down the bundle of Kent and back up the AV node (**antidromic AVRT**), or may conduct in the other direction, that is, down the AV node and retrogradely up the bundle of Kent (**orthodromic AVRT**), to produce a self-perpetuating circus pathway and tachycardia (Figure 5.15). The sensation of palpitations is frightening, and the truncated diastolic filling interval reduces the cardiac output, leading to light-headedness. Conduction down the bundle of Kent is sometimes observed on the normal sinus rhythm ECG, manifesting as a short PR interval with a Δ (delta) wave as ventricular excitation occurs more rapidly. If a patient with an accessory pathway develop AF, there is a small risk that this will be conducted via the bundle of Kent down to the ventricles and initiate VF and sudden cardiac death. The risk of this is around 1:1000 per year, although it also depends on how well the accessory pathway conducts. Treatment is with pharmacological agents that block the pathway rather than the AV node (such as flecainide or sotalol) or by the destruction of the bundle of Kent via a percutaneous ablation procedure.

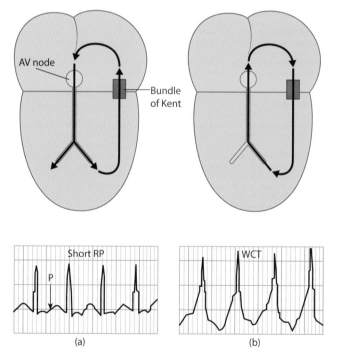

AV node

Bundle of Kent

Short RP

P

WCT

(a)

(b)

**Figure 5.15** An atrioventricular (AV) re-entry tachycardia (AVRT) results from an extra electrical connection across the annulus fibrosus (the bundle of Kent), additional to the AV node and bundle of His. The re-entry circuit can form with conduction down the AV node and then retrogradely up the bundle of Kent (orthodromic AVRT, as shown in **(a)**), to produce a self-perpetuating re-entry pathway and tachycardia. This produces a narrow complex tachycardia with a short RP interval. It can also occur with anterograde conduction down the bundle of Kent and retrogradely back up the AV node (antidromic AVRT, as shown in **(b)**) which produces a wide complex tachycardia (WCT).

## Atrial flutter

Typical atrial flutter is a macro re-entry tachycardia around the right atrium in which a wave of excitation passes counterclockwise down the lateral wall of the right atrium, across the cavotricuspid isthmus (between the inferior vena cava and tricuspid valve), up the interatrial septum and across the roof of the right atrium (Figure 5.16). This circuit produces a characteristic saw-tooth pattern on the ECG with AV conduction occurring every other circuit (2:1 block) or less frequently (3 or 4:1 block). As with AT, the rapid atrial rate can cause palpitations, breathlessness and light-headedness, and carries a **thromboembolic risk**. Atrial flutter can be difficult to rate control with AV blocking drugs. Percutaneous ablation of the cavotricuspid isthmus is highly successful (>90%) in blocking the re-entry circuit and preventing reoccurrence.

## Atrial fibrillation

AF is the most common pathological arrhythmia. The pulmonary veins appear to play a key role in its initiation (being a source of ectopic beats) and maintenance (by providing regions of conduction block around which re-entry can occur). It is also associated with infections (especially respiratory), thyrotoxicosis, electrolyte disturbances and mitral valve disease, but often there appears to be no underlying condition triggering the arrhythmia, so-called lone AF. AF can be paroxysmal or persistent, and with prolonged episodes structural and electrophysiological remodelling of the atria can occur so that AF becomes easier to sustain, hence the saying that "**AF begets AF**". Like atrial flutter and tachycardia, the rapid ineffective atrial contraction can produce symptoms of palpitations, breathlessness and light-headedness, although some patients are asymptomatic. AF also carries a significant **thromboembolic stroke risk**. Excitation is transmitted sporadically through the AV node to the ventricles (Figure 5.17), resulting in a characteristic, easily diagnosed **irregularly irregular** radial pulse of variable amplitude. Small, irregular 'f' waves replace the P wave in the ECG. Treatment is via a rate or rhythm control strategy depending on patients' symptoms. Percutaneous ablation involves isolation of the pulmonary veins. This is most successful for paroxysmal AF and has a success rate of ~70%, although up to 40% of patients requiring more than one procedure.

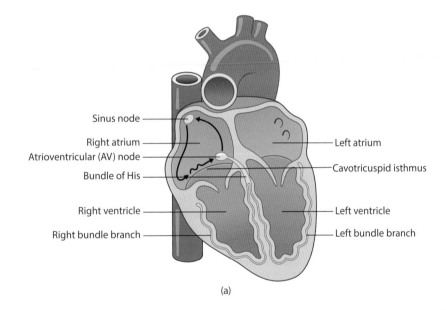

(a)

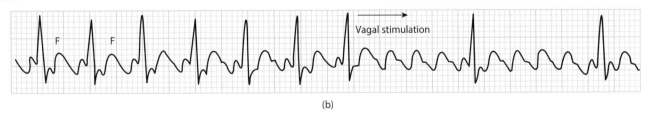

(b)

**Figure 5.16** Typical atrial flutter is a re-entry tachycardia around the right atrium in which a wave of excitation passes counterclockwise down the lateral wall of the right atrium, across the cavotricuspid isthmus (between the inferior vena cava and tricuspid valve), up the interatrial septum and across the roof of the right atrium, as shown in **(a)**. This circuit produces a characteristic sawtooth pattern with an F (or flutter) wave on the ECG with atrioventricular (AV) conduction occurring every other circuit (2:1 block) or less frequently if there is AV nodal block, for example, during vagal stimulation or administration of intravenous adenosine, as shown in **(b)**.

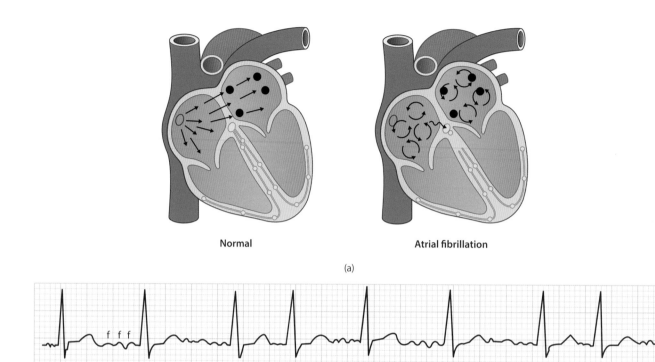

Normal                                    Atrial fibrillation

(a)

(b)

**Figure 5.17** Atrial fibrillation usually involves the four pulmonary veins in the left atria, which appear to play a key role in its initiation (being a source of ectopic beats) and maintenance (by providing regions of conduction block around which re-entry can occur), as shown in **(a)**. Excitation is transmitted sporadically through the atrioventricular node to the ventricles, resulting in characteristic, irregularly irregular QRS complexes. Small irregular fibrillation 'f' waves replace the P wave on the ECG, as shown in **(b)**.

## Ventricular tachycardia

VT is a dangerous arrhythmia that originates within the ventricle, usually when there is an abnormal structural substrate (such as ischaemia or infarction, dilated cardiomyopathy, hypertrophic cardiomyopathy or arrhythmogenic right ventricular cardiomyopathy) or an abnormal electrophysiological substrate (such as LQT syndrome, or Na$^+$ channel [*SCN5A*] mutations causing Brugada syndrome). The ECG shows a characteristic **regular broad complex tachycardia** (Figure 5.18). The atria are not involved in the circuit although they can be activated retrogradely through the AV node in up to 10% of cases. Occasionally, P waves can be observed on the ECG but they are completely dissociated from the broad complex rhythm. Sometimes, a P wave may conduct through the AV node to give a narrow complex **capture** beat, or collide with the VT circuit to form a **fusion** beat. At slower rates, VT may cause palpitations but if the rate is more rapid so that cardiac output falls significantly, then symptoms such as breathlessness and chest pain can occur. If the rate is more rapid still, then VT can lower blood pressure and reduce cerebral perfusion, so that loss of consciousness may occur, or cardiac output may fall to nothing and a cardiac arrest ensue. VT can also change from a single re-entry circuit into multiple wavelets and fibrillation if wavebreak occurs. VT should therefore be treated with emergency cardioversion either pharmacologically or, if there is any haemodynamic compromise, electrically.

Clinical trials have also identified patients who have survived a cardiac arrest from VT or VF, or patients with severely impaired ventricular function or an inherited cardiac condition who are at high risk of VT/VF and sudden cardiac death, who may benefit from an implantable cardioverter defibrillator (ICD). Sometimes, VT can be cardioverted by rapid **overdrive** or **anti-tachycardia pacing**, that is, pacing the ventricle with a burst of beats at a rate faster than the VT in the hope of making enough ventricular tissue refractory so that the re-entry circuit will be broken. This can be successful in up to 90% of VT although it may also accelerate the VT in up to 5% of cases. ICDs use this approach first before resorting to electrical cardioversion to save on battery life and reduce painful shocks if the patient is conscious during the arrhythmia.

In some situations, VT can be incessant despite antiarrhythmic medication, recurrent overdrive pacing and multiple electrical cardioversions. This **electrical storm** is perhaps one of the most challenging clinical presentations for cardiologists. Ultimately, many patients require general anaesthesia and an emergency percutaneous ablation of their VT, although success is limited. Procedures that reduce cardiac sympathetic drive may also be useful in such patients given that adrenergic stimulation can trigger and sustain ventricular arrhythmias. Even sedation or general anaesthesia can be antiarrhythmic because sympathetic hyperactivity during the electrical storm is often worsened by chest pain from VT and ICD shocks received while still conscious. Recent studies have

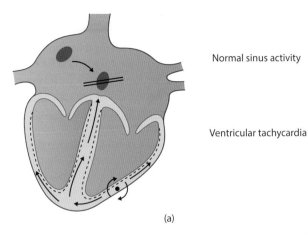

Normal sinus activity

Ventricular tachycardia

(a)

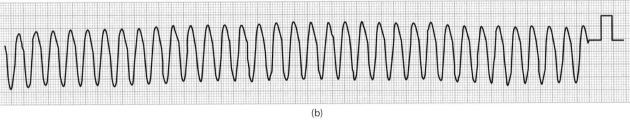

(b)

**Figure 5.18** Ventricular tachycardia is a dangerous arrhythmia that originates from a re-entry circuit within the ventricles (as seen in **(a)**), usually when there is an abnormal structural substrate (such as ischaemia or infarction, dilated cardiomyopathy, hypertrophic cardiomy-opathy or arrhythmogenic right ventricular cardiomyopathy) or an abnormal electrophysiological substrate (such as long QT or Brugada syndrome). The ECG shows a characteristic regular broad complex tachycardia, as shown in **(b)**. The atria are not involved in the circuit although they can occasionally be activated retrogradely through the atrioventricular node.

used thoracic epidural anaesthesia as a method to block the stellate ganglia and stabilize the patient long enough for consideration of heart transplantation. Stellectomy may also be a useful long-term intervention in patients with ischaemic cardiomyopathies or some LQTS (e.g. type 1 LQTS) and recurrent VT despite medical therapy and ICD implantation.

## Ventricular fibrillation

VF is the most feared cardiac arrhythmia because numerous uncoordinated electrical waves within the ventricle results in no cardiac output, and death follows within minutes (Figure 5.19).

Without effective cardiopulmonary resuscitation the chance of successful electrical defibrillation falls by around 10% per minute of VF. Early defibrillation is therefore essential and the reason behind rapid response resuscitation teams in hospitals, placing automated external defibrillators in public places such as airports and shopping centres, and training the public in basic life support (especially effective chest compressions). Although clinical trials have identified patients at high risk of VT/VF and sudden cardiac death who may benefit from a primary prevention ICD, most patients who have a VT/VF arrest do not fall into these categories, and most people in whom ICDs are implanted never have a shock from their device.

---

**CONCEPT BOX 5.2**

### AFTERDEPOLARIZATION AND RE-ENTRY CAUSE ARRHYTHMIAS

- In an ischaemic heart, the overloaded SR $Ca^{2+}$ store may discharge in early diastole. This increases $Ca^{2+}$ expulsion by the $3Na^+/1Ca^{2+}$ exchanger. The net positive charge ($Na^+$) transferred into the cell by the exchanger causes an afterdepolarization.
- A DAD can reach threshold, triggering an action potential and poorly co-ordinated ectopic beat (extra systole).
- In the latter half of the T wave ('vulnerable window'), ectopic activation readily triggers re-entry-based arrhythmias.
- During the vulnerable window, local circus pathways can develop because some myocytes have repolarized while others have not. An ectopic excitation propagating slowly through a circus pathway will re-excite myocytes emerging from their refractory period (re-entry). This re-excites the circus pathway, a self-perpetuating process.
- Ischaemia slows myocardial conduction, due to the inactivation of some $Na^+$ channels. Slow conduction allows the return of circus excitation after the refractory period, and thus favours re-entry-based arrhythmias. Re-entry underlies ventricular tachycardia.

**Normal heart**

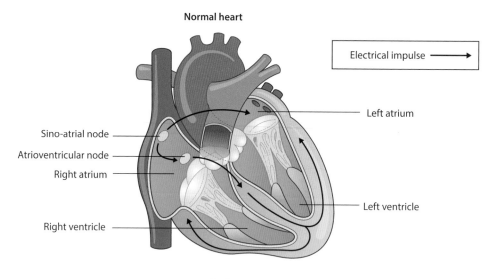

Electrical impulse ⟶

Left atrium

Sino-atrial node

Atrioventricular node

Right atrium

Left ventricle

Right ventricle

**Ventricular fibrillation**

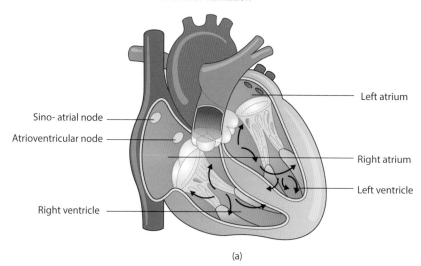

Left atrium

Sino- atrial node

Atrioventricular node

Right atrium

Left ventricle

Right ventricle

(a)

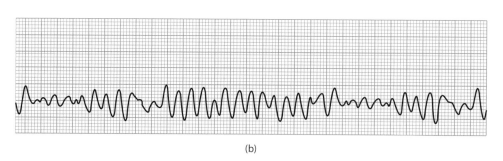

(b)

**Figure 5.19** Ventricular fibrillation arises from numerous uncoordinated electrical waves (black arrows) within the ventricle, as shown in **(a)**, which produces no cardiac output. There may be multiple small wandering wavelets, or a 'mother rotor', that is a stable re-entry circuit from which many unstable smaller wavelets arise. The ECG shows chaotic, irregular deflections of varying amplitude, as seen in **(b)**. Unless advanced life support and defibrillation are initiated rapidly, this rhythm is fatal.

## SUMMARY

- The 12-lead ECG is a recording of small potential differences (~1 mV) in the frontal plane (3 bipolar limb leads and 3 unipolar limb leads) and transverse plane (6 precordial leads).

- The P wave is caused by atrial depolarization, the QRS complex by ventricular depolarization and the T wave by ventricular repolarization.

- The PR interval is a delay caused chiefly by slow transmission through the AV node. The delay allows atrial systole to precede ventricular systole. It should not exceed 0.2 s in humans. If the PR interval is beyond 0.2 s, this is called first-degree heart block.

- Second-degree heart block is characterized by a lengthening PR interval until a P wave is not conducted (type I Mobitz (Wenckebach) phenomenon), or with several P waves for every QRS complex (type II Mobitz). With complete heart block, there is no association between P waves and QRS complexes and the ventricular rate is very slow, with risk of pauses or asystole. This usually requires the implantation of a permanent pacemaker.

- The isoelectric ST segment corresponds to the plateau of the ventricular action potential. It can be displaced by injury currents during myocardial ischaemia.

- The T wave is upright (pointing in the same direction as the R wave) in most leads because repolarization occurs in reverse sequence to depolarization, due to the short action potentials of subepicardial and apical myocytes.

- At any instant during the spread of ventricular excitation, negative and positive extracellular charges create an electrical dipole.

- The QRS complex differs between leads because each lead detects the dipole from a different angle. Lead I (left arm–right arm) is horizontal (0°). Lead II (left leg–right arm) is at 60° and Lead III (left leg–left arm) at 120° in the frontal plane. These three leads form Einthoven's triangle.

- The components Q (down), R (up) and S (second down wave) result from changes in the dipole over <0.12 s. Excitation spreads first into the left interventricular septum, then out through the subendocardium to the subepicardium and base. The resulting dipole, which is dominated by the left ventricle, rotates anticlockwise in the frontal plane, waxing and waning as it does so.

- The angle of the largest QRS dipole in the frontal plane, usually −30° to +90°, is called the electrical axis of the heart.

- The ECG can be used to diagnose ventricular hypertrophy, cardiac ischaemia and arhythmias.

- Pathological arrhythmias requires a trigger (such as EADs or DADs) or abnormal automaticity, and a substrate (which may be fixed or dynamic). If the substrate sets up a re-entry circuit, subsequent wavebreak can lead to multiple wavelets and fibrillation.

- Clinical arrhythmias can be benign (sinus arrhythmia and ectopic beats) or pathological. Some carry a risk of left atrial thrombus formation and thromboembolic stroke (atrial tachycardia, atrial flutter and atrial fibrillation). Ventricular arrhythmias (ventricular tachycardia and ventricular fibrillation) can be life-threatening and require emergency electrical cardioversion or defibrillation.

## FURTHER READING

Ajijola OA, Lux RL, Khahera A, et al. Sympathetic modulation of electrical activation in normal and infarcted myocardium: implications for arrhythmogenesis. *American Journal of Physiology (Heart and Circulatory Physiology)* 2017; **312**(3): H608–21.

Kirchhof P, Benussi S, Kotecha D, et al. 2016 ESC Guidelines for the management of atrial fibrillation developed in collaboration with EACTS. *European Heart Journal* 2016; **37**(38): 2893–962.

Fukuda K, Kanazawa H, Aizawa Y, et al. Cardiac innervation and sudden cardiac death. *Circulation Research* 2015; **116**(12): 2005–19.

Priori SG, Blomström-Lundqvist C, Mazzanti A, et al. 2015 ESC Guidelines for the management of patients with ventricular arrhythmias and the prevention of sudden cardiac death: The Task Force for the Management of Patients with Ventricular Arrhythmias and the Prevention of Sudden Cardiac Death of the European Society of Cardiology (ESC). Endorsed by: Association for European Paediatric and Congenital Cardiology (AEPC). *European Heart Journal* 2015; **36**(41): 2793–867.

Allessie M, de Groot N. CrossTalk opposing view: rotors have not been demonstrated to be the drivers of atrial fibrillation. *The Journal of Physiology* 2014; **592**(15): 3167–70.

Narayan SM, Jalife J. CrossTalk proposal: rotors have been demonstrated to drive human atrial fibrillation. *The Journal of Physiology* 2014; **592**(15): 3163–6.

Pandit SV, Jalife J. Rotors and the dynamics of cardiac fibrillation. *Circulation Research* 2013; **112**(5): 849–62.

Rudy Y. Noninvasive electrocardiographic imaging of arrhythmogenic substrates in humans. *Circulation Research* 2013; **112**(5): 863–74.

Zipes DP, Jalife J. *Cardiac Electrophysiology: from Cell to Bedside*, 6th edn. Philadelphia, PA: Saunders; 2013.

John RM, Tedrow UB, Koplan BA, et al. Ventricular arrhythmias and sudden cardiac death. *Lancet* 2012; **380**(9852): 1520–9.

Myles RC, Bernus O, Burton FL, et al. Effect of activation sequence on transmural patterns of repolarization and action potential duration in rabbit ventricular myocardium. *American Journal of Physiology – Heart and Circulatory Physiology* 2010; **299**(6): H1812–22.

Herring N, Paterson DJ. ECG diagnosis of acute ischaemia and infarction: past, present and future. *Quarterly Journal of Medicine* 2006; **99**(4): 219–30.

Nash MP, Mourad A, Clayton RH, et al. Evidence for multiple mechanisms in human ventricular fibrillation. *Circulation* 2006; **114**(6): 536–42.

Haïssaguerre M, Jaïs P, Shah DC, et al. Spontaneous initiation of atrial fibrillation by ectopic beats originating in the pulmonary veins. *New England Journal of Medicine* 1998; **339**(10): 659–66.

Echt DS, Liebson PR, Mitchell LB, et al. Mortality and morbidity in patients receiving encainide, flecainide, or placebo. The Cardiac Arrhythmia Suppression Trial. *New England Journal of Medicine* 1991; **324**: 781–8.

January CT, Riddle JM. Early afterdepolarizations: mechanism of induction and block. A role for L-type $Ca^{2+}$ current. *Circulation Research* 1989; **64**(5): 977–90.

Marban E, Robinson SW, Wier WG. Mechanisms of arrhythmogenic delayed and early afterdepolarizations in ferret ventricular muscle. *Journal of Clinical Investigation* 1986; **78**(5): 1185–92.

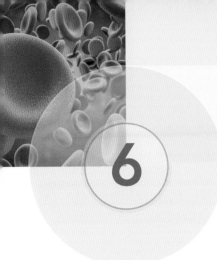

# 6

# Control of stroke volume and cardiac output

## LEARNING OBJECTIVES

*After reading this chapter you should be able to:*

- sketch the length–tension relation and give its probable mechanism (6.2, 6.3);
- describe the Frank–Starling mechanism and its importance for stroke volume regulation (6.4);
- draw a ventricular function (Frank–Starling) curve and define stroke work (6.4, 6.5);
- list the chief factors influencing central venous pressure (6.6);
- state the roles of the Frank–Starling mechanism in man (6.7);
- use Laplace's law to explain why cardiac distension is harmful in heart failure (6.8);
- state the direct and secondary effects of arterial pressure on stroke volume (6.9);

- define contractility and draw a graph to show how altered contractility affects the Frank–Starling curve (6.10);
- list the effects of sympathetic stimulation on cardiac performance (6.10);
- draw a ventricular pressure–volume loop and sketch the effect of: (1) increased filling pressure (preload); (2) increased contractility; (3) increased arterial pressure (afterload); and (4) exercise (6.5, 6.10);
- name two important inotropic hormones and two classes of inotropic drugs (6.11);
- outline the negative inotropic and arrhythmogenic effects of myocardial ischaemia (6.12);
- outline the co-ordinated cardiac response to exercise (6.13);
- explain the close link between myocardial performance and coronary blood flow (6.14).

## 6.1 OVERVIEW

In a resting adult, each ventricle pumps out 4–7 L of blood per minute – the cardiac output. The **cardiac index**, which relates resting output to body size, is 3 L/min per m² of body surface area (~1.8 m² for a 70 kg adult). However, cardiac output is not fixed but is continually adjusted to meet changes in demand. For example, cardiac output is reduced by ~10% during sleep, and is increased by 20%–30% during excitement, stress or a heavy meal. It rises by up to 40% during pregnancy

and four- to sixfold during hard exercise, though less than this in ischaemic hearts (Table 6.1). These changes are brought about by changes in both heart rate and stroke volume. The control of **heart rate** by autonomic nerves was described in Chapter 4. In this chapter, we focus initially on the control of stroke volume, followed by the co-ordinated regulation of stroke volume, heart rate and peripheral vascular tone when cardiac output is raised.

**Stroke volume** is influenced by two opposing factors, namely the **energy of contraction** of the ventricles and the **aortic/pulmonary artery pressure** that must be overcome

**Table 6.1** Output of an adult human heart in L/min (mean and standard deviation)

|  | Rest | Exercise |
|---|---|---|
| Normal adult | 6.0 (1.3) | 17.5 (6.0) |
| Coronary artery disease | 5.7 (1.5)[a] | 11.3 (4.3)[b] |

*Source:* After Rerych SK, Scholz PM, Newman GE, et al. *Annals of Surgery* 1978; 187: 449–58.

[a] The output of the diseased heart was within the normal range at rest.

[b] The output of the diseased heart became inadequate during exercise at 85% of maximum heart rate or at onset of angina.

before any blood can be expelled (Figure 6.1). A highly energetic contraction produces a large stroke volume. A high arterial pressure, on the other hand, opposes ejection and reduces the stroke volume, unless there are compensatory changes.

The **energy of contraction** can be raised by two mechanisms: (1) stretching the myocardium in diastole by raising the end-diastolic pressure enhances the contractile energy (known as the **Frank–Starling mechanism**); (2) the strength of contraction at a given degree of stretch can be increased by sympathetic nerves and circulating adrenaline (i.e. an increase in **contractility**).

**Arterial pressure** depresses stroke volume because ejection cannot begin until ventricular pressure exceeds aortic pressure. If arterial pressure is high, much of the contractile energy of the heartbeat is needed to raise ventricular blood pressure (BP) during the isovolumetric contraction phase, so less energy remains for the ejection phase. The presence of valvular stenosis will also influence the pressure needed to expel blood from the chamber.

Stroke volume thus depends on the interplay of three factors:

- diastolic stretch, which depends on venous filling pressure;
- contractility, which is regulated by sympathetic fibres and hormones and is reduced by cardiac disease;
- arterial pressure, which opposes ejection.

This chapter describes first the effect of diastolic stretch (Sections 6.2–6.8), then arterial pressure (Section 6.9) and then contractility (Sections 6.10–6.12).

## 6.2 CONTRACTILE PROPERTIES OF ISOLATED MYOCARDIUM

Isolated strips of myocardium, such as an isolated papillary muscle, have been studied as an aid to understanding the behaviour of the more complex intact heart. These studies *in vitro* have demonstrated the importance of 'preload' and 'afterload' in contractile performance, as follows.

### Preload enhances contractile force: the isometric length–tension relation

A relaxed strip of myocardium can be stretched to a set length by hanging a weight from it, called the **preload** (Figure 6.2). If the ends of the muscle are then anchored to rigid points and the muscle is stimulated electrically, it develops active tension (force) but cannot shorten. This is called an **isometric contraction** (from the Greek *isos* = equal; *metric* = length). Remarkably, the greater the initial stretch, the greater the contractile force upon stimulation (Figures 6.2a and 6.3). This important effect is called the **length–tension relation**. Translating this to the intact ventricle, the stretch of the muscle fibres is set not by a weight but by the **diastolic filling pressure**; the ensuing **isovolumetric contraction** is roughly equivalent to an isometric contraction, and the increase in contractile energy with stretch is called the **Frank–Starling mechanism** (Section 6.4).

### Afterload impairs shortening: the isotonic afterload–shortening relation

To study shortening, as opposed to tension development, one end of the isolated myocardial strip is left free to move

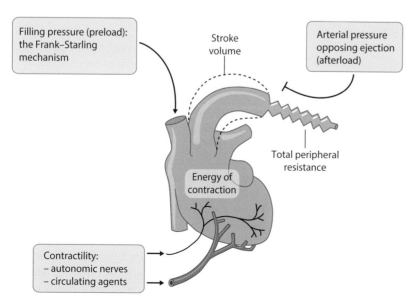

**Figure 6.1** Factors that regulate stroke volume. Total peripheral resistance, which arises mainly in the arterioles and terminal arteries, is represented here by the narrow tube in series with the aorta.

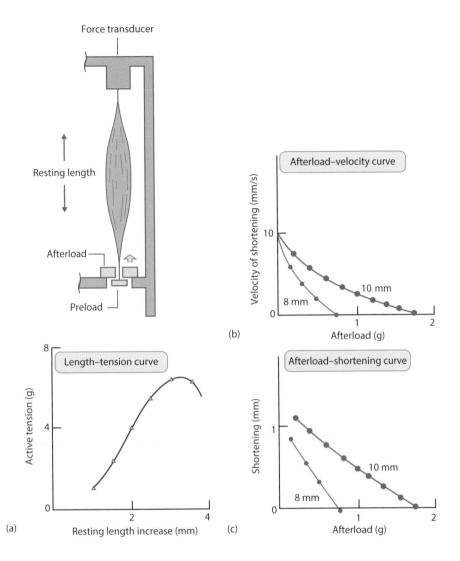

**Figure 6.2** Contractile behaviour of isolated cat papillary muscle. The preload weight sets the resting length. If preload is clamped, shortening is prevented and the electrically stimulated contraction is isometric. **(a)** Effect of resting length on isometric contractile force. **(b,c)** If the muscle is allowed to shorten, it lifts a constant weight, the afterload, and the contraction is isotonic. Isotonic contractions starting from 10-mm resting length (high preload) are stronger than from an 8-mm resting length (low preload). (After Sonnenblick EH. *American Journal of Physiology* 1962; 202: 931–9, with permission from the American Physiological Society.)

on stimulation; however, as it begins its contraction, it lifts a constant weight, the **afterload** (Figure 6.2, top left). This compels the muscle to shorten while exerting a fixed, known force; this is a mode of contraction called **isotonic contraction** (*isos* = equal; *tonic* = force). If the afterload is increased, both the rate and degree of shortening decrease, unsurprisingly (Figure 6.2b,c). This is called the **afterload–shortening relation**; however, if the starting length is increased by raising the preload, the speed and degree of shortening increase because stretch increases the contractile force (Figure 6.2b,c, red curves).

The moment when an isolated strip begins to pick up the afterload corresponds, in an intact heart, to the moment when the tensing ventricle opens the outlet valve by slightly exceeding arterial pressure. Therefore, **arterial pressure** determines afterload *in vivo*; the **ejection phase** is roughly equivalent to isotonic shortening; and the cardiac **pump function curve** (Section 6.9) is roughly equivalent to the afterload–shortening relation. The qualifier 'roughly' is used because the afterload is not constant in a contracting heart; it waxes and wanes as arterial pressure peaks and

falls. This form of contraction is called **auxotonic** (from the Greek *auxo* = increase, growth). The afterload–shortening relation is important clinically because it underlies the use of arterial pressure-reducing drugs to improve the output of failing hearts.

## 6.3 MECHANISMS UNDERLYING THE LENGTH–TENSION RELATION

### Stretching the sarcomere increases contractile energy

When the myocardium is stretched by a preload, every sarcomere in the myocyte is lengthened, as shown by laser diffraction measurements. A plot of contractile force versus relaxed sarcomere length forms a curve. Maximum force is attained at a sarcomere length of 2.2–2.3 μm (Figure 6.3), and stretch beyond this point reduces contractile force; but such lengths are probably never reached *in vivo* because myocytes become very stiff above 2.3 μm. In intact hearts at normal end-diastolic

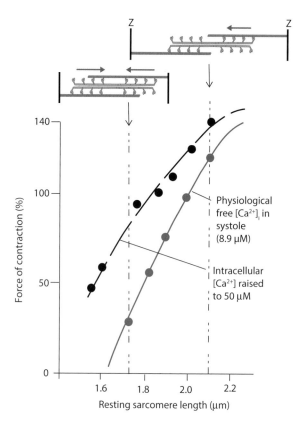

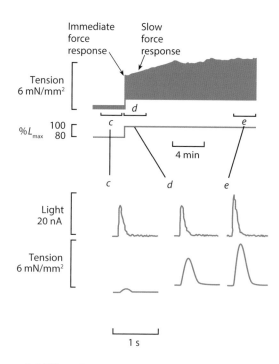

**Figure 6.3** Effect of resting sarcomere length on contractile force in 'skinned' myocardium. The sarcolemm has been permeabilized by a detergent, then exposed to a near-physiological systolic Ca$^{2+}$ concentration (8.9 µM), or a saturating one that causes maximal contraction (50 µM). The lower but steeper curve is like intact cardiac muscle. Sketches at the top show how stretch reduces interference by myosin heads (red) that are pulling in the 'wrong' direction beyond the sarcomere mid-point. (Adapted from Kentish JC, ter Keurs HEDJ, Ricciardi L, et al. *Circulation Research* 1986; 58: 755–68, with permission.)

**Figure 6.4** Effect of stretch on isometric contractile force and Ca$^{2+}$ transients in isolated papillary muscle. The muscle was stretched from 80% of optimum length ($L_{max}$) to 100%. Note the immediate, large increase in force at *d*, then a smaller, slow force response. Light signal from the Ca$^{2+}$-sensitive protein, aequorin, shows that the big initial response, *d*, does not require an increased Ca$^{2+}$ transient, whereas the slow force response at *e* does (Anrep effect). (After Allen DG, Nichols CG, Smith GL. *The Journal of Physiology* 1988; 406: 359–70, with permission from Wiley-Blackwell.)

pressure, the sarcomere length is ~1.8–2.0 µm, so **myocytes normally operate on the ascending part of the length–tension curve.**

## Stretch can raise contractile force without raising intracellular calcium

The reader may have come away from Chapters 3 and 4 with the impression that a stronger heartbeat must always be due to a rise in cytoplasmic Ca$^{2+}$; but this is not so. Figure 6.4 shows the effect of diastolic stretch on twitch force and the cytoplasmic Ca$^{2+}$ transient. Stretch causes an **immediate force increase**, with no increase in the systolic Ca$^{2+}$ transient, unlike the Ca$^{2+}$-mediated effect of catecholamines (Sections 3.8 and 4.5). If the stretch is maintained, there is a further slow increase in force over ~5 min, which is due to increased Ca$^{2+}$ transients. The immediate force increase accounts for 60% of the eventual response and is the basis of the length–tension relation. The subsequent Ca$^{2+}$-mediated **slow force response** underlies the **Anrep effect** in intact hearts (Section 6.9).

## Stretch reduces filament overlap and raises calcium sensitivity

How is the immediate force increase achieved? Two mechanisms contribute to it, namely changes in actin/myosin filament overlap and increased sensitivity to Ca$^{2+}$. The latter mechanism is the more important one in cardiac muscle, unlike skeletal muscle.

- **Filament overlap and interference**. When the sarcomere is <2.0 µm long, the actin filaments (1 µm long) extend across the midline into the 'wrong' half of the sarcomere (Figure 6.3, top left). Consequently, a fraction of the myosin crossbridges are pulling in the opposite direction to the majority, reducing the net tension generated. Moreover, in sarcomeres <1.6 µm long, the myosin filament hits the Z lines. Stretch between 1.6 and 2 µm reduces these interference problems and thus increases the net contractile force. However, this explanation is clearly incomplete because it applies equally to skeletal muscle, yet **cardiac muscle is much more sensitive to stretch than skeletal muscle**, that is, the length–tension curve is much steeper for cardiac than skeletal muscle (Figure 6.5). An additional, more important mechanism must therefore operate in cardiac muscle.

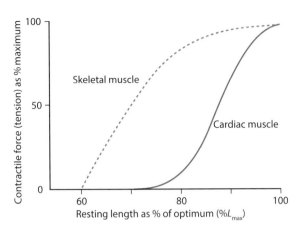

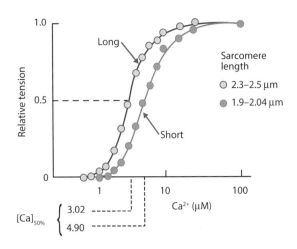

**Figure 6.5** Length–tension relation of cardiac muscle compared with skeletal muscle. Cardiac muscle has a much steeper curve than skeletal muscle at physiological lengths (80%–100%; $L_{max}$), even though the filament overlap is the same. This is because stretch increases the $Ca^{2+}$ sensitivity of cardiac myocytes. (Adapted from Fuchs F, Smith SS. *News in Physiological Science* 2001; 16: 5–10, with permission from the American Physiological Society.)

**Figure 6.6** Contractile tension developed by chemically permeabilized rat ventricular muscle in response to bathing solution $Ca^{2+}$ concentration, at two different resting sarcomere lengths. The $Ca^{2+}$ concentration needed to generate a 50% maximum contraction, $[Ca]_{50\%}$, was reduced by stretch; that is, $Ca^{2+}$ sensitivity was increased by stretch (From Hibberd MG, Jewell BR. *The Journal of Physiology* 1982; 329: 527–40, with permission from Wiley-Blackwell.)

- **Increased sensitivity to $Ca^{2+}$.** If all possible crossbridges at a given sarcomere length are activated *in vitro*, by raising cytoplasmic $Ca^{2+}$ to supranormal levels, there is still a length–tension relation, but it is less steep than normal (Figure 6.3, upper curve). The relation now resembles that for skeletal muscle and is explained by the filament interference effect. At a more physiological $Ca^{2+}$ level (Figure 6.3, lower curve), the active tension is lower because only a fraction of the potential crossbridges is activated; however, the force increases much more steeply with stretch, approaching closer and closer to the line for full activation. This experiment shows that **stretch increases the fraction of crossbridges activated by a given $Ca^{2+}$ level**. Stretch thus increases the sensitivity of the contractile machinery to $Ca^{2+}$. This has been confirmed by plotting contractile force against $Ca^{2+}$ concentration at two different sarcomere lengths; stretch shifts the curve to the left (Figure 6.6). In other words, a stretched myocyte needs less $Ca^{2+}$ to produce a given contractile force.

## The cause of length-dependent calcium sensitivity remains controversial

The mechanism underlying length-dependent $Ca^{2+}$ sensitivity is still not fully established, but the **lattice spacing hypothesis** holds sway at present. In a myocyte of fixed volume, any increase in length is associated with a fall in cross-sectional diameter. This reduces the side-to-side separation of the actin and myosin filaments, which may allow crossbridges to form more readily. In support of this hypothesis, reducing the myocyte diameter by immersing it in a hyperosmotic solution

increases its contractile force. The magnitude of this effect may be too small to fully explain the physiological $Ca^{2+}$ sensitization. Recent evidence has also implicated the giant elastic protein titin as a potential length-dependent sensor. Titin may be important in mediating a reduction in lattice spacing, induce stronger crossbridge formation or induce conformational changes in cardiac troponin C to increase $Ca^{2+}$ sensitivity. While all of these actions could potentially contribute, it is safe to say that the Frank–Starling mechanism is not fully understood!

Having defined the properties of isolated cardiac muscle, we can now turn to the intact organ, and consider how stretch affects ventricular performance.

## 6.4 THE FRANK–STARLING MECHANISM

### The isovolumetric contracting heart: Frank's experiment

The isometric length–tension relation of Figure 6.5 operates also in intact hearts, as shown by the German physiologist Otto Frank in 1895. Frank ligated the aorta of a frog's heart, so that each contraction was purely isovolumetric, like an isometric contraction. When the ventricle wall was stretched in diastole, by increasing the diastolic fluid volume (preload), a greater pressure was generated by the systolic contractions (Figure 6.7a). Therefore, **the energy of contraction of the intact heart increases as a function of diastolic distension** (Figure 6.7b, red curve). We will see later that this isovolumetric contraction curve sets an upper limit to ventricular pressure–volume loops (Section 6.5).

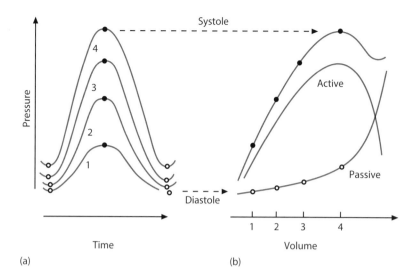

**Figure 6.7** Pressure generated by isovolumetric contraction of frog ventricle (aorta ligated), over a range of diastolic volumes. **(a)** The 'active' pressure generated between diastole (open circles) and systole (closed circles) increased as ventricular volume was raised from 1 to 4 (arbitrary units). **(b)** Effect of volume on pressure. The bottom curve is the passive compliance curve, showing the effect of volume on the diastolic pressure of the relaxed ventricle. Note the increasing stiffness (upswing) as the ventricle is distended. The top curve shows the corresponding systolic pressures. The red curve shows the pressure generated actively; that is, the systolic pressure minus the diastolic pressure. (After Otto Frank's seminal experiment of 1895.)

## The ejecting heart: Starling's experiment

A more physiological situation, namely ventricular ejection, was studied by Ernest Starling and his co-workers in London in the early 20th century. In their classic experiment, the isolated heart and lungs of a dog were perfused with warm oxygenated blood from a venous reservoir (Figure 6.8). The height of the reservoir controlled the central venous pressure (CVP). CVP is the pressure at the entrance to the right atrium; it is important because it determines the right ventricular end-diastolic pressure (RVEDP) and hence the stretch of the resting chambers. In other words, **the CVP determines the preload experienced by right ventricular muscle**. Similarly, pulmonary vein pressure governs left ventricle end-diastolic pressure and preload. A useful term encompassing these various pressures is **filling pressure**.

Since aortic pressure influences afterload, Starling kept it constant by means of a variable resistance. The combined stroke volume of the two ventricles was recorded with a bell cardiometer. Being isolated and denervated, the heart–lung preparation was free from any extrinsic nervous or hormonal influences, so any response was a property of the heart itself. The chief findings were as follows.

### Raising central venous pressure increases stroke volume

When CVP is raised, the RVEDP and ventricular volume increase. This stretches the right ventricle fibres. As a result, the ventricle develops a greater contractile energy and ejects a greater stroke volume. The left ventricle quickly follows suit because the increased right ventricular output raises the pressure in the pulmonary circulation. This increases the filling

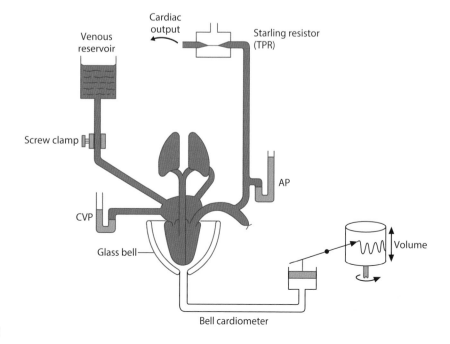

**Figure 6.8** Starling's isolated dog heart–lung preparation. The height of the venous reservoir and the screw-clamp control the central venous pressure (CVP). CVP and arterial pressure (AP) were measured by the manometers. AP was held constant by a variable resistance equal to the total peripheral resistance (TPR). Ventricular volume was measured with a Henderson bell cardiometer, an inverted glass bell attached to the atrioventricular groove by a rubber diaphragm. Beat-by-beat volume changes were recorded on a rotating smoked drum. (After Knowlton FP, Starling EH. *The Journal of Physiology* 1912; 44: 206–19.)

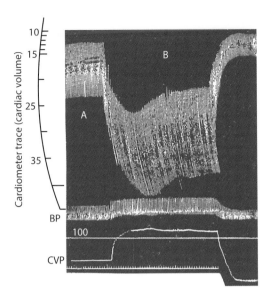

**Figure 6.9** Beat-by-beat recording of ventricular volume in the isolated heart–lung preparation. Note the inverted volume scale (mL): diastolic volume is at the bottom, systolic volume at the top. Stroke volume is the top-to-bottom distance. Raising central venous pressure (CVP) from 9 cmH₂O (period A) to 15 cmH₂O (period B) distends the ventricles in both diastole and systole, and increases stroke volume by 64%. The later modest reduction in ventricular distension with no fall in stroke volume indicates a small rise in contractility (the Anrep effect). (From the original smoked drum recordings of Patterson SW, Piper H, Starling EH. *The Journal of Physiology* 1914; 48: 465–511, with permission.)

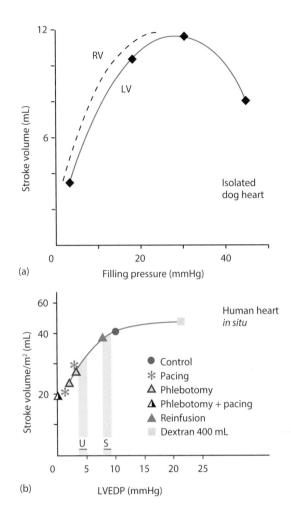

**Figure 6.10** Ventricular function curves of **(a)** dog and **(b)** human. **(a)** Effect of filling pressure on stroke volume of isolated dog heart pumping against a constant arterial pressure. Solid line shows Starling's results for effect of left atrial pressure on left ventricular (LV) stroke volume. Dashed line shows effect of central venous pressure on right ventricular (RV) stroke volume. **(b)** Human ventricular function curve. LV end-diastolic pressure (LVEDP) was varied *in vivo* by phlebotomy (venous bleeding) and other maneuvers. Stroke volume is expressed per unit body surface area (stroke index). Grey bands mark normal human LVEDP when supine (S) and upright (U). Human stroke volume reaches a plateau at filling pressures above ~10 mmHg. (After Parker JD, Case RB. *Circulation* 1979; 60: 4–12, with permission.)

pressure and distension of the left ventricle, raising contractile energy in the left heart. Thus, a rise in CVP increases the output of both ventricles (Figure 6.9).

## The human ventricular function curve reaches a plateau

A plot of stroke volume versus filling pressure is called a ventricular function curve or Starling curve (Figure 6.10). At filling pressures between zero (atmospheric) and 10 mmHg, the stroke volume increases as a curvilinear function of pressure. This is called the **ascending limb**. Above 10 mmHg, the human ventricle reaches a **plateau** (Figure 6.10b). To put this into an everyday context, a standing or sitting human has a left ventricular end-diastolic pressure (LVEDP) of 4–5 mmHg, and is thus on the ascending limb of the Starling curve. A supine human has a higher LVEDP, 8–9 mmHg, due to the redistribution of blood from the lower body, and the heart is close to the plateau of the Starling curve.

In the isolated dog hearts studied by Starling and co-workers, the stroke volume declined when the CVP was raised above 25 mmHg. This produced a **descending limb** on the ventricular function curve (Figure 6.10a). However, it is unlikely that human hearts ever reach such extreme filling pressures. The stroke volume declines in overdistended hearts for two reasons. One is that the atrioventricular valves begin to leak. The other is that the reduced curvature of the wall impairs the conversion of wall tension into BP (Laplace's law; see Figure 6.14).

Ventricular function curves appear in a bewildering variety of guises. Any plot whose ordinate (y-axis) is a measure of contractile energy and whose abscissa (x-axis) is an index of resting fibre length is called a ventricular function curve. The abscissa is often CVP because human CVP is easily measured through a catheter; other indices include RVEDP, LVEDP and using echocardiography to measure ventricle diameter. For the ordinate, stroke volume is a reasonable index of contractile energy if mean arterial pressure is constant, as in Starling's heart–lung preparation. However, it obviously takes more energy to raise a given stroke volume to a high pressure than a low pressure; so, stroke volume × mean arterial pressure, or **stroke work**, is a better measure of contractile energy (Section 6.5).

## The 'law of the heart'

The results in Figure 6.10 prove that **the greater the stretch of the ventricle in diastole, the greater the stroke work achieved in systole**. As Patterson, Piper and Starling concluded in 1914, "the energy of contraction of a cardiac muscle fibre, like that of a skeletal muscle fibre, is proportional to the initial fibre length at rest". This statement is now honoured as the **Frank–Starling mechanism**, although, as so often in science, Starling's definitive studies built on evidence from many previous workers, including that of the great German physiologist Carl Ludwig in 1856. The physiological and pathophysiological roles of the Frank–Starling mechanism in humans are described in Section 6.7. But first, we need to consider the concept of stroke work a little more fully.

## 6.5 STROKE WORK AND THE PRESSURE–VOLUME LOOP

### Stroke work depends on stroke volume and arterial pressure

The energy expended by the myocardium in systole is converted partly into heat and partly into useful mechanical work.

The latter takes the form of an increase in the pressure and volume of blood in the arteries. To calculate how much useful work is achieved, we must first define work and pressure. Work ($W$) is force ($F$) × distance moved ($L$): $W = F \times L$. For example, 1 J of work is 1 N of force moved 1 m. Pressure ($P$) is force per unit area ($A$): $P = F/A$. From the latter definitions, we see that the active force $F$ exerted by a contracting ventricle equals the rise in pressure $\Delta P$ times the wall area $A$. If the wall then contracts over a distance $L$, the volume $\Delta V$ displaced into the aorta is $L \times A$, as illustrated by the top manikin in Figure 6.11. So, applying our definition of work, the work per stroke $W$ is given by:

$$W = F \times L = \Delta P \times A \times L = \Delta P \times \Delta V$$

In other words, the stroke work equals the systolic increase in ventricular BP multiplied by the stroke volume.

### Stroke work is the area inside the pressure–volume loop

The ventricle pressure–volume loop, introduced in Section 2.2, is a useful graphical way of depicting stroke work, which we will use later to illustrate changes in cardiac performance. Each side of the roughly rectangular loop represents one

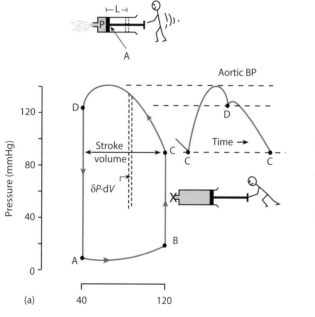

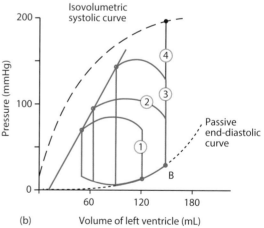

**Figure 6.11** Pressure–volume loops for the human left ventricle. **(a)** Relation to aortic pressure wave: A, the mitral valve opens; AB, filling phase; B, mitral valve closes at onset of systole; BC, isovolumetric contraction; C, aortic valve opens; CD, ejection phase; D, aortic valve closes; DA, isovolumetric relaxation. Stroke work is the sum of all $\Delta P \cdot dV$ strips inside the loop, that is, the total loop area. Sketches illustrate high energy expenditure and O$_2$ consumption by the myocardial manikin during isovolumetric contraction, achieving no external work, followed by the lower energy cost of ejection. The patient is probably middle-aged/old, since aortic pressure was 130/85 mmHg. **(b)** Set of pressure–volume loops for a constant contractility. The lower boundary is the passive pressure–volume curve of the relaxed ventricle (compliance curve). The upper boundary is the systolic pressure of a purely isovolumetric contraction at increasing end-diastolic volumes (Frank–Starling mechanism). Loop 1 is basal. Raising the end-diastolic volume to B increases stroke volume (loop 2), due to Starling's law. Note that end-systolic volume also increases. Raising peripheral resistance increases arterial pressure but reduces stroke volume (loop 3), due to the 'pump function' effect (Figure 6.15). A purely isovolumetric contraction (line 4) reaches the upper boundary line. A line joining the end-systolic points is almost straight (diagonal red line). Its slope, the end-systolic elastance, is an index of contractility. BP, blood pressure. (Based in part on Burkhoff D, Mirsky I, Suga H. *American Journal of Physiology* 2005; 289: H501–12.)

phase of the cardiac cycle, and each corner represents the opening or closing of a valve (Figure 2.6). The width of the loop is the stroke volume and its height is the systolic increase in pressure. Since stroke work is stroke volume × pressure increase, **stroke work equals the area inside the ventricular pressure–volume loop** (Figure 6.11). During the isovolumetric contraction phase B-C, the ventricle is 'working' in the everyday sense (i.e. it is consuming $O_2$ and generating force) but no blood is entering the aorta, so the ventricle is accomplishing no external work. This phase is like someone trying to push over a house; they consumes a lot of $O_2$, but achieves no external work! At point C the aortic valve opens, because diastolic arterial pressure has been reached. The ejection phase C-D is loosely equivalent to an isotonic contraction, or more strictly an auxotonic contraction, and this is the phase during which mechanical work is accomplished.

## The pressure–volume loop is confined inside active and passive boundary curves

The loop is constrained by two boundaries (Figure 6.11b). The lower boundary is the **passive compliance curve** of the ventricle, which shows the end-diastolic pressure at increasing end-diastolic volumes. Every contraction starts from this line. This 'compliance curve' is not linear, because the ventricle is relatively stretchy (compliant) at low pressures and stiff at high pressures, rather like a bicycle tyre. Thus, changes in CVP in the physiological range, 0–10 mmHg, evoke bigger changes in filling than do changes above ~10 mmHg.

The upper boundary is set by the **isovolumetric pressure relation**, that is, the systolic pressure that would be generated if ejection were prevented, as in Frank's experiment (Figure 6.7). This curve has an ascending limb and plateau, due to the Frank–Starling mechanism; the greater the end-diastolic volume, the greater the contractile energy, and hence the greater the isovolumetric pressure generation. In an ejecting heart, the systolic pressure never reaches the isovolumetric boundary curve because some of the contractile energy is used to eject the blood.

Figure 6.11b illustrates how preload and afterload alter the loop within the above boundaries. Loop 1 represents a human left ventricle ejecting a stroke volume of 70 mL at a low pressure. Loop 2 shows the effect of increasing the **preload**. The end-diastolic volume and pressure have been raised, for example, by lying down, so corner B has moved up the passive compliance curve (lower boundary). The increased stretch raises the contractile energy via the Frank–Starling mechanism, so the stroke volume and loop area (stroke work) increase. Note that the Frank–Starling mechanism involves the ventricle getting bigger both at end-diastole (side B/C) and at end-systole (side D/A).

Loop 3 shows the deleterious effect of increasing the **afterload**, for example, by raising arterial BP with a vasoconstrictor drug. In our example, loop 3 starts from the same end-diastolic stretch as loop 2, but more energy is consumed in raising the ventricle pressure to a high enough level to open the aortic valve, leaving less energy available for ejection. As a result, the stroke volume declines. If ejection were prevented totally, as

in line 4, the ventricle would generate maximum systolic pressure and touch the upper boundary; however, stroke volume and useful work would be zero, so the loop has no width.

The top left corner of the loop shows the myocardium at the instant of greatest shortening, that is, end-systole. When a set of pressure–volume loops is plotted as in Figure 6.11b, the end-systolic points fall on a nearly straight line, the **end-systolic pressure–volume relation**. The slope of this line, called the end-systolic 'elastance', has been used as a measure of ventricular **contractility** (Section 6.10). For example, adrenaline, which increases ventricular contractility, steepens the end-systolic pressure–volume line.

## 6.6 CENTRAL VENOUS PRESSURE AND CARDIAC FILLING

Any event that changes the CVP, such as a blood transfusion or haemorrhage, changes the stroke volume via the Frank–Starling mechanism. The CVP depends partly on the total volume of blood in the circulation and partly on the distribution of blood between the central and peripheral veins. Volume distribution is affected by five main factors: gravity (posture); peripheral venous tone; the skeletal muscle pump; the pumping action of the heart; and breathing pattern.

### Low blood volume reduces filling pressure

About 60%–70% of the entire blood volume is in the venous system (Figure 1.12). Consequently, a fall in blood volume (hypovolaemia), resulting from a **haemorrhage** or **dehydration**, lowers the CVP. This reduces the stroke volume via the Frank–Starling mechanism and can cause hypotension in patients with severe hypovolaemia. Conversely, a blood transfusion raises CVP and thereby improves the stroke volume and arterial BP after a haemorrhage.

### Gravity: standing reduces central venous pressure

In a standing human, the drag of gravity redistributes ~500 mL of blood from the thorax into the veins of the lower limbs. This **venous pooling** reduces the CVP. As a result, human stroke volume is reduced in the standing or sitting position. Conversely, lying down redistributes venous blood from the lower body to the thorax, raising the CVP and stroke volume (Figure 6.10b).

### Sympathetic nerves regulate peripheral venous tone

The veins of the skin, kidneys and splanchnic (gastrointestinal) system are innervated by sympathetic venoconstrictor fibres, and peripheral venoconstriction shifts blood into the central veins (Figures 14.5 and 14.14). The central nervous system can thus regulate cardiac filling pressure to some degree. Peripheral venoconstriction occurs during exercise, stress, deep respiration, haemorrhage and shock, and contributes significantly to the raised filling pressure of heart failure. Conversely, cutaneous venodilatation in a hot climate (for temperature regulation) coincidentally reduces CVP and stroke volume; hence, the greater propensity of humans to dizziness and fainting in hot weather.

## The venous muscle pump boosts central venous pressure in exercise

During rhythmic exercise, skeletal muscle contraction repeatedly compresses the deep veins of the limbs. Since the limb veins have semilunar valves, the compression displaces the blood centrally (Figure 8.27). This raises the CVP and stroke volume moderately during dynamic exercise. Conversely, soldiers standing at attention for long periods in hot weather have an inactive muscle pump, leading to an embarrassing tendency to faint on parade. The combination of gravitational venous pooling, heat-induced venodilatation and lack of muscle pump activity reduces the CVP and stroke volume, leading to cerebral hypoperfusion and fainting.

## An increase in cardiac pumping reduces filling pressure

The heart is a pump; that is, it removes blood from the venous system and transfers it into the arterial system. It is easy to forget that pumping not only increases the volume and pressure of blood in the arterial system but also **reduces the volume and pressure of blood in the central veins** (Figure 6.12). Stimulation of the cardiac output, for example, by the sympathetic system, speeds

up the transfer of blood from the central veins to the arteries, so the central venous filling pressure and preload tend to fall, while the arterial pressure and afterload rise. Both changes have an adverse effect on the stroke volume unless compensatory changes are brought into play, as they often are (Section 6.13). Conversely, **if cardiac output is suddenly reduced by acute cardiac failure, for example, a heart attack, the filling pressure rises**. This rise is exacerbated by a reflex sympathetic peripheral venoconstriction, as noted earlier.

## Respiration and coughing affect cardiac extramural pressure and output

Ventricular filling in diastole depends not only on the internal BP but also on the external pressure on the heart. The true filling pressure is the difference between the internal and external pressures, or **transmural pressure** (trans = across; mural = wall). The external pressure on the heart is the subatmospheric intrathoracic pressure, namely $-5$ cmH$_2$O at end-expiration and $-10$ cmH$_2$O at end-inspiration. Since intrathoracic pressure becomes more negative during inspiration, and at the same time intra-abdominal pressure becomes more positive (due to the descent of the diaphragm), inspiration boosts the filling of the thoracic venae cavae and right ventricle (Figure 8.24, top). Consequently, **inspiration raises right ventricular stroke volume**. However, at the same time, the expansion of the lungs during inspiration increases the pulmonary blood pool, which temporarily reduces the return of blood to the left ventricle. So, **inspiration reduces left ventricular stroke volume by the Frank–Starling mechanism**. This is the reason why murmurs associated with right-sided heart valves become louder on inspiration, while those associated with left-sided heart valves become louder during expiration. The reduction in left ventricular output is partly offset by sinus arrhythmia, the tachycardia associated with inspiration (Section 5.11); nevertheless, left ventricular output falls during inspiration. Expiration reverses these effects. As a result, breathing causes synchronous oscillations in arterial pressure, called **Traube–Hering waves**.

Coughing, and other forms of forced expiration, such as the Valsalva manoeuvre (Section 17.2), raise intrathoracic pressure to positive values; up to 400 mmHg has been recorded during coughing! This reduces or even reverses the ventricular transmural pressure in diastole. The resulting fall in ventricular filling and cardiac output contributes to the dizziness associated with a severe bout of coughing.

## Disorders of the pericardium impair filling

Cardiac extramural pressure can also be raised by diseases of the pericardium, the fibrous, fluid-filled sac that encloses the heart. **Pericardial effusions** and **constrictive pericarditis** both raise the pressure around the heart. This impairs ventricular filling and can reduce the cardiac output severely, requiring surgical intervention. During inspiration, there can be a dramatic fall in left ventricular filling that leads to a substantial fall in systolic BP. This is known as 'pulsus paradoxus',

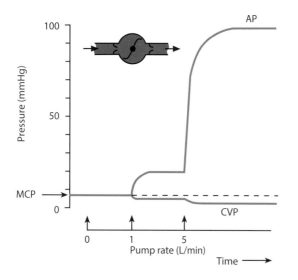

**Figure 6.12** Effect of a pump on input and output pressure. At zero pumping rate, the central venous pressure (CVP) and arterial pressure (AP) equalize (mean circulatory pressure [MCP]). When the pump starts, it removes fluid from the input line, so it reduces input pressure and CVP, as well as raising output pressure (AP). CVP changes less than AP, because venous compliance (volume accommodated per unit pressure change) is greater than arterial compliance. (Based in part on Berne RM, Levy MN. *Cardiovascular Physiology*. St Louis, MO: Mosby; 1997, with permission from Elsevier.)

but it is essentially an exaggerated Traube–Hering wave (see Section 8.4). It is often accompanied by a rise in the jugular venous pulse during inspiration because right ventricular filling is also impaired; this is known as 'Kussmaul's sign'.

## 6.7 OPERATION OF THE FRANK–STARLING MECHANISM IN HUMANS

The single most important role of the Frank–Starling mechanism is to **balance the outputs of the right and left ventricles** (see below). It also contributes to the **increased stroke volume of exercise** (Section 17.3); mediates **postural hypotension** (fall in cardiac output and BP on standing; Section 17.1); mediates **hypovolaemic hypotension** following a haemorrhage or dehydration (Section 18.2); and accounts for the **fall in stroke volume during forced expiration** (Valsalva manoeuvre; Section 17.2).

### The Frank–Starling mechanism equalizes right and left ventricular outputs

It is essential that right ventricular output equals left ventricular output over any period longer than a few beats. Imagine a right ventricular output that is merely 1% greater than the left ventricular output. The pulmonary blood volume, normally 0.6 L, would increase with each heartbeat and reach 2 L within half an hour, causing catastrophic pulmonary congestion and oedema. In heavy exercise, with outputs around 25 L/min, catastrophic congestion would build up within minutes. Conversely, a sustained excess of left ventricular output would quickly drain the pulmonary vessels dry.

The Frank–Starling mechanism prevents such catastrophes by equalizing the two outputs. If right ventricular output begins to exceed left ventricular output, the increase in pulmonary blood volume raises the pressure in the pulmonary veins, which increases the filling of the left ventricle. By the Frank–Starling mechanism, this raises the left ventricular output until balance is restored. The opposite happens if left ventricular output transiently exceeds right ventricular output. The two outputs are thus automatically equalized in the long term.

Imbalances do occur, but they are transient. On standing up, the right output is less than the left output for a few beats, due to venous pooling. Also, as noted earlier, the different effects of respiration on right and left outputs cause a regular, alternating imbalance, synchronous with the respiratory cycle.

### Central venous pressure, not 'venous return', is the true determinant of stroke volume

Students sometimes get into an awful muddle by trying to explain the control of cardiac output in terms of 'venous return' rather than filling pressure. 'Venous return' is the flow of blood into the right atrium. When the circulation is in a steady state, the venous return equals the cardiac output because the

circulation is a closed system of tubes; any inequality can only be transient. Under steady-state conditions, the **venous return is simply the cardiac output observed in veins**, rather than arteries. The popular notion that venous return 'controls' cardiac output is an unhelpful, literally circular viewpoint, because venous return **depends** on cardiac output. By contrast, CVP is an **independent** variable; it can be adjusted independently of cardiac output, for example, by changes in venoconstrictor tone or blood volume. CVP is thus an independent determinant of stroke volume, unlike venous return.

### Guyton's cross plot highlights the role of central venous pressure

The pivotal role of CVP is illustrated by an ingenious cross plot devised by the American physiologist Arthur Guyton (Figure 6.13). The **cardiac output curve** on the Guyton's cross plot represents the positive effect of CVP on stroke volume, via the Frank–Starling mechanism. The other line, the **venous return curve**, shows a negative effect of CVP on venous return, as defined by Darcy's law of hydraulics (Section 1.5). That is, a rise in CVP reduces the pressure gradient driving blood from the capillaries to the central veins, and thus tends to reduce venous flow. The venous return curve reaches zero at ~7 mmHg

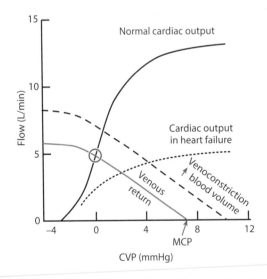

**Figure 6.13** Guyton's graphical analysis of the circulation. The cardiac output curve reflects the increase in ventricular output as central venous pressure (CVP) increases (the Frank–Starling mechanism). The 'venous return curve' shows the fall in blood flow from the capillaries into the central veins as CVP rises (Darcy's law of flow). At zero venous return (circulatory arrest), CVP equals the mean circulatory pressure (MCP). Cardiac output must equal venous return in the steady state, so where the two lines cross is the steady state (open red circle). Heart failure depresses the output curve (reduced contractility, short dashes), but raises the venous return curve (long dashes) because MCP is increased by venoconstriction and increased plasma volume. The new steady state, where the dashed lines cross, occurs at a raised CVP but almost normal cardiac output. Hypovolaemia shifts the venous return curve downwards (not shown). Increased contractility (exercise) shifts the output curve upwards (not shown). (After Guyton AC, Jones CE, Coleman TG. *Circulatory Physiology: Cardiac Output and its Regulation.* Philadelphia, PA: WB Saunders; 1973, with permission from Elsevier.)

CVP, because 7 mmHg is the **mean circulatory pressure**, the pressure of blood when all flow has stopped in the circulation and pressures have equalized. In the steady state *in vivo*, **the cardiac output and venous return must be equal**, and this happens at only one point on the plot, namely where the two curves cross. The stable intersection occurs at a CVP that generates an identical cardiac output and venous return.

## The Starling curve is depressed in heart failure

Guyton's cross plot provides insights into many pathophysiological states, including cardiac failure (Figure 6.13). In cardiac failure, the output curve (Starling curve) is depressed by a fall in contractility. At the same time, there is a rise in mean circulatory pressure, due to sympathetic peripheral venoconstriction and renal fluid retention. This displaces the venous return curve upwards. The new steady state for the failing heart occurs at the new intersection. The failing output is, surprisingly, only slightly below normal, because the CVP has increased. These are the characteristic features of moderate ventricular failure (Chapter 18).

## 6.8 LAPLACE'S LAW AND DILATED HEARTS

### Radius links wall tension and pressure

The radius of the ventricle determines how effectively the active wall tension raises BP. This consideration is particularly important in failing hearts, which become very dilated and have an abnormally large radius. The degree of curvature of any hollow chamber (heart, football, soap bubble) links the wall tension to the internal pressure, as pointed out by the French mathematician, Pierre Simon Marquis de Laplace, in his *Traité de mécanique celeste* (*Celestial Mechanics*) (1798–1827)! Laplace's law states that, for a hollow sphere, the internal pressure $P$ is proportional to the wall tension $T$ and is inversely proportional to the internal radius $r$:

$$P = \frac{2T}{r} \qquad (6.1)$$

(A simple proof for a cylinder appears in Figure 8.17. The factor '2' in the sphere formula can be explained by the fact that a sphere has two planes of curvature, compared with one for a cylinder.) **Tension** is a force, equal to wall stress ($S$) × wall thickness ($w$). **Wall stress** is defined as the force per unit cross-sectional area of the wall, so Laplace's law can also be written as:

$$P = \frac{2Sw}{r} \qquad (6.2)$$

The involvement of the radius is readily understood by considering the curvature of the wall (Figure 6.14). As radius

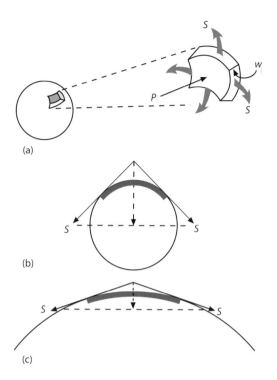

**Figure 6.14** Effect of curvature of a hollow sphere on the conversion of wall stress $S$ into internal pressure $P$ (Laplace's law). **(a)** Hollow sphere with an 'exploded' segment, showing the two circumferential wall stresses. Stress is force per unit cross-sectional area, of thickness $w$. The wall stress in the ejecting heart equals the afterload on the myocytes. **(b)** Cross-section showing how the wall stresses (tangential arrows) give rise to an inwardly directed stress equal and opposite to the pressure. The thick red line represents a muscle segment exerting tension. The arrow length is proportional to stress magnitude. **(c)** Increasing the radius reduces the curvature, and therefore the inward component of the wall stress; therefore, pressure falls (Laplace's law).

increases, curvature decreases. Consequently, a smaller component of the wall tension is angled towards the cavity, generating less pressure. The curvature of the ventricle wall thus determines how effectively the active wall tension is converted into intraventricular pressure.

Laplace's law affects cardiac performance in several ways, as described in the following sections.

### The Laplace effect facilitates late ejection

Wall stress equals the afterload against which the myocytes must shorten during ejection (Figure 6.2). Laplace's law tells us that the afterload $S$ is not simply the ejection pressure (a common but loose assumption), but is the ejection pressure $P$ × radius/$2w$ (equation 6.2). In other words, **afterload depends on chamber radius, as well as arterial pressure**. The bigger the radius, the bigger the afterload, for a given arterial pressure. Since the radius of the chamber falls as ejection proceeds, afterload falls too, facilitating the late phase of ejection; in other words, ejection gets easier as it proceeds. The decreasing chamber radius likewise contributes to the peaking of aortic pressure after ejection has been under way for a little while (Figure 2.5).

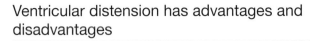

## Ventricular distension has advantages and disadvantages

The Laplace effect and the Frank–Starling mechanism clearly have opposite effects on ventricular performance. Distension of the ventricle raises its force of contraction, due to the Frank–Starling mechanism; however, distension also reduces the pressure generated by a given contractile force, due to Laplace's law. Fortunately, in a healthy heart the gain in contractile energy resulting from moderate distension (the Frank–Starling mechanism) greatly outweighs the fall in pressure-generating efficiency (Laplace's law). However, this is not so in the grossly dilated, failing heart (in the following section; see also Section 6.14).

---

**CONCEPT BOX 6.1**

### VENTRICULAR 'PRELOAD' AND 'AFTERLOAD'

- Preload is the wall stress $S$ (force per unit cross-sectional area) in the resting myocardium. It can be adjusted *in vitro* by suspending a weight from a muscle strip.
- In the intact ventricle, the preload (diastolic wall stress) depends on the end-diastolic pressure $P$, chamber radius $r$ and wall thickness $w$ (Laplace's law); $S = Pr/2w$. The end-diastolic pressure itself is often referred to, inaccurately, as the preload.
- Afterload is the force per unit cross-sectional area (stress) that opposes the shortening of an isotonically contracting muscle strip. It can be adjusted *in vitro* by making a muscle pick up a weight as it begins to shorten.
- In the intact ventricle, the afterload (systolic wall stress) depends on arterial pressure, chamber radius and wall thickness (Laplace's law). Arterial pressure itself is often referred to, inaccurately, as the afterload.

---

## The dilated, failing heart operates at low mechanical efficiency

The failing heart is often grossly dilated (Figure 18.17), making the Laplace effect the dominant one. An increase in radius in an already swollen heart causes little to no increase in contractile force because the ventricle is on the plateau of the Starling curve; but the increase in radius impairs the generation of systolic pressure and hence ejection (Laplace's law). **Reduction of cardiac distension is an important therapeutic goal in heart failure** because it improves the conversion of contractile force into intraventricular pressure. Distension is usually reduced by lowering the cardiac filling pressure, using diuretics to reduce plasma volume.

## Summary of the Frank-Starling mechanism and laplace's laws in man

Few summaries of the operation of the Frank–Starling mechanism in man could be more memorable than

Professor Alan Burton's rhyme, *What Goes in, Must Come Out*:

*The great Dr. Starling, in his Law of the Heart*
*Said the output was greater if, right at the start,*
*The cardiac fibres were stretched a bit more,*
*So their force of contraction would be more than before.*
*Thus, the larger the volume in diastole,*
*The greater the output was likely to be.*

*If the right heart keeps pumping more blood than the left,*
*The lung circuit's congested; the systemic bereft.*
*Since no one is healthy with pulmo-congestion,*
*The Law of Doc. Starling's a splendid suggestion.*
*The balance of outputs is made automatic*
*And blood–volume partition becomes steady–static.*

*When guardsmen stand still and blood pools in their feet*
*Frank–Starling mechanics no longer seem neat.*
*The shift in blood volume impairs C–V–P,*
*Which shortens the fibres in diastole.*
*Contractions grow weaker and stroke volume drops,*
*Depressing blood pressure; so down the guard flops.*

*But when the heart reaches a much larger size,*
*This leads to heart failure, and often demise.*
*The relevant law is not Starling's, alas,*
*But the classical law of Lecompte de Laplace.*
*Your patient is dying of decompensations,*
*So reduce his blood volume or call his relations.*

(From Burton AC. *Physiology and Biophysics of the Circulation.* Chicago, IL: Year Book Medical Publishers; 1972. By courtesy of the publishers. Apologies to Alan Burton's spirit for the addition of verse 3.)

---

## 6.9 MULTIPLE EFFECTS OF ARTERIAL PRESSURE ON THE HEART

Arterial BP affects cardiac output through several opposing mechanisms. Overall, a high arterial pressure has an adverse effect, depressing the output in the short term and leading to ventricular hypertrophy and eventually cardiac failure in the long term.

## Increasing the afterload reduces stroke volume: the pump function curve

Let us remember that the greater the afterload on a strip of myocardium *in vitro*, the less it shortens (Figure 6.2c). In the intact heart, the afterload is often increased by a rise in arterial pressure and this reduces shortening during systole. Thus, **a rise in arterial BP impairs stroke volume**, as shown in Figure 6.11b (loop 3). **Pulmonary embolism** provides a clinically important example. A large venous thrombus becomes detached, often from a deep leg vein, it is swept along (embolizes) through the right heart and into the pulmonary arterial tree, where it lodges in a branch. This raises pulmonary vascular resistance, pulmonary arterial pressure and right ventricular afterload. The increased afterload causes a sharp fall in right ventricular output and the patient may collapse.

The deleterious effect of arterial pressure on stroke volume is shown graphically by the **pump function curve** (Figure 6.15). For any pump operating at a fixed power, be it the heart or a laboratory roller pump, the maximum stroke volume occurs at zero outflow pressure. As the pressure opposing outflow is raised, the stroke volume declines (point W to point 1; Figure 6.15). Maximum pressure is generated at zero stroke volume, as in line 4 of Figure 6.11b. If the energy of the pump is increased, for example, through the Frank–Starling mechanism, the pump function curve is shifted upwards (e.g. from point 1 to point 2; Figure 6.15). If the contractile energy is reduced by heart failure, the pump function curve is shifted downwards (point W to point 3).

Since the resistance of the peripheral circulation is a major determinant of mean arterial pressure, it also affects stroke volume. This is put to practical use in the treatment of heart failure; **the stroke volume of a failing heart can be improved by lowering the peripheral resistance**, using vasodilator drugs. The fall in peripheral resistance reduces arterial pressure, which reduces ventricular afterload and

enhances stroke volume (as in point 4 [Figure 6.15] or loop 3 to loop 2 [Figure 6.11b]).

A raised arterial pressure evokes these secondary effects:

1. **Compensation through the Frank–Starling mechanism**. If arterial pressure is raised acutely, ejection is at first reduced (point 1; Figure 6.15). Then, as returning blood begins to accumulate in the left ventricle, the end-diastolic volume expands over a few beats (Figure 6.16). This raises the contractile energy of the ventricle through the Frank–Starling mechanism. As a result, the pump function curve is shifted to a higher level and stroke volume improves, though at the expense of cardiac dilatation (point 2; Figure 6.15).

2. **Compensation through the Anrep effect**. Over the next 5–10 min, there is a further adaptation (Figure 6.16). The contractility of the ventricle increases, and this enables the ventricle to maintain the stroke volume from a lower, near-normal end-diastolic volume. This is called the Anrep response and it is equivalent to the **slow force response** in the isolated myocardium (Figure 6.4). It arises from at least three mechanisms:

   a. Inotropic (strengthening) agents are produced within the myocardium, namely myocardial angiotensin II (Ang II) and endothelin 1. These act in an autocrine/paracrine fashion to increase the myocyte $Ca^{2+}$ store and $Ca^{2+}$ transient.

   b. Activation of the $Na^+/H^+$ exchanger raises the intracellular $Na^+$, which slows the expulsion of $Ca^{2+}$ by the $Na^+/Ca^{2+}$ exchanger.

   c. Stretch-activated channels increase the entry of extracellular $Ca^{2+}$, boosting the $Ca^{2+}$ store.

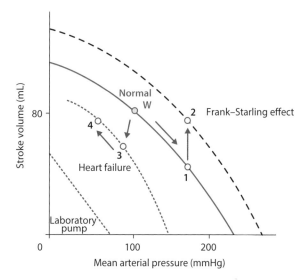

Figure 6.15 Pump function curves for normal heart, failing heart and laboratory roller pump. W, normal work point. Raising the peripheral resistance raises pressure but depresses stroke volume (point 1), if end-diastolic volume is held constant (as in loop 3, Figure 6.11). Ventricular distension can restore the stroke volume by shifting the pump function curve to a higher energy level (point 2) (the Frank–Starling mechanism). Impaired contractility (heart failure) shifts the curve to a lower energy level (point 3). The stroke volume of a failing heart can be improved with pressure-reducing drugs (point 4). (Based on concepts from Elzinga G, Westerhof N. *Circulation Research* 1979; 32: 178–86; and Nichols WW, O'Rourke MF. *McDonald's Blood Flow in Arteries*, 5th edn. London: Arnold; 2005.)

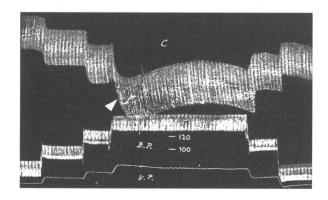

Figure 6.16 Three effects of raising peripheral resistance and arterial blood pressure (BP) (middle trace, B.P.) on stroke volume (excursion of upper trace) and ventricular end-diastolic volume (EDV, lower border of upper trace), in the Starling heart–lung preparation. Volume record is inverted as in Figure 6.9; the time scale is the same. The white arrowhead marks the immediate reduction in stroke volume on raising arterial BP, due to the pump function relation. As returning blood accumulates in the heart, venous pressure (V.P.) and EDV increase, restoring stroke volume (length–tension or Frank–Starling mechanism). Thereafter, around C, contractility increases gradually, as shown by a fall in EDV with no reduction in stroke volume (the Anrep effect). (From Patterson SW, Piper H, Starling EH. *The Journal of Physiology* 1914; 48: 465–511, with permission.)

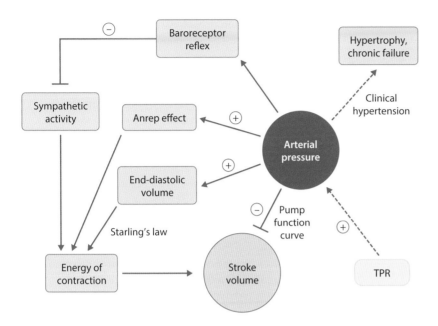

**Figure 6.17** An acute rise in arterial pressure (AP), resulting from a rise in total peripheral resistance (TPR), affects stroke volume through two negative and two positive mechanisms. TPR may be increased acutely by sympathetic vasomotor activity, or chronicaly by clinical hypertension. Chronic hypertension introduces additional factors: ventricular hypertrophy and eventual failure. On the right side, pulmonary resistance may be increased acutely by pulmonary embolism, raising pulmonary AP.

3. **Depression of output by the baroreflex**. In an intact animal, as opposed to an isolated heart, an acute rise in arterial pressure also triggers a neurophysiological reflex, the baroreceptor reflex (Chapter 16). This reduces cardiac sympathetic nerve activity, which reduces ventricular contractility, stroke volume and heart rate to return the arterial pressure to normal (Figure 6.17).

The **overall effect** of an acute rise in arterial pressure on stroke volume thus depends on the interplay between two negative influences (increased afterload and the baroreflex) and two compensatory changes (the Starling and Anrep effects) (see Figure 6.17). In general, the depressor influences predominate. That is, a high vascular resistance usually depresses the stroke volume, as in the case of pulmonary embolism described earlier.

## Chronic hypertension causes concentric ventricular hypertrophy

In patients with clinical hypertension, the long-standing (chronic) elevation of the arterial pressure has additional, slow effects on the heart. The left ventricle gradually undergoes concentric hypertrophy; that is, the wall grows thicker without any increase in chamber size. This contrasts with the response in endurance-trained athletes, where chamber size increases. The hypertrophy is driven by local growth factors, such as Ang II and endothelin 1. These trigger a kinase pathway, the mitogen-activated protein kinase cascade, which activates nuclear transcription factors; these in turn activate hypertrophy genes. Hypertrophy helps the ventricle cope with the persistent high afterload, at least for a while. However, in the long term the overloaded ventricle can go into failure. This is one of several reasons why clinical hypertension should always be treated, despite being asymptomatic.

## 6.10 SYMPATHETIC REGULATION OF CONTRACTILITY

### The meaning of contractility

Up to this point, the chapter has focused on changes in contractile energy brought about by changes in resting fibre length (intrinsic regulation). However, contractile energy is also regulated by neurohumoral factors (extrinsic regulation). **A change in contractile energy that is caused by neurohumoral factors, not altered fibre length, is called a change in contractility**. The term 'contractility' thus specifically excludes changes brought about by the Frank–Starling mechanism. The most important inotropic (strengthening), neurohumoral agent, physiologically, is the sympathetic neurotransmitter noradrenaline. Other inotropic agents include circulating adrenaline, Ang II, extracellular $Ca^{2+}$ ions, inotropic drugs and reduced beat interval.

### Sympathetic stimulation produces a stronger, shorter beat

Cardiac sympathetic nerve activity increases during exercise, orthostasis (standing up), stress and haemorrhage. The sympathetic terminal varicosities release noradrenaline, which activates myocyte $\beta_1$ adrenergic receptors. The receptors activate the $G_s$–$\alpha_s$–adenylate cyclase–cyclic adenosine monophosphate (cAMP)–protein kinase A (PKA) phosphorylation cascade shown in Figure 4.10. The ensuing rise in membrane $Ca^{2+}$ current, $i_{Ca}$, increases the sarcoplasmic reticulum (SR) $Ca^{2+}$ store and boosts the amount of trigger $Ca^{2+}$ at the start of each contraction. As a result, the magnitude of the **cytosolic free $Ca^{2+}$ transient increases**, causing more crossbridge formation and force development (Figure 4.9). At the same time, the $Ca^{2+}$

## CONTRACTILITY

- Contractility is the force of contraction achieved from a given initial fibre length.
- Contractile force can be increased either by increased contractility and/or by increasing the resting fibre length through the end-diastolic stretch (the Frank–Starling mechanism).
- Positive inotropic agents are factors that increase contractility. They include the sympathetic neurotransmitter noradrenaline, circulating adrenaline, $\beta_1$ adrenergic receptor agonist drugs, phosphodiesterase inhibitors and digoxin.
- Negative inotropes include acute myocardial ischaemia (acting through intracellular acidosis), chronic cardiac failure, anaesthetics, parasympathetic fibre activity (a minor effect), $\beta_1$ adrenergic receptor antagonists and $Ca^{2+}$ channel blockers.

uptake pumps of the SR (SERCA) are stimulated through the phosphorylation of phospholamban, and the increased rate of removal of cytoplasmic $Ca^{2+}$ by the pumps **shortens the $Ca^{2+}$ transient** and hence the duration of systole. Sympathetic stimulation thus causes a shorter, more forceful contraction of the individual myocytes, with the following effects on ventricular performance (additional to tachycardia; see Figure 4.7):

- **Ventricular pressure** climbs more rapidly in systole and reaches a higher level because the elastic arteries receive an increased volume of blood in a shorter time (Figure 6.18a). The maximum rate of pressure increase, $dP/dt_{max}$, has been used as an index of contractility, although it is also increased by the Frank–Starling mechanism (Figures 6.2b and 6.7).

- **Ejection fraction** rises above two thirds, which is the resting fraction. This is a popular clinical measure of contractility because it is readily estimated by echocardiography.
- **Diastolic volume** falls because the ejection fraction has increased. Note that a rise in contractility makes the ventricle **smaller in both diastole and systole** (Figure 6.18b), whereas increased filling pressure through the Frank–Starling mechanism makes the ventricle bigger in both diastole and systole.
- **Stroke volume** increases. In an isolated preparation, the increase is attenuated by the concomitant fall in end-diastolic volume (which reduces the Frank–Starling effect) and increase in arterial pressure (the afterload effect). The full increase in stroke volume is only achieved when these adverse changes are prevented or minimized by reflex changes in the peripheral circulation, as happens in intact animals. During exercise, for example, peripheral vascular adjustments minimize the fall in end-diastolic volume and rise in arterial pressure, thus allowing an optimal increase in stroke volume.
- The **duration of systole** shortens (Figure 6.18a). This prevents excessive shortening of the diastolic filling time as the heart rate increases. Increased contraction velocity enables the stroke volume to be ejected during the shortened systole.

The net effect of sympathetic nerve stimulation, therefore, is to increase the arterial pressure, stroke volume, ejection fraction and heart rate, and to reduce the ejection time, end-diastolic pressure and ventricle size.

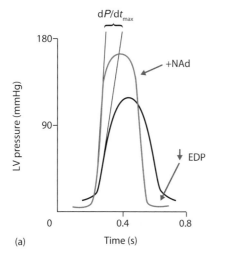

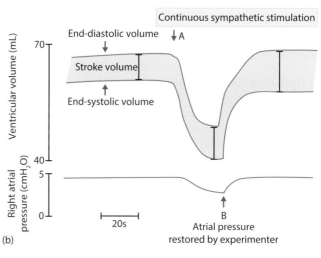

(a)

(b)

**Figure 6.18** Effect of sympathetic stimulation or noradrenaline (+NAd) on cardiac performance. **(a)** Left ventricular (LV) pressure climbs faster ($dP/dt_{max}$), systolic pressure increases, systole shortens, relaxation is quicker and end-diastolic pressure (EDP) falls. **(b)** Combined stroke volume recorded by a cardiometer at a constant, paced heart rate. The left cardiac sympathetic nerves were stimulated continuously from point A. The increased ejection fraction reduced right atrial pressure and ventricular volumes. However, the Frank–Starling mechanism, operating at reduced end-diastolic volume (EDV), attenuated the increase in stroke volume. The enhanced contractility is evident from the fact that stroke volume increased slightly despite the much-reduced EDV. At B, the filling pressure was artificially restored to its previous level, allowing the effect of contractility on stroke volume to emerge fully. The vertical bar represents the size of control stroke volume. (Adapted from Linden RJ. *Anaesthesia* 1968; 23: 566–84, with permission from Wiley-Blackwell.)

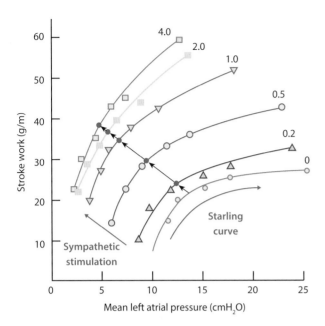

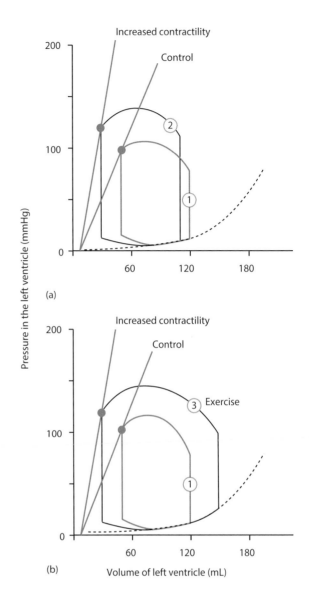

**Figure 6.19** Family of ventricular function curves (Starling curves) generated by graded sympathetic stimulation of dog heart. Sympathetic activity in range 0–4 s$^{-1}$ increased contractility in a graded fashion. The arrows to red points show how enhanced contractility reduces filling pressure, as well as raising stroke volume. (From Sarnoff SJ, Mitchell JH. *Handbook of Physiology Cardiovascular System*. Vol. 1. Baltimore, MD: American Physiological Society; 1962. pp. 489–532, with permission.)

## Graded sympathetic activity generates a family of ventricular function curves

Since sympathetic stimulation increases the contractile energy produced at a given end-diastolic volume, it shifts the entire Starling curve upwards (Figure 6.19). In the 1960s, Sarnoff showed that the shift is graded and proportional to the level of sympathetic activity. The heart therefore operates not on a single Starling curve but on an entire family of curves. Stroke volume can be altered by moving along a curve (i.e. by changing contractile energy through the Frank–Starling mechanism) or by moving from one curve to a higher or lower one (i.e. by changing the contractility). A combination of both changes is common *in vivo*. For example, during upright exercise increased filling pressure shifts the ventricles along a Starling curve, and increased ventricular contractility shifts the curve upwards.

## Sympathetic stimulation widens the pressure–volume loop and shifts it leftwards

Sympathetic stimulation raises the upper limit of the pressure–volume loop, that is, the isovolumetric systolic pressure line. Peak pressure (loop height), stroke volume (loop width) and stroke work (loop area) all increase, within the confines of the raised boundary (Figure 6.20a, loop 2). Cardiac sympathetic

**Figure 6.20** Effect of increased left ventricular contractility on human pressure–volume loop. The slope of the straight line through each end-systolic point, the end-systolic elastance, is an index of contractility, as in Figure 6.11b. **(a)** Loop 1 is the baseline state. Loop 2 shows the effect of increased contractility per se. Ejection fraction is increased, so end-diastolic volume (EDV) falls. The loop area (stroke work) is increased. **(b)** During exercise (loop 3), contractility is raised by sympathetic activity; in addition, EDV is raised by peripheral venoconstriction and the skeletal muscle pump. The increase in stroke volume is now greater.

stimulation alone also shifts the loop to the left because it reduces end-diastolic volume (unless compensatory mechanisms are brought into play); so, the Frank–Starling mechanism attenuates the increase in stroke volume. However, in an intact animal the end-diastolic volume is prevented from falling, or is even raised, by peripheral venoconstriction and the muscle pump, for example, during upright exercise. Consequently, the loop widens in both directions, resulting in a bigger increase in stroke volume and stroke work (Figure 6.20b, loop 3).

## 6.11 OTHER POSITIVE INOTROPIC INFLUENCES

### Adrenaline and other β adrenergic receptor agonists

The human adrenal medulla secretes adrenaline and noradrenaline in the ratio of approximately 4:1. Adrenaline activates cardiac $\beta_1$ adrenergic receptors; therefore, it has the same direct effects on the heart as noradrenaline. The plasma concentrations of both substances increase ~20 times during maximal exercise. Even so, the cardiac response to exercise is normally dominated by the powerful cardiac sympathetic nerves.

β adrenergic receptor agonist drugs, such as **isoprenaline**, **dopamine** (a precursor of adrenaline) and the synthetic analogue **dobutamine**, have similar inotropic and chronotropic effects. β adrenergic receptor agonists can be used to support an acutely failing heart for a short period.

Broad-spectrum phosphodiesterase inhibitors, such as **caffeine** and **theophylline**, and selective phosphodiesterase type III inhibitors such as **milrinone**, raise intracellular cAMP and thus mimic the effects of β adrenergic receptor agonists (Figure 4.10). This action of caffeine probably accounts for the tendency of strong coffee to cause palpitations in some individuals.

### Angiotensin II

The circulating concentration of the hormone Ang II increases during exercise and heart failure (Section 14.8). Much of its positive inotropic effect results from neuromodulation; Ang II receptor type 1 (AT1R) receptors on central neurons and sympathetic ganglia increase sympathetic activity, while AT1R receptors on sympathetic nerve terminals facilitate noradrenaline release (Figure 14.2). Ang II also acts directly on cardiac myocyte receptors to enhance the membrane $Ca^{2+}$ current, $i_{Ca}$.

### Other circulating inotropes

The hormones levothyroxine (Section 14.5), insulin, glucagon and corticosteroids all have a long-term, positive inotropic effect. The inotropic drug **digoxin** partially inhibits the sarcolemmal $Na^+/K^+$ pump, leading to a rise in intracellular $Ca^{2+}$ (Section 3.9).

### Effects of beat interval on contractile force

The American physiologist Henry Pickering Bowditch first observed in 1871 that shortening the interval between heartbeats causes a gradual increase in contractile force. If the frequency of electrical stimulation is suddenly raised, there is a

single weaker beat, then the beats grow progressively stronger in a 'staircase' pattern, until a new steady state is reached. Conversely, if the beat interval is increased (reduced frequency), there is one stronger beat, then the contractions become weaker (Figure 6.21a). The Bowditch staircase effect, or interval–tension relation, occurs in amphibians and some mammals, including man; however, it is blunted or even negative in failing hearts.

The increase in contractility with heart rate is caused by an increase in the SR $Ca^{2+}$ store, leading to bigger systolic $Ca^{2+}$ transients (Figure 6.21a). The store is increased by (1) the reduced diastolic period for $Ca^{2+}$ expulsion and (2) a rise in intracellular $[Na^+]$, caused by the increased action potential frequency. The rise in intracellular $Na^+$ slows $Ca^{2+}$ expulsion by the $Na^+/Ca^{2+}$ exchanger. Although the Bowditch rate effect is an interesting phenomenon, it contributes only a little to the increased contractility of exercise. The latter is due chiefly to increased $\beta_1$ adrenergic receptor activation.

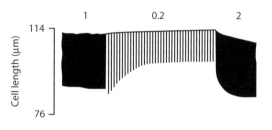

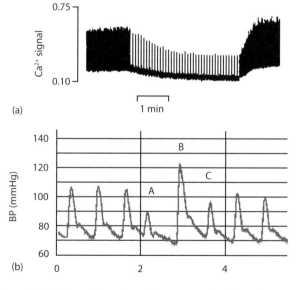

**Figure 6.21** Effect of beat interval on contractility. **(a)** Twitches of an isolated rat ventricular myocyte stimulated at 1, 0.2 and 2 beats/s. Intracellular $Ca^{2+}$ was monitored with the fluorescent dye Fura-2. **(b)** In a patient with heart failure, a premature systole (beat A) is feeble and beat B after the compensatory pause is stronger than usual (post-extrasystolic potentiation). **(a)** From Frampton JE, Orchard CH, Boyett MR. *Journal of Physiology* 1991; 437: 351–75, with permission; **(b)** from Voss A, Baier V, Schumann A, et al. *Journal of Physiology* 2002; 538: 271–78, with permission from Wiley-Blackwell.)

After an interval reduction, the first beat is weaker rather than stronger, unlike all the subsequent beats. Similarly, a **premature ectopic beat** in a patient produces a weak beat, even when excitation follows the normal conduction pathway (Figure 6.21b; beat A). The premature beat is weak because the SR $Ca^{2+}$ release channels recover relatively slowly from their inactivated state, so they are partially refractory during a premature beat.

After a premature ectopic beat, there is a compensatory pause and the next beat is stronger than normal (Figure 6.21b; beat B). This is called **post-extrasystolic potentiation**. The patient may feel the post-extrasystolic potentiation and complain "My heart gives a jump, Doctor". The increased filling time occasioned by the compensatory pause raises the end-diastolic volume and thus contributes to post-extrasystolic potentiation in a patient. However, post-extrasystolic potentiation also occurs in isolated myocardium, where it is attributed to the increased filling of the SR $Ca^{2+}$ store during the prolonged beat interval.

## 6.12 NEGATIVE INOTROPISM, ISCHAEMIA AND ARRHYTHMIA

Negative inotropic influences are factors that reduce myocardial contractility. Aside from parasympathetic activity, negative inotropic effects are usually non-physiological, and often a component of cardiac disease. They include:

- parasympathetic (vagal) activity and cholinergic agonists;
- β-blocker drugs, such as propranolol, metoprolol and bisoprolol (Section 4.9);
- $Ca^{2+}$ channel blockers, such as verapamil (Section 4.9);
- hyperkalaemia (Section 4.8);
- barbiturates and many general anaesthetics;
- acidosis and hypoxia, often the result of ischaemic heart disease;
- cronic cardiac failure (Section 18.5).

## Parasympathetic fibres have only a weak effect on ventricular contractility

Vagal parasympathetic fibres innervate the pacemaker–conduction system and atrial myocardium. They markedly reduce heart rate, but have a relatively small effect on ventricular contractility. The human ventricles receive only a scanty parasympathetic innervation; even maximal vagal stimulation reduces ventricular contraction by only 15%–38%. Interestingly, there is a concomitant fall in noradrenaline in the coronary venous blood because some parasympathetic fibres terminate close to sympathetic fibres and inhibit the sympathetic terminals. Conversely, sympathetic fibres release not only noradrenaline but also neuropeptide Y and galanin,

which inhibit acetylcholine release from vagal fibres. In the sino-atrial node, this **cross-inhibition** facilitates an increase in heart rate (see Section 4.7).

## Ischaemia impairs contractility and causes arrhythmia

Ischaemia is an inadequate tissue oxygenation, resulting usually from an inadequate blood flow. In the heart, atheromatous narrowing of one or more coronary arteries is usually responsible (Figure 15.6). The reduced blood supply causes local hypoxia, leading to anaerobic glycolysis and intracellular lactic acidosis (Section 6.14). These metabolic changes impair contractility and cardiac output, especially during exercise, so exercise capacity is reduced (Table 6.1). Cardiac ischaemia also causes chest pain (angina/myocardial infarction) and can precipitate an arrhythmia. The ECG shows the characteristic changes illustrated in Figure 5.11. The multiple effects of ischaemia are described in a little more detail in the next sections; they are summarized in Figure 6.22.

### Impaired contractility

The fall in mitochondrial oxidative metabolism leads to a fall in the phosphocreatine energy reserve, a rise in inorganic phosphate and adenosine diphosphate (ADP), and eventually a fall in adenosine triphosphate (ATP). Pyruvate oxidation is diverted into lactic acid formation, causing intracellular acidosis. **Acidosis has a strongly negative inotropic effect** (Figure 6.23), probably because $H^+$ ions act on the troponin I subunit to cause a conformational change and reduce the affinity of the troponin C subunit for Ca2+. The rise in inorganic phosphate likewise impairs contractility, though less strongly.

### Arrhythmia

The ischaemic heart is prone to impaired electrical conduction and arrhythmia. These changes are the result of multiple mechanisms, as follows (Figure 6.22):

- resting membrane potential depolarizes, because interstitial $[K^+]$ increases as the $Na^+/K^+$ ATPase runs down;
- action potential size (phase 0) and duration (phase 2) are reduced; phase 0 is impaired because the low resting membrane potential traps some of the $Na^+$ channels in the inactivated state (Figure 3.13, top right), while phase 2 duration is reduced by $K_{ATP}$ channel activation (Figure 3.10);
- connexon conductivity is reduced, impairing the electrical coupling between cells; ventricular fibrillation is especially likely to arise at moderate levels of uncoupling because a mix of slow conduction

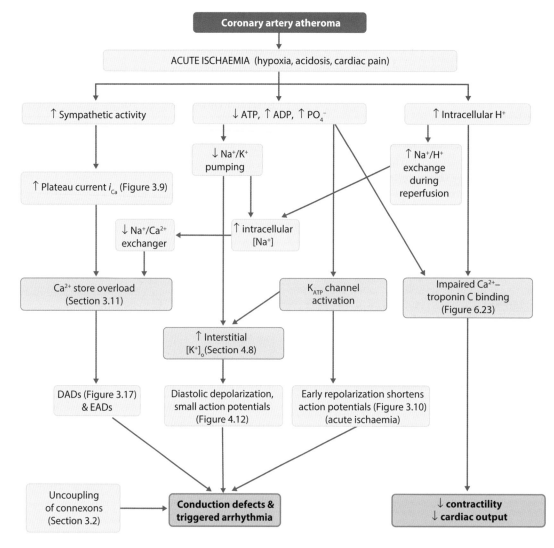

**Figure 6.22** Summary of the multiple mechanisms by which acute ischaemia impairs contractility and causes arrhythmia. Acute myocardial ischaemia is usually caused by coronary artery disease. For chronic heart failure, see Section 18.5. ADP, adenosine diphosphate; ATP, adenosine triphosphate; DAD, delayed afterdepolarization; EAD, early afterdepolarization; $PO_4^-$, phosphate.

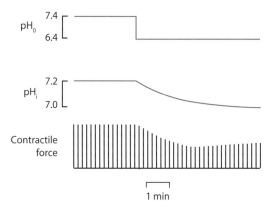

**Figure 6.23** Negative inotropic effect of intracellular acidosis. Intracellular pH, $pH_i$, was changed by adding extracellular acid ($pH_o$). Reduction of $pH_i$ by only 0.2 units halves the contractility. (Based on Hongo K, White E, Orchard CH. *Experimental Physiology* 1995; 80: 701–12, with permission from Wiley-Blackwell; and Bountra C, Vaughan-Jones RD. *Journal of Physiology* 1989; 418: 163–87, with permission from Wiley-Blackwell.)

and blocked conduction favours circus formation (Figure 5.12);

• intracellular [Na⁺] increases, because Na⁺/K⁺ ATPase activity declines and intracellular acidosis stimulates the Na⁺/H⁺ exchanger (Figure 3.14). The rise in $[Na^+]_i$ reduces the Na⁺ gradient that drives Ca²⁺ expulsion by the Na⁺/Ca²⁺ exchanger. Consequently, acidosis causes intracellular Ca²⁺ loading

• the SR Ca²⁺ store becomes overloaded, partly for the above reason and partly because there is an increase in extracellular Ca²⁺ influx $i_{Ca}$, due to a reflex increase in sympathetic activity.

The overloaded Ca²⁺ store may discharge spontaneously in early diastole, stimulating the 3Na⁺/1Ca²⁺ exchanger to generate a delayed afterdepolarization, which may trigger an ectopic beat (Figure 3.17). Re-entry circuits may then develop, because the reduced action potential size and reduced connexon conductivity slow conduction, and the abnormalities are not uniformly distributed (Figure 5.12). Thus, an **ectopic beat** triggered by an **afterdepolarization** during the **vulnerable period** (late T wave, when some myocytes are repolarized and others are not) can initiate a **re-entry arrhythmia** such as fibrillation (Figure 5.19).

## The paradox of myocardial ischaemia/reperfusion injury

An adequate $O_2$ supply is essential for a healthy myocardium. Yet, paradoxically, the reperfusion of ischaemic myocardium with oxygenated blood increases the amount of cell damage. Two factors cause the damage:

1. Reperfusion restores extracellular pH to normal, thus disinhibiting the $Na^+/H^+$ exchanger, causing intracellular Na+ to rise. This quickly corrects the intracellular acidosis and thereby restores contractility; however, if the intracellular $Ca^{2+}$ overload has not yet been corrected, the restored contractility results in a severe, sustained **contracture**. Contracture can damage the cytoskeleton, disrupt cell membranes and cause **necrosis** (cell death).
2. The myocytes are also damaged by the formation of toxic **$O_2$-derived free radicals**, as described in Section 13.9. The $O_2$-derived free radicals damage the sarcolemma, leading to arrhythmia.

The $Na^+/H^+$ exchange inhibitor, amiloride, greatly reduces reperfusion injury in experimental animals. It prolongs the duration of intracellular acidosis and depressed contractility. This gives the myocyte sufficient time to restore its normal, low free $Ca^{2+}$ concentration and avoid contracture.

## Myocardial stunning and ischaemic preconditioning

If coronary blood flow remains low after a coronary thrombosis, myocardial contractility remains low (**hibernation**). If coronary blood flow is then restored, and the ischaemia was not too severe, there may be little cellular necrosis yet cardiac performance remains depressed for days. This is called **myocardial stunning**. 'Stunning' is decreased contractile function despite normal $Ca^{2+}$ transients, normal energetic status and restored perfusion. It is caused by troponin I degradation, leaving the thin filament troponin complex less responsive to $Ca^{2+}$.

In animal experiments, prior exposure to sublethal ischaemia has a protective effect, in that there is less cardiac damage during a second episode of ischaemia. This is called **ischaemic preconditioning**. The protection lasts up to 3 days. Ischaemic preconditioning is thought to be mediated by the release of certain chemicals (adenosine, nitric oxide and others) that activate intracellular kinase cascades (protein kinase C and others). These promote the transcription of cardioprotective genes (inducible *nitric oxide synthase*, *cyclooxygenase 2* and others), which increases the production of the cardioprotective agents nitric oxide and prostaglandins.

## 6.13 CO-ORDINATED CONTROL OF CARDIAC OUTPUT

### An uncoordinated stimulus is relatively ineffective

To achieve an effective regulation of cardiac output in humans, as opposed to isolated hearts, the cardiac changes must be co-ordinated with changes in the arterial and venous systems. It is illuminating to see how ineffective an uncoordinated change in a single cardiac factor can be. The relatively trivial change in stroke volume on sympathetic stimulations of an isolated heart provides one example (Figure 6.18b). Another example is the relatively small increase in cardiac output when the pacing frequency is raised in a patient with an artificial pacemaker; there is remarkably little increase in cardiac output at paced rates above 100 min⁻¹, and output declines at high pacing rates, due to the reduced diastolic filling time. Thus, changes in a single cardiac variable are relatively ineffective. Co-ordinated, cooperative changes in both cardiac and vascular function are required for cardiac output to increase effectively. This is well illustrated by the response to exercise.

### Exercise involves co-ordinated cardiac and vascular changes

Human cardiac output increases by ~6 L/min for every extra litre of $O_2$ consumed per minute. The increased output is brought about by increases in heart rate and stroke volume. Tachycardia is generally the major factor; the human heart rate increases in proportion to $O_2$ consumption, to a maximum 180–200 beats/min–roughly 220 beats/min minus the individual's age (in years). Studies using echocardiography and aortic Doppler flowmetry show that the contribution of increased stroke volume depends on posture, exercise intensity and age. During upright exercise, stroke volume can increase by 50%–100% (Table 6.2 and Figure 6.24). However, in the supine position stroke volume is already high at rest, so it increases relatively less during exercise. The co-ordinated cardiac and peripheral changes that underlie the increase output are as follows:

1. Cardiac sympathetic stimulation and reduced vagal activity **raise the heart rate** and **shorten systole**. The **reduced diastolic filling interval** is offset by a sympathetic-mediated rise in **atrial contractility**, which enhances the atrial contribution to ventricular filling.
2. Cardiac sympathetic stimulation, and to a lesser degree circulating adrenaline, increase ventricular contractility. This **raises stroke volume** and ejection fraction, by **reducing end-systolic volume** (Figure 6.24).
3. Sympathetic vasomotor nerves cause **venoconstriction** in the splanchnic circulation, and the **skeletal muscle pump** compresses limb veins. The resulting transfer of blood into the central veins prevents the **CVP** from falling, which is otherwise an effect of increased

**Table 6.2** Typical cardiac response to upright exercise in a non-athlete

|  | Rest | Hard exercise[a] |
|---|---|---|
| O$_2$ consumption (L/min) | 0.25 | 3.0 |
| Cardiac output (L/min) | 4.8 | 21.6 |
| Heart rate (beats/min) | 60.0 | 180.0 |
| Stroke volume (mL) | 80.0 | 120.0 |
| End-diastolic volume (mL) | 120.0 | 140.0 |
| End-systolic residual volume (mL) | 40.0 | 20.0 |
| Ejection fraction | 0.67 | 0.86 |
| Cycle time (s) | 1.0 | 0.33 |
| Duration of systole (s) | 0.35 | 0.2 |
| Duration of diastole (s) | 0.65 | 0.13 |

*Source:* After Rerych SK, Scholz PM, Newman GE, et al. *Annals of Surgery* 1978; 187: 449–58.

[a] Exercise intensity: ~85% of maximum increase in heart rate.

cardiac pumping (Figure 6.12). The CVP can increase by 1 mmHg or so during exercise in the upright position, **raising end-diastolic volume** (Figure 6.24). As a result, the **Frank–Starling mechanism** contributes to the increase in stroke volume. This contribution is most marked during sudden, intense, upright exercise and in older people.

4. **Vasodilatation** in the exercising skeletal muscle reduces peripheral vascular resistance, and thus prevents arterial pressure from rising excessively as the cardiac output increases. In this way, stroke volume is not restrained by a big increase in afterload.

The increased cardiac output of exercise thus involves a co-ordinated interaction between changes within the heart (rate, contractility) and vascular changes that adjust the CVP (preload) and vascular resistance (afterload).

## Transplanted and artificially paced hearts respond to exercise

Cardiac transplantation necessarily entails cutting the autonomic nerves to the heart (denervation). Rather surprisingly, exercise performance is only moderately impaired. Indeed, racing greyhounds with denervated hearts experienced only a 5% reduction in track speed (Figure 17.7). This is due to a **redundancy of cardiac control mechanisms**. Although the denervated heart does not show the usual, immediate tachycardia at the start of exercise, stroke volume increases rapidly because the CVP increases (effect of leg muscle pump), raising preload; the arterial pressure dips (effect of muscle resistance vessel dilatation), reducing afterload. Moreover, the heart rate and contractility increase over the next 1–2 min, due to increases in circulating adrenaline and Ang II. Greyhound track performance only deteriorates substantially if the heart is denervated and the adrenergic backup is blocked by a β antagonist (Figure 17.7).

Like the denervated greyhound, a patient with a transplanted heart or artificial pacemaker benefits from the redundancy of cardiac control systems. Even at a fixed pacing rate, exercise increases the stroke volume, due to the skeletal muscle pump, peripheral vasodilatation and adrenaline-enhanced contractility. Most modern pacemakers contain a programmable 'rate response' function, such that during exercise heart rate can increase appropriately, although not all patients (even those who depend on their pacemaker all of the time) require this.

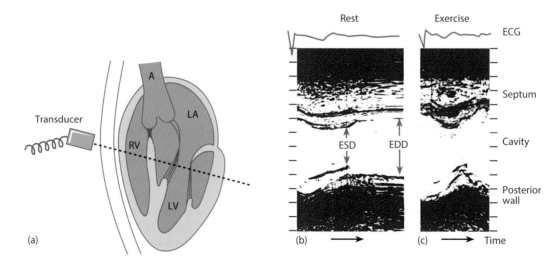

**Figure 6.24** Effect of exercise on ventricular dimensions and contraction. **(a)** Ultrasound beam directed across the ventricle (sagittal section). **(b,c)** M-mode echocardiograms of human left ventricle during **(b)** rest and **(c)** upright exercise. The end-diastolic dimension (EDD) increased by 2 mm on average. End-systolic dimension (ESD) fell by 5 mm. The EDD–ESD difference, an index of stroke volume, increased by 24%. A, aorta; LA, left atrium; LV, left ventricle; RV, right ventricle. (From Amon KW, Crawford MH. *Journal of Clinical Ultrasound* 1979; 7: 373–76.)

## 6.14 CARDIAC ENERGETICS AND METABOLISM

### Ventricular systole adds potential energy and kinetic energy to arterial blood

Part of the energy expended in ventricular systole is 'useful' in the sense that it accomplishes mechanical work on the arterial system; the rest is dissipated as heat. The useful, mechanical work takes the form of an increase in the pressure of the ejected blood (potential energy) and an increase in its velocity (kinetic energy).

### Pressure work (stroke work) predominates

As explained in Section 6.5, the work done by the ventricle in pressurizing and shifting the stroke volume into the arteries is called the stroke work. Stroke work equals stroke volume $\Delta V$ multiplied by the mean increase in pressure $\Delta P$. Stroke work is therefore the area inside the ventricle pressure–volume, $\Delta V \cdot \Delta P$ (Figure 6.11). If the left ventricle raises BP by 100 mmHg ($1.33 \times 10^4$ N/m$^2$) and adds 75 cm$^3$ of this blood to the arterial system ($0.75 \times 10^{-4}$ m$^3$), it performs ~1 N · m of work (1 J). The arterial system gains 1 J of potential energy.

### Kinetic work is low in a resting human

The ventricle also imparts velocity to the ejected blood; that is, it adds **kinetic energy** $KE$. Kinetic energy, the energy of motion, is proportional to velocity squared ($v^2$) and moving mass $m$. Total ventricular work $W$ equals the pressure work plus the kinetic work, that is:

$$W = \Delta V \Delta P + KE = \Delta V \Delta P + mv^2/2$$

Under resting conditions, ~0.08 kg (80 mL) of blood is ejected at a mean velocity of 0.5 m/s during systole, so the kinetic energy imparted by either ventricle is 0.01 kg m$^2$s$^{-2}$, or 0.01 J. This is only 1% of the left ventricular stroke work and ~5% of right ventricular stroke work (stroke work being lower on the right side because of the low ejection pressure).

### Kinetic work increases substantially during exercise

During heavy exercise, the ejection velocity of each ventricle increases around fivefold, to ~2.5 m/s. Pressure and stroke volume, by contrast, increase only moderately. As a result, kinetic energy accounts for 14% of left ventricular work and 50% of right ventricular work during heavy exercise.

### Cardiac power

Power is rate of working, so cardiac power equals ventricular work × heart rate. Cardiac power ranges from ~1.2 J/s (1.2 W) at rest to ~8 W during heavy exercise. The latter is about one-eighth of the power of a traditional household light bulb.

### Emotional stress and high blood pressure increase cardiac work

A raised arterial BP increases stroke work, and therefore myocardial O$_2$ consumption. An angry, emotional scene causes a large rise in BP, so it greatly increases the myocardial O$_2$ demand. This is clearly something to be avoided by patients with **coronary artery insufficiency**. As the celebrated 18th century anatomist John Hunter observed in relation to his own ischaemic heart, "My life is at the mercy of any rascal who chooses to annoy me"; the couch on which Hunter died after a stormy committee meeting can still be seen in the library of St George's Hospital Medical School in London.

### Cardiac efficiency improves during exercise

Gross mechanical efficiency is the amount of external work achieved per unit energy expended. Cardiac efficiency is only 5%–10% in a resting human, partly because the ion pumps consume about a quarter of the energy, and partly because tension generation during isovolumetric contraction consumes a lot of energy. Myocardial O$_2$ consumption is in fact dominated by internal work rather than external mechanical work, and correlates well with the active tension multiplied by the period for which it is maintained (the **tension-time index**). This may seem odd, until one recalls that the O$_2$ consumption of a tug-of-war team depends mainly on the huge tension they exert, rather than on the external work involved in shifting the opposition over a metre or so. In cardiology, the tension-time index is estimated as heart rate × systolic pressure.

During dynamic exercise, cardiac efficiency improves markedly to ~15%, because flow increases much more than arterial pressure; there is relatively little increase in the energy-expensive isovolumetric phase. This is helpful to patients with cardiac disease. By contrast, isometric exercise, such as weightlifting, is best avoided by cardiac patients, because it greatly raises arterial pressure and hence O$_2$ demand.

### Cardiac efficiency is reduced by dilatation in heart failure

When treating heart failure, it is important to improve cardiac efficiency as much as possible. Heart failure leads to cardiac dilatation (Figure 18.16), which impairs efficiency. **Laplace's law** tells us that to maintain a normal systolic pressure $P$, a heart of enlarged radius $r$ must exert a greater contractile tension $T$, because $P = 2T/r$ (Section 6.8). To generate a given pressure, a dilated ventricle consumes more O$_2$ and has a lower mechanical efficiency than a ventricle of normal radius. Since **excessive cardiac dilatation impairs efficiency**, it must be reduced with diuretic drugs.

## Myocardial metabolism and Oxygen consumption

### High-energy phosphate

Myocardial metabolism is normally aerobic. The immediate energy source for the myosin head is the high-energy third phosphate bond of ATP, which is generated by oxidative phosphorylation in the abundant cardiac mitochondria. There is a small backup store of high-energy phosphate bonds in the form of **phosphocreatine**, but this is only sufficient for ~15 beats. Consequently, cardiac performance depends entirely on mitochondrial ATP production increasing in proportion to myosin ATP consumption. This coupling is remarkably good; myocardial $O_2$ consumption increases linearly with myocardial work without any measurable change in ATP or phosphocreatine concentration; this is a phenomenon called the **metabolic stability paradox**. So how is mitochondrial ATP production coupled so tightly to myosin ATP consumption? The traditional answer was that $Ca^{2+}$ not only triggers contraction but also stimulates mitochondrial oxidative phosphorylation; it now appears that **creatine kinase** has a key role. Creatine kinase is present in the myosin filaments and in the mid-membrane space of the mitochondria, and it transfers high-energy phosphate from phosphocreatine to ADP to keep up a constant cellular ATP level.

### Oxygen

Cardiac myocytes have only a small reserve of $O_2$, bound to myoglobin, so a continuous supply of $O_2$ is necessary to maintain mitochondrial ATP production. In a resting human, the myocardial $O_2$ consumption, ~10 mL/min/100 g of heart tissue, represents 65%–75% of the $O_2$ delivered in the coronary arterial blood, leaving little in reserve. Consequently, during exercise the **increased myocardial $O_2$ demand can only be met by increased coronary blood flow**. In other word, myocardial performance is critically dependent on coronary blood flow. Since the heart, unlike skeletal muscle, cannot stop for a rest, coronary perfusion must keep pace with mitochondrial demand. The 'engine out of fuel' hypothesis proposes that inadequate myocardial ATP production or delivery to the myofilaments may contribute to the poor performance of the heart in systolic heart failure.

### Metabolic substrates

The substrates consumed by the myocardium have been worked out by comparing coronary sinus (venous) and arterial plasma concentrations. Broadly speaking, **free fatty acids** normally supply 60%–90% of cardiac energy. The other 10%–40% is supplied by **glucose** and **lactate**. In contrast to skeletal muscle, well-oxygenated myocardium can oxidize blood lactate. This is a useful asset during hard exercise, since lactate is released into the bloodstream by the active skeletal muscle. During 25 min of cycling at moderate intensity (30%–55% maximal), glucose consumption by the human heart approximately doubles; however, at higher exercise intensities glucose consumption falls as the plasma lactate level increases. If the myocardium becomes hypoxic, it switches from lactate consumption to **anaerobic lactate production**, leading to intracellular acidosis and impaired contractility.

## Myocardial enzymes appear in plasma after a heart attack

Lactate is normally oxidized by the heart through the enzyme **myocardial lactic dehydrogenase** (LDH), an isoform specific to the heart. When myocytes undergo ischaemic damage after a coronary thrombosis, LDH and other intracellular enzymes, such as **creatine kinase** (MB) and **aspartate aminotransferase**, escape into the circulation. Their plasma levels can be used as a laboratory test for myocardial infarction. The plasma levels of **troponin T or I** are now the gold standard for detecting myocardial infarction because they are highly sensitive and highly specific for cardiac damage; plasma troponin T or I increase 2–4 h after an infarct and persists for up to a week.

---

### SUMMARY

- Cardiac output equals heart rate × ventricular stroke volume. Stroke volume is influenced by three physiological factors: (1) diastolic stretch increases contractile force; (2) noradrenaline and adrenaline increase contractility; (3) arterial pressure opposes ejection.
- Ventricular diastolic stretch is determined by filling pressure, that is, CVP on the right, pulmonary venous pressure on the left. Stretch increases the $Ca^{2+}$ sensitivity of myocytes and, therefore, contractile force and stroke work (stroke volume × pressure). This is called the length–tension relation/Frank–Starling mechanism.
- The Frank–Starling mechanism equalizes right and left stroke volumes and helps increase stroke volume during upright exercise and after transfusions. It reduces stroke volume during orthostasis (standing) and hypovolaemia.
- Human CVP, and therefore stroke volume, is influenced by blood volume, posture, sympathetic-mediated peripheral venous tone, the skeletal muscle pump and breathing.
- In heart failure, an excessively high CVP overdistends the heart. The increased radius $r$ impairs the conversion of active wall tension $T$ into internal pressure $P$, because $T = (r \times P)/2$ (Laplace's law). Treatment therefore aims to reduce CVP with diuretics.
- An increase in force mediated not by stretch but by neurohumoral agents is called an increase in contractility. Ventricular contractility is raised by the sympathetic neurotransmitter

noradrenaline and by circulating adrenaline. These activate the myocyte $\beta_1$ adrenergic receptor adenylate cyclase–cAMP–PKA cascade. The cascade enhances the action potential $Ca^{2+}$ current, boosts the SR $Ca^{2+}$ store and cytoplasmic $Ca^{2+}$ transient amplitude, and stimulates $Ca^{2+}$ reuptake into the store to speed up relaxation. The result is a stronger, shorter contraction, a bigger stroke volume, ejection fraction and systolic pressure and a reduced end-systolic volume. The pressure-volume loop becomes wider, taller and is shifted leftwards.

- Increased contractility steepens the Starling curve (stroke work versus filling pressure). The effect is graded, that is, proportional to sympathetic activity. The heart thus operates on a 'family of ventricular function curves'.

- Other positive inotropic influences include $\beta$ adrenergic receptor agonist drugs (isoprenaline, dobutamine), phosphodiesterase inhibitors (caffeine, milrinone), $Na^+/K^+$ pump inhibitors (digoxin, ouabain) and increased beat frequency (Bowditch effect). Premature beats (extra systoles) are weaker than normal and the beat after the compensatory pause is stronger than normal, due to the effect of time on $Ca^{2+}$ store restocking.

- Negative inotropic influences include myocardial ischaemia (causing hypoxia and acidosis) and chronic heart failure. Arrhythmias, a common complication, can result from reduced membrane potentials, increased intracellular $[Na^+]$ and premature discharge of overloaded SR $Ca^{2+}$ stores in early diastole, triggering afterdepolarization.

- An acute rise in arterial pressure increases the 'afterload' on ventricular myocytes, which reduces the stroke volume (the afterload–shortening relation, or pump function curve). Therefore, reduction of arterial pressure by vasodilator drugs is used to improve stroke volume in failing hearts.

- An acute rise in arterial pressure also evokes multiple, conflicting secondary effects. The subsequent diastolic distension raises contractile force (Starling's law) and, more slowly, contractility (Anrep effect). However, the baroreflex reduces sympathetic drive and contractility. Chronic hypertension evokes concentric ventricular hypertrophy and eventually heart failure.

- During exercise, changes in the peripheral circulation and heart cooperate to raise cardiac output. Peripheral venoconstriction and the skeletal muscle pump maintain or raise the CVP (preload) and end-diastolic volume, activating the Frank–Starling mechanism. End-systolic volume is reduced by sympathetic stimulation. Stroke volume can double. Vasodilatation in active muscle minimizes the rise in arterial pressure and afterload. Sympathetic stimulation raises the heart rate.

- Myocardial performance is tightly coupled to $O_2$ delivery by the coronary arteries. Much of the $O_2$ is consumed in raising ventricular pressure. Since emotional stress raises pressure, it should be avoided by patients with coronary artery insufficiency.

## FURTHER READING

Sequeira V, van der Velden J. The Frank–Starling Law: a jigsaw of titin proportions. *Biophysical Reviews* 2017; **9**(3): 259–67.

Ait-Mou Y, Hsu K, Farman GP, et al. Titin strain contributes to the Frank–Starling law of the heart by structural rearrangements of both thin- and thick-filament proteins. *Proceedings of the National Academy of Sciences* 2016; **113**(8): 2306–11.

Hausenloy DJ, Yellon DM. Ischaemic conditioning and reperfusion injury. *Nature Reviews. Cardiology* 2016; **13**(4): 193–209.

Heusch G, Rassaf T. Time to give up on cardioprotection? A critical appraisal of clinical studies on ischemic pre-, post-, and remote conditioning. *Circulation Research* 2016; **119**(5): 676–95.

Neves JS, Leite-Moreira AM, Neiva-Sousa M, et al. Acute myocardial response to stretch: what we (don't) know. *Frontiers in Physiology* 2016; **6**: 408.

Cingolani HE, Pérez NG, Cingolani OH, et al. The Anrep effect: 100 years later. *American Journal of Physiology. Heart and Circulatory Physiology* 2013; **304**(2): H175–82.

Coote JH. Myths and realities of the cardiac vagus. *The Journal of Physiology* 2013; **591**(17): 4073–85.

Kharbanda RK, Nielsen TT, Redington AN. Translation of remote ischaemic preconditioning into clinical practice. *Lancet* 2009; **374**(9700): 1557–65.

Neubauer S. The failing heart: an engine out of fuel. *New England Journal of Medicine* 2007; **356**(11): 1140–51.

Lewis ME, Al-Khalidi AH, Bonser RS, et al. Vagus nerve stimulation decreases left ventricular contractility in vivo in the human and pig heart. *The Journal of Physiology* 2001; **534**(Pt. 2): 547–52.

Patterson SW, Piper H, Starling EH. The regulation of the heartbeat. *The Journal of Physiology* 1914; **48**(6): 465–513.

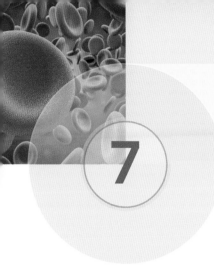

# Assessment of cardiac output and arterial pulse

## 7

### LEARNING OBJECTIVES

*After reading this chapter you should be able to:*

- define Fick's principle (cf. Fick's law of diffusion) (7.1);
- apply Fick's principle to estimate pulmonary blood flow from measurements of $O_2$ uptake (7.1);
- draw a typical concentration or temperature versus time plot for the indicator or thermal dilution method, and explain how cardiac output is derived from it (7.2);

- outline three modern 'high-tech' methods for estimating human stroke volume (7.3, 7.5);
- describe the relationship between central arterial pulse and cardiac output (7.4);
- define arterial compliance and state three major factors affecting it (7.4).

Cardiac output is the volume of blood ejected by one ventricle in 1 min, and equals the stroke volume × number of beats per minute. The need to measure human cardiac output arises in many areas of research, for example, evaluating the cardiac adaptation to physical training, and in clinical practice, to quantify the severity of cardiac disease and its response to treatment.

Cardiac output can be measured as a single entity in humans using **Fick's principle** or the **dilution method**. Alternatively, stroke volume can be measured separately by **Doppler ultrasound**, **radionuclide counting**, two-dimensional (2-D) **echocardiography** or cardiac magnetic resonance imaging, and the result multiplied by the heart rate to give cardiac output. The heart rate is obtained by counting the radial pulse, by electrocardiogram (ECG) or by a pulse oximeter (see Section 7.4). All of these cardiac output methods require complex technology. A much simpler and more convenient estimate, albeit rather indirect, is to feel a central **arterial pulse**. We will begin here with the gold standard but invasive method, Fick's principle, then move in the direction of less direct but less invasive methods. Fick's principle has a wider physiological importance besides cardiac output measurement. It is a general

principle describing the transport of any solute across a capillary bed, and is thus crucial to understanding a core role of the cardiovascular system, namely the uptake of $O_2$ in the lungs.

## 7.1 FICK'S PRINCIPLE AND PULMONARY OXYGEN TRANSPORT

In 1870, Adolf Fick, a German-born physician and physiologist, pointed out that the rate at which the pulmonary capillaries take up $O_2$ in the lungs must equal the increase in $O_2$ concentration in the blood multiplied by the pulmonary blood flow. Since the pulmonary blood flow is the right ventricular output, it follows that cardiac output can be calculated by measuring $O_2$ transport.

### Fick's principle quantifies oxygen uptake in the lungs

Fick's principle is more than just a method. It is basic to understanding $O_2$ uptake in the lungs, $CO_2$ elimination and many other physiological exchanges (Figure 7.1). The amount of $O_2$

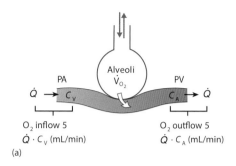

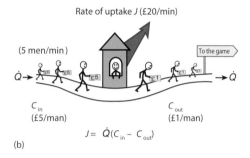

**Figure 7.1** Fick's principle. **(a)** Applied to measure pulmonary blood flow ($\dot{Q}$). PA, pulmonary artery containing venous blood; PV, pulmonary vein containing arterialized blood. For other symbols, see text. **(b)** Applied to measure flow ($\dot{Q}$) of football supporters through a gate, based on the rate of takings ($J$) and the 'concentration' of money in the supporters' pockets before and after the gate. In other scenarios, each individual could be a red cell giving up $CO_2$ to the lungs, or a volume of plasma giving up glucose to the brain. The principle has wide application.

carried into the lungs per minute in venous blood = pulmonary blood flow $\dot{Q}$ × venous $O_2$ concentration $C_V$:

$$O_2 \text{ in venous blood entering lungs per minute} = \dot{Q}C_V$$

Similarly, the amount of $O_2$ carried away from the lungs per minute in the oxygenated blood equals the pulmonary blood flow $\dot{Q}$ × the arterial $O_2$ concentration $C_A$:

$$O_2 \text{ in arterialized blood leaving lungs per minute} = \dot{Q}C_A$$

The amount of $O_2$ taken up by the blood as it passes through the lungs is the difference between the amount of $O_2$ entering and the amount leaving, that is:

$$O_2 \text{ uptake by pulmonary blood per minute} = \dot{Q}C_A - \dot{Q}C_V$$

In the steady state, the amount of $O_2$ taken up by the blood per minute must equal the amount of $O_2$ removed from the lung alveolar gas per minute, $\dot{V}_{O_2}$, so we can write:

$$O_2 \text{ removal from alveolar gas} = O_2 \text{ uptake by pulmonary blood}$$

or in symbols:

$$\dot{V}_{O_2} = \dot{Q}C_A - \dot{Q}C_V$$

Re-expressing this in terms of the $O_2$ arteriovenous concentration difference $C_A - C_V$:

$$\dot{V}_{O_2} = \dot{Q}(C_A - C_V) \qquad (7.1)$$

This is **Fick's equation**. It tells us that the rate of $O_2$ uptake from the inspired air, in mL $O_2$/min, equals pulmonary blood flow (in L/min) multiplied by the arteriovenous difference in $O_2$ concentration (in mL $O_2$/L of blood).

Since the pulmonary blood flow is the right ventricular output, we can rearrange the Fick's equation to work out the cardiac output, thus:

Cardiac output $\dot{Q}$ (L/min) =

$$\frac{O_2 \text{ uptake rate } \dot{V}_{O_2} \text{ (mL/min)}}{\text{Arterial } O_2 \text{ concentration } C_A - \text{Venous } O_2 \text{ concentration } C_V \text{ (mL/L)}}$$

An example should make this clear. A resting human absorbs ~250 mL $O_2$ per minute from the alveolar gas ($\dot{V}_{O_2}$). Arterial blood contains 195 mL $O_2$ per litre and the mixed venous blood entering the lungs contains 145 mL $O_2$ per litre; so, each litre of blood takes up 50 mL $O_2$ as it passes through the alveoli; that is, $(C_A - C_V) = 50$ mL/L. To take up 250 mL $O_2$, 5 L of blood are required (250/50). This amount of $O_2$ is taken up in 1 min. Right ventricular output at rest is therefore 5 L/min.

## Fick's method requires cardiac catheterization

Fick's method only became practicable in humans in the 20th century, when the advent of cardiac catheterization enabled **mixed venous blood** sampling from the right ventricle/pulmonary trunk. Mixed venous blood analysis tells us the average $O_2$ concentration entering the lungs. Because peripheral venous $O_2$ concentration varies markedly between tissues, for example, renal venous $O_2$ 170 mL/L, coronary venous $O_2$ 70 mL/L, peripheral venous blood is no good for this purpose. The different streams of venous blood only become fully mixed in the right ventricle. The difficult problem of sampling mixed venous blood in humans was solved by the German physician Werner Forssman, who in 1929 passed a ureteric catheter up his own arm vein into the right heart, watching its progress on an X-ray screen. This brave act founded human cardiac catheterization, won Forssman the disapproval of his head of department and, later, a Nobel prize.

The Fick method is now applied as follows. The subject's resting $O_2$ consumption, $\dot{V}_{O_2}$, is measured for 5–10 min by spirometry, or by collecting expired air in a Douglas bag. During this period, an arterial blood sample is taken from the brachial, radial or femoral artery, and a mixed venous sample is taken from the right ventricle outflow tract/pulmonary trunk, using a cardiac catheter introduced through the femoral or jugular vein. The $O_2$ concentration in each blood sample is measured and the cardiac output is calculated as described earlier.

## Fick's method has several limitations

Although Fick's method is the gold standard by which new methods are judged, it has its limitations. The $O_2$ uptake measurement takes 5–10 min to perform, so beat-by-beat changes in stroke volume cannot be resolved. Also, the method is only valid in the steady state, so a rapidly changing cardiac output cannot be measured. Being invasive, the method is inadvisable during hard exercise because the cardiac catheter may trigger an arrhythmia in a vigorously beating heart. The **indirect Fick's method** avoids cardiac catheterization and estimates $C_V$ indirectly, by the analysis of rebreathed gas, an approach used recently in an orbiting space laboratory.

## Fick's principle has many applications

Fick's principle is an important, general physiological principle that applies to the exchange of any material in any perfused organ, for example, glucose transport from blood to skeletal muscle or the brain (Section 10.10). Fick's principle even applies to heat exchange in a water-perfused radiator, or money turnover at the turnstile of a football ground (Figure 7.1b). In general terms, the transfer rate, $J$, of any substance between a flowing body and its surroundings equals the flow $\dot{Q}$ multiplied by the concentration difference between the incoming fluid, $C_{in}$, and the outgoing fluid, $C_{out}$:

$$J = \dot{Q}\left(C_{out} - C_{in}\right) \tag{7.2}$$

Fick's principle has therefore been used to work out the rate at which an organ consumes a metabolite, such as glucose, based on measurements of local blood flow and arteriovenous concentration difference.

## 7.2 INDICATOR AND THERMAL DILUTION METHODS

The thermal dilution method has been much used, but we will first consider its parent, the indicator dilution method, which is easier to understand. Both methods are also applications of Fick's principle, but ones in which $J = 0$ in equation 7.2, as it is assumed there is no transfer of temperature or indicator between the blood and tissues.

## Indicator dilution method

A known mass of a foreign substance, the indicator, is injected rapidly into a central vein or the right heart. The indicator must be confined to the bloodstream and easy to assay, such as dyes that bind to plasma albumin (Evans blue, indocyanine green), radiolabelled albumin or radiolabelled red cells. The indicator becomes diluted in the venous bloodstream, then carried through the heart and lungs and ejected into the systemic

arteries (Figure 7.2a). Systemic arterial blood is sampled from the radial or femoral artery, and its indicator content is plotted against time.

For simplicity, let us first suppose that the ejected bolus of arterial blood has a uniform concentration of the indicator (Figure 7.2b). The concentration versus time plot tells us two things: the time $t$ taken by the labelled bolus to pass a given point and the average concentration of indicator in the bolus. Concentration $C$ is the injected mass $m$ divided by the volume of plasma in which the indicator has become distributed, $V_D$; in other words, $C = m/V_D$. The distribution volume of the indicator is thus:

$$V_D = m/C$$

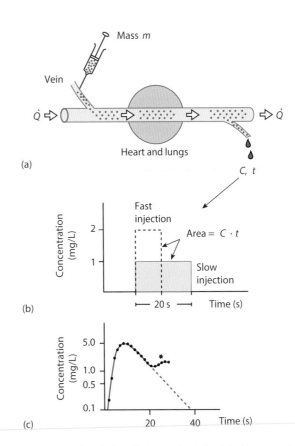

(a)

(b)

(c)

**Figure 7.2** Hamilton's dye dilution method. **(a)** Arterial concentration $C$ depends on the mass of indicator injected ($m$) and the volume of blood in which it became diluted. **(b)** Idealized plot of $C$ against time. Area $C \times t$ is 20 mg s $L^{-1}$ here. Height and duration depend on injection rate, but area is not affected; an increase in concentration produced by a fast injection is offset by the shorter duration of the bolus, due to a smaller distribution volume. If $m$ is 1 mg, the cardiac output of plasma is 1 mg/20 mg s $L^{-1}$ = 0.05 L/s, or 3 L/min. For a haematocrit of 0.4, the cardiac output of blood is 5 L/min. **(c)** The grim reality is that the concentration peaks and decays over time, then shows a recirculation hump. Fortunately, when $C$ is plotted on a logarithmic scale, the early decay is linear. This allows extrapolation past the recirculation hump (asterisk). The area under the extrapolated curve is used to calculate the cardiac output. (After Asmussen E, Nielsen M. *Acta Physiologica Scandinavica* 1953; 27(2–3): 217, with permission from Wiley-Blackwell.)

For example, if 1 mg of indicator produced a mean plasma concentration of 1 mg/L, its volume of distribution must be 1 L. If this volume takes $t$ seconds to pass the sampling point, the left ventricle must be ejecting plasma at the rate $V_D/t$. In Figure 7.2b, the rate is 1 L in 20 s, or 3 L/min. Thus, the plasma output is:

$$\text{Cardiac output (plasma)} = \frac{V_D}{t} = \frac{\text{Mass of indicator, } m}{\text{Mean concentration } C \times \text{passage time } t}$$

The output of blood is the plasma output divided by $1 -$ haematocrit; the haematocrit is the fraction of the blood that is made up of red cells (0.40–0.45).

Since the denominator $C \times t$ is the area under the plot of concentration versus time, we can simplify the previous expression to:

$$\text{Cardiac output (plasma)} = \frac{\text{Mass of indicator, } m}{\text{Area under the } C \text{ versus } t \text{ plot}}$$

This simplification is very helpful because the arterial concentration is not constant (Figure 7.2c; cf. Figure 7.2b); however, we can still measure the area under the curve. The concentration rises to a peak, after which it decays exponentially because the ventricle only ejects about two-thirds of its contents per systole. The residual indicator in the ventricle is diluted by indicator-free venous blood returning during the next diastole, and the diluted blood is in turn only partially ejected during systole, and so on.

After about 15 s the concentration decay curve is interrupted by a recirculation hump, the asterisk in Figure 7.2c. This is caused by blood with a high indicator content returning to the heart after one complete transit of the myocardial circulation, which is the shortest, quickest circulation in the body. To use the area equation, we need to work out the area under the curve excluding the recirculation hump. To this end, the pre-hump part of the decay curve is extrapolated underneath the recirculation hump. A semi-logarithmic plot converts the exponential decay into a straight line, which can then be extrapolated under the hump to a negligible concentration (usually 1% of the peak), as shown in Figure 7.2c. The area under the corrected $C$ versus $t$ curve is used to calculate the cardiac output.

A modern, computerized version of the method is based on intravenous **lithium ion** injection. The lithium can be detected in the arterial blood with an ion-sensitive electrode. It appears that lithium loss during passage through the lungs is negligible.

## Pros and cons of the indicator dilution method

The indicator dilution method agrees with the Fick's method to within 5%. The dilution method has a better time resolution (30 s) than the Fick's method (5–10 min). Also, it can be used during exercise because there is no need for ventricular catheterization. However, the error involved in extrapolating the decay curve is a drawback, and becomes a serious limitation in diseased hearts, where the initial part of the decay curve may be short and distorted.

## Thermal dilution method

This variant method has been used widely in cardiac departments, owing to its greater convenience. Instead of a soluble indicator, temperature is used. A thermistor (temperature sensor) at the tip of a Swan–Ganz catheter is advanced into the pulmonary trunk/artery. A known mass of cold saline is then injected quickly into the right atrium, right ventricle or proximal pulmonary trunk. The distal thermistor records the dilution of the cold saline by the warm pulmonary bloodstream. Cardiac output is calculated as the injected amount of heat (i.e. cold) divided by the area under the temperature/time plot.

## Pros and cons of thermal dilution

The major advantage of thermal dilution over indicator dilution is that it circumvents the recirculation hump problem. The cold saline has warmed up to body temperature by the time it recirculates to the right ventricle. Heat transfer across the walls of the right ventricle and pulmonary artery can cause an overestimation of the distribution volume and hence cardiac output, but a computed correction is made for this.

## 7.3 AORTIC FLOW BY PULSED DOPPLER METHOD

To estimate left ventricular stroke volume, pulses of ultrasound (US) are directed down the ascending aorta from a transmitter crystal placed over the suprasternal notch (Figure 7.3, top). The moving red cells alter the frequency of the US reflected off them, and the frequency shift is proportional to the red cell velocity. This is called the Doppler shift; it is analogous to the change in pitch of a police car siren as it speeds past. The reflected US is recorded and used to compute the mean blood velocity across the aorta, millisecond by millisecond. The aortic blood velocity is plotted against time (Figure 7.3, bottom) and interpreted (see the following section).

## Stroke distance is distance advanced along the aorta per ejection

Since distance is velocity × time, the distance that blood advances along the aorta during one systole, the **stroke distance**, equals the area under the aortic velocity–time curve. To convert stroke distance into stroke volume, the cross-sectional area of the aorta is measured by 2-D echocardiography (see Section 2.6). The area, in $cm^2$, multiplied by stroke

## Stroke volume and pulse pressure are linked by arterial compliance

The relationship between left ventricular stroke volume and systemic arterial pressure is one of the key haemodynamic relationships of the circulation. It is introduced here and is analysed in more detail in Chapter 8. During ejection, most of the stroke volume (70%–80% at rest) is accommodated in the elastic arteries because the ventricle ejects blood faster than it can drain away through the resistance vessels. The increase in arterial volume distends the arteries, and the arterial wall tension raises the blood pressure (BP) (Figure 7.4). Therefore, the magnitude of the increase in pressure, or pulse pressure, depends on the **stroke volume** and the **compliance** (distensibility) of the arterial system. Compliance is defined as change in volume per unit change in pressure:

$$\text{Arterial compliance} = \frac{\text{Increase in arterial blood volume}}{\text{Increase in arterial pressure}} \quad (7.3)$$

Arterial compliance in a young adult is ~2 mL per mmHg at normal BP. The increase in arterial blood volume during systole equals stroke volume minus the volume that drains away during the ejection period (run-off). Inserting this statement into the top line of equation 7.3 and rearranging, we see that

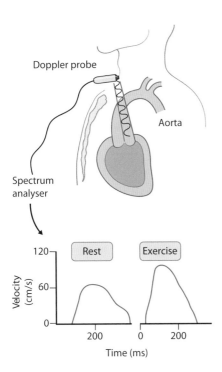

**Figure 7.3** Transaortic pulsed Doppler ultrasound (US) method. The Doppler shift in the frequency of reflected US is used to compute the mean velocity of blood across the aorta at successive moments during systole. Stroke distance is the area under curve. (From Innes JA, Simon TD, Murphy K, et al. *Quarterly Journal of Experimental Physiology* 1988; 73(3): 323–41, with permission from Wiley-Blackwell.)

distance in cm, gives stroke volume in cm³, less the volume drained off by the coronary arteries.

## Pros and cons of the doppler method

The Doppler method is difficult to calibrate and has noise problems. However, it has two enormous advantages: (1) it is non-invasive; (2) it has an extremely high temporal resolution, recording every instant of ejection, unlike Fick's method or dilutional techniques.

## 7.4 CENTRAL ARTERIAL PULSE AND ITS RELATION TO CARDIAC OUTPUT

The oldest, cheapest, quickest and easiest way to assess human cardiac output is to palpate a central pulse, such as at the carotid artery in the neck. **Heart rate** can be counted and the **strength of the pulse** can be estimated subjectively. A strong pulse is the result of a large stroke volume, for example, during exercise; a weak pulse is the result of a low stroke volume, for example, after a haemorrhage. What the finger detects is the expansion of the artery as pressure rises during systole. The rise in pressure, or **pulse pressure**, equals systolic minus diastolic pressure. Pulse pressure is easily quantified by sphygmomanometry usually at the brachial artery (Section 8.5), and is closely related to stroke volume.

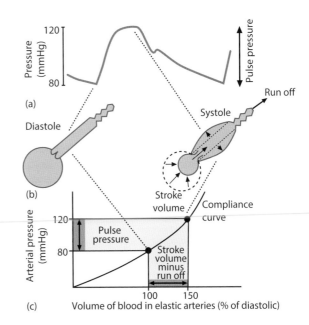

**Figure 7.4** Relationship between pulse pressure and stroke volume. Dotted lines link coincident points in time. **(a)** Aortic pressure wave. **(b)** Ejection of left ventricle stroke volume into elastic arteries. **(c)** Pressure/volume relationship (compliance curves) of young human aorta. Note the increase in stiffness (steeper slope) with pressure. (Based on Nichols WW, O'Rourke MF. *McDonald's Blood Flow in Arteries: theoretical, experimental and clinical principles*, 5th edn. London: Hodder Arnold, 2005.)

the increase in arterial pressure per heartbeat, the **pulse pressure**, is related to stroke volume as follows:

$$\text{Pulse pressure} = \frac{\text{Stroke volume} - \text{Runoff in systole}}{\text{Arterial compliance}} \quad (7.4)$$

Changes in pulse pressure can thus serve as a guide to changes in stroke volume. In hospitals, systolic and diastolic blood pressure (and therefore pulse pressure) is monitored non-invasively with sphygmomanometry and recorded regularly as part of the patient's nursing 'observations'. In high dependency and intensive care units, continuous direct recording of arterial pressure is often required using an automatic flushing pressure catheter placed directly into an artery (e.g. brachial, femoral or radial).

## Arterial compliance is not a fixed quantity

A significant problem when interpreting pulse pressure is that arterial compliance does not have a unique, unchanging value; its magnitude varies, as follows:

- Arterial compliance falls (stiffness increases) as pressure and volume increase; so, the arterial pressure/volume plot is a steepening curve (Figure 7.4c).
- Arterial compliance is reduced by high ejection velocities, because the artery wall is a viscoelastic material and takes time to relax. During exercise, the pulse pressure increases relatively more than the stroke volume because there is less time for viscous relaxation of the wall during a fast ejection.

---

**CONCEPT BOX 7.1**

**ARTERIAL COMPLIANCE LINKS PULSE PRESSURE AND STROKE VOLUME**

- Compliance is a measure of distensibility; it is the inverse of stiffness. Arterial compliance $C$ is defined as the increase in blood volume in the arterial system, $\Delta V$, that results from a given increase in arterial pressure, $\Delta P$. Thus $C = \Delta V / \Delta P$.
- Pulse pressure is the increase in pressure between diastole and systole.
- From the above definitions, pulse pressure $\Delta P$ = stroke volume (minus the run-off during ejection)/arterial compliance). Pulse pressure can thus be increased by a rise in stroke volume (e.g. exercise) or a fall in arterial compliance (e.g. ageing).
- Arterial compliance falls as pressure increases, due to the tensing of collagen in the artery wall. Consequently, a rise in mean arterial pressure also causes a rise in pulse pressure.
- Arterial compliance declines with age due to arteriosclerosis, a diffuse stiffening of the media of elastic vessels. As a result, pulse pressure can double between youth and old age.

---

- Arterial compliance declines with age, due to a degenerative stiffening of elastic arteries called **arteriosclerosis**. Consequently, pulse pressure increases with age, and this increases stroke work (Sections 8.4 and 17.7). Arteriosclerosis is the diffuse stiffening of ageing elastic arteries, due primarily to changes in the tunica media. It should not be confused with **atheroma**, which is primarily a cholesterol-related disease of the tunica intima (Table 17.4).

## Pros and cons of pulse method

The variable nature of arterial compliance can introduce some ambiguity, as can run-off during ejection, since run-off increases when peripheral resistance falls. Nevertheless, changes in pulse pressure, recorded with nothing more sophisticated than a wrist watch and sphygmomanometer cuff, offer a convenient, instant bedside indication of changes in cardiac output in an individual from hour to hour, for example, during recovery from an acute haemorrhage. At a more sophisticated level, computer models make reasonably accurate computations of acute changes in stroke volume from continuous recordings of arterial pressure. The latter can be measured continuously by an electronic, finger volume-clamp method (see Finapress, Section 8.5).

## Pulse oximetry monitors pulse rate

The heart rate can be measured using a watch and palpation of the radial artery, or a miniaturized ECG that transmits the heart rate to a wrist monitor, or a **pulse oximeter**. An oximeter is a small device that shines a light through superficial tissue, usually an earlobe or finger, and measures the transmitted light using a photoelectric cell. Red cells absorb some of the light, and oxyhaemoglobin absorbs a different wavelength to deoxyhaemoglobin. As the arterial system expands with each pulse, the light transmission changes. From this, the pulse rate and blood $O_2$ saturation are computed.

## 7.5 RADIONUCLIDE VENTRICULOGRAPHY, 2-D ECHOCARDIOGRAPHY, CARDIAC MAGNETIC RESONANCE IMAGING AND OTHER METHODS

### Radionuclide ventriculography

A gamma-emitting radionuclide, usually a technetium-99 compound bound to red cells, is injected intravenously, and a precordial gamma camera records the gamma counts emanating from the ventricles. The difference between the radioactive content of the ventricles in diastole and systole is used to calculate the ejection fraction and stroke volume. The method requires the services of a nuclear medicine department.

## 2-D echocardiography and cardiac magnetic resonance imaging

2-D echocardiography is non-invasive, and can measure the end-diastolic and end-systolic dimensions of the ventricle (Figures 2.9 and 6.24) in both long axis and short axis views. The three-dimensional stroke volume and ejection fraction are then computed from the linear dimensions, using an assumed chamber geometry (known as Simpson's biplane method). Typical values are listed in Table 2.2. **Magnetic resonance imaging** of the cardiac chambers can be used in a similar way but is more accurate because it has superior 'edge detection' between the myocardium and the blood inside the chamber.

## Impedance cardiography

Chest and neck leads pass a small current through the thorax to measure its cyclically changing electrical resistance (impedance). Aortic blood volume increases and decreases over each cardiac cycle, and because blood is a better conductor than air, the electrical impedance of the thorax oscillates likewise. Aortic stroke volume can be estimated, albeit rather indirectly, from the impedance oscillation. The method is non-invasive, but very indirect.

## Electromagnetic 'flowmeter'

This method is invasive and is only used in laboratory animals for research purposes. Under general anaesthesia, a miniature, semicircular magnet is surgically implanted, with its magnetic poles on either side of the blood vessel of interest, for example, the pulmonary artery. Blood is an electrical conductor, and as it cuts through the magnetic field it induces an electrical potential, which is measured. The potential is proportional to the blood velocity (cm/s), not flow. To convert mean velocity to flow, the internal diameter of the vessel is required. Being small, an electromagnetic flowmeter can be left inside a conscious animal, transmitting a signal by telemetry (radio waves). In this way, much has been learned about the regulation of stroke volume in unfettered, conscious animals, such as dogs running on a treadmill.

## SUMMARY

- The gold standard method for measuring human cardiac output is **Fick's principle**. This states that solute transfer rate = blood flow × concentration difference between incoming and outgoing blood. $O_2$ uptake in the lungs is measured over 5–10 min by spirometry or expired air collection. The $O_2$ content of mixed venous blood is measured in a blood sample taken from the right ventricle by cardiac catheterization. Arterial blood is sampled from a systemic artery. Pulmonary blood flow, that is, right ventricular output, is then calculated from Fick's equation.

- **Indicator dilution** and **thermal dilution** methods have a better time resolution. A known mass of dye or cold saline is injected quickly into the right heart, and the concentration or temperature is recorded at a point downstream. Concentration or temperature is plotted versus time. Knowing the injected mass $m$, and the average downstream concentration $C$ (or temperature), the volume of blood in which the indicator has distributed can be calculated: $V_D = m/C$. Volume $V_D$ is divided by the time taken for the labelled blood to pass the sampling point. This equals the cardiac output.

- **Pulsed Doppler US** measures the average blood velocity across the aorta, millisecond by millisecond. The area under the velocity/time plot gives the distance advanced per ejection (stroke distance). Stroke volume is stroke distance × aortic area, which is measured by US.

- **Radionuclide ventriculography** measures the radioactive counts present in the ventricle during end-diastole and end-systole. The stroke volume and ejection fraction are calculated from the difference between counts.

- **2-D echocardiography and cardiac magnetic resonance imaging** record the changes in ventricular dimensions between diastole and systole, to estimate stroke volume and ejection fraction.

- With all methods that estimate stroke volume, the cardiac output is calculated as heart rate × stroke volume. The pulse rate can be monitored by **pulse oximetry** or **ECG**.

- **Arterial pulse examination** is the simplest bedside method for assessing cardiac output. Heart rate is determined by counting the pulse. Sphygmomanometry measures the pulse pressure (systolic minus diastolic pressure). **Pulse pressure** is proportional to stroke volume, although the relationship is complicated by run-off, non-linear aortic compliance, dependence on ejection rate and age-related arterial stiffening (arteriosclerosis). A computerized, continuous display of cardiac output based on finger pulse monitoring is used in intensive care units.

## FURTHER READING

Thiele RH, Bartels K, Gan TJ. Cardiac output monitoring: a contemporary assessment and review. *Critical Care Medicine* 2015; **43**(1): 177–85.

Chandra S, Skali H, Blankstein R. Novel techniques for assessment of left ventricular systolic function. *Heart Failure Reviews* 2011; **16**(4): 327–37.

Mor-Avi V, Sugeng L, Lang RM. Real-Time 3-dimensional echocardiography: an integral component of the routine echocardiographic examination in adult patients? *Circulation.* 2009; **119**(2): 314–29.

Bogert LW, van Lieshout JJ. Non-invasive pulsatile arterial pressure and stroke volume changes from the human finger. *Experimental Physiology* 2005; **90**(4): 437–46.

Band DM, Linton RA, O'Brien TK, et al. The shape of indicator dilution curves used for cardiac output measurement in man. *The Journal of Physiology* 1997; **498**(Pt 1): 225–9.

Schelbert HR, Verba JW, Johnson AD, et al. Nontraumatic determination of left ventricular ejection fraction by radionuclide angiocardiography. *Circulation* 1975; **51**(5): 902–9.

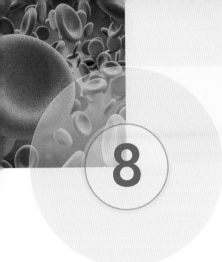

# Haemodynamics: flow, pressure and resistance

# 8

## LEARNING OBJECTIVES

*After reading this chapter you should be able to:*

- use Darcy's law of flow to link mean arterial pressure, cardiac output and peripheral resistance (8.1);
- sketch laminar and turbulent flow patterns and state where they occur (8.2);
- state the relationship between arterial pulse pressure, arterial compliance and stroke volume (8.4, 7.4);
- draw an arterial pressure pulse, label and scale it, and explain its main features (8.4);
- explain how arterial stiffening raises cardiac work (8.4);
- explain the cuff method for measuring human blood pressure (8.5);
- use Poiseuille's law to explain how arteriolar radius regulates flow and arterial pressure (8.7);

- show how Laplace's law contributes to aneurysm progression (8.7);
- state the factors governing blood viscosity and their clinical significance (8.8);
- draw a graph showing blood flow as a function of arterial pressure in the absence and presence of autoregulation (8.9);
- list the key factors determining the volume of blood in peripheral veins (8.10);
- explain how human central venous pressure can be estimated by inspecting neck veins (8.10);
- explain how gravity affects arterial and venous pressures on standing (8.11);
- describe the skeletal muscle pump and its three beneficial effects (8.12).

## 8.1 HYDRAULIC PRINCIPLES: THE LAWS OF DARCY AND BERNOULLI

The science of haemodynamics concerns the relationship between blood flow, blood pressure and hydraulic resistance. The simplest guide to these issues is Darcy's law, which was introduced in Chapter 1.

### Darcy's law relates flow to pressure difference

Henry Darcy was a French civil engineer who studied the flow of water through the gravel beds of the fountains in Dijon. In 1856, Darcy reported that flow in the steady state, $\dot{Q}$, is linearly proportional to the pressure difference between two points, $P_1 - P_2$. That is to say:

$$\dot{Q} = K(P_1 - P_2) = \frac{(P_1 - P_2)}{R} \qquad (8.1a)$$

The proportionality coefficient $K$ is called the hydraulic conductance, which is in effect the ease of flow. Its reciprocal is called the hydraulic resistance, $R$ – the difficulty of flow. Darcy's law serves as a way of defining what we mean by 'resistance' and can be applied to channels or tubes of any geometry, including blood vessels. For example, blood flow through the kidney is equal to the pressure in the renal artery minus the pressure in the renal vein, divided by renal vascular resistance.

The flow through the systemic circulation is the cardiac output, $CO$, and the pressure difference driving it equals mean aortic pressure $\bar{P}_a$ minus the central venous pressure (CVP). The systemic resistance is called the total peripheral resistance (TPR). Putting these symbols into Darcy's law, we have:

$$CO = \frac{(\bar{P}_a - CVP)}{TPR} \qquad (8.1b)$$

All blood pressures are conventionally expressed as pressure above atmospheric pressure, and since CVP is close to atmospheric pressure, $CVP \cong 0$. Equation 8.1b therefore simplifies to $CO \cong \bar{P}_a / TPR$. This can be rearranged to answer the fundamental question: **What determines mean arterial blood pressure?** The answer is that mean arterial pressure is determined by $CO$ and $TPR$:

$$\bar{P}_a \simeq CO \times TPR$$

or in words,

**Mean arterial blood pressure ≈ cardiac output**

**× total peripheral resistance**

## Bernoulli's theory includes additional kinds of fluid energy

Darcy's law deals with pressure, but this is only one of three kinds of mechanical energy that affect flow. The other two are gravitational potential energy and kinetic energy, as recognized by Bernoulli, an 18th-century Swiss mathematician and physicist, who became a professor of mathematics at the age of 25. Bernoulli's theory states that the energy loss between points A and B, in the steady state, is the difference in the mechanical energy of the fluid; and the mechanical energy is the sum of the pressure energy, potential energy and kinetic energy:

- **Pressure energy** equals pressure × volume, $P \times V$.
- **Potential (gravitational) energy** is the capacity of a mass to do work in a gravitational field by virtue of its height. The potential energy of blood relative to the heart is the blood mass (volume $V$ × density $\rho$) × height above the heart $h$ × acceleration due to gravity $g$.
- **Kinetic energy** is the energy of movement. It depends on mass and velocity, increasing in proportion to velocity squared ($v^2$). The kinetic energy of flowing blood is $\rho V v^2 / 2$, where $V$ is blood volume.

Adding the three energies together we have:

Energy loss per unit volume of blood (from A to B)

$$= (\Delta P + \rho g h + \rho v^2) \qquad (8.2)$$

Note that both Darcy's law and Bernoulli's law apply to steady-state flow, that is, flow that is not varying with time. If the flow is pulsatile, as in arteries, the laws still apply to the mean flow, but they do not tell us how the flow varies instant by instant.

## Application of Bernoulli's theory to the circulation

### Pressure falls inside a stenosed artery

If blood passing along an artery encounters a stenosed (narrowed), atheromatous segment, blood velocity increases in the narrow segment (Figure 8.1), just as water velocity in a river increases when the banks narrow. Since $v$ increases, some of the fluid energy is converted into kinetic energy, leaving less energy in the form of pressure (Bernoulli's theory). Consequently, the pressure gradient across the vascular wall falls within the stenosis and this may exacerbate the narrowing if the segment is compliant. At the exit, blood flows into the wider segment despite a contrary pressure gradient, consistent with the fact that flow occurs down a gradient of total energy rather than pressure alone.

### A kinetic energy gradient aids cardiac filling

Kinetic energy accounts for ~12% of the total mechanical energy of venous blood in a resting human. On entering the ventricle, blood velocity and hence kinetic energy fall virtually to zero. There is therefore a kinetic energy gradient between the central veins and ventricle, which aids ventricular filling. To put it another way, the momentum of the returning blood contributes to ventricular expansion.

### Gravitational 'puzzles' in humans

Although Darcy's law is adequate for many purposes in vascular physiology, the more comprehensive Bernoulli's theory can resolve several apparent puzzles. For example, during

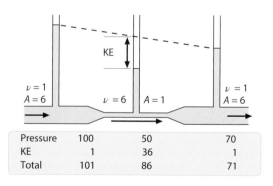

**Figure 8.1** Basic Bernoulli hydraulics: flow is driven by the total mechanical energy gradient. For a given volume flow, velocity $v$ increases where the cross-sectional area $A$ narrows (e.g. arterial atheroma). Pressure energy is converted into kinetic energy KE at this point. Where the tube widens, KE is reconverted to pressure. Flow from the narrow to the wide section is against the pressure gradient but down the total energy gradient.

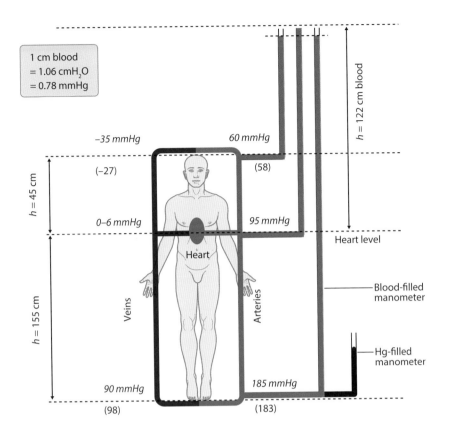

**Figure 8.2** Effect of gravity on arterial and venous pressure in a standing human. Red manometers are filled with blood, the black one (lower right) with mercury. Pressures in italics are central pressure plus pressure due to vertical fluid column. Pressures in brackets represents actual values for flowing blood, which are modified slightly by the arterial and venous resistances.

standing the mean arterial pressure is ~95 mmHg in the proximal aorta and 183 mmHg in the dorsalis pedis artery of the foot (Figure 8.2); yet, blood flows from the aorta to the foot, seemingly in defiance of Darcy's law. The explanation is that the total energy of arterial blood per unit volume is the same (or very slightly less) at the foot than in the proximal aorta and the apparent difference is due to the gravitational potential energy at the two sites, equivalent to a pressure of 90 mm Hg. The energy per unit volume of blood at the aortic root is 95 + 90 = 185 mm Hg, compared with the foot's 183 mmHg. The small difference, 2 mmHg, suffices to drive flow from the aorta to the dorsalis pedis artery, because large arteries offer little resistance to flow.

## 8.2 PATTERNS OF BLOOD FLOW: LAMINAR, TURBULENT, SINGLE-FILE

Three patterns of flow occur in the circulation: laminar flow; turbulent flow; and single-file or bolus flow (Figures 8.3 and 8.4). Laminar flow occurs in normal arteries, arterioles, venules and veins. Turbulent flow occurs in the ventricles and stenosed arteries. Single-file flow occurs in capillaries.

### Laminar flow has smooth, parallel streamlines

When a liquid flows through a smooth cylindrical tube at not too high a velocity, the liquid behaves like a set of infinitesimally thin concentric shells (laminae) that slide past each other (Figure 8.3a, right). The lamina in contact with the vessel wall has zero velocity due to molecular cohesive forces – the **zero-slip condition**. The adjacent lamina slides slowly past the zero-slip lamina. The third lamina slides past the second lamina, and because the second lamina is itself moving, the third lamina has a higher velocity relative to the tube wall, and so on, until maximum velocity is reached in the centre of the tube. Blood in the centre of the vessel therefore has a higher velocity than blood near the wall. You can see the same effect during any riverside stroll; the current is faster in the centre than near the banks. For a simple fluid such as water, **the velocity profile across a cylindrical tube is a parabola**. For a particulate suspension, such as blood, the profile is more blunted (Figure 8.3a, red line). At the **entrance** to a tube, where there has been insufficient time for the parabolic profile to develop, the velocity profile is almost flat (Figure 8.3a, left). This is the situation in the **ascending aorta**, where the flat profile simplifies the estimation of aortic flow by Doppler ultrasound (US) (Section 7.3).

### Laminar shearing of blood creates a marginal plasma layer

The sliding motion of one lamina past another – like one hand rubbing over the other – is called **shear**. Shear causes the red cells to orientate preferentially in the direction of flow and drift a little towards the central axis (**axial flow of**

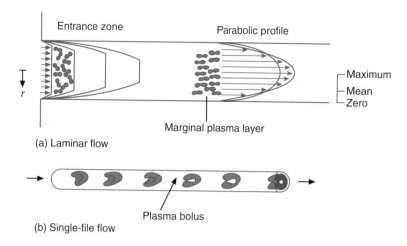

(a) Laminar flow

Marginal plasma layer

Entrance zone

Parabolic profile

Maximum
Mean
Zero

Plasma bolus

(b) Single-file flow

**Figure 8.3** Blood flow pattern in **(a)** a large vessel or **(b)** capillary. In **(a)**, the arrow length indicates the velocity of each lamina. For a Newtonian (one in which viscosity is constant) fluid in fully developed laminar flow, velocity $\nu$ is a parabolic function of radial position $r$, namely $\nu = \nu_{max}(1 - r^2/R^2)$, where $R$ is tube radius. For non-Newtonian blood, the velocity profile is blunter (red line). The gradient of the velocity curve, called the 'shear rate', is greatest at the margins. In capillaries **(b)**, the red cells deform into parachute/slipper configurations (left) and folded shapes (right). (After Chien S. *Microvascular Research* 1992; 44(3): 243–54, with permission from Elsevier.)

red cells). This leaves a thin, cell-deficient layer of plasma next to the vessel wall called the **marginal plasma layer**, which is 2–4 µm thick. The marginal plasma layer is important because it greatly facilitates the flow of blood through narrow resistance vessels (Fåhræus–Lindqvist effect, Section 8.8). It also contributes to the low haematocrit in microvessels (Fåhræus–effect, Section 8.8).

## Laminar shear stress tugs on the endothelium

The friction between the molecules in adjacent laminae causes each lamina to exert a dragging, tugging force on its neighbour, called **shear stress**. The shear stress increases with **shear rate** (rate of sliding) and fluid viscosity. At the vessel wall, the **wall shear stress** tugs on the glycocalyx, a polymer coat rooted in the endothelium (Figure 9.2). This stresses the endothelium, with a mean shear stress of 0.5–1.5 Pa in human arteries, which stimulates the endothelium to secrete regulatory, vasoactive agents such as nitric oxide (Chapter 9). In some individuals with hypertension, atheroma or Marfan's syndrome, the high wall shear stresses in the proximal aorta (peak >4 Pa) can even tear the vessel wall, creating a **dissecting aortic aneurysm**. Blood passes through the endothelial tear and tracks along the aortic wall in the subintimal plane, with potentially fatal results. An interim measure, before emergency surgery, is to reduce CO and hence shear stress with cardioinhibitory drugs.

## Turbulence

If the pressure driving fluid through a tube is progressively increased, a point is reached where flow no longer increases linearly with pressure, but increases as the square root of pressure (Figure 8.4). This marks the transition from laminar flow to a disorganized, turbulent flow. In turbulent flow, chaotic cross-currents dissipate more of the pressure energy as heat. The conditions that provoke turbulence were defined in 1883 by the engineer Sir Osborne Reynolds, who visualized turbulence using dyes. Turbulence is encouraged

by a high fluid velocity $\nu$, a large tube diameter $D$ and a high fluid density ($\rho$, rho) because these factors increase fluid momentum and encourage the persistence of flow distortions. Turbulence is discouraged by a high viscosity ($\eta$, eta), which damps out flow deviations. The dimensionless ratio of the pro- to antiturbulence factors is called the **Reynolds number**, $Re$:

$$Re = \frac{\nu D \rho}{\eta}$$

The critical Reynolds number for the onset of turbulence is ~2000 for steady flow down a rigid, straight, uniform tube, and <2000 in blood vessels where the flow is pulsatile and the vessels are neither rigid nor straight. Even so, $Re$ in most blood vessels is well below the critical value; for example, $Re$ is ~0.5 in resistance vessels.

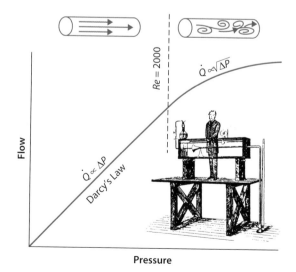

$Re = 2000$

$\dot{Q} \propto \sqrt{\Delta P}$

$\dot{Q} \propto \Delta P$
Darcy's Law

Flow

Pressure

**Figure 8.4** Pressure–flow relation for a Newtonian fluid in a rigid tube. Darcy's law is the straight line through the origin. This breaks down when turbulence begins. The inset shows the apparatus devised by Sir Osborne Reynolds to study the onset of turbulence. The flow pattern (top) was visualized by injecting dye into the fluid.

Turbulence occurs normally in the ventricles, and can also occur in the human aorta and pulmonary artery during peak flow, creating an **innocent systolic ejection murmur** (Section 2.5). In the human aortic root, during peak ejection, $Re$ reaches ~4600 (peak velocity $v$ = 70 cm/s, diameter $D$ = 2.5 cm, blood density $\rho$ = 1.06 g/cm³, blood viscosity $\eta$ = 0.04 gcm⁻¹s⁻¹, or 4 mPa.s). An innocent ejection murmur may develop during exercise (because ejection velocity increases) and during pregnancy/anaemia (because blood viscosity falls).

Pathological turbulence can occur in leg arteries roughened by atheromatous plaques. The turbulence can cause a local murmur, audible through the stethoscope (a **bruit**), and sometimes a palpable **thrill**. By contrast, normal laminar blood flow is silent.

## Single-file (bolus) flow occurs in capillaries

A capillary, diameter 5–6 μm, is narrower than a human red cell (8 μm). Consequently, red cells must bend into a folded, parachute-like configuration to pass through capillaries – a cartoon-like spectacle when seen *in vivo*. Since the deformed red cell spans the full width of the capillary, the cells are compelled to travel single-file. The plasma trapped between each pair of red cells travels as a bolus at uniform velocity (bolus flow). This eliminates much of the internal friction associated with laminar flow, so bolus flow is a very low resistance type of flow. At the capillary wall, red cell friction is reduced by the 'shagpile' of biopolymers coating the endothelium, that is, the glycocalyx (Figure 9.2).

As explained earlier, capillary flow depends on the **deformability of red cells**. In **sickle cell anaemia**, red cells contain an abnormal haemoglobin that polymerizes in hypoxic situations. The polymerization causes the red cells to become sickle-shaped, rigid and adhesive to endothelium and each other. These changes impair the passage of the red cells through microvessels, leading to tissue ischaemia, painful 'sickling crises' and strokes.

**White cells** (leukocytes) are rounder and much stiffer than red cells. Therefore, a leukocyte moves less freely along a microvessel, and often creates a little traffic jam of red cells behind it. During inflammation, the leukocytes adhere to the endothelium, particularly in small venules, raising the resistance to flow and impairing tissue perfusion. This happens in inflammation, ischaemia, severe haemorrhagic hypotension and venous leg ulcers.

## 8.3 MEASUREMENT OF BLOOD FLOW

It is often necessary to measure blood flow for research or for clinical evaluation, for example, in an ischaemic or ulcerated leg. The assessment of human coronary blood flow and other specialized circulations is covered in Chapter 15.

In *anaesthetized animals*, the velocity of blood in large vessels can be measured by a surgically implanted **electromagnetic velocity flowmeter** (Section 7.5), or by **hot-wire anemometry**, in which the cooling of a heated wire in the bloodstream is proportional to blood velocity. Blood flow in smaller regions can be assessed by giving a brief intra-arterial injection of **radiolabelled microspheres**, with a diameter of ~15 μm. The microspheres are washed into the tissue in proportion to local blood flow, and lodge in some of the terminal arterioles. The distribution of flow within the tissue is then assessed by excising the tissue, dicing it into small pieces and counting the radioactivity.

In *humans*, the method used to measure blood flow depends on the vessel or tissue of interest, as follows.

## Doppler ultrasound measures large artery blood velocity

The use of pulsed Doppler US to measure human aortic blood flow was described in Section 7.3. This non-invasive approach is also widely used to assess placental perfusion in pregnancy, carotid artery blood flow, middle cerebral artery blood flow and arterial blood flow in the legs of patients with ischaemic or ulcerative limb disease. A variant of the method, the **laser Doppler fluxmeter**, employs a laser light beam rather than US to record the flux of red cells through the superficial dermis.

## Fick's method measures organ blood flow

Fick's principle was introduced in Section 7.1 as a way of measuring pulmonary blood flow; but it can also be used to measure blood flow in several other organs. To measure **renal blood flow**, para-aminohippuric acid (PAH) is injected intravenously. PAH is almost completely cleared from the renal blood into urine, so the renal venous concentration is taken as zero and the arteriovenous concentration difference equates with the measured arterial concentration. Blood flow is calculated as PAH excretion rate in urine (mg/min) divided by PAH arterial concentration (mg/mL) to measure renal plasma flow (Fick's principle) and then adjusting according to the haematocrit to measure renal blood flow.

## Venous occlusion plethysmography measures limb blood flow

Plethysmography is a non-invasive technique that measures blood flow in a human limb, foot or digit (Figure 8.5). To measure forearm blood flow, an inflatable cuff is wrapped around the upper arm, overlying the brachial vein, and is inflated suddenly to 40 mmHg. This arrests the venous drainage out of the arm, but not the arterial inflow; so, the forearm begins to swell with blood. The initial rate of swelling equals arterial inflow. The swelling is measured by recording the limb circumference, using an electronic strain gauge device wrapped around the forearm. In former years, limb swelling was measured by

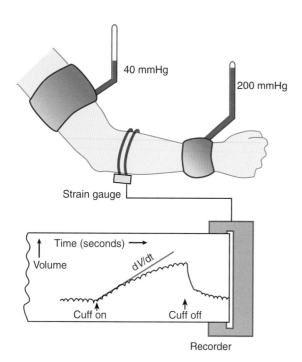

**Figure 8.5** Venous occlusion plethysmography. The 'congesting cuff' (upper arm) occludes venous return; the wrist cuff eliminates hand blood flow from the measurement. The extension of the strain gauge records the increase in forearm circumference due to the continuing arterial inflow; the pulsatile flow can be seen in the trace. The initial swelling rate (tangent to curve, dV/dt) measures forearm blood flow. Swelling rate tails off as venous backpressure rises. After a few minutes, venous pressure exceeds cuff pressure, so venous outflow resumes and forearm blood volume stabilizes.

displacing air or water out of a rigid jacket around the limb, called a plethysmograph ('fullness record'), hence the method's gargantuan name.

## Kety's tissue clearance method measures microvascular blood flow

Microvascular blood flow in a small region of human tissue can be estimated from the rate of washout of a locally injected radioisotope. A rapidly diffusing, radioactive solute is injected as a local, interstitial depot (Figure 8.6). The solute is gradually cleared from the depot by diffusion into the neighbouring capillaries, which carry the solute away. Removal is recorded by a gamma-counter over the depot. If the solute diffusion rate is fast enough, clearance is limited solely by the capillary blood flow and is directly proportional to the blood flow ('Flow-limited exchange', Section 10.10). A small, lipid-soluble radioisotope, such as xenon-133 or krypton-85, is used to achieve the necessary high diffusion rate. In 1949, Kety pointed out that, given flow-limited exchange, the solute concentration declines exponentially with time, so a plot of the natural logarithm of concentration $C$ against time $t$ is linear (Figure 8.6). Its slope, $k$, is called the removal rate constant:

$$\log_e C = \log_e C_0 - kt$$

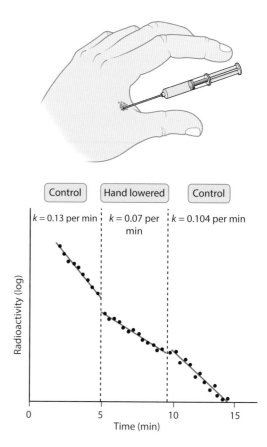

**Figure 8.6** Kety's tissue clearance method. Xenon-133 was injected into the skin. With the hand at heart level, the washout slope $k$ was 13% per min (half-life = 0.693/$k$ = 5.3 min), from which blood flow was calculated to be 9 mL min$^{-1}$ 100 mL$^{-1}$. Lowering the hand 40 cm below heart level reduced blood flow to 7 mL min$^{-1}$100 mL$^{-1}$, due to arteriolar constriction (see Chapter 13). (After Lassen NA, Henriksen U, Sejrsen P. In: Shepherd JT, Abboud FM, eds. *Handbook of Physiology: a Critical, Comprehensive Presentation of Physiological Knowledge and Concepts. Section 2, The Cardiovascular System. Vol. 3: Peripheral Circulation and Organ Blood Flow.* Bethesda, MD: American Physiological Society, 1983: 21–64, with permission.)

where $C_0$ is concentration at time zero. The removal rate constant $k$ is proportional to the microvascular flow $\dot{Q}$:

$$k = \dot{Q}/V_D \lambda \qquad (8.3)$$

where $V_D$ is the volume in which the solute is distributed and $\lambda$ (lambda) is the solute equilibrium partition coefficient between blood and tissue. Microvascular blood flow per unit volume, $\dot{Q}/V_D$, is calculated from slope $k$.

## 8.4 THE ARTERIAL PRESSURE PULSE

## Basic shape of the pulse wave in central systemic arteries

The ventricle ejects blood into the proximal elastic arteries, namely the aorta and subclavian vessels, faster than the blood can drain away. The resulting expansion of these elastin-rich vessels causes

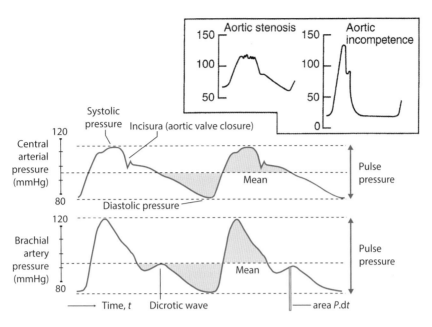

**Figure 8.7** Pressure wave in the human subclavian artery (similar to the aorta) compared with brachial artery, recorded by electronic transducer over two cardiac cycles. Mean pressure is, formally, $\int(P.dt)/t$, meaning the sum of (integral sign $\int$) the thousands of thin rectangular strips of individual area $P.dt$, divided by time $t$; $dt$ is an infinitesimally small unit of time (bottom right). The pressure–time product above the mean pressure (pink area above central dashed line) equals that below the mean. In central arteries, mean pressure is halfway between systolic and diastolic pressures. In the brachial artery, the mean is diastolic + one-third pulse pressure, due to the altered shape of the wave. Mean pressure falls by ~2 mmHg between the central artery and brachial artery, providing a mean pressure gradient for flow, even though systolic pressure is higher in the brachial artery. (**Insets**) Abnormal waveform in aortic valve stenosis (slow rise, prolonged plateau) and aortic incompetence (excessive pulse pressure, low diastolic pressure). (After Mills CJ, Gale IT, Gault JH, et al. *Cardiovascular Research* 1970; 4(4): 405–17, by permission of Oxford University Press; and Nichols WW, O'Rourke MF. *McDonald's Blood Flow in Arteries: Theoretical, Experimental and Clinical Principles*, 5th edn. London: Hodder Arnold, 2005.)

a steep increase in arterial pressure during systole (Figures 8.7 and 8.8). Around 67%–80% of the stroke volume is temporarily stored in the elastic arteries during systole, while 20%–33% runs off through the peripheral resistance. The mechanical energy stored in the stretched elastin serves to maintain the blood pressure during diastole (known as the Windkessel effect).

As ventricular ejection wanes, run-off begins to outpace ejection, so blood volume and pressure in the proximal arteries begin to fall. When ejection ceases, a slight backflow closes the aortic valve. Valve closure produces a notch, the **incisura**, in the descending limb of the arterial pressure trace, followed by a brief, high-frequency wavelet due to vibration of the tensed aortic valve cusps. In more peripheral arteries, such as the brachial artery, there is a pronounced notch, the **dicrotic notch** (Greek *dikrotos* = beating twice) resulting from a diastolic reflected wave (Figure 8.7), as explained later in the chapter. As the arterial blood continues to run off through the peripheral resistance vessels, central arterial pressure gradually decays towards its diastolic minimum. Since diastolic decay is slower than the systolic rise, the arterial pressure wave is asymmetrical.

## Pulse pressure depends on stroke volume and arterial stiffness

The **pulse pressure** is the difference between diastolic and systolic pressure. The factors governing pulse pressure were explained in Section 7.4, but to recap briefly, the primary determinants are: **stroke volume**, minus the run-off during the ejection phase; and **arterial stiffness (elastance)**, which is 1/compliance (Concept box 7.1).

Thus, the greater the stroke volume, the bigger the pulse pressure (Figure 8.8, top); also, the greater the stiffness of the artery wall, the bigger the pulse pressure (Figure 8.8, bottom). Arterial stiffness increases with mean pressure, ejection velocity and age. As **mean pressure** rises, the arterial compliance curve gets steeper (stiffer), so a rise in mean pressure increases the pulse pressure, even if the stroke volume is unchanged (Figure 8.8, middle). Increased **ejection velocity** also raises pulse pressure because the viscoelastic artery wall has less time to undergo viscous relaxation. This contributes to the increase in pulse pressure during exercise. Ageing is accompanied by **arteriosclerosis**, which increases artery wall stiffness and hence pulse pressure (Figure 8.8, bottom). The pulse in **chronic hypertension** is described in Section 18.4.

## The proximal pulse is transmitted rapidly to the peripheral arteries

If arteries had rigid walls, blood pressure would rise virtually instantaneously throughout the arterial system during systole. However, arteries are not rigid so the proximal pressure rise takes a finite time to spread to distal arteries, such as the radial artery. The pulse travels at around 4–5 m/s in young people

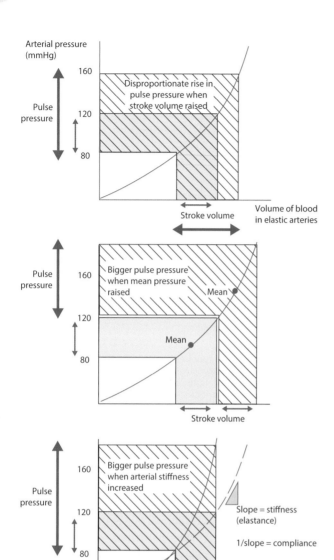

**Figure 8.8** Non-linear pressure–volume relation of elastic arteries and effect on pulse pressure. (**Top**) A moderate increase in stroke volume increases pulse pressure disproportionately because the artery gets stiffer with stretch; that is, the curve gets steeper. (**Middle**) The same stroke volume ejected at a higher mean pressure (filled circles) causes a bigger pulse pressure, because distension increases the arterial stiffness (elastance). (**Bottom**) An increase in stiffness (e.g. arteriosclerosis of ageing) markedly increases the pulse pressure. Arterial compliance is the reciprocal of the slope.

and 10–15 m/s in older people – one of the few things older people do faster than the young!

The pulse transmission velocity, 4–15 m/s, is much faster than the blood velocity, which averages ~0.2 m/s in the ascending aorta. The difference between pulse transmission velocity and blood velocity is difficult to understand, but not impossible (Figure 8.9). Since blood is incompressible, blood ejected into the proximal aorta must create space for itself.

It does this partly by distending the proximal aorta (which raises the blood pressure) and partly by pushing forwards the blood previously occupying the space. As the displaced blood moves forwards, it too must make space for itself, which it does partly by distending the wall downstream (which raises the pressure there) and partly by displacing the blood ahead. This shunting sequence repeats itself in rapid succession along the arterial tree. The process can be likened to a railway engine shunting trucks; the engine may only be moving at 3 mph, but the shunting shock wave travels down the line of wagons much faster. The pulse is thus transmitted by a wave of wall distension at 4–15 m/s, while the ejected blood itself advances just 20 cm (the **stroke distance**) in 1 s.

Since pulse propagation involves wall deformation, the stiffness of the wall affects the transmission velocity; **transmission velocity increases with wall stiffness**. As noted earlier, arterial stiffness increases with blood pressure and ageing. Consequently, pulse transmission is faster in hypertensive and older patients. The pulse lag time between central and peripheral arteries can be used to estimate human arterial distensibility.

## The shape of the pulse alters with ageing and pathophysiological status

Depending on age and pathophysiological status, the pressure wave in a human proximal artery may show two additional features, namely a **diastolic wave** or a **systolic inflection** (Figure 8.10). These features can affect cardiac performance, as explained later in the chapter.

## Reflection causes a diastolic wave in the young

In children, young adults and many mammals, the decay of pressure in diastole is interrupted by a small bump, that is, a transient rise in pressure, called a diastolic or dicrotic wave. This is not present in older people, in whom pressure falls off exponentially after the incisura. The diastolic wave is caused by **wave reflection**. The initial systolic pressure wave travels rapidly down the arterial tree and reaches the major branches and resistance vessels in a fraction of a second. The branch points and resistance vessels partially reflect the wave, sending an attenuated pressure wave back up the arterial tree (inset, Figure 8.10). Since the wave velocity is ~4 m/s in young humans, and the distance to major reflection sites such as the aortic bifurcation is ~0.5 m, and the cardiac cycle lasts ~1 s, the reflected wave returns to the proximal arteries in time to interact with the initiating or **incident wave**. This creates the diastolic wave in young people (Figure 8.10b). An everyday analogy is the reflection of an incoming sea wave by a harbour wall; as the reflected

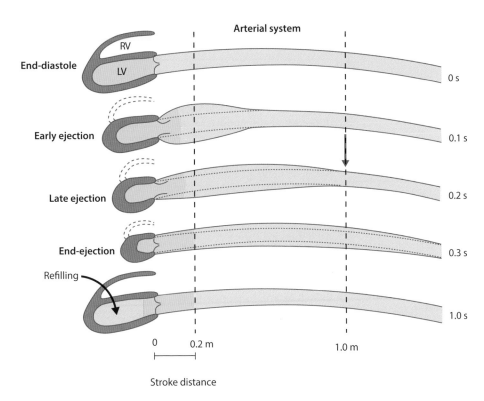

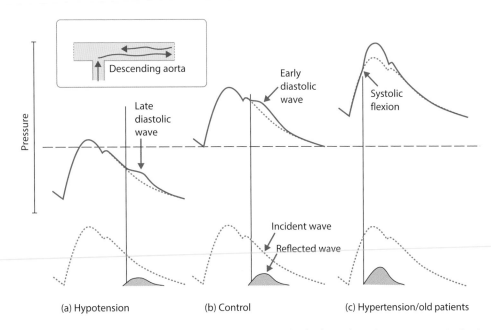

**Figure 8.9** Transmission of pressure pulse along human arterial system at 5 m/s. In this example, the left ventricle (LV) ejects 100 cm³ blood into an aorta of cross-sectional area 5 cm². The blood advances 20 cm in one beat (stroke distance). The wall distension, that is, the arterial pulse, travels much faster (1 m in 0.2 s), as marked by the red arrow.

**Figure 8.10** Changes in aortic pulse due to wave reflection. The observed pulse (red) consists of two components: the basic or 'incident' wave and the reflected wave. The time from the foot of the incident wave to the arrival of the reflected wave depends on transmission velocity. **(a)** In hypotension, or after a vasodilator drug, the low pressure reduces arterial stiffness (Figure 8.8, middle). This slows pulse wave propagation, so the reflected wave occurs in late diastole. **(b)** At normal pressure and arterial stiffness in a young human or rabbit, faster pulse transmission causes an early diastolic reflected wave. **(c)** In hypertensive or older patients, or a normal patient after a vasoconstrictor drug, the raised arterial stiffness and transmission velocity cause a systolic reflected wave, which creates a systolic inflection. Pattern **(b)** can be generated from **(c)** by vasodilator drugs, for example, glyceryl trinitrate. (**Inset**) Model of arterial system as an asymmetric T-tube. The short limb on the left represents all arteries of the upper body; the long limb on the right represents the lower body; the ends represent the average of all the reflection sites in the upper and lower body, respectively. (After Nichols WW, O'Rourke MF. *McDonald's Blood Flow in Arteries: Theoretical, Experimental and Clinical Principles*, 5th edn. London: Arnold, 2005.)

wave travels back out to sea, it meets an incoming wave and the two waves summate briefly into a tall peak. The time interval between the foot (start) of the incident wave and the inflection marking arrival of the reflected wave can be used to estimate wave velocity, and hence arterial stiffness, in humans.

## Reflection causes a systolic inflection in older or hypertensive patients

The central arteries of ageing humans and hypertensive patients are stiffer than in young subjects, so the incident and reflected waves travel faster. As a result, the reflected wave arrives back in the aorta in late systole rather than diastole (Figure 8.10c). Consequently, older humans lack a diastolic wave. Instead, the reflected wave adds to the late part of the incident systolic wave, raising the peak systolic pressure and creating a kink or **flexion** in the systolic wave.

## The waveform alters in pathophysiological states

Whether the central pulse has a diastolic wave or a systolic inflection depends on: (1) the degree of reflection by peripheral vessels, which is increased by vasoconstriction and reduced by vasodilatation; and (2) pulse transmission velocity, which increases with ageing and mean blood pressure. Since clinical hypotension and vasodilator drugs lower blood pressure, and therefore artery wall stiffness (Figure 8.8), the reflected waves travel more slowly (Figure 8.10a). As a result, the systolic inflection of middle-aged/older humans is replaced by a diastolic wave during hypotension. This is also one of the effects of the anti-angina vasodilator, **glyceryl trinitrate** (GTN). Conversely, raising blood pressure with a vasoconstrictor drug causes the reflected wave to return faster, which can transform a pulse with a low systolic pressure and diastolic wave (Figure 8.10a,b) into one with a high systolic pressure, a systolic inflection and no diastolic wave (Figure 8.10c).

## Why wave reflection matters

Reflected waves are important because they affect coronary blood flow and cardiac work. In young humans and many animals, the slow return of the reflected wave augments the diastolic pressure, which boosts coronary artery perfusion. By contrast, in older individuals or hypertensive patients the early return of the reflected wave increases systolic pressure (**systolic pressure augmentation**). Therefore, the left ventricle must eject blood against an increased afterload, which increases cardiac work and $O_2$ demand. The properties of the artery wall thus affect cardiac $O_2$ demand.

## Aortic stiffness increases cardiac oxygen demand

In young humans, the high distensibility of the aorta and proximal arteries keeps systolic pressure low, which in turn reduces cardiac work and $O_2$ demand. In older individuals, the stiff arterial system raises systolic pressure, both directly and through systolic pressure augmentation (Figure 8.10c), and this increases cardiac work and $O_2$ demand. It has been shown experimentally that the $O_2$ consumption of a dog heart ejecting through a rigid plastic tube is much higher than when ejecting through the aorta. The therapeutic benefit of **GTN**, a vasodilator used to treat angina (cardiac pain due to $O_2$ demand exceeding supply), is partly because it relaxes large arteries and veins, and to a lesser degree, resistance vessels. Large artery relaxation increases arterial compliance and reduces systolic augmentation by wave reflection. The resulting fall in systolic pressure reduces afterload and cardiac $O_2$ demand, and so contributes to the relief of angina (Section 15.1).

## The shape of the pulse changes as it travels into the peripheral arteries

As the pressure wave passes from the aorta into the peripheral arteries, its shape changes in a surprising way; the wave becomes taller in the larger proximal arteries of young humans and dogs, rather than damping out as one might imagine (Figure 1.10, top; Figures 8.7 and 8.11). For example, systolic pressure is higher in the brachial artery than in the aorta in young to middle-aged humans. Four features of the pressure wave change:

- The systolic pressure wave grows taller, rather like a sea wave approaching the beach. This **pressure amplification** can be as much as 60% in the femoral artery of young humans. Pressure amplification is less marked in middle-aged humans and is absent in older individuals (Figure 8.11).
- The incisura is damped out and disappears.
- The mean pressure falls only slightly, by ~2 mmHg between the ascending aorta and radial artery, showing that large arteries account for only ~2% of *TPR*.
- A new pressure wave appears in late diastole, the dicrotic wave, preceded by a pronounced dicrotic notch (Figures 8.7 and 8.11).

These complex changes are caused by a combination of factors: increased arterial stiffness with distance; faster transmission of the higher-pressure components; aortic taper (the abdominal aorta is roughly half as wide as the ascending aorta); and wave reflection. The pulse pressure continues to increase as far as third- or fourth-generation arteries, such as the radial artery. Beyond this, the pulse becomes progressively damped out by the viscous properties of the vessel wall and blood (Figure 1.10, top). The pressure oscillations dwindle and the flow becomes more continuous as the blood enters the resistance vessels.

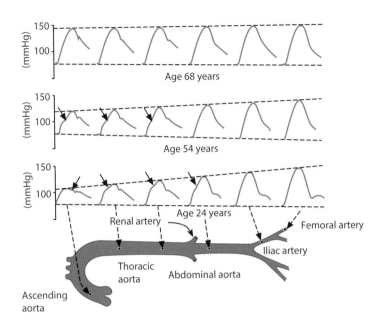

**Figure 8.11** Pressure wave amplification along the human arterial tree, and its dependence on age. Distal pressure amplification is ~60% in the young but is negligible in the old. Arrows show systolic inflection, marking the arrival of the reflected wave. (After Nichols WW, O'Rourke MF. *McDonald's Blood Flow in Arteries: Theoretical, Experimental and Clinical Principles*, 5th edn. London: Hodder Arnold, 2005.)

## Clinical abnormalities of the pulse

### Aortic valve stenosis

Narrowing of the aortic valve by fibrosis results in a slow, prolonged ejection phase. Arterial pressure rises sluggishly and has an abnormal plateau (Figures 2.8, top and 8.7, top).

### Aortic valve incompetence

Diastolic reflux into the ventricle causes the arterial pressure to decay abnormally quickly. As a result, the pulse pressure may be twice normal, causing relaxed limbs to jerk in time with the throbbing pulse (Figures 2.8, bottom and 8.7, top).

### Pulsus paradoxus

This is a condition in which pulse pressure falls by more than 10 mmHg during each inspiration. This is not really a 'paradox' at all; it is an exaggeration of the normal inspiratory fall (see 'Traube–Hering waves', next section). Pulsus paradoxus >20 mmHg is generally caused by **cardiac tamponade** (pressure around the heart), due to an accumulation of fluid in the pericardial cavity. Tamponade sets a fixed limit to the combined volume of the two ventricles inside the pericardial sac. During inspiration, the fall in intrathoracic pressure increases the flow of venous blood into the right ventricle, increasing the right ventricular volume. Since the total volume is limited by the tamponade, the rise in right ventricular volume reduces the left ventricular volume. Thus, left ventricular stroke volume and systolic pressure decline excessively during inspiration. Pulsus paradoxus can also be caused by severe bronchospasm during an asthma attack.

### Pulsus alternans

This is a pulse that is alternately strong and weak; the pulse pressure is reduced every other beat. This is caused by

oscillation of the size of the myocyte $Ca^{2+}$ store, and is generally a sign of severe left ventricular failure.

## 8.5 MEAN ARTERIAL PRESSURE AND PRESSURE MEASUREMENT

### What does 'mean' pressure mean?

The time-averaged mean is the area under the pressure wave ($\int P.dt$) divided by time. However, in routine clinical practice only systolic and diastolic pressures are measured, usually in the brachial artery rather than aorta. In the aorta, mean pressure is approximately halfway between systolic and diastolic pressures; that is, it is the arithmetic average (Figure 8.7, middle trace). However, in the brachial artery the narrowing of the systolic peak, caused by distal transmission, shifts the time-averaged mean in the diastolic direction (Figure 8.7, bottom trace), and the mean pressure is approximately the diastolic pressure plus one third of the pulse pressure:

$$\text{Mean brachial artery pressure } \bar{P}_a \simeq P_{\text{diastolic}} + \frac{P_{\text{systolic}} - P_{\text{diastolic}}}{3}$$

(8.4)

For example, if the brachial artery pressure is 110/80 mmHg, the pulse pressure is 30 mmHg and the mean pressure is 90 mmHg. In the aorta, where the wave is less 'peaky', the mean is simply $(P_{\text{diastolic}} + P_{\text{systolic}})/2$.

### What determines mean arterial blood pressure?

As explained in Section 8.1, Darcy's law tells us that two factors determine the mean arterial pressure, namely *CO* and *TPR*:

| Mean blood pressure $\bar{P}_a$ | $\approx$ | Cardiac output × Total peripheral resistance *TPR* | (8.5) |

This is called the **mean blood pressure equation**. The mean blood pressure equation can be combined with the pulse pressure equation 7.4 and brachial pressure equation 8.4 to tell us how high the systolic pressure rises and how low the diastolic pressure falls for a given CO and peripheral resistance. For example, the brachial systolic pressure is given by:

$$P_{systolic} = (SV \times HR \times TPR) + 2(SV - R_{off})/3C$$

where *SV* is stroke volume, *HR* is heart rate, $R_{off}$ is volume run-off during ejection and *C* is arterial compliance.

## Direct measurement of arterial pressure

### Principle of manometry

Arterial pressure was first measured by Stephen Hales, an English clergyman and vicar of Teddington, near London, in 1733. Hales connected a 3m vertical glass tube to the carotid artery of a horse via a goose trachea, and noted the height to which the blood rose in the tube (manometry). A century later, the Parisian physicist and physiologist Jean Léonard Marie Poiseuille developed the smaller **U-tube mercury manometer**, which remained in routine use until recently. The principle of manometry is that the column of fluid in a vertical tube exerts a downward pressure at the base, which is connected to the pressure source that is being measured (Figures 8.1 and 8.2). When the column height *h* is stable, the pressure at the bottom of the fluid column must be equal to the pressure to which it is connected. The pressure at the bottom of a column of fluid is $\rho g h$ (fluid density $\rho$ × force of gravity $g$ × *h*). Since mercury is very dense, 13.6 g/mL, a column ~100 mm high is sufficient to balance the mean arterial blood pressure at heart level. Using his new mercury manometer, Poiseuille was the first to show that there is little change in mean pressure along the arterial system, and therefore little resistance to flow along proximal macroscopic arteries.

### Electronic pressure transducers

A mercury column has too much inertia to follow the rapidly changing waveform of a single pulse; it just records average pressure. To record the waveform, a fast-responding, electronic pressure transducer is connected, via a stiff, fluid-filled tube, to an intra-arterial cannula. The electronic pressure transducer was developed by American scientists Lambert and Wood during aviation research in World War II. The transducer contains a thin metal diaphragm, which deforms slightly under pressure, changing the electrical resistance.

The thin diaphragm can follow fast changes in pressure. However, the electrical signal must be calibrated against a column of liquid, so blood pressure is still reported in mmHg rather than pascal.

## Indirect measurement of human blood pressure using the sphygmomanometer

Human blood pressure is usually measured in the brachial artery, using a non-invasive method called **sphygmomanometry**. This is based on the principle that a soft, healthy artery is readily compressed by external pressure (Figure 8.12). An inflatable rubber sac inside a cotton sleeve, called a **Riva Rocci sphygmomanometer cuff**, is wound around the upper arm. The inflatable sac must be located medially over the brachial artery and the artery must be at heart level, with the subject seated. The cuff is inflated progressively, squeezing the soft tissues of the upper arm, until the brachial artery is occluded, as judged by the disappearance of a palpable radial pulse. This might require a pressure of >180 mmHg in an older individual. Until recently the cuff pressure was measured by a mercury manometer, but this has been replaced in modern instruments by a dial gauge, calibrated in mmHg by the manufacturer. A stethoscope is then placed over the brachial artery in the antecubital fossa (hollow of the elbow). No sound is heard at this stage, because no blood is flowing. Cuff pressure is then gradually lowered, using a screw valve, until the following sequence of sounds is heard.

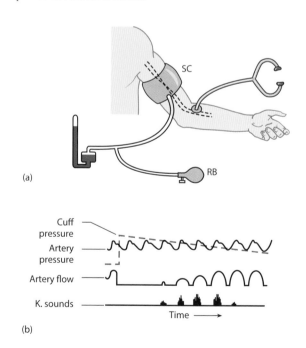

**Figure 8.12** Measurement of human blood pressure.
**(a)** The dashed line shows compression of the brachial artery by sphygmomanometer cuff (SC). Cuff pressure is controlled by the rubber bulb (RB). Cuff pressure was measured for generations by a mercury column, but recent instruments use a dial gauge.
**(b)** Korotkoff (K) sounds begin when cuff pressure is reduced to just below systolic pressure. They cease when cuff pressure is below diastolic pressure.

1. When cuff pressure falls just below systolic pressure, the artery opens briefly during each systole. The transient spurts of blood vibrate the artery wall, creating a dull tapping noise called a **Korotkoff sound**. The pressure at which the Korotkoff sound first appears is conventionally accepted as systolic pressure, although it is ~10 mmHg below the true value.
2. As the cuff pressure is lowered further, the Korotkoff sounds grow louder, because the intermittent spurts of blood grow stronger.
3. When cuff pressure is close to diastolic pressure, the artery remains patent for most of the cardiac cycle and the vessel vibration diminishes. This causes a rapid diminution of the Korotkoff sounds. The cuff pressure at which this happens used to be the accepted measure of the diastolic pressure, although it is ~8 mmHg higher than true diastolic pressure. A faint Korotkoff sound may persist below this and complete silence may not be attained until 8–10 mmHg below the true diastolic pressure. The British Hypertension Society currently recommends the point of silence as the reported diastolic pressure.

In some hypertensive patients there is a silent period within the systolic–diastolic pressure range, which could cause systolic hypertension to be missed. Therefore, it is important when first inflating the cuff, to palpate the radial artery and note the pressure at which the pulse disappears. This is a good measure of systolic pressure and guards against failure to diagnose a case of systolic hypertension.

## The measured brachial artery pressure may differ from the aortic pressure

As noted earlier, the pulse pressure is amplified as it travels along the arterial tree, except in the elderly (Figure 8.11). Consequently, brachial artery systolic pressure overestimates aortic systolic pressure, by up to 20 mmHg in resting, young to middle-aged individuals (Figure 8.7). When the blood pressure is altered by drugs, brachial artery measurements may underestimate the aortic pressure response, owing to changes in wave reflection.

## Ankle–brachial pressure index assesses ischaemic leg disease

Human leg arteries are a common site for atheroma, leading to peripheral ischaemia. To assess the state of the leg arteries, blood pressure is measured in the foot. A Riva Rocci cuff above the ankle is inflated to occlude the tibial artery, and blood flow in a distal artery such as the dorsalis pedis (foot) is recorded by Doppler US as cuff pressure is lowered. The pressure at which distal flow restarts in the tibial artery is called the ankle systolic pressure. Ankle systolic pressure divided by brachial artery systolic pressure, the ankle–brachial pressure index (ABPI), is normally ≥1. An ABPI of <0.8 indicates

substantial upstream arterial stenosis by atheroma. This leads to poor peripheral perfusion, pallor, **intermittent claudication** (pain on walking that is relieved by rest) and **arterial ulcers**. An ABPI of ≤0.4 is associated with pain at rest and eventually **gangrene**. The ABPI is important for distinguishing between arterial ulcers and venous ulcers (ABPI ~1), since venous ulcers are treated by compression bandaging, which would be harmful in the presence of an impaired arterial supply. If the tibial artery is hardened, as with **diabetes**, a higher-than-normal cuff pressure must be applied to compress the stiff artery, resulting in false high estimates of tibial artery pressure and an ABPI of >1.2.

## Indirect, automated measurement of human blood pressure

**Automated oscillometric cuff systems**, such as the Dinamap, report brachial artery diastolic, systolic and mean pressure. An electronic system records not the Korotkoff sounds but the pulsing air pressure in the Riva Rocci cuff, caused by the pulsation of the underlying brachial artery. An electrical pump first inflates the cuff to above systolic pressure. Since the artery is completely occluded, there is little oscillation in cuff pressure. The cuff is then automatically deflated. As the cuff pressure falls just below systolic pressure, the artery under the cuff begins to pulse, causing cuff pressure to oscillate. As cuff pressure is reduced further, the oscillation increases, reaching a maximum at the mean arterial pressure. The pulsation drops to a minimum at the diastolic pressure. These **oscillation criteria** are used to record the pressures electronically.

A different principle, called **volume clamp**, is used to record digital artery pressure continuously and non-invasively (the Finapress). The finger is enclosed in an inflatable cuff and changes in finger volume are monitored by infrared light transmission. Finger volume normally oscillates slightly with each arterial pulse. The volume signal is fed back to a pump, which increases its output to the finger cuff each time the artery pulses, just enough to 'clamp' the volume at a constant level. The cuff pressure is thus enslaved

---

**CONCEPT BOX 8.1**

### WHAT DETERMINES ARTERIAL PRESSURE?

- Mean arterial pressure is determined by *CO* and *TPR*. From Darcy's law (Concept box 1.1), mean pressure = *CO* × *TPR*.
- Systolic and diastolic pressures are determined by the size of the oscillation about the mean pressure.
- The size of the oscillation, or pulse pressure, is determined by the stroke volume *SV* and arterial compliance *C*. See Concept box 7.1.
- In the long-term, the kidneys are crucial regulators of mean blood pressure, because they regulate the plasma volume and hence the cardiac filling pressure.

to the arterial pressure. The enslaved pressure is measured electronically and displayed continuously on a monitor, along with an estimate of CO by the pulse pressure method (Section 7.4).

## What is the 'normal' blood pressure?

That mythological polymath, 'every schoolboy', knows that 'normal' human blood pressure is 120/80 mmHg. For the brachial artery of a young adult under certain conditions, he would be right; but it is wrong to adopt 120/80 mmHg as the normal standard for a resting child, a pregnant woman in midterm or an older man. Blood pressure is quite labile over 24 h (Figure 8.13), and the factors affecting it include the following.

### Age

Human blood pressure increases with age, averaging 105/65 mmHg at 10 years, 120/70 mmHg at 30 years and 140/75 mmHg at 70 years (Figure 17.10). The large increase in pulse pressure with age is caused by arteriosclerosis (not to be confused with atheroma; see Table 17.4).

### Activity, sleep and exercise

Blood pressure can fall as low as 80/50 mmHg during sleep (Figure 8.13). Conversely, in heavy, dynamic exercise, mean pressure increases by 10–40 mmHg. In heavy, resistive exercise, such as weightlifting, the pressure can increase by over 100 mmHg.

### Gravity and standing: the giraffe's nightmare

Pressure increases equally in arteries and veins below heart level, due to the weight of the column of blood between the heart and blood vessel (Figure 8.2). For a fluid column of height $h$, the increase in pressure is $\rho gh$ (see 'Principle of manometry' earlier). In the human foot ~115 cm below heart level, arterial blood pressure will increase by 122 cmH$_2$O (blood being 1.06 times denser than water). This is 90 mmHg (mercury is 13.6 times denser than water). Therefore, if mean aortic pressure at heart level is 95 mmHg, arterial pressure in the foot will be almost 90 + 95 = 185 mmHg; it will be ~2 mmHg less than this, due to the slight arterial resistance to flow. Conversely, pressure falls in arteries above heart level, and is only 60 mmHg in the human brain during standing. However, our gravitational problems are small compared with the giraffe. Because the giraffe head is so far above heart level, the heart must generate an aortic pressure of ~200 mmHg to ensure adequate cerebral perfusion.

### Gravity and standing: indirect effects

On moving from lying to standing, changes in CO and peripheral resistance lead to changes in arterial pressure. An initial, transient fall in arterial pressure can produce a passing dizziness (postural hypotension). This is followed by a small but sustained reflex rise in pressure (Section 17.1).

### Emotion and stress

Anger, apprehension, fear, stress and sexual excitement are all potent 'pressor' stimuli; that is, they elevate blood pressure (Figure 8.13). A formal meeting, such as a visit to the doctor, can raise blood pressure by 20 mmHg ('white coat hypertension'), so a solitary high value is not diagnostic of clinical hypertension; the measurement must be repeated later, with the patient relaxed. The pressor effect of stress is particularly harmful to patients with ischaemic heart disease, as the cautionary tale of John Hunter in Section 6.14 illustrates.

### Regular oscillations in mean arterial blood pressure

Mean blood pressure oscillates in time with breathing (**Traube–Hering waves**). Pressure falls by a few mmHg during each inspiration, because left ventricular stroke volume declines as the lung vascular bed expands. Although inspiration also raises the heart rate (sinus arrhythmia; see Section 5.11), this compensates only partially for the fall in stroke volume, so human CO and blood pressure fall during

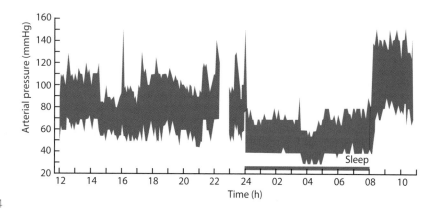

**Figure 8.13** Continuous record of human arterial blood pressure over 24 h. Sleep (red period) reduced blood pressure. A painful stimulus at 16.00 h and sexual intercourse at 24.00 h markedly raised pressure. (From Bevan AT, Honour AJ, Scott FH. *Clinical Science* 1969; 36: 329, by permission.) © The Biochemical Society.

inspiration. In dogs, by contrast, the pressure rises during inspiration, because the inspiratory tachycardia outweighs the fall in stroke volume.

In addition to respiration-related oscillations, arterial pressure may show regular oscillations at a lower frequency of ~6/min (0.1 Hz), called **Mayer waves**. These are due to synchronous oscillations in sympathetic vasoconstrictor activity. The sympathetic oscillation is thought to result from a slow feedback by the baroreflex (Chapter 16).

## Other factors

The **Valsalva manoeuvre**, which is a forced expiration against a closed or narrowed glottis, triggers a complex sequence of raised blood pressures (Section 17.2). In **pregnancy**, blood pressure falls to a minimum at ~6 months, due to the expansion of the uterine and other vascular beds. Consequently, in obstetrical practice a pressure of 130/90 mmHg at 6 months' gestation would cause concern. Many **pathological processes** also alter arterial pressure, such as dehydration, haemorrhage, shock, syncope (loss of consciousness), chronic hypertension, acute heart failure and valvular lesions, such as aortic incompetence.

It is clear from this survey that the criteria for assessing whether blood pressure is normal must be adjusted for the individual's age, and their physiological and psychological condition.

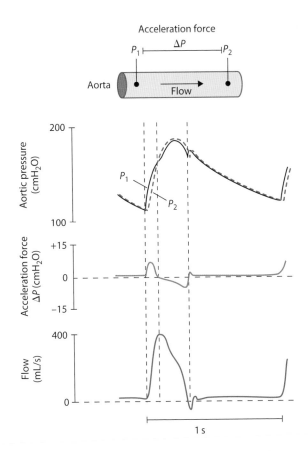

**Figure 8.14** Flow, acceleration and pressure gradients in the human ascending aorta. The pressure difference $\Delta P$ at first accelerates flow along the aorta, then reverses and decelerates flow until a brief backflow closes the aortic valve. Proximal aortic flow is almost zero during diastole. (After Snell RE, Clements JM, Patel DJ, et al. *Journal of Applied Physiology* 1965; 20(4): 691–5, with permission from the American Physiological Society.)

## 8.6 PULSATILE FLOW

Blood flow is almost stop–go in the major arteries and aorta (Figure 8.14). Darcy's law cannot predict the flow at a given instant in the cardiac cycle because Darcy's law is a steady-state expression; it can only describe mean flow over many cardiac cycles. When flow is pulsatile, the flow at a given instant is governed by Newton's second law of motion, namely acceleration = force/mass. During systole, the pressure (force per unit area) rises first in the proximal aorta, creating a pressure gradient from the proximal aorta to the peripheral arteries (Figure 8.14, top trace). This accelerates the blood (Figure 8.14, middle trace). The pressure pulse then spreads distally, reaching the radial artery in ~0.1 s. At this moment in time, the distal pressure is transiently higher than the proximal pressure, which is tailing off. As a result, the pressure gradient is now reversed, and decelerates the flow. Thus, flow in the major arteries first accelerates and then decelerates over the initial third of the cardiac cycle. Proximal aortic flow reverses briefly as the aortic valve closes, and is very low throughout diastole (Figure 8.14, bottom trace).

The period of near zero flow gradually shortens as blood enters the smaller arteries, and in the smallest arteries the flow becomes continuous, albeit still pulsatile (Figure 1.10, middle trace).

## 8.7 PERIPHERAL RESISTANCE, POISEUILLE'S LAW AND LAPLACE'S WALL MECHANICS

The resistance of the systemic circulation to flow is located chiefly in the tiny terminal arteries and arterioles (Section 1.7; Concept box 1.1). *TPR* is the pressure drop required to drive unit flow through the systemic circulation (equation 8.1b), namely ~1 mmHg per mL/s in a resting adult, or 1 peripheral resistance unit. But what factors determine the resistance to flow?

### Poiseuille's law describes the hydraulic resistance of a tube

Resistance to flow arises exclusively from the internal friction within the fluid rather than friction at the tube wall. Resistance is nevertheless greatly affected by tube radius, because the rate at which one lamina slides past the adjacent one (the shear rate) is greater in narrow tubes than wide tubes, for a given flow. High shear rates require more force and thus a bigger pressure gradient, and resistance is the pressure gradient required to produce unit flow.

The factors governing tube resistance were first elucidated by Jean Léonard Marie Poiseuille, around 1840, in a meticulous study of water flowing through glass capillary tubes. By studying the steady laminar flow of a Newtonian fluid (one in which viscosity is constant, such as water, plasma) along a straight cylindrical tube, Poiseuille established that the **resistance R is inversely proportional to tube radius raised to the fourth power, $r^4$**. Also, resistance is directly proportional to fluid viscosity $\eta$ and tube length $L$:

$$R = \frac{8\eta L}{\pi r^4} \tag{8.6}$$

R represents the energy-loss per unit volume in the full Bernoulli equation 8.2. Combining this expression with Darcy's law of flow (equation 8.1a), and recalling that conductance $K$ is $1/R$, we get an expression for flow through a tube called **Poiseuille's law**:

$$\dot{Q} = (P_1 - P_2)K = (P_1 - P_2)\frac{\pi r^4}{8\eta L} \tag{8.7}$$

Poiseuille's law tells us that tissue blood flow is extremely sensitive to the radius of the resistance vessels, namely the terminal arteries and arterioles. Since these smooth muscle-rich vessels can change their radius actively, they can employ the powerful Poiseuille relation to regulate local tissue perfusion.

## Resistances in series versus in parallel

Poiseuille's law describes flow along a single tube. When several tubes are joined together in **series** (end-to-end), for example, a terminal artery and an arteriole, their total resistance $R_{total}$ is the sum of the individual resistances (Figure 8.15, top). The sum of resistance is written as $\Sigma R$ (Greek capital sigma $\Sigma$ means 'the sum of all individual values'). Thus, in a series array, $R_{total}$ equals $\Sigma R$.

If several tubes are arranged in **parallel**, as in a capillary bed, a given driving pressure will produce more flow than it would through a single tube because the conducting capacities of the tubes summate (Figure 8.15, bottom). The net conductance is the sum of the individual conductances, $\Sigma K$. Because resistance is the reciprocal of conductance, the net resistance is $1/\Sigma K$. Therefore, in parallel arrays $R_{total} = 1/\Sigma K$. To summarize the rule, 'For series arrays, add the resistances; for parallel arrays, add the conductances'. The summation of huge numbers of conductances in parallel contributes to the surprisingly low hydraulic resistance of the capillary bed.

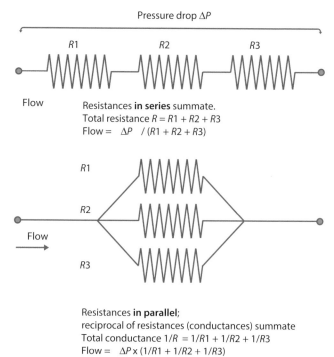

**Figure 8.15** Basic rules of hydraulics. When vessels are linked in series (e.g. feed artery–terminal artery–arteriole), each adds to the resistance to the flow; net resistance is high. When vessels are linked in parallel, as in a capillary bed, their flow-transmitting capabilities (conductances) add up, so the net resistance is low.

Armed with Poiseuille's law, plus the basic rules for vessels in series and in parallel, we can now consider the systemic resistance that resides chiefly in the arterioles and tiniest arteries.

## Arteriolar radius regulates both local blood flow and central arterial pressure

Vascular resistance is exquisitely sensitive to radius, due to the $r^4$ relation in Poiseuille's law. The difference in radius between the human aorta (1 cm) and a single arteriole (0.01 cm) represents a 100-millionfold increase in resistance. Therefore, the arterioles and terminal arteries are the main sites of resistance. Because of the $r^4$ effect, a mere 19% increase in the radius of the resistance vessels will double the low blood flow.

The radius of a resistance vessel is actively regulated by the tunica media smooth muscle. Contraction narrows the lumen (vasoconstriction) and relaxation widens it (vasodilatation). When constriction occurs throughout the body, *TPR* increases, raising **arterial blood pressure** at a given CO (Figure 8.16). Conversely, widespread vasodilatation, as in septic shock, lowers blood pressure. Widespread changes in resistance vessel tone are thus a powerful way of regulating arterial blood pressure (equation 8.5). By contrast, if the changes in vessel tone are confined to a single organ or tissue, the **local blood flow** to that organ is altered (equation 8.1a), without greatly affecting *TPR* or blood pressure. For example, during eating, a 1.8-fold dilatation of the salivary gland resistance vessels increases their perfusion tenfold (the $r^4$ effect); but, since the salivary glands account for only a tiny fraction of the *TPR*, there is no significant change in *TPR* or arterial blood pressure.

Capillaries are even narrower than arterioles, so the resistance of a single capillary is bigger than that of an arteriole. Yet the pressure drop across the whole capillary network, 20–30 mmHg, is less than that across the arteriolar network, 40–50 mmHg (Figure 8.16); that is, the capillary network has the smaller resistance. How can this be? The low net capillary resistance is due to: (1) the vast number of capillaries arranged in parallel ($R_{total} = 1/\Sigma K$; Figure 8.15); (2) the shortness of capillaries, ~500 μm (length *L* in equation 8.7); and (3) bolus flow in capillaries, which reduces the effective blood viscosity ($\eta$ in equation 8.7).

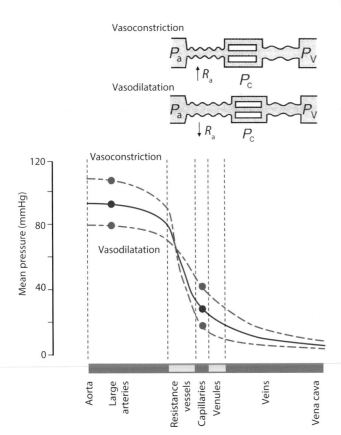

**Figure 8.16** Changes in pressure distribution across the circulation caused by widespread vasoconstriction/vasodilatation of resistance vessels (terminal arteries and arterioles, resistance $R_a$). At a given cardiac output, vasoconstriction raises arterial pressure ($P_a$) because blood escapes less easily from the upstream arteries through the raised downstream resistance. Vasoconstriction reduces capillary pressure $P_C$, because more pressure is lost as blood traverses the raised precapillary resistance $R_a$; less pressure 'gets through'. Conversely, a widespread vasodilatation tends to lower arterial pressure and raise capillary pressure.

---

**CONCEPT BOX 8.2**

### FLOW THROUGH A TUBE: POISEUILLE'S LAW

- The conductance of a tube is the flow per unit pressure drop.
- Poiseuille's law states that the conductance of a tube of radius *r* is proportional to $r^4$, and inversely proportional to fluid viscosity $\eta$ and vessel length *L*. The conductance is $\pi r^4/8\eta L$.
- For tubes connected in parallel, the conductances add up. Thus, the conductance of the capillary bed is high.
- The inverse of conductance is resistance. Resistance is $8\eta L/\pi r^4$. For tubes connected in series, the resistances add up, for example, small arteries and arterioles.
- Due to the $r^4$ relation, active changes in arteriolar calibre have a very powerful effect on local blood flow, and on *TPR* and mean arterial pressure.
- Blood viscosity $\eta$ depends chiefly on the haematocrit. The effective viscosity falls in microvessels (the Fåhræus–Lindqvist effect), which reduces microvascular resistance and conserves cardiac energy.

## Laplace's law links radius, wall tension and pressure

The radius of a distensible tube depends on three mechanical factors (Figure 8.17):

- the **internal pressure** distending it ($P_i$);
- the **outside pressure** compressing it ($P_o$);
- the **circumferential wall tension**, that is, force per unit length of vessel (*T*).

When the radius is stable (a state called mechanical equilibrium), the circumferential wall tension exactly counteracts the transmural pressure difference, $P_i - P_o$ (Figure 8.17). The equilibrium wall tension is given by **Laplace's law**, which we met earlier in relation to ventricular wall tension (Section 6.8). For a thin-walled tube, Laplace's equation is:

$$T = (P_i - P_o)r \qquad (8.8)$$

Laplace's law thus states that **the bigger the vessel radius, the bigger the wall tension** needed to counter a given transmural pressure difference. For example, wall tension is higher in the aorta than in smaller arteries with a similar pressure, and capillary wall tension is very low (Figure 8.18). Laplace's law helps us understand why an **aortic aneurysm** (bulging of a weak aortic wall) progresses inexorably, once started. The increase in *r* raises the tension *T* in the aneurysm wall; the high tension thins and weakens the wall. This increases *r*, and so on. The positive feedback eventually leads to wall rupture, with catastrophic consequences.

A slightly more elaborate version of Laplace's law, called Love's equation, takes into account wall thickness, *w*. Wall thickness is important because it affects the **wall stress**, *S*,

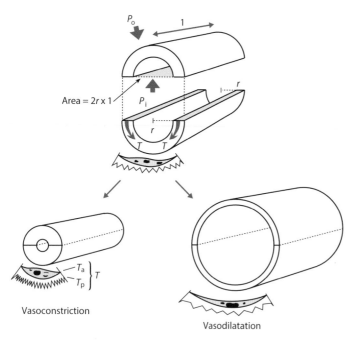

**Figure 8.17** Wall mechanics in a tube of unit length. (**Upper panel**) Pressure equals force per unit area. Internal pressure $P_i$ pushes outwards on area $2r$, driving the two halves of the cylinder apart with force $P_i 2r$. External pressure $P_o$ exerts force $P_o 2r$ in the opposite direction. The net distending force, $P_i 2r - P_o 2r$, is countered by the wall tension $T$ on each side of the cylinder. Thus $2T = P_i 2r - P_o 2r$, or $T = (P_i - P_o)r$ (Laplace's law). (**Lower panels**) Tension $T$ is the sum of active tension in smooth muscle, $T_a$, and passive tension in elastin/collagen fibres, $T_p$, shown as a spring. The spring on the left is in its relaxed state and that on the right is stretched and tense. $T_a$ and $T_p$ change in opposite directions during vasoconstriction to achieve mechanical stability.

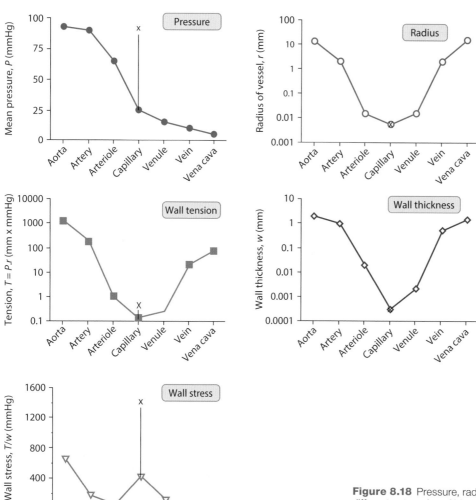

**Figure 8.18** Pressure, radius, wall tension and stress in different categories of blood vessel at heart level (Laplace's law). Vessel wall thickness affects stress, which is tension/thickness. The crosses represent capillaries in the foot during quiet standing, when gravity raises capillary pressure to ~90 mmHg.

which is the force per unit wall area; $S = T/w$ for unit length of vessel. The aorta has a thick wall, so although the wall tension is high, it is shared between many cells, collagen and elastin fibres, reducing the stress on them. By contrast, the capillary wall is only ~0.3 μm thick, so capillary wall stress approaches that in many arteries, despite the low capillary blood pressure and wall tension (Figure 8.18, bottom). Indeed, capillary wall stress in the human foot during standing exceeds that in the aorta, highlighting the extraordinary strength of the capillary wall.

## Changes in wall tension bring about constriction and dilatation

The total tension $T$ in the artery wall has two components: the passive tension of the elastin and collagen fibrils, and the active tension exerted by smooth muscle cells. When the smooth muscle contracts, its immediate effect is to raise the wall tension $T$. This produces a temporary mechanical disequilibrium, so the radius begins to decrease. Laplace's law tells us that, if the transmural pressure $P_i - P_o$ is constant and radius $r$ falls, a new mechanical equilibrium can only be attained by reducing the **net** (total) wall tension $T$. A fall in net wall tension is achieved by unloading the passive fibrils; the tension in the collagen and elastin fibres falls as the vessel radius is reduced (Figure 8.17). There is in effect a transfer of tension from the passive fibres to the active muscle cells. Without this, vasoconstriction would be an extremely unstable process.

Conversely, vasodilatation is brought about by smooth muscle relaxation. This reduces the active tension, creating a temporary mechanical disequilibrium. The internal distending pressure then pushes the wall out to a bigger radius, until a point is reached where the increased tension of the stretched collagen and elastin re-establishes mechanical equilibrium (Figure 8.17).

## 8.8 VISCOUS PROPERTIES OF BLOOD

Poiseuille's law tells us that vascular resistance depends not just on vessel geometry but also on the viscosity of the perfusing liquid, blood. Blood viscosity is altered in many haematological diseases, leading to changes in blood flow and pressure.

## Viscosity represents the internal friction in a fluid

The word viscosity stems from *viscum*, Latin for mistletoe, because mistletoe berries contain a thick, glutinous fluid. Viscosity was defined by Isaac Newton as *defectus lubricitatis*, lack of slipperiness, because viscosity is really the internal friction within a moving fluid, analogous to the friction between two moving solid surfaces. Viscosity is defined formally as the shear stress required to generate one unit of shear rate. **Shear stress** is the sliding force applied to a unit area

of contact between two laminae of fluid, and is proportional to the pressure gradient along the vessel. **Shear rate** is the change in fluid velocity per unit distance across the tube, that is, the slope of the velocity profile in Figure 8.3. (To visualize these terms, imagine pushing one sheet of paper across the surface of another. The shear stress is the sliding force you apply, per unit area, and the shear rate is the speed with which the top paper slides over the lower one.) The absolute unit of viscosity is $N.s/m^2$ or $Pa.s$. However, it is often more convenient to cite **relative viscosity**, which is dimensionless. The relative viscosity of blood or plasma is the viscosity divided by that of water.

## Plasma viscosity is dominated by plasma proteins

The voluminous albumin and globulin molecules of plasma raise plasma viscosity to 1.7 times that of water. In **myeloma**, a cancer of globulin-secreting cells, an increase in globulin concentration raises plasma viscosity and can cause the red cells to agglutinate (attach to each other) under cool conditions. The latter can raise blood viscosity to such a degree that tissue perfusion is badly impaired, leading to necrosis (tissue death) of the fingertips.

## Blood viscosity is dominated by haematocrit

The haematocrit is red cell volume as a percentage of blood volume. Red cells greatly increase the internal friction of blood, so blood viscosity is an increasing function of the haematocrit (Figure 8.19). The relative viscosity of human blood is ~4 at a haematocrit of 47%. The haematocrit of a species represents a compromise between high $O_2$-carrying capacity

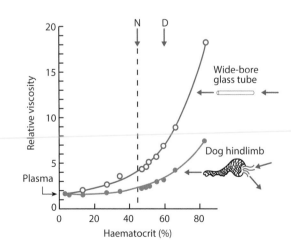

**Figure 8.19** Effect of the haematocrit on the viscosity of blood relative to water. Open circles: viscosity in a high-velocity, wide-bore glass viscometer. Closed circles: lower effective viscosity in an isolated, perfused dog hindlimb, due to the Fåhræus–Lindqvist effect. N, normal haematocrit; D, haematocrit at which cells are packed so tightly that they deform even at rest. (After the classic experiment of Whittaker SR, Winton FR. *The Journal of Physiology* 1933; 78(4): 339–69.)

and high viscosity, which impairs flow and raises blood pressure. In humans, the normal haematocrit is 40% (female) to 45% (male). In camels, the red cells are less flexible, so their viscous effect is greater and the camel's compromise haematocrit is lower, 27%. Abnormalities of haematocrit have serious consequences, as follows.

## Polycythaemia

Poly-(many)-cythaemia (blood cells) is a condition in which the haematocrit is higher than normal. In people living at **high altitude**, polycythaemia is a physiological adaptation to chronic hypoxia; however, in the disease **polycythaemia rubra vera** red cell overproduction by the bone marrow can raise the haematocrit excessively, to 70%. At a haematocrit of 63%, the red cells are packed so closely that viscosity and resistance are doubled. As a result, polycythaemia rubra vera causes hypertension and a sluggish blood flow that predisposes to cerebral or coronary thrombosis (strokes and heart attacks).

## Anaemia

Anaemia reduces blood viscosity, and therefore *TPR*. To maintain the arterial blood pressure, CO increases (equation 8.5). If the anaemia is prolonged, a form of cardiac failure called high-output failure can ensue. Thus, **homeostasis of blood viscosity is important for normal cardiovascular function**.

## Blood viscosity is non-Newtonian: I. Flow through narrow tubes

The viscosity of a simple fluid, such as water or plasma, is unaffected by the radius of the conducting tube or shear rate. Such a fluid is called a **Newtonian fluid**. By contrast, whole blood shows bizarre, but physiologically helpful, non-Newtonian behaviour, as follows.

### Viscosity decreases in microvessels (the Fåhræus–Lindqvist radius effect)

In 1931, Fåhræus and Lindqvist measured blood viscosity in a viscometer, consisting of a fine glass tube in which flow can be timed accurately. They discovered a strange phenomenon; blood viscosity is lower in a narrow-bore tube than a wide-bore tube (Figure 8.20a). The dependence of blood viscosity on tube radius evidently also occurs in the circulation because the effective viscosity of blood perfused through a dog hindlimb is half that of blood in a wide-bore viscometer (Figure 8.19). Blood viscosity begins to fall in tubes <1 mm wide (small arteries), and falls to ~2.5 in tubes of 30–40 μm arteriolar width. In tubes of capillary width, ~6 μm, blood viscosity reaches a minimum, almost as low as plasma viscosity. This 'Fåhræus–Lindqvist effect' accounts for the surprisingly low effective viscosity of blood in the circulation (Figure 8.19). The Fåhræus–Lindqvist effect is important because it greatly reduces microvascular resistance, and therefore the arterial pressure needed to perfuse the microcirculation. Without this effect, arterial pressure and cardiac work would be much higher.

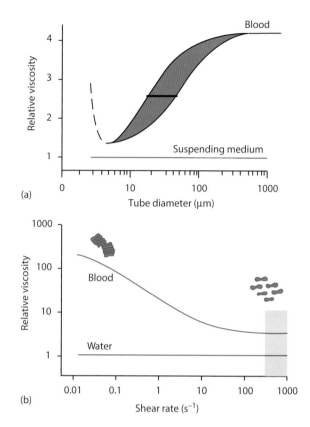

**Figure 8.20** Anomalous viscosity of blood, demonstrated in glass tubing. **(a)** Blood viscosity falls as tube diameter is reduced (Fåhræus–Lindqvist effect), but water viscosity is unchanged. The effective viscosity of blood in the circulation is ~2.5 (black bar), implying that the functional diameter of the resistance vessels is ~30 μm (arterioles). At diameters smaller than a blood capillary, viscosity rises again (dashed line). **(b)** Viscosity falls with increasing shear rate. The pink region shows typical shear rates *in vivo*. Sketches show red cell aggregation into rouleaux at low shear rates and disaggregation at high rates. (**(a)** After Gaetghens P. In: Gross DR, Wang NHC, eds. *The Rheology of Blood, Blood Vessels and Associated Tissues*. Amsterdam: Sijthoff & Noordhoff, with permission from Elsevier; **(b)** from Chien S. *Microvascular Research* 1992; 44(3): 243–54, with permission.)

Several mechanisms underlie the Fåhræus–Lindqvist effect. In capillaries, **bolus flow** reduces the effective viscosity (Section 8.2). In arterioles, the viscosity is reduced by the **peripheral plasma stream** generated by axial flow (Figure 8.3). Since shear rates are highest close to the vessel wall, a reduction in friction close to the wall has a marked, beneficial effect on net viscosity. The Fåhræus–Lindqvist effect is not noticeable in tubes wider than 1 mm because the thickness of the marginal plasma layer, 2–4 μm, becomes negligible relative to the tube width.

### Haematocrit decreases in microvessels (Fåhræus effect)

Robin Fåhræus described an additional curious effect in narrow tubes. The concentration of red cells in flowing blood inside a narrow tube, the **dynamic** or **tube haematocrit**, is lower than the 'central' haematocrit in the feeding and draining vessels. If a tube of radius 15 μm is fed from a reservoir with a central haematocrit of 40%, the dynamic haematocrit of flowing blood in the tube is only ~24%. This is a little hard to digest at first acquaintance! The phenomenon is the result of the difference between axial and marginal stream velocity (Figure 8.3). Suppose, for example, that blood of central haematocrit 50% feeds an arteriole, in which the red cells have twice the velocity of the plasma, owing to their more axial location. This blood drains into a vein. If the haematocrit in the parent artery and vein is to remain the same, 50% (which must be the case, since the circulation is in a steady state), equal volumes of plasma and red cells must pass through the arteriole in a given time. Because cell velocity is twice plasma velocity in our example, equal volume flows are only possible if the concentration of red cells in the arteriole is half that in the parent blood. This is achieved by the red cells speeding away from the plasma at the tube entrance, thinning out like traffic entering a fast road from a congested slip road.

The dynamic haematocrit is particularly low in capillaries, because the glycocalyx makes the effective radius of the tube even narrower than its apparent radius.

## Blood viscosity is non-Newtonian: II. Shear thinning

The viscosity of blood changes not only with vessel radius but also with flow velocity, or more accurately shear rate (Figure 8.20b). Shear rate, you may recall, is the change in fluid velocity per unit distance normal to the direction of flow, and it has the curious units of $s^{-1}$ (m/s per m). Blood viscosity falls as flow and shear rate increase. This is called shear thinning, the same phenomenon as in non-drip paint.

The shear thinning of blood is attributed to the deformation and lining up of red cells along the laminar flow lines, and to a tank-tread motion of the red cell membrane around its interior. At low flows in horizontal tubes, partial sedimentation of the cells within the tube also contributes to the rise in viscosity.

Shear rates are normally high in the circulation (~1000 $s^{-1}$), so blood is normally in a shear-thinned state. However, abnormally low flow allows the red cells to adhere to each other to form **rouleaux**, resembling stacks of coins. It is thought that such changes probably occur in veins *in vivo* if blood flow is sluggish. The tendency of red cells to aggregate in this way is related to the concentration of **fibrinogen** in the plasma.

## 8.9 PRESSURE–FLOW RELATIONSHIPS AND AUTOREGULATION

Poiseuille's law applies to a steady flow (cf. pulsatile) of Newtonian fluid (cf. non-Newtonian blood) through a long, straight vessel (cf. branching, curved blood vessels) with rigid walls (cf. distensible blood vessels). Not surprisingly, therefore, blood flow through tissues can deviate from Poiseuille's law (Figure 8.21). For example, in perfused lungs, or a perfused dog hindlimb with little vascular tone, the pressure–flow relationship is curved at low pressures, though nearly linear in the

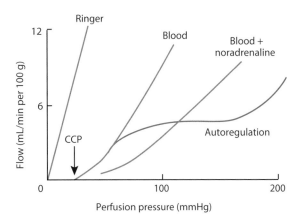

**Figure 8.21** Pressure–flow curves in perfused skeletal muscle (canine). The 'autoregulation' curve applies under physiological conditions because arterioles respond myogenically to pressure changes (see text). The 'blood' curve is observed if autoregulation is abolished. Near-zero flow occurs at a positive critical closing pressure (CCP), probably because of increased blood viscosity at low shear rates. The 'blood + noradrenaline' curve is less steep, because noradrenaline-induced vasoconstriction raises vascular resistance. Perfusion with Ringer's solution ('Ringer' line), a physiological salt solution of low Newtonian viscosity, produces a steep line that is almost straight because the anomalous viscous effect of blood is absent. (From Pappenheimer JR, Maes JP. *American Journal of Physiology* 1942; 137: 187–99; and Stainsby WN, Renkin EM. *American Journal of Physiology* 1961; 201: 117–22, with permission from the American Physiological Society.)

physiological range (Figure 8.21, 'blood' curve). The curvature at low pressures shows that resistance falls as pressure is raised. This is caused by the shear thinning of blood and, to a lesser degree, vessel distension. Shear thinning seems to be the chief factor, since the pressure-flow relationship is almost linear when a dog hindlimb is perfused with a physiological salt solution (Ringer's solution) rather than blood (Figure 8.21).

Many vascular beds with a high physiological level of arteriolar tone show a very different, physiologically important shape of pressure–flow relationship, called an **autoregulation curve**, which deviates wildly from Poiseuille behaviour. Blood flow increases with perfusion pressure up to a certain point, beyond which the flow changes surprisingly little with pressure (the plateau), until pressure exceeds ~160 mmHg. An almost constant flow in the face of a changing pressure (autoregulation) is due to the vascular resistance changing in the opposite direction to pressure. For example, a rise in pressure triggers resistance vessel constriction, which prevents flow from rising (Section 13.6). Autoregulation is important because it helps to stabilize the blood flow to an organ, such as the brain, in the face of fluctuating arterial pressures. Autoregulation occurs to a greater or lesser degree in most organs, except the lungs.

## 8.10 VENOUS PRESSURE AND VOLUME

Peripheral veins and venules are thin-walled, contractile, voluminous vessels that contain about two thirds of the blood pool. Due to their large, variable volume, the peripheral vessels act as an adjustable reservoir of blood; that is, they can contract and expel some of their blood to top up the central veins, and hence boost the CVP, stroke volume and arterial pressure. The volume of blood in the peripheral veins depends on the **venous blood pressure** and **smooth muscle tone** in the tunica media, as follows (Figure 8.22).

## The venous pressure–volume curve is sigmoidal due to changes in vessel profile

Blood pressure is ~12–20 mmHg in venules at heart level, falling to ~8–10 mmHg in more central veins, such as the antecubital or femoral vein. Since venous resistance is small, 8–10 mmHg is enough to drive the CO back to the right ventricle, where diastolic pressure is 0–6 mmHg.

Venous pressure depends very much on the position of the vein relative to heart level, because of gravity (Figure 8.2). Moreover, since the vein wall is thin and collapsible, the cross-sectional profile and volume change markedly with pressure (Figure 8.22). This results in large changes in peripheral venous blood volume with changes in body posture. When venous pressure is below zero (atmospheric pressure), as in a hand above heart level, the vein collapses into a dumb-bell shaped profile, and flow is confined to the narrow marginal channels. At a transmural pressure of +1 mmHg, the vein assumes a narrow elliptical cross section. As pressure rises towards 10 mmHg, the elliptical profile becomes progressively rounder. These changes in profile enable peripheral veins to accommodate a large volume of blood in response to relatively small changes in pressure. The maximum distensibility (compliance) occurs at ~4 mmHg and is ~100 mL/mmHg for the human systemic venous system. This is some 50 times greater than arterial compliance.

Above 10–15 mmHg, the vein profile is fully circular, and since the collagen in the wall is relatively inextensible, venous volume becomes less sensitive to pressure. Because of the collapse of veins at low pressure and their relative stiffness at high pressure, the venous pressure–volume curve is sigmoidal (S-shaped).

## Venous smooth muscle tone regulates venous volume

In the gastrointestinal tract, liver, kidneys and skin, the venous tunica media is richly innervated by sympathetic vasomotor nerves. Sympathetic venoconstriction greatly reduces venous capacitance in these tissues, and the displaced blood moves into the thoracic compartment (Figure 8.22). In this way, the central nervous system can exert a degree of control over the filling pressure of the heart.

## Human central venous pressure can be estimated by inspecting the neck veins

CVP can be monitored directly in intensive care units by a catheter inserted into the internal jugular vein. However, during routine clinical examination CVP is assessed indirectly by inspection of the neck veins (Figure 8.23). The external jugular vein runs over the sternocleidomastoid muscle and the internal jugular vein runs deep to the muscle. When a human is semi-supine, the lower part of the jugular vein is normally distended but the upper part is collapsed because blood in the upper part is at subatmospheric pressure, because of gravity (Figure 8.2). From the sigmoidal pressure–volume curve of veins, we know that **at the point of venous collapse, the transmural pressure is approximately zero**. Therefore, the CVP must equal the pressure exerted by the vertical column of blood between the point of jugular vein collapse and the right atrium.

A numerical example should make this clearer. Suppose that the point of jugular vein collapse, where venous blood pressure equals atmospheric pressure, is a 7 cm vertical distance above the right atrium. The CVP must therefore be 7 cm of blood, which is 7.4 $cmH_2O$. The atrium is not visible, of course, but it is known to be ~5 cm lower than the manubriosternal angle, which can be palpated. Thus, by measuring the vertical distance between the point of jugular vein collapse and the manubriosternal angle (2 cm in our example), and adding 5 cm, human CVP can be roughly estimated.

Although the accuracy of the inspection method is only about ±2 cm, it is good enough to detect the grossly elevated CVP that characterizes right ventricular failure (Chapter 18).

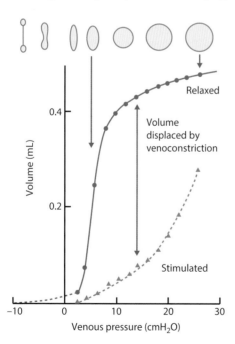

**Figure 8.22** Venous pressure-volume curves, when veins are relaxed (circles) or maximally venoconstricted (triangles). Change in venous cross section with pressure in relaxed state shown above. Volume $V$ at a given pressure $P$, called venous capacitance, is reduced by venoconstriction. Compliance (distensibility) is the slope $dV/dP$. (Canine saphenous vein; from Vanhoutte PM, Leusen I. *Pflügers Archiv: European Journal of Physiology* 1969; 306(4): 341–53, with kind permission from Springer Science and Business Media.)

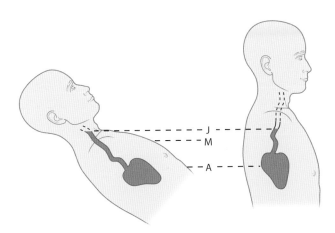

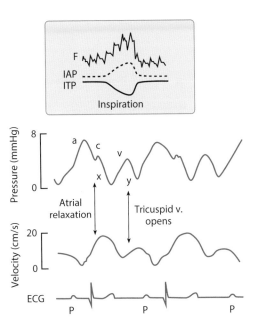

**Figure 8.23** How to estimate central venous pressure (CVP) in a semi-recumbent (45 degrees) human. CVP is vena cava blood pressure at the junction with the right atrium. It equals the vertical distance J–A, between the point of collapse of the jugular vein (J, blood at atmospheric pressure) and right atrium (A). Since A is not visible, the vertical height of J above the manubriosternal angle (M) is measured in cm, and an average vertical distance M–A (~5 cm) is added on. Thus CVP = (J − M) cm + 5 cm, in cm blood (almost same as cmH$_2$O). In the upright position, the entire jugular vein is normally collapsed, so it is not visible.

**Figure 8.24** Pressure and flow in the human superior vena cava over two cardiac cycles. (**Inset**) Effect of breathing on venous return. a, c, v, x, y as in Figure 2.5. F, flow in the thoracic inferior vena cava; IAP, intra-abdominal pressure; ITP, intrathoracic pressure. (Data from Brecher GA. *Venous Return*. New York: Grune & Stratton, 1956; and Wexler L, Bergel DH, Gabe IT, et al. *Circulation Research* 1968; 23(3): 349–59.)

In right ventricular failure, the CVP may be so high that the jugular venous pulse is visible even when the patient is upright. A normal patient must be semi-supine (at 45 degrees) for the jugular pulse to be visible, because in the upright position the transition point between collapse and distension is below the level of the clavicle.

## Central venous pressure waves are visible in jugular veins in recumbent humans

The superior vena cava and jugular veins form a relatively direct tube into the right atrium, with no venous valves. Consequently, jugular venous pressure mirrors the pulsatile pressure wave in the right atrium (Section 2.3 and Figure 8.24). Although the jugular pulse pressure is only a few mmHg, it is sufficient to move the overlying skin. The 'x' and 'y' descents of the wave are normally visible as inward flickers of the skin in a semi-recumbent human. Palpation readily distinguishes the jugular venous pulse (too weak to feel) from the carotid arterial pulse (easily felt). Unlike the arterial pulse, the level of the jugular venous pulse above the clavicle can be increased by pressing on the right side of the abdomen just below the diaphragm to compress the liver. This forces blood into the vena cava and raises jugular venous pressure (hepatojugular reflux).

## 8.11 EFFECTS OF GRAVITY ON THE VENOUS SYSTEM

A change in posture from supine to standing triggers extensive changes in the human cardiovascular system (Section 17.1). The primary event that initiates these changes is the effect of gravity on venous blood distribution.

## Orthostasis distends veins below heart level

In the standing position (**orthostasis**), pressure increases in all the blood vessels below heart level and falls in all the vessels above heart level, due to the pull of gravity on the vertical column of fluid between heart and vessel (Figures 8.2 and 8.25). This particularly affects the distribution of blood in the venous system, owing to its steep, sigmoidal pressure–volume curve (Figure 8.22).

On tilting a human from the supine to upright position, a transitory closure of the venous valves in the limbs prevents any substantial venous backflow. Pressure in the dependent (below heart) veins then rises steadily over 30–60 s, as blood flows into them from the arterial system. As venous pressure rises, flow recommences up the limb veins and pushes open the venous valves. This re-establishes an uninterrupted column of blood. The weight of the continuous fluid column between heart and feet raises venous pressure in the feet ninefold, from ~10 mmHg supine to ~90 mmHg in orthostasis (Figures 8.2, 8.25 and 8.27).

There is no counterbalancing rise in extramural pressure during orthostasis (unless the patient is immersed in water), so the dependent veins become greatly distended. Check for yourself. The effect is plainly visible in the back of the hand as the hand is moved above and below heart level. In a human adult, about 500 mL of blood accumulates in the distended veins below heart level during orthostasis, over ~45 s (Figure 8.25). This is widely referred to as venous 'pooling', though the imagery here is misleading; a pool is static whereas

143

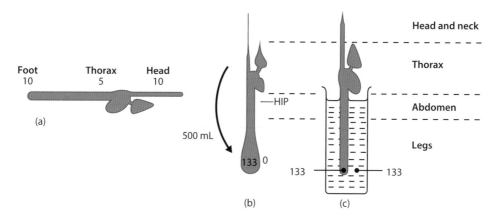

**Figure 8.25** Venous blood displacement (red) on moving from **(a)** supine to **(b)** standing. The thoracic compartment includes the central veins, heart and pulmonary blood. Numbers indicate cmH$_2$O pressure above atmospheric. The pressure surrounding the extrathoracic veins is approximately atmospheric (zero baseline). The hydrostatic indifferent point (HIP) is the point where pressure does not change on tilting. **(c)** Upright immersion in water raises pressure outside the veins, displacing 'pooled' blood centrally and raising the central venous pressure. (After Gauer OH, Thron HL. In: Hamilton WF, Dow P, eds. *Handbook of Physiology, a Critical, Comprehensive Presentation of Physiological Knowledge and Concepts. Section 2. Circulation*, Vol. 3. Bethesda, MD: American Physiological Society, 1963: 2409–40.)

**venous blood flows continuously** in the steady state. Most of the redistributed blood comes ultimately from the intrathoracic compartment, via arterial flow (not via venous backflow, since valves prevent this). The loss of blood from the intrathoracic veins reduces the CVP, which impairs the stroke volume through the Frank–Starling mechanism. This causes a transitory arterial hypotension and sometimes dizziness, called **postural hypotension** (Section 17.1). A hand count among medical students indicates that nearly all healthy individuals occasionally experience orthostatic dizziness, especially when warm and venodilated.

## Gravity does not affect flow directly: the siphon principle

This short section deals with a common student misconception, namely that venous blood flow must decrease in the leg during standing 'because the blood has to go uphill against gravity'. This concept is wrong because it ignores the fact that gravity exerts an equal and opposite 'downhill' pull on the arterial column. Gravity acts equally on the venous and arterial fluid columns, so the **pressure difference** between artery and vein at any level is not affected by orthostasis (Figures 8.2 and 11.5). Since flow is proportional to pressure difference, blood flow in the steady state is not directly affected by standing. The circulation through the leg or brain in fact resembles flow through a U-tube siphon (Figure 8.26). Flow through a rigid siphon is totally unaffected by the orientation of the siphon; flow is the same whether the siphon is horizontal, vertical or upside down, for the reason given above. Similarly, if blood vessels were completely rigid, gravity would have no effect whatsoever on venous or arterial flow in the steady state.

Limb blood flow declines in the steady state during dependency (Figure 8.6), but this is not because 'blood has to go

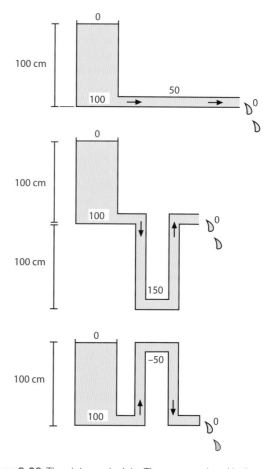

**Figure 8.26** The siphon principle. The pressure head in the feed tank, 100 cmH$_2$O, drives flow through the open-ended tube. Pressure is 50 cmH$_2$O halfway along the tube when horizontal. If the tube is bent into a U shape, the pressure difference driving flow from tank to outlet is the same, so the flow is identical, irrespective of which way up the U tube is. Only the intermediate pressures are changed (numbers, cmH$_2$O); see Bernoulli principle. The middle sketch is equivalent to the situation in the leg vasculature during standing.

uphill in the veins'. The reduction is caused by an active arteriolar contraction, which is partly a local response to the rise in pressure and partly a baroreceptor reflex.

## Extracranial veins collapse above heart level

Gravity reduces the pressure of blood in vessels above heart level. When the transmural pressure falls to zero or less, unsupported superficial veins collapse (Figures 8.22, 8.23 and 8.25), as is easily observed in the back of one's hand. Deeper veins are better supported and do not collapse completely. Veins inside the cranial cavity are a special case. They do not collapse during orthostasis, despite their subatmospheric blood pressure, because gravity also reduces the pressure of the cerebrospinal fluid surrounding them. Thus, the **transmural pressure** across the vein wall hardly changes. However, in the **venous sinuses of the dura mater** the subatmospheric pressure creates one potential hazard. The walls of these sinuses are attached to the rigid interior of the skull and are therefore not collapsible. Consequently, if they are breached by an accident or surgery in the upright position, air can be sucked into the veins by the subatmospheric venous pressure, causing **air embolism**.

## Immersion and other gravitational effects

When a human is partially immersed vertically in water, gravity acts on the water as well as the blood, so the extramural pressure at any point below heart level rises by almost the same amount as the intramural blood pressure. Consequently, transmural venous pressure barely changes in the lower limbs, unlike the situation in air. Upright immersion thus prevents venous pooling and maintains the intrathoracic blood volume and cardiac filling pressure. Due to the operation of the Frank–Starling mechanism, the stroke volume increases by ~50% on upright immersion to the neck.

Aeroplane pilots experience altered $g$ forces during aerobatics. A pilot pulling out of a steep dive can experience 13–14 $g$ along the body axis. Venous pooling in the lower body is then so severe that CVP and stroke volume fall rapidly, leading to cerebral hypoperfusion and a blackout. To prevent this, an antigravity suit is worn; bags inflate automatically around the legs to raise extramural pressure and minimize venous distension during turns, mimicking immersion in water (Figure 8.25). Conversely, in an inverted 'loop-the-loop', a high negative $g$ force is experienced; that is, gravity is directed towards the head. This distends the retinal vessels and causes vision 'red-out'.

In space travel, the circulation is subjected to zero gravity for long periods. Unlike water immersion (Figure 8.25), CVP has been measured to fall when going into space due to the changed mechanics of the whole thorax. This presents no special problem for the cardiovascular system, until the return to positive gravity.

Venous blood flow is influenced by two accessory pumps, the exercise skeletal muscle pump and the respiratory pump.

## The skeletal muscle pump has multiple roles

When a skeletal muscle contracts, it compresses the local veins and displaces their blood proximally, towards the central veins (Figure 8.27, top). The venous valves prevent retrograde flow and ensure that the emptied segments refill from the periphery when the muscle relaxes. Thus, rhythmic exercise has a pumping effect on venous flow. Although this is not essential for venous return, it has the following beneficial effects:

- By redistributing venous blood from the periphery into the central veins, the muscle pump prevents CVP from falling during exercise, counteracting the cardiac pump effect of Figure 6.12. The muscle pump can even increase CVP slightly, shifting the ventricle up the Starling curve.
- Like any other pump, the skeletal muscle pump reduces pressure in its feed line (Figure 6.12). Each time the leg muscles relax, blood drains rapidly from the distal veins into the empty muscle veins, lowering venous pressure in the foot and ankle. At the same time, closure of the proximal valves interrupts the vertical column of blood between limb and heart. In this way, the leg muscle pump can reduce venous pressure in the lower leg from 70–90 mmHg during immobile standing to 20–40 mmHg during walking, running and cycling (Figure 8.27, bottom). This increases the arteriovenous pressure gradient driving blood through the calf muscle by 50%–60% (Figure 15.8).
- Since capillary pressure is close to venous pressure, the muscle pump lowers capillary pressure too, reducing fluid filtration into the feet and ankles. This helps prevent the feet and ankles from becoming swollen and oedematous (fluid-filled) in the upright position.

## Valvular incompetence leads to varicose veins and venous leg ulcers

The venous valves of the leg often become incompetent with ageing. As a result, the vertical column of venous blood cannot be broken up by the now ineffective muscle pump, and the distal leg veins are subjected to a chronically elevated pressure load during orthostasis (Figure 8.27, red recording). This leads to a permanent dilatation of the veins, the familiar **varicose veins**. Chronic venous hypertension also causes leukocytes to adhere in the dependent microcirculation, through mechanisms that are still being explored. The microvascular changes lead to trophic skin changes, namely discoloration and induration (hardening), followed by skin ulceration. **Venous leg ulcers**

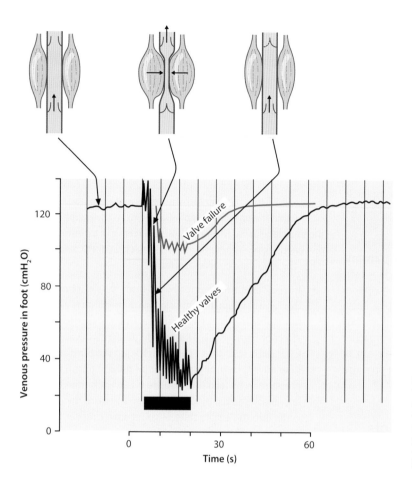

**Figure 8.27** The skeletal muscle pump. The trace shows pressure in the dorsal vein of the foot (solid line), initially standing still, then rhythmically when the calf muscles were contracted (black bar). Insets show how the muscle pump operates. The red line shows the effect of failure of the venous valves, as in varicose veins. (Levick JR, Michel CC. Unpublished results.)

usually develop just above the medial malleolus of the ankle. They are common in older individuals, difficult to heal and a great expense for national health services. Since venous ulcers are treated by compression bandaging while arterial ulcers are not, the ABPI is used to distinguish between arterial and venous disease before treatment (Section 8.5).

## The respiratory pump and coughing

Inspiration increases blood flow into the thoracic venae cavae by two mechanisms (Figure 8.24, inset). The fall in intrathoracic pressure expands the intrathoracic veins, and the descent of the diaphragm compresses the abdominal contents, raising the abdominal venous pressure and hence flow into the thorax. Conversely, expiration reduces flow into the thoracic venae cavae. The latter effect is greatly exaggerated during forced expiration, such as the **Valsalva manoeuvre** (Chapter 17) or coughing. **Coughing** can elevate intrathoracic pressure transiently to 400 mmHg, greatly impeding venous return. Indeed, **paroxysmal coughing** can impede venous return to such an extent that fainting ensues.

The respiratory pump has a dwindling effect on flow in more peripheral veins, though a small effect is still detectable in the femoral vein.

## Flow is pulsatile in the great veins

Flow in the great veins is pulsatile because there are no valves separating them from the right atrium. There are two venous spurts per cycle (Figure 8.24). **Peak flow** occurs during the $x$ descent of the atrial pressure wave, as the atria begin to relax. Peak flow is aided by ventricular systole, which has a suction effect on the atria and central veins. As right ventricular systole shoots a mass of blood up into the pulmonary trunk, the ventricle itself is propelled downwards, like the ballistic recoil of a gun (Newton's law of action and reaction). This causes the annulus fibrosus (base of ventricle) to descend (Figure 2.3), stretching the atria and sucking blood into them. A **second flow-spurt** occurs during the $y$ descent of the atrial pressure wave, due to the opening of the tricuspid valve in diastole. The second spurt is boosted by a second suction effect, mediated by the elastic recoil of the ventricular walls, especially when end-systolic volume is low during exercise. Thus, flow through the great veins is driven primarily by the upstream (distal) pressure of ~8 mmHg (pressure from behind or *vis a tergo*) and is boosted by two transient reductions in downstream pressure due to the motion of the heart (suction from in front, *vis a fronte*).

## SUMMARY

- The **pattern of blood flow** is **laminar** in healthy arteries and veins, **turbulent** in the ventricles and atheromatous arteries, and **bolus** (single-file) in capillaries.

- **Darcy's law** states that laminar flow is proportional to the pressure drop along a tube, $P_1 - P_2$ and inversely proportional to resistance $R$. **Bernoulli's theory** takes account of kinetic energy and gravitational potential energy as well as pressure energy. **Poiseuille's law** defines the factors governing $R$ in a tube.

- **Human blood flow** is measured in major arteries by Doppler US; in certain organs by Fick's principle (e.g. renal blood flow using PAH); in limbs by venous occlusion plethysmography; and in the microcirculation by Kety's radioisotope clearance method.

- **Human arterial pressure** is usually measured by brachial artery sphygmomnomery. It varies with age, exercise, emotional stress, sleep, pregnancy, orthostasis, gravity, hypovolaemia, hypertension and many other pathological conditions. The ankle–brachial pressure ratio tests for leg arterial disease.

- **Mean arterial pressure** equals $CO \times TPR$. Mean pressure in the brachial artery is calculated as diastolic pressure + one third of the pulse pressure.

- **Pulse pressure** is systolic minus diastolic pressure. Pulse pressure and systolic pressure depend on stroke volume, arterial stiffness (1/compliance) and wave reflection. Wave reflection adds a diastolic wave after the incisura in young individuals, but a systolic inflection before the incisura in older individuals, raising systolic pressure and cardiac work.

- The pressure wave **propagates** rapidly along the arterial tree. The propagation rate increases as ageing stiffens the artery wall (**arteriosclerosis**). Arterial stiffening also raises systolic pressure, hence cardiac work and $O_2$ demand.

- **Vascular resistance** is located chiefly in terminal arteries and arterioles, across which the pressure falls from ~80 mmHg to 35 mmHg. **Poiseuille's law** states that resistance depends on blood viscosity $\eta$, vessel length $L$ and (inversely) radius

$r^4$; $R = 8\eta L/\pi r^4$. Vascular radius is regulated by smooth muscle. Due to the $r^4$ effect, a small reduction in vascular tone increases local blood flow greatly. A widespread rise in vascular tone raises the $TPR$ and therefore arterial pressure.

- In many organs *in vivo*, flow is almost independent of arterial pressure in the physiological range, contrary to the classic laws of physics, because the arterioles actively regulate their resistance (**autoregulation**).

- **Laplace's law** shows that wall tension $T$ in a thin tube at mechanical equilibrium increases with radius and transmural pressure; $T = \Delta Pr$. Therefore, wall tension and stress are high in the aorta, which can lead to aneurysm formation.

- **Blood viscosity** $\eta$ depends on the haematocrit. This is raised in polycythaemia, leading to hypertension, strokes and heart attacks. Viscosity is reduced in anaemia. Blood viscosity falls in microvessels, facilitating microvascular perfusion (Fåhræus–Lindqvist effect). Viscosity increases at low shear rates.

- **Venous pressure** is 8–10 mmHg in peripheral veins at heart level. CVP is 0–7 mmHg and can be estimated by inspection of the jugular veins.

- **Peripheral venous blood volume** is variable, and affects CVP and stroke volume. It depends on (1) venous smooth muscle tone, which is regulated by sympathetic fibres in the renal, splanchnic and cutaneous circulations; and (2) venous pressure, which depends on position of the vein relative to heart level (gravity). The venous pressure–volume curve is sigmoidal, due to vein profile changes.

- During **orthostasis**, gravity raises the venous and arterial pressures in the legs (principle of manometry, $\rho gh$). Venous 'pooling' in distended leg veins reduces CVP and stroke volume, leading to transient postural hypotension. The muscle pump counteracts venous pooling during walking. Venous valve incompetence leads to chronic venous hypertension, varicose veins and venous leg ulcers.

## FURTHER READING

Tanaka K, Nishimura N, Kawai Y. Adaptation to microgravity, deconditioning, and countermeasures. *The Journal of Physiological Sciences* 2017; **67**(2): 271–81.

Elder A, Japp A, Verghese A. How valuable is physical examination of the cardiovascular system? *British Medical Journal* 2016; **354**: i3309.

Nichols WW, O'Rourke MF. *McDonald's Blood Flow in Arteries: Theoretical, Experimental and Clinical Principles*, 6th edn. London: Hodder Arnold, 2011.

Fung YC. *Biomechanics*. New York: Springer, 2010.

Julien C. The enigma of Mayer waves: facts and models. *Cardiovascular Research* 2006; **70**(1): 12–21.

Pickering TG, Shimbo D, Haas D. Ambulatory blood-pressure monitoring. *New England Journal of Medicine* 2006; **354**(22): 2368–74.

Lipowsky HH. Microvascular rheology and hemodynamics. *Microcirculation* 2005; **12**(1): 5–15.

Vowden KR, Goulding V, Vowden P. Hand-held doppler assessment for peripheral arterial disease. *Journal of Wound Care* 1996; **5**(3): 125–8.

Dormandy JA. Microcirculation in venous disorders: the role of the white blood cells. *International Journal of Microcirculation, Clinical and Experimental* 1995; **15**(Suppl 1): 3–8.

Secomb T. Mechanics of blood flow in the microcirculation. In: Ellington CP, Pedley TJ, eds. *Biological Fluid Dynamics*. Cambridge: Company of Biologists; 1995. pp. 305–21.

Goldsmith HL, Cokelet GR, Gaehtgens P. Robin Fåhræus: evolution of his concepts in cardiovascular physiology. *American Journal of Physiology* 1989; **257**(3 Pt 2): H1005–15.

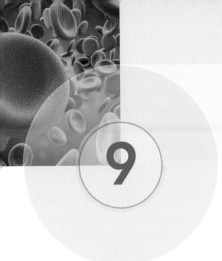

# Endothelium

## 9

## LEARNING OBJECTIVES

*After reading this chapter you should be able to:*

- outline the structure of the glycocalyx, intercellular junction, vesicle system and actin cytoskeleton (9.2);
- name the endothelial $Ca^{2+}$-conducting ion channels, and the role of endothelial $Ca^{2+}$ (9.3);
- list four vasoactive endothelial secretions (9.4, 9.5);
- give the actions of endothelial nitric oxide (NO) and the factors regulating its production (9.4);
- state the effect of the endothelium on blood (9.6);

- outline how the endothelium captures leukocytes during inflammation (9.8);
- describe the other roles of the endothelium in inflammation (9.8);
- outline the factors that regulate capillary permeability (9.7);
- state the role of the endothelium in angiogenesis (9.9);
- describe the contribution of endothelial dysfunction to atheroma (9.10);
- describe the role of platelets and the coagulation cascade in thrombus formation (9.11).

Endothelium is the monolayer of endothelial cells that lines the blood interface throughout the cardiovascular system, including the cardiac chambers. Its aggregate mass is several hundred grams in a human adult. The active nature of the endothelium is much less obvious than that of cardiac myocytes, yet endothelial cells make numerous and remarkably varied contributions to cardiovascular function. The enormous surface area of the endothelium (~280 m² in human skeletal muscles; ~90 m² in the lungs) facilitates the transfer of respiratory gases, nutrients and white cells between blood and tissue; the transfer of regulatory signals to vascular smooth muscle (VSM); and the modification of plasma composition (Figure 9.1).

## 9.1 OUTLINE OF ENDOTHELIAL FUNCTIONS

### Endothelium regulates blood–tissue exchange

The primary role of the endothelium is to form a semipermeable membrane in order to retain plasma and blood cells inside the circulation, yet permit nutrient transfer into the tissues. Specialized, regulated intercellular junctions confer permeability to water and nutrients such as glucose, while an internal coating of biopolymers, the glycocalyx, restricts plasma protein escape.

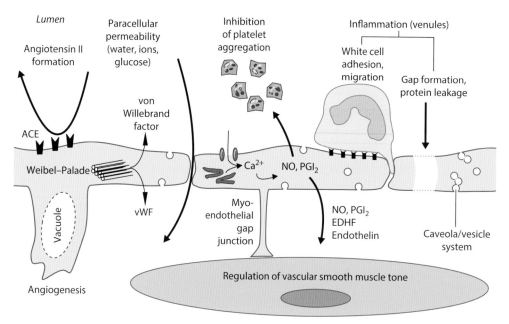

**Figure 9.1** Multiple functions of the endothelial cell; the lumen is at the top. ACE, angiotensin-converting enzyme; NO, nitric oxide; PGI₂, prostacyclin; EDHF, endothelium-derived hyperpolarizing factor; vWF, von Willebrand factor.

## Paracrine secretions regulate vascular tone

Arterial endothelial cells express receptors for many vasoactive agents, such as acetylcholine (ACh), and it can also sense the shear stress generated by flowing blood. It responds to these signals by secreting vasoactive agents, namely nitric oxide (NO), endothelium-derived hyperpolarizing factor (EDHF), prostacyclin (PGI₂) and endothelin. These agents act in a paracrine fashion (i.e. locally) on adjacent VSM cells to adjust local blood flow, for example, flow-induced arterial dilatation in exercising muscle (Section 13.7). Emerging evidence suggests that local cardiac endothelial NO and endothelin may influence cardiac contractility. Vasodilatation to EDHF involves not only the release of a paracrine factor, but also spread of endothelial cell hyperpolarization, so the overall mechanism is now referred to as endothelium-dependent hyperpolarization (EDH). Nevertheless, the hyperpolarizing 'factor' remains to be identified.

## Endothelial cell surface enzymes modify vasoactive peptides in the bloodstream

The luminal surface of the endothelium possesses an enzyme, angiotensin-converting enzyme (ACE), which chemically modifies circulating vasoactive peptides. The large surface area of the endothelium ensures the efficient conversion of substrate.

## Endothelium secretes both antithrombotic and pro-clotting factors

NO and prostacyclin are not only vasodilators but also inhibitors of platelet aggregation. This prevents circulating blood from clotting (thrombosis). The endothelium also secretes von Willebrand factor (vWF), a component of the clotting cascade.

## Endothelium participates in the inflammatory defence against pathogens

In an inflamed tissue, venular endothelium inserts adhesion molecules into its surface membrane to capture circulating leukocytes and promote their migration to the source of the inflammation. Also, the endothelial cells change shape, forming large gaps that allow circulating immunoglobulins to access the inflamed tissue.

## Endothelium initiates new blood vessel formation

The sprouting of endothelial cells is the starting point for the development of all new blood vessels (angiogenesis). Angiogenesis is essential for tissue growth, pregnancy, wound repair and the growth of cancers. Antiangiogenic drugs are now used to inhibit cancer growth.

## Endothelial dysfunction contributes to atheroma

The impairment of endothelial function appears to contribute to the development of arterial atheroma, the single biggest cause of morbidity and mortality in westernized societies. Plasma-derived cholesterol and fibrin become trapped between the endothelium and tunica media, leading to the formation of the atheromatous plaque.

The roles of endothelium are thus many, diverse and vitally important. This chapter describes the cell biology underlying these roles. Solute exchange and fluid movement across the endothelium are covered in Chapters 10 and 11, respectively. The regulation of vascular tone by endothelial secretions is integrated with the numerous other vascular control mechanisms in Chapter 13.

## 9.2 STRUCTURE OF ENDOTHELIUM

Endothelium is a thin monolayer of polygonal, flattened endothelial cells. The cells are 0.2–0.3 μm thick, and are joined edge-to-edge in a 'crazy paving' pattern (Figures 1.11 and 9.2). Each cell contains a small store of $Ca^{2+}$ in the endoplasmic reticulum, which can be as little as 8 nm or so from the surface. Endothelial cells also have a unique storage organelle, the Weibel–Palade body (Section 9.6).

### The actin/myosin cytoskeleton provides shape and anchorage

Endothelial cell shape is maintained by an actin cytoskeleton, which is organized into three distinct systems: the cortical web, the junctional band and the basal stress fibres (Figure 9.2). The **cortical web** is a thin layer of actin filaments under the cell membrane, linked to membrane glycoproteins by filamin and other proteins. The cortical web helps anchor surface molecules, such as the glycocalyx and leukocyte-capturing selectins. The **junctional band** is a prominent ring of actin running around the cell perimeter (Figure 9.2). It is attached to the intercellular junction proteins via α-actinin and anchors them in place (Figure 9.3); if the junctional actin band is disassembled,

using cytochalasin, gaps appear between the cells. **Basal stress fibres** are prominent in arterial endothelium and resist the shearing effect of the bloodstream. They comprise interdigitating myosin and actin filaments organized into 2–4 μm long, sarcomere-like units. The ends of the stress fibre are attached via a protein complex (α-actinin, vinculin, talin) to transmembrane dimers, called **integrins**. The integrins bind to extracellular laminin, collagen and fibronectin at **focal contacts** (adhesion plaques), thus gluing the cell down (Figures 9.2 and 9.3).

### Intercellular clefts provide a pathway for water and nutrient transfer

Water and small, lipid-insoluble solutes, such as glucose, amino acids and drugs, can cross the endothelial barrier via the intercellular clefts, chiefly in capillaries. The clefts are 20 nm wide and occupy only 0.2%–0.4% of the capillary surface (Figure 9.2, top). Rows of protein particles in the cell membrane facing the cleft form **junctional strands**. Two or three junctional strands run around the cell perimeter. The strands on neighbouring cells meet across the intercellular cleft to form **tight junctions** (Figure 9.3). However, the tight junctions do not continue unbroken around the entire cell perimeter; there are occasional 150–200 nm long **breaks in the junctional strands**, which provide a continuous, albeit tortuous, permeable pathway across the capillary wall (Figures 9.4 and 10.3). The number and width of the breaks greatly influence capillary permeability; postcapillary venules, for example, have

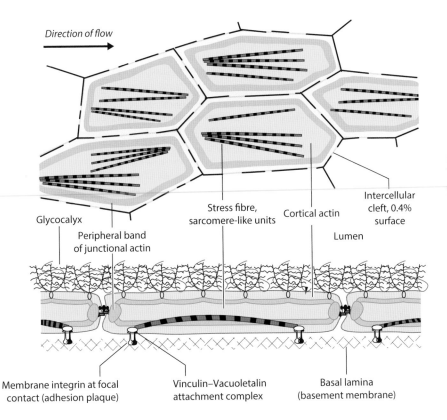

Figure 9.2 Organization of the endothelial cytoskeleton and intercellular junctions, viewed face on (top) and in cross section (bottom). Black intercellular lines viewed face on represent sealed region of cleft (~90%); the grey lines are the open, permeable parts of the cleft, at breaks in the junctional strands. Glycocalyx molecules form hairy tufts attached to the cell membrane and linked to the cortical actin cytoskeleton at ~100 nm intervals. (Adapted from Drenckhahn D, Ness W. In: Born GVR, Schwartz CJ, eds. *Vascular Endothelium: Physiology, Pathology and Therapeutic Opportunities*. Stuttgart: Schattauer, 1997; and Weinbaum S, Tarbell JM, Damiano ER. *Annual Review of Biomedical Engineering* 2007; 9: 121–67.)

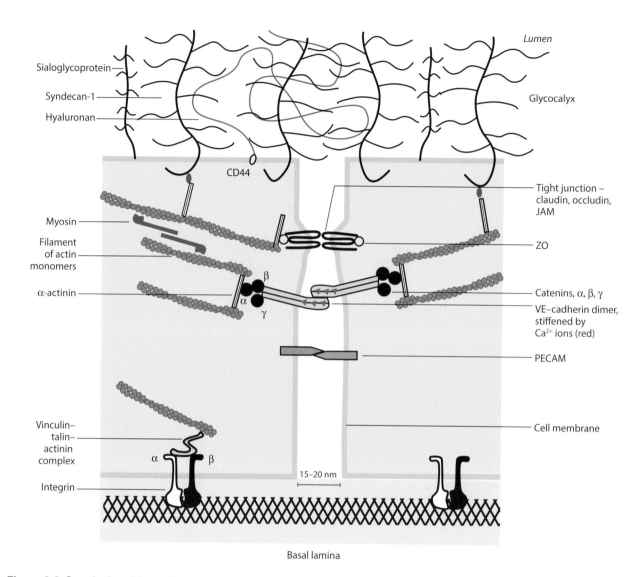

**Figure 9.3** Organization of the endothelial intercellular junction and glycocalyx. The cadherin extracellular domain requires $Ca^{2+}$ ions (red triangles) for stiffness. Homocellular gap junctions in the arterial endothelium are not shown. The glycocalyx comprises linear core proteins to which are attached long heparan sulphate (and some chondroitin sulphate) side chains (e.g. syndecan-1) or short sialic acid residues (sialoglycoproteins). Hyaluronan is an acetylglucosamine-glucuronic acid polymer with no core protein. JAM, junctional adhesion molecule; PECAM, platelet endothelial cell adhesion molecule; VE–cadherin, vascular endothelial cadherin; ZO, zonula occludens-1. (Based on Waschke J, Drenckhahn D, Adamson RH, et al. *American Journal of Physiology. Heart and Circulatory Physiology.* 2004; 287(2): H704–11 with permission from the American Physiological Society; and Weinbaum S, Tarbell JM, Damiano ER. *Annual Review Biomedical of Engineering* 2007; 9: 121–67.)

fewer junctional strands and wider breaks than capillaries, so they have a higher permeability to water; whereas brain capillaries have numerous, complex junctional strands with no breaks, so their permeability is very low.

An additional, specialized transendothelial pathway, the **fenestrae** (windows), occurs in the capillaries of certain tissues, as described in Section 10.2.

## Junctional proteins form a dynamic, regulated complex

In an epithelium, a tight or 'occludens' junction forms close to a distinct, separate anchoring or 'adherens' junction. The endothelial junction contains proteins associated both with occludens-type junctions (claudin-5, occludin, junctional adhesion molecule, linker molecule ZO-1) and adherens-type junctions (vascular endothelial [VE]–cadherin, catenins) (Figure 9.3). VE–cadherin is a membrane-spanning glycoprotein whose extracellular domain binds to the VE–cadherin of the adjacent cell. Its intracellular domain binds to a complex of α, β and γ catenin, which is tethered by α-actinin to the junctional band of actin. A further junctional protein, platelet endothelial cell adhesion molecule (PECAM), promotes leukocyte emigration.

The junctional complex is a dynamic structure that can be regulated rapidly via intracellular messengers. For example, agents that increase endothelial cyclic adenosine monophosphate (cAMP), such as isoprenaline, increase the number of

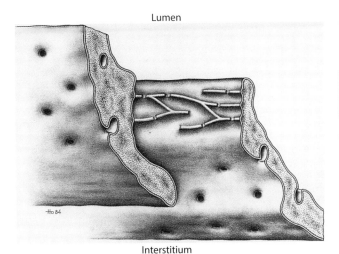

Lumen

Interstitium

**Figure 9.4** Three-dimensional reconstruction of capillary intercellular cleft, based on serial electron micrographs. The cleft is 500–1000 nm long (top to bottom) and 15–20 nm wide, except at the tight junctions. Water and small lipophobic solutes follow the tortuous pathway through the breaks in the junctional strands. (From Bundgaard M. *Journal of Ultrastructure Research* 1984; 88(1): 1–17, with permission from Elsevier.)

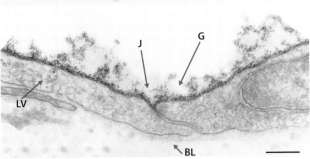

**Figure 9.5** Electron micrograph of capillary after perfusion with cationized ferritin (i.e. ferritin with added positive charges). Each black dot is a ferritin molecule bound to the negatively charged glycocalyx (G). Binding causes a fall in permeability (Chapter 10.6, 'the protein effect'). Ferritin is excluded from the intercellular junction (J), but some enters the caveola/vesicle system (LV, labelled vesicle). Neutral ferritin does not bind to the glycocalyx and does not reduce permeability. BL, basal lamina. Bar = 0.2 μm. (From Turner MR, Clough G, Michel CC. *Microvascular Research* 1983; 25(2): 205–22, with permission from Elsevier.)

junctional strands and thus reduce permeability. Conversely, during inflammation the phosphorylation of β-catenin and breakdown of junctional actin rapidly weaken the junction, leading to gap formation.

## Gap junctions in arterial endothelium transmit signals

The arterial endothelium has numerous gap junctions, as well as tight junctions. The gap junctions comprise connexins 37 and 40 assembled as aligned, conducting hemichannels, as in Figure 3.1 (bottom). **Homocellular gap junctions** are junctions between neighbouring endothelial cells; they transmit ions, membrane potentials and small chemical messengers (<1000 Da) along the endothelial sheet. **Heterocellular** or **myoendothelial gap junctions** convey signals between the endothelium and underlying VSM cells. Together the homo- and heterocellular gap junctions can conduct signals along small arteries, causing ascending vasodilatation (Section 13.7).

## The glycocalyx is a negatively charged barrier to macromolecules

The luminal surface of the endothelium is coated with a 60–570 nm thick, hydrated gel, the glycocalyx (Figures 9.2 and 9.5). The glycocalyx comprises negatively charged carbohydrate polymers, usually attached to a core protein, for example, sialoglycoprotein, syndecan 1 (a heparan sulphate and chondroitin sulphate proteoglycan with a transmembrane 'root'; Figure 9.3) and glypican (a membrane-attached heparan sulphate proteoglycan). The long glycosaminoglycan, hyaluronan,

is bound to the membrane receptor CD44. These various polymers protrude into the lumen in hairy, bush-like tufts and are connected intracellularly to the actin cytoskeleton at ~100 nm intervals. The functions of the glycocalyx are as follows:

- The luminal polymers, aided by bound albumin and orosomucoid, form a size-selective, charge-selective molecular sieve that is permeable to water and small solutes, but not to plasma proteins or atherogenic, low-density lipoproteins (LDLs). The glycocalyx thus creates the all-important **semipermeability of the endothelium**.
- The glycocalyx lubricates the deformed red cells as they squeeze in single file along a capillary.
- The glycocalyx is a **mechanosensor**, sensing changes in blood flow. For example, the flow-stimulated secretion of NO by the endothelium is impaired if the glycocalyx is degraded by protease, heparinase or hyaluronidase.
- The glycocalyx can be **degraded and shed** into the bloodstream in response to ischaemia–reperfusion injury (reactive $O_2$ species), atrial natriuretic peptide, atherogenic oxidized LDL and atheroma. Similar damage at the renal glomeruli can also lead to albuminuria or nephrotic syndrome. This results in hyperpermeability, protein leakage, oedema, increased capillary dynamic haematocrit and leukocyte adhesion.

## Caveolae and vesicles: specialized microdomains and transcytosis

Up to a quarter of the endothelial cell is occupied by membrane-bound **vesicles** with a diameter of ~70 nm. Although they look like detached spheres in a single section, serial sections show that 99% are connected to each other, and ultimately to the luminal/abluminal endothelial surface (Figure 9.6a). The surface vesicle resembles a little flask or

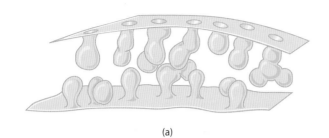

(a)

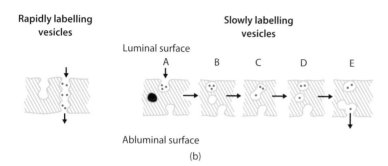

**Rapidly labelling vesicles**

**Slowly labelling vesicles**

Luminal surface

A      B     C     D     E

Abluminal surface

(b)

**Figure 9.6** The caveola/vesicle system. **(a)** Reconstruction of serial sections show that most vesicles connect, directly or indirectly, with a surface via the caveolae (flask-shaped surface invaginations). Detached vesicles are rare. **(b)** Frames A–E show how transcytosis of macromolecules (red dots, ferritin) may occur by transient vesicular fusion and mixing of contents. Occasional abluminal vesicles that label unusually rapidly may be part of a multivesicular, transendothelial channel (left frame). (**(a)** From Frøkjaer-Jensen J. *Progress in Applied Microcirculation* 1983; 1: 17–34, by permission; and **(b)** from Clough G, Michel CC. *The Journal of Physiology* 1981; 315: 127–42, with permission from Wiley-Blackwell.)

cave (**caveola**) because the interior is connected to the plasma or interstitial fluid via a 20–30 nm wide neck (Figures 9.1 and 9.5). The vesicle system is thus a set of racemose invaginations of the cell membrane, resembling bunches of grapes dangling from each surface.

The caveolar membrane is a highly specialized 'microdomain' of different composition to the rest of the cell membrane. The cytoplasmic face is covered by a striated coat of protein, caveolin, and the lipid membrane is enriched in NO synthase (NOS), cholesterol, sphingomyelin and receptors for albumin (albondin), insulin, transferrin and caeruloplasmin. The concentration of so many proteins in a small lipid raft may facilitate local biochemical signalling.

The caveola/vesicle system can take up plasma macromolecules and transport them into the cell (**endocytosis**, the transfer of receptor-bound materials to endosomes). The vesicles can also transport small amounts of albumin, immunoglobulins and lipoproteins across the cell, from plasma to interstitium (**transcytosis**); however, the quantitative significance of this is controversial. Vesicular transcytosis appears to involve the transient fusion of vesicles and transfer of contents (Figure 9.6). Also, very occasionally, a row of fused vesicles and caveolae creates a continuous channel through the cell (Figure 9.6b, left). These rare 'multivesicular transendothelial channels' may likewise contribute to macromolecular permeation.

## Capillary fragility: the basal lamina normally prevents rupture

The 50–100 nm thick basal lamina comprises a layer of lightly staining extracellular matrix next to the cell, the **lamina rara**, surrounded by a denser layer, the **lamina densa**. A major component is **type IV collagen**, which confers great mechanical

strength. **Laminin**, an adhesive glycoprotein, and perlecan, a negatively charged heparan sulphate proteoglycan, are the other major constituents. The endothelial cell is attached to the collagen and laminin by $\beta_1$ **integrins** at the focal contact points (Figures 9.2 and 9.3). In most tissues, the basal lamina is not a barrier to solutes, even those as large as plasma proteins.

Since capillaries lack a tunica media or adventitia, most of their mechanical strength resides in the basal lamina. The basal lamina prevents capillary rupture by blood pressure. **Tension** itself is low in the capillary wall, due to the small radius (Laplace's law), but the tension per unit wall thickness, **wall stress**, is high, due to the extreme thinness of the wall. Indeed, capillary wall stress is comparable to artery wall stress (Figure 8.18). In **Goodpasture syndrome**, autoantibodies against type IV collagen weaken the basal lamina, and the fragile capillaries bleed into the lung alveoli and renal glomeruli.

## Endothelium differs between vessels

Not all endothelium is the same; it differs between types of blood vessel and between tissues. In **arteries**, where haemodynamic stresses are high, the endothelial cells are elongated in the direction of flow and have prominent stress fibres. **Postcapillary venules** have extensive breaks in the junctional strand, raising their permeability. Venular endothelium also abundantly expresses receptors to inflammatory mediators and has a large reserve of leukocyte 'glue' (P-selectin); so, venular endothelium is the primary site of the inflammatory response. In **lymph nodes**, postcapillary venules have unusually tall endothelial cells, called 'high endothelium', which entice lymphocytes to recycle from blood to lymph node. In **glandular tissues, intestinal mucosa and the kidney**, the capillary endothelium is perforated by circular windows

## THE ENDOTHELIUM IS A SELECTIVELY PERMEABLE MEMBRANE

- The lipid membrane of endothelial cells permits the rapid permeation of lipid-soluble molecules such as $O_2$, carbon dioxide and anaesthetics between blood and tissue.
- The endothelial intercellular cleft is an aqueous, paracellular pathway that transmits water and small lipophobic solutes such as glucose – except in the brain, where there are no breaks in the intercellular junctional strands.
- The permeability of the intercellular cleft is reduced by the β adrenergic receptor–cAMP pathway, which enhances junctional strand formation. Intercellular permeability is increased by flow and by atrial natriuretic peptide, acting through cyclic guanosine monophosphate (cGMP).
- The glycocalyx, a coating of biopolymers on the luminal surface, forms a semipermeable layer; it reflects plasma proteins, but permits the passage of smaller solutes and water.
- Cytoplasmic vesicles transfer plasma proteins slowly across the endothelium by a poorly understood process.
- In inflammation, wide gaps form between and through venular endothelial cells. The rapid transfer of plasma proteins and water through the gaps causes inflammatory swelling.

# 9.3 ION CHANNELS, CALCIUM AND ENDOTHELIAL FUNCTION

Endothelial cells express a variety of ion channels, many of which influence intracellular $Ca^{2+}$ ion concentration. $Ca^{2+}$ ions regulate several endothelial functions, including NO synthesis, EDH activation and the hyperpermeability of inflammation. Basal cytosolic $Ca^{2+}$ concentration, 30–100 nM, is much lower than extracellular $Ca^{2+}$ concentration, ~1 mM, and can be increased five- to tenfold (e.g. by histamine), partly by the influx of extracellular $Ca^{2+}$ through ion channels, and partly by the release of $Ca^{2+}$ stored in the endoplasmic reticulum (Figure 9.1). In the following account, it is assumed that the reader is familiar with the electrophysiological concepts introduced in Chapter 3.

## Membrane potential affects endothelial responses

Endothelial cells are not excitable; that is, they cannot generate action potentials because they do not express voltage-gated $Na^+$ or $Ca^{2+}$ channels. They do, however, have a regulated, negative intracellular potential that varies between approximately −20 mV in isolated cells to values close to the VSM membrane potential *in situ*, that is, up to approximately −60 mV. The membrane potential is influenced by the outward movement of $K^+$ ions through **inward rectifying $K^+$ channels ($K_{IR}$), when these channels are present, and by $K_{Ca}$ channels** (Figure 9.7), and by the electrogenic $3Na^+/2K^+$ pump, which may contribute about ~8 mV. Membrane potential magnitude is important because it affects the electrochemical force driving extracellular $Ca^{2+}$ into the endothelial cell; abolition

called fenestrae, which boost permeability (Figure 10.2). At the other extreme, **brain microvessels** have no fenestrations, no breaks in the junctional strands and few vesicles, creating a blood–brain barrier to many solutes (Section 15.4).

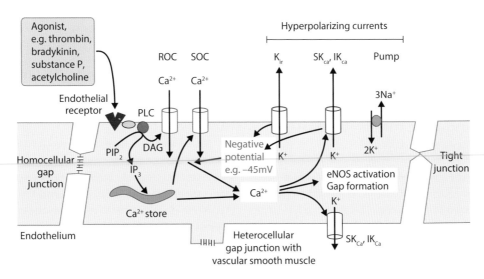

**Figure 9.7** Endothelial electrophysiology and $Ca^{2+}$ regulation. The coupling between receptor and membrane phospholipase C (PLC) differs between receptors. Classic G-protein-coupled receptors are heptahelical proteins (seven transmembrane loops) that on activation cause the dissociation of the trimeric G protein $G_{q/11}$. The released $G\alpha$ component diffuses in the membrane to activate the PLC-β isoform. Other receptors (e.g. to growth factors) are dimeric transmembrane proteins called receptor protein tyrosine kinases, which activate the PLC-γ isoform. Either PLC isoform generates intramembrane diacyl glycerol (DAG) and cytosolic inositol trisphosphate ($IP_3$). eNOS, endothelial nitric oxide synthase; $IK_{Ca}$, intermediate conductance $Ca^{2+}$-activated $K^+$ channel; $SK_{Ca}$ small conductance $Ca^{2+}$-activated $K^+$ channel; $K_{ir}$, inwardly rectifying $K^+$ channel; $PIP_2$, phosphatidylinositol bisphosphate (an inner membrane phospholipid); PLC, phospholipase C in the membrane, linked by G protein (grey) to agonist receptor; ROC, receptor-operated $Ca^{2+}$ channel; SOC, store-operated $Ca^{2+}$ channel.

of the potential greatly attenuates $Ca^{2+}$-mediated responses in venules. (Figure 11.29). Also, changes in endothelial membrane potential can be conducted through gap junctions to serve as a signal, as in ascending vasodilatation (Section 13.7).

## Endothelium expresses transient receptor potential calcium-conducting channels

Although the endothelium lacks voltage-gated $Ca^{2+}$ channels, the surface membrane has two other types of $Ca^{2+}$-conducting channel: receptor-operated and store-operated channels. When the cell is stimulated by an agonist, such as histamine, these $Ca^{2+}$ channels are activated and raise the intracellular free $Ca^{2+}$ concentration five- to tenfold.

**Receptor-operated channels (ROCs)** are cation-conducting channels that are activated via a biochemical cascade when an extracellular agent, the 'agonist', binds to its specific membrane receptor. Endothelial agonists include histamine, bradykinin, thrombin, serotonin, adenosine triphosphate (ATP) and ACh. The agonist receptor activates a $G_{q/11}$ protein, which activates the membrane-bound enzyme phospholipase C (PLC) (Figure 9.7). PLC splits the phospholipid, phosphatidylinositol bisphosphate, into **diacylglycerol (DAG)** and **inositol 1,4,5 trisphosphate (IP$_3$)**. DAG activates the ROC ion channel, and $IP_3$ releases $Ca^{2+}$ from the endoplasmic reticulum. ROCs are poorly selective cation channels that conduct $Ca^{2+}$ and some $Na^+$ and $K^+$. Since there is a large electrochemical gradient for $Ca^{2+}$ influx, ROC activation causes a rapid rise in cytosolic $[Ca^{2+}]$. The ROC constituent proteins were recently identified as members of the transient receptor potential (TRP) C (TRPC) and V (TRPV) families (canonical and vanilloid subtypes).

**Store-operated channels (SOCs)** are again $Ca^{2+}$-conducting channels in the surface membrane, but their activation is associated with $Ca^{2+}$ store release. Endothelial SOCs may be TRP channels since TRPC1 is found in human endothelium. Furthermore, a role for TRPC4 and TRPC6, and possibly heteromeric channel complexes of these proteins, have also been suggested to underlie SOC $Ca^{2+}$ entry (Figure 9.7). However, this remains a controversial area, to the extent that an involvement of TRPs as SOCs in native endothelium has been questioned. Of note, much of the experimental work in the area has studied cultured endothelial cells, conditions known to increase TRP protein expression. A second type of SOC is composed of Orai proteins. This channel is exquisitely $Ca^{2+}$-selective, and is activated by an endoplasmic reticulum protein, stromal interaction molecule 1, following $Ca^{2+}$ store release; so, it is also called the $Ca^{2+}$-release activated Ca2+ (CRAC) channel. SOC activation leads to an influx of extracellular $Ca^{2+}$, called either capacitive or store-operated $Ca^{2+}$ entry. This raises the free $Ca^{2+}$ level, as well as restocking the sarcoplasmic reticulum store. SOCs are thought to be more abundant than ROCs in many types of endothelium.

Because of these multiple pathways, an agonist usually evokes a biphasic change in endothelial $Ca^{2+}$ concentration. There is an initial high spike in free $Ca^{2+}$ concentration, brought about by $IP_3$-mediated store release and DAG-mediated ROC activation. This is followed by a lesser, but more sustained, $Ca^{2+}$ elevation due to SOC activation. Endothelial cells may also possess **stretch-activated channels**, which allow $Ca^{2+}$ entry in response to shear stress. Another TRP channel, TRPV4, is thought to underlie stretch-activated $Ca^{2+}$ entry in the endothelium.

## Calcium-activated potassium channels ($K_{Ca}$) can hyperpolarize endothelial cells

A rise in endothelial free $Ca^{2+}$ activates a special type of $K^+$ channel, the $Ca^{2+}$-activated $K^+$ channel $K_{Ca}$ (Figure 9.7). This increases the membrane permeability to $K^+$, leading to hyperpolarization, that is, a more negative potential (equation 3.4). Hyperpolarization serves two functions: (1) it increases the electrochemical force drawing extracellular $Ca^{2+}$ into the cell; and (2) it can be transmitted through myoendothelial gap junctions to induce arteriolar relaxation (Sections 9.5 and 13.7). There are three subtypes of $K_{Ca}$ channel: small conductance (**SK$_{Ca}$**); intermediate conductance (**IK$_{Ca}$**); and big (usually called large) conductance (**BK$_{Ca}$**). $SK_{Ca}$ and $IK_{Ca}$ occur exclusively in the endothelium (Figure 9.7), while $BK_{Ca}$ occurs in VSM. The channels are pharmacologically distinguishable: $SK_{Ca}$ is blocked by apamin, a constituent of bee venom; $IK_{Ca}$ and $BK_{Ca}$ are blocked by charybdotoxin, a constituent of scorpion venom; and $BK_{Ca}$ is blocked by iberiotoxin, another component of scorpion venom.

## 9.4 NITRIC OXIDE PRODUCTION BY ENDOTHELIAL CELLS

NO is a freely diffusible, dissolved gas with vasodilator properties. It is generated continuously by arterial endothelium at a low (often subthreshold) basal rate. The discovery that the endothelium secretes vasoactive agents was a relatively late one, and arose as follows.

## The discovery that endothelium can modulate vascular tone

### Prostacyclin

The role of the endothelium as a regulator of vascular tone began to emerge in 1976, when Vane and colleagues discovered that blood vessels secrete prostacyclin (PGI$_2$). $PGI_2$ can induce dilatation as illustrated in Figure 9.8 (lower panels), but this action does not seem to be of widespread physiological significance. The importance of $PGI_2$ seems to be its ability to inhibit platelet activation and prevent blood clot formation.

### Nitric oxide

A second, and very important, endothelium-derived vasodilator agent was discovered in 1980 by Furchgott and Zawadzki, who noted that the vasodilatation of large arteries by an ACh analogue, carbachol, changed into vasoconstriction when the endothelial lining was rubbed away (Figure 9.8, upper panels).

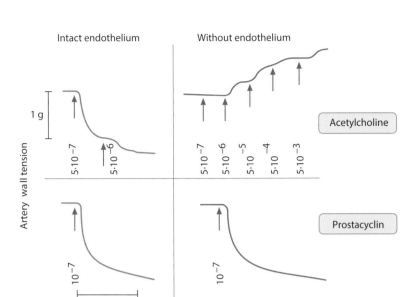

**Figure 9.8** Recording of force exerted by a strip of canine artery *in vitro*. Addition of acetylcholine (ACh) or prostacyclin (PGI₂) caused relaxation (left panels). When the endothelium was rubbed away, the response to ACh changed to contraction (top right). Thus, the relaxation was endothelium-dependent. In the unrubbed vessel, the response depends on the balance between endothelium-mediated relaxation (dominant) and the direct constrictor action of ACh on smooth muscle. The response to added PGI₂ was not endothelium-dependent (bottom right). (Redrawn and modified using data from Altura BM. *Microcirculation, Endothelium and Lymphatics* 1988; 4(2): 91–111, by permission.)

It emerged that agonists, such as ACh, stimulate the endothelium to secrete a vasodilator substance, initially dubbed 'endothelium-derived relaxing factor'. In the late 1970s the Murad group demonstrated that organic nitrates release NO and relax vascular smooth muscle via activation of guanylyl cyclase. The similarities between NO and 'endothelial derived relaxing factor' were noted, and the identification of EDRF as NO came independently in 1987 from both the Ignarro and Moncada groups. Furchgott, Ignarro and Murad were awarded the 1998 Nobel Prize in Medicine or Physiology, and Moncada was unlucky not to be included as only three recipients can be named.

## Endothelium-derived hyperpolarizing factor

A third vasodilator influence, EDHF, was discovered when it was realized that endothelium-dependent vasodilatation persists in small vessels after blocking NO and PGI₂ synthesis. The response involves smooth muscle hyperpolarization (Figure 9.9). EDHF, or EDH as it is now known, is a major influence in small arteries, which depend principally on voltage-dependent $Ca^{2+}$ influx to cause vasoconstriction such that membrane hyperpolarization would significantly oppose this.

## Endothelin

A fourth endothelial secretion, a vasoconstrictor peptide called endothelin, was discovered in 1989 by a Japanese group using molecular biology techniques.

All four substances (PGI₂, NO, EDH and endothelin) are released as they are produced, rather than being stored for later secretion.

## Endothelial nitric oxide has multiple functions

NO is soluble in both lipid and water, so it diffuses freely from the endothelium into the neighbouring VSM and bloodstream, with multiple local effects:

- NO **lowers vascular tone in veins, and in large muscular arteries**, such as the coronary artery (Figure 9.9a). NO also dilates small resistance vessels,

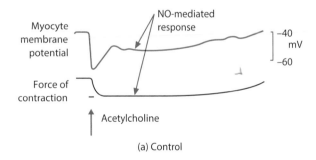

(a) Control

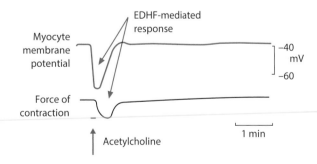

(b) NAME + indomethacin

**Figure 9.9** **(a)** Endothelium-dependent relaxation of guinea pig coronary artery (black line) in response to acetylcholine (bar). The relaxation is mediated partly by hyperpolarization of the vascular smooth muscle (red line). **(b)** Blockage of nitric oxide (NO) production, using nitroarginine methyl ester (NAME), and prostacyclin, using indomethacin, abolishes the late part of the response. The early phase of hyperpolarization and relaxation, which is mediated by endothelium-derived hyperpolarizing factor (EDHF), persists. (From Parkington HC, Tonta MA, Coleman HA, et al. *The Journal of Physiology* 1995; 484(Pt 2): 469–80 with permission from Wiley-Blackwell.)

though EDH is relatively more important in these vessels. Arterial NO production is stimulated by shear stress, leading to **flow-induced dilatation in large arteries**, which helps increase the blood flow to exercising muscles (Sections 13.3 and 13.7). NO production is also stimulated by inflammatory mediators such as bradykinin, leading to the characteristic **vasodilatation of inflammation**. The NO-releasing drug **glyceryl trinitrate** (GTN) relieves angina partly through venous dilatation, which reduces central venous pressure and therefore cardiac work, and partly through large artery relaxation, which reduces wave reflection and therefore systolic pressure and cardiac work (Figure 8.10). Since basal NO production is continuous, inhibitors of NO production cause vasoconstriction.

- NO contributes to **gap formation in venules during inflammation**.
- NO **inhibits vascular myocyte proliferation**, a component of atheroma.
- NO **inhibits platelet aggregation** and thus protects blood vessels from thrombosis.
- NO **inhibits the transcription of leukocyte-binding adhesion molecules**, such as endothelial vascular cell adhesion molecule 1 (VCAM-1).

The inhibition of smooth muscle proliferation, platelet activation and leukocyte adhesion by NO are all anti-atheroma actions, and reduced NO availability is thought to contribute to atheroma formation (Section 9.10).

## Nitric oxide is generated from L-arginine by endothelial nitric oxide synthase (eNOS)

NO is generated continuously and survives only seconds before degradation. It is produced by a constitutively expressed enzyme, endothelial NOS (eNOS). eNOS is a haem-containing enzyme located on the inner surface of the caveolar membrane, in a complex with caveolin, high-density lipoprotein (HDL) and oestrogen receptors. eNOS cleaves the nitrogen group from the amino acid L-arginine and combines it with molecular $O_2$ to form NO (Figure 9.10). The process is driven by electrons, derived from nicotinamide adenine dinucleotide phosphate (NADPH), and requires flavin adenine dinucleotide (FAD), flavin mononucleotide (FMN), tetrahydrobiopterin ($BH_4$) and calmodulin as additional cofactors. In the absence of $BH_4$, the eNOS enzyme can become 'uncoupled' and produce superoxide, rather than NO. This may contribute to oxidative stress and endothelial dysfunction. Inactive analogues of arginine, such as nitroarginine methyl ester, compete with normal arginine for the eNOS binding site, and therefore act as eNOS blockers.

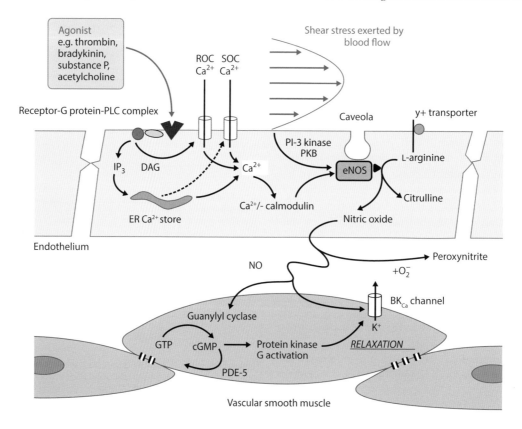

**Figure 9.10** Regulation of nitric oxide production and its effect on neighbouring vascular smooth muscle. $BK_{Ca}$, large-conductance $Ca^{2+}$-activated $K^+$ channel; cGMP, cyclic guanosine 3′,5′-monophosphate; DAG, diacylglycerol; eNOS, endothelial nitric oxide synthase; ER, endoplasmic reticulum; GTP, guanosine triphosphate; $IP_3$, inositol trisphosphate; NO, nitric oxide; PDE-5, phosphodiesterase 5 (inhibited by sildenafil); PI-3 kinase, phosphatidylinositol-3 kinase; PKB, protein kinase B; PLC, phospholipase C in the membrane, linked by G protein (grey) to agonist receptor; ROC, receptor-operated $Ca^{2+}$ channel; SOC, store-operated $Ca^{2+}$ channels.

There are also non-endothelial isoforms of NOS (inducible iNOS, neural nNOS), as described in Section 13.3.

## Nitric oxide production is stimulated by shear stress and agonists

As noted earlier, eNOS activity is stimulated tonically by the shear stress exerted by flowing blood, and can be enhanced by agonists such as ACh and inflammatory mediators.

### Shear stress stimulates eNOS via phosphatidylinositol-3 kinase

Basal shear stress (Figure 8.3) provides an important, tonic drive for NO production. Moreover, during exercise, increased blood flow in the arteries feeding the active skeletal muscles raises the shear stress and NO production. This results in **flow-induced vasodilatation** in large conduit arteries supplying active muscle groups (Section 13.4). The shear stress is probably transduced into a biochemical signal by the glycocalyx, since glycocalyx-degrading enzymes reduce NO production. Transduction activates the enzyme **phosphatidylinositol-3 kinase**, leading to the activation of protein kinase B (PKB), which phosphorylates eNOS (Figure 9.10). Phosphorylation renders eNOS more sensitive to background $Ca^{2+}$/calmodulin, the intracellular activator of eNOS.

### Agonists stimulate eNOS via calcium-calmodulin

Agonists such as ACh raise endothelial free $Ca^{2+}$ concentration via the PLC–ROC/SOC pathway (Figure 9.7). Some of the $Ca^{2+}$ binds to an intracellular $Ca^{2+}$-binding protein, calmodulin. The $Ca^{2+}$-calmodulin complex enhances eNOS activity and hence NO production (Figure 9.10). Agonists that act in this way include bradykinin, thrombin, substance P, ATP, adenosine diphosphate (ADP), ACh (via muscarinic $M_3$ receptors), vasoactive intestinal polypeptide, insulin and in some tissues/species histamine. Several of these agents are released during inflammation, so NO contributes to the characteristic redness (vasodilatation) of inflamed tissue.

### Nitric oxide causes vasodilatation by two mechanisms

Endothelial NO diffuses rapidly into neighbouring VSM cells, where it binds to the haem group of a soluble enzyme, guanylyl cyclase (Figure 9.10). NO is the chemical cousin to $O_2$, hence its high affinity for haem. The activated guanylyl cyclase catalyses the production of **cGMP** from guanosine triphosphate; cGMP activates kinases (enzymes that phosphorylate other proteins to alter their activity) that promote vascular relaxation, as detailed in Section 12.7. High concentrations of NO directly activate large conductance **$BK_{Ca}$ channels** in the smooth muscle membrane (Figure 9.10). This hyperpolarizes the smooth muscle, leading to vascular relaxation (Figure 9.9a).

## Nitric oxide is inactivated rapidly

NO is inactivated within seconds by two mechanisms. First, NO reacts with a by-product of oxidative metabolism, the superoxide anion $O_2^-$, to form peroxynitrite, $ONOO^-$. Then, peroxynitrite is converted into ordinary nitrite ($NO_2^-$) and nitrate ($NO_3^-$) for excretion in the urine. Some NO diffuses into the bloodstream, where its similarity to $O_2$ causes it to bind to red cell haemoglobin.

## 9.5 OTHER VASOACTIVE ENDOTHELIAL PRODUCTS: ENDOTHELIUM-DERIVED HYPERPOLARIZATION, PROSTACYCLIN AND ENDOTHELINS

### Endothelium-derived hyperpolarization

NO exerts its main physiological effects in large vessels, where eNOS is abundant. If NO and $PGI_2$ production is blocked in **small arteries and arterioles**, agonists such as ACh and bradykinin still evoke endothelium-dependent dilatation, which is mediated by smooth muscle hyperpolarization (Figure 9.9b). Also, in some tissues, saline washed through agonist-stimulated vessels picks up a chemical that can hyperpolarize isolated vascular muscle – an EDHF.

Any influence that raises endothelial cell $Ca^{2+}$ will activate the EDHF pathway. Stimuli include the classical parasympathetic transmitter ACh, inflammatory agents such as bradykinin and possibly shear stress. Furthermore, genetic modification to remove either of the endothelial $SK_{Ca}$ or $IK_{Ca}$ channels mediating EDHF leads to a significant rise in blood pressure, indicating that this mechanism has a continuous and important physiological role.

Apart from an influence on blood pressure, other **roles of EDHF** include:

- to help increase blood flow to exercising muscle, by dilating small feed arteries (ascending, conducted vasodilatation; see Section 13.7) and generally co-ordinate blood flow within the microcirculation;
- to contribute to the cholinergic vasodilatation of small resistance vessels in the small number of tissues with a cholinergic autonomic innervation (Sections 14.2 and 14.3);
- to contribute to the vasodilatation of inflammation.

Although EDH can indeed be brought about by the release of chemical factor(s), hence the term EDHF, EDH can also be caused by hyperpolarization spreading to the VSM via direct, electrical coupling due to the presence of myoendothelial gap junctions. Electrical transmission may be the primary hyperpolarizing mechanism, with released, soluble EDHFs serving to boost myocyte hyperpolarization.

## Direct electrical transmission of endothelial hyperpolarization to vascular myocytes

This has been demonstrated in arterioles and small arteries (diameter 50–300 μm), where myoendothelial gap junctions are abundant (Figure 1.11). When an agonist raises the endothelial free $Ca^{2+}$ concentration, the activated SKCa and $IK_{Ca}$ channels hyperpolarize the endothelial cell (Figure 9.7). The endothelial hyperpolarization then spreads through the myoendothelial (heterocellular) gap junctions to hyperpolarize and relax the vascular myocytes by reducing the open probability of voltage-dependent $Ca^{2+}$ channels. This form of 'EDH' is inhibited by gap junction blockers, and by apamin and charybdotoxin, toxins that block endothelial $SK_{Ca}$ and $IK_{Ca}$ channels.

## Released chemical factors

Activated endothelial $SK_{Ca}$ and $IK_{Ca}$ channels release **K⁺ ions** into the interstitial spaces around neighbouring VSM cells. The rise in extracellular K⁺ reinforces myocyte hyperpolarization by stimulating the VSM $3Na^+/2K^+$ pump and by activating myocyte $K_{IR}$ channels (Section 13.4). Also, in small coronary, renal and skeletal muscle arteries, epoxyeicosatrienoic acid (EET) may act as an additional EDHF. In these vessels, the agonist bradykinin activates endothelial phospholipase $A_2$ ($PLA_2$), which generates arachidonic acid. Arachidonic acid is converted by endothelial cytochrome P450 epoxygenase to diffusible EET. Myocyte EET receptors trigger a pathway that activates $BK_{Ca}$ channels, located on the VSM, not on the endothelial cells, leading to hyperpolarization and vasodilatation (Section 12.7).

## Prostacyclin

Like NO, $PGI_2$ causes vasodilatation and inhibits platelet aggregation. It is produced by endothelium constitutively (i.e. without needing stimulation), and in response to agonists such as thrombin. **Phospholipase $A_2$** converts membrane phospholipids into the unsaturated fatty acid, **arachidonic acid**. Arachidonic acid is then converted by **cyclooxygenases** into $PGI_2$. $PGI_2$ production is greatly increased in inflammation and contributes to the associated vasodilatation. It also contributes to the cutaneous vasodilatation associated with sweating. Under normal conditions, however, it seems not to have a significant role in causing vasodilatation.

## Endothelins

Endothelins are a family of peptides related to the snake venom sarafotoxin. Endothelin 1 (ET-1), the main isoform secreted by the endothelium, causes a powerful, unusually sustained vasoconstriction, lasting 2–3 h. ET-1 activates myocyte $ET_A$ receptors, which are coupled via a G protein to the myocyte $PLC/IP_3$ system. The resulting rise in myocyte $Ca^{2+}$ triggers vasoconstriction. Over a longer timescale, ET also stimulates vascular and cardiac myocyte proliferation.

ET is produced continuously and makes a small contribution to basal vascular tone in humans. Its production can be increased by vibration, hypoxia, angiotensin II, vasopressin and thrombin. Plasma ET levels are raised in pre-eclamptic toxaemia (the hypertension of pregnancy) and heart failure. ET also contributes to cerebral artery vasospasm in patients with haemorrhagic strokes.

## 9.6 ACTIONS OF ENDOTHELIUM ON BLOOD

## Endothelium catalyses angiotensin II production

Angiotensin I (Ang I) is a relatively inactive, circulating decapeptide formed in renal plasma (Section 14.8). It is converted into Ang II, an octapeptide with strong vasoconstrictor properties, by **angiotensin-converting enzyme** (ACE), a zinc carboxypeptidase expressed on the luminal surface of the endothelium (Figure 9.1). Conversion occurs mainly in the lungs, the first large area of endothelium encountered by Ang I after its production in renal venous plasma. ACE inhibitors, such as captopril, reduce Ang II levels and are widely used to treat hypertension and heart failure (Chapter 18).

Lung ACE also rapidly degrades the circulating vasoactive agents bradykinin and serotonin. These are pro-inflammatory substances, so occasional side effects of ACE inhibitors are oedema formation and cough.

## Endothelium prevents thrombosis

The endothelial lining of blood vessels is now recognized to be central to preventing thrombosis in undamaged vessels by several mechanisms (Figure 9.11):

- It presents a physical barrier that separates platelets and coagulation factors in the blood from stimulatory collagen in the subendothelial layers of the blood vessel.
- Secretion of heparan sulphate on the luminal surface activates antithrombin III and prevents the activation of the clotting factors.
- Powerful inhibitors of platelet activation are synthesized. $PGI_2$ and NO act synergistically to prevent the increase in intra-platelet $Ca^{2+}$ essential for activation.
- The enzyme CD39 is expressed on the luminal surface to convert the platelet activator, ADP, to inactive AMP.
- Tissue plasminogen activator (tPA) is released to convert plasminogen to plasmin, which cleaves fibrin strands, earning tPA the title of 'clot-buster'.

Damage to the endothelium compromises some or all of these protective effects and leads to the release of the platelet

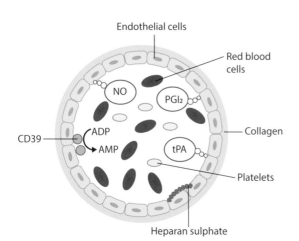

**Figure 9.11** Antiplatelet and anticoagulation properties of the endothelium. The endothelial lining of undamaged blood vessels prevents thrombosis via the secretion of heparan sulphate on the luminal surface, by synthesizing inhibitors of platelet activation, such as prostacyclin ($PGI_2$), and nitric oxide (NO), and expressing the enzyme CD39 on the luminal surface to convert the platelet activator, adenosine diphosphate (ADP), to inactive adenosine monophosphate (AMP), and by releasing tissue plasminogen activator (tPA) to convert plasminogen to plasmin. (Adapted from the *Oxford Handbook of Medical Sciences*, 2nd edn. Oxford: Oxford University Press; 2011. p. 467.)

activator, vWF, and the tPA inhibitor, plasminogen activator inhibitor-1.

## The endothelium secretes a haemostatic agent, von willebrand factor

Endothelial cells contain a unique, rod-shaped, storage organelle, the Weibel–Palade body, which consists of numerous, stacked tubules composed of a glycoprotein, vWF (Figure 9.1). The vWF protein is secreted constitutively into the bloodstream and has two roles in blood clotting (see Section 9.11): (1) vWF is a carrier for clotting factor VIII; (2) during blood clotting, plasma prothrombin is converted into thrombin. Thrombin not only converts fibrinogen into insoluble fibrin (a crucial step in blood clotting), but also activates endothelial thrombin receptors, which triggers a rapid, local exocytosis of vWF (Figure 9.1). Some of the vWF binds to subendothelial collagen and promotes platelet adhesion, another crucial step in blood clotting. **Von Willebrand disease**, which is a common, inherited failure to synthesize vWF, is characterized by prolonged bleeding after injury.

The Weibel–Palade body also contains a store of the leukocyte-adhesive protein **P-selectin**. When the endothelium is activated by an inflammatory agonist, P-selectin is translocated to the surface and initiates the capture of passing leukocytes (Figure 9.12).

Platelet aggregation, an important step in thrombosis and blood clotting, is inhibited by NO and $PGI_2$. When blood clots, activated endothelial thrombin receptors not only cause vWF exocytosis, but also stimulate NO and $PGI_2$ production. This limits the spread of platelet aggregation. The endothelial

secretions thus contribute to a limited, well-regulated haemostatic process, rather than a runaway vascular thrombosis (see Section 9.11).

## 9.7 ENDOTHELIAL PERMEABILITY AND ITS REGULATION

The endothelial intercellular cleft of capillaries is the main pathway for the transfer of water and nutrients from blood to tissue (Figures 9.3 and 9.4). The permeability of this pathway is not fixed; it can be modulated by blood velocity and by chemical messengers, as outlined here. For a fuller account, see Chapters 10 and 11.

### Increased permeability

An increase in **plasma velocity** raises capillary intercellular permeability, which facilitates the transfer of glucose from blood into exercising muscle (Section 10.11). The increased permeability is mediated by flow-stimulated NO production, since it is blocked by eNOS inhibitors. Permeability can also be increased by **atrial natriuretic peptide**, a hormone involved in the regulation of plasma volume (Section 14.9). Both NO and atrial natriuretic peptide raise endothelial cGMP, which activates pathways that raise intercellular permeability. **Endothelial cGMP** also has a key role in raising permeability during inflammation (Sections 9.8 and 11.11). **Vascular endothelial growth factor A** (VEGF-A, originally called 'vascular permeability factor') is a protein secreted by growing or healing tissues that increases endothelial permeability and stimulates microvessel growth (Section 9.9).

### Reduced permeability

**β2 adrenergic receptor agonists**, such as isoprenaline and terbutaline, reduce basal capillary permeability. These agents raise **endothelial cAMP**, which activates pathways that enhance junctional strand formation. Thus, cAMP is a barrier-enhancing messenger and cGMP is a barrier-reducing messenger. cGMP may act in part by activating a phosphodiesterase that degrades cAMP (Section 11.11).

## 9.8 ENDOTHELIUM AND THE INFLAMMATORY RESPONSE

### Endothelium contributes to the classic signs of inflammation

Inflammation is a group of defensive responses to infection, burns, trauma and autoimmune diseases, such as rheumatoid arthritis. Celsus (30BC–38AD) defined inflammation as a combination of redness (*rubor*), heat (*calor*), swelling (*tumor*)

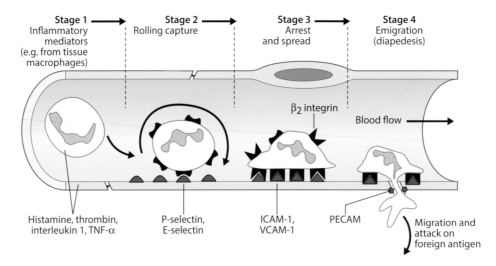

**Figure 9.12** Rolling capture, arrest and extravasation of leukocyte during the inflammatory response. ICAM-1, intercellular adhesion molecule; PECAM, platelet endothelial cell adhesion molecule; TNFα, tumour necrosis factor α; VCAM-1, vascular cell adhesion molecule.

and pain (*dolor*), to which Galen (130–200AD) added a fifth criterion, loss of function. This definition remains lucid and valid today, and the endothelium has a central role in the redness, heat and swelling.

The **redness** and **heat** are the results of vasodilatation, which is induced by a host of inflammatory mediators (histamine, bradykinin, $PGI_2$, substance P, platelet-activating factor (PAF), superoxide radicals and cytokines). Most of these agonists produce vasodilatation by raising endothelial $[Ca^{2+}]$, which stimulates NO and EDHF production.

The characteristic **swelling** of inflammation is caused by the rapid escape of plasma from the circulation through the newly formed gaps in venular endothelium. These inflammatory gaps are triggered by the agonist-induced rise in endothelial $[Ca^{2+}]$ and NO (Figures 9.7 and 11.30).

A sixth fundamental feature of inflammation, discovered by Addison (1843) and Waller (1846), is the **emigration of leukocytes**, which in its most gross form leads to pus formation. The endothelium has a crucial role in leukocyte emigration, as follows.

## Venular endothelium induces circulating leukocytes to emigrate (diapedesis)

During acute inflammation, polymorphonuclear neutrophils migrate from the bloodstream into the inflamed tissue, followed by monocytes and eventually lymphocytes. Leukocyte migration involves three sequential steps: rolling capture; arrest; and emigration.

### Rolling capture

The capture of circulating leukocytes begins in the venular endothelium, where inflammatory agonists, such as histamine and thrombin, trigger the transfer of **P-selectin** from the Weibel–Palade body to the surface membrane. P-selectin is a

carbohydrate-binding protein ('lectin') that renders the surface sticky to leukocytes. The leukocyte itself has microvilli that penetrate the glycocalyx, and oligosaccharides on the microvilli bind loosely to the P-selectin. Since the adhesion is weak, the 'marginated' leukocyte continues to roll slowly over the endothelium, driven by the bloodstream. Rolling, marginated leukocytes appear within minutes of applying an inflammatory stimulus.

The inflamed tissue produces not only acute inflammatory agonists such as histamine, but also the cytokines IL-1, TNFα and interferon γ, which act more slowly. These cytokines stimulate the endothelium to produce a second type of leukocyte glue, **E-selectin**, which can maintain rolling margination for several hours.

---

### CONCEPT BOX 9.2

**ENDOTHELIUM MEDIATES MANY ASPECTS OF INFLAMMATION**

- Inflammation is characterized by redness, heat, swelling, pain, loss of function and leukocyte migration. The endothelium has key roles in these changes.
- The redness and heat are caused by vasodilatation. Many mediators of inflammation (bradykinin, substance P, thrombin and cytokines) increase endothelial production of the vasodilator, NO.
- The swelling is due to the formation of large gaps in venular endothelium. The gaps allow a rapid efflux of water and plasma proteins, including immunoglobulins.
- Leukocyte capture occurs when specific 'glue' molecules (P-selectin, E-selectin, intercellular adhesion molecule 1 [ICAM-1], VCAM-1) are inserted into the luminal membrane of venular endothelium under the influence of cytokines (interleukin-1 beta [IL-1β], tumour necrosis factor α [TNFα]). The arrested leukocytes migrate through the intercellular junctions to attack the cause of the inflammation.

## Arrest

Tight-binding proteins are then activated on both the endothelium and leukocyte. The endothelial binding proteins are ICAM-1 and VCAM-1. ICAM-1 and VCAM-1 bind firmly to $\beta_2$ **integrins**, which appear on the surface of slowly rolling leukocytes. This brings the leukocytes to a halt, "like so many pebbles or marbles over which a stream runs without disturbing them", as Waller vividly reported in 1846. In the rare genetic condition of **leukocyte adhesion deficiency**, a lack of $\beta_2$ integrins results in a failure of leukocyte arrest, leading to a life-threatening susceptibility to bacterial infection.

## Emigration

Once arrested, the leukocyte inserts a thin foot into the endothelial intercellular junction and squeezes through into the tissue (diapedesis). This process depends on a high local concentration of ICAM-1 and platelet endothelial cell adhesion molecule (PECAM-1). In genetically engineered, knockout mice lacking PECAM-1, leukocytes become trapped at the basal lamina, reducing emigration. This indicates that PECAM-1 is needed to activate the leukocyte to break through the basal lamina.

The intercellular junction reseals rapidly, in seconds, after leukocyte migration. Not infrequently, leukocytes also migrate through holes in the endothelial cell itself, rather than the intercellular junctions. These transcellular holes likewise reseal quickly.

## 9.9 ENDOTHELIUM AND ANGIOGENESIS

The endothelial cell has a lifespan of months to years, so cell division is normally infrequent. However, when there is a need for new vessels (angiogenesis), endothelial cells can multiply rapidly, forming a simple endothelial tube in a few days. The tube then matures into an artery, vein or capillary. In adults, angiogenesis is essential for tissue growth, adaptation (e.g. increased number of capillaries in trained muscle) and wound healing. The endothelium also grows over the artificial grafts used in vascular surgery. On the downside, angiogenesis contributes to cancer growth, rheumatoid arthritis and diabetic eye disease.

## New vessels arise from capillary sprouts and splits

New vessel formation begins with the degradation of the endothelial basement membrane by proteases in an existing capillary or venule. This is followed by an outward **sprouting** of the endothelial cells (Figure 9.1). Vacuolation of the cell interior creates a lumen, and further cell division extends the tube, until it connects with another new vessel. The new vessels are hyperpermeable at first, and allow fibrinogen to extravasate into the tissues. This creates an oedematous, fibrin-rich vascular matrix called **granulation tissue**, which is a favourable environment for cell growth and wound healing. With maturity, microvessel permeability declines to normal,

probably due to an increase in the cAMP-to-cGMP ratio. In addition to sprouting, new vessels can be formed by **splitting**. In this process, an endothelial septum grows inwards along a length of a capillary, partitioning the lumen into two.

The maturation of new endothelial tubes into arterioles and venules is brought about by the recruitment of smooth muscle cells and connective tissue cells, driven by **platelet-derived growth factor** (PDGF) and **angiopoietins**. The final fate of the vessel, that is, whether it becomes an artery or vein, is determined by the expression of the protein **ephrin-B** and its receptor.

## Angiogenesis is initiated by vascular endothelial growth factor and other growth factors

Angiogenesis is initiated by tissue growth factors that induce endothelial gene expression. The principal endothelial growth factors are the vascular endothelial growth factors (VEGF-A for capillary sprouting; VEGF-C for lymphatic sprouting) and acidic and basic fibroblast growth factors. VEGF is abundant wherever tissues are forming new vessels, for example, fetus, placenta, healing wounds, tumours, psoriatic plaques, rheumatoid pannus, myocardium adjacent to infarcts and the diabetic retina (a leading cause of blindness in the West). The endothelial VEGF receptor is linked to a tyrosine kinase that activates a cascade of mitogen-activated protein kinases. This activates nuclear transcription factors, which switch on the angiogenesis genes.

What regulates VEGF secretion in such a way as to produce a capillary within 20–50 μm of most cells, and the highest capillary density in the most active tissues? The answer is that a shortage of $O_2$ stimulates cells to produce **hypoxia-inducible factor (HIF1)**, a gene-regulating protein (transcription factor). During normoxia, the α subunit of HIF1 is hydroxylated by HIF prolyl-hydroxylases and targeted for degradation by **von Hippel–Lindau tumor suppressor** (pVHL) protein. During hypoxia, the HIF1α and β subunits are stabilized. HIF binds to HIF responsive elements (HREs) in a gene promoter to stimulate the transcription of the *VEGFA*. gene, which in turn leads to angiogenesis. When sufficient new vessels have formed, the $O_2$ supply becomes adequate, so HIF levels fall and VEGF production is switched off. If VEGF production fails to switch off, the result is a haemangioblastoma, a tumour composed largely of a dense mass of blood vessels.

## Angiogenesis is restrained by thrombospondin and angiostatin

Endothelial growth is normally held in check by the antiangiogenic proteins thrombospondin and angiostatin. For angiogenesis to occur, the levels of thrombospondin and angiostatin must fall, as well as VEGF rising. The discovery of antiangiogenic factors has led to antiangiogenic drugs to restrict cancer growth. Once a tumour grows above ~1 mm in size, it depends on angiogenesis for an adequate nutrient supply. Antiangiogenic drugs are therefore now used to complement cytotoxic drugs in the treatment of some cancers.

## 9.10 ENDOTHELIUM AND ATHEROMA

Atheroma, the most common cause of serious morbidity and death in westernized societies, is a patchy, cholesterol-rich deposit in the subendothelial intima of large arteries. Atheroma is known alternatively as atherosclerosis, a rather self-contradictory term meaning 'gruel-like hardening'. The atheroma forms a plaque that narrows the artery lumen, leading to tissue ischaemia and thrombosis. In the heart, this results in **angina** and **myocardial infarctions**; in the brain, **transient ischaemic attacks** and **ischaemic strokes**; and in the legs, **intermittent claudication** (ischaemic pain on walking), **arterial ulcers** and **gangrenous necrosis** (tissue death, requiring amputation). The chief predisposing factors are high plasma levels of LDL (cholesterol bound to a carrier protein, $\sim 3 \times 10^6$ Da), high plasma fibrinogen, smoking, diabetes and hypertension. Shear stress disturbances are also atherogenic, since atheroma commonly develops at branches and bends. A moderate, regular intake of any alcoholic drink reduces the incidence of ischaemic heart disease by 20%–30%, and red wine may be particularly beneficial.

## Atheroma is rich in plasma-derived cholesterol

The atheromatous plaque begins as an intimal, subendothelial accumulation of LDL (mainly cholesterol) and fibrin, both derived from the plasma. The early lesion is also characterized by foam cells, which are lipid-laden macrophages derived from circulating monocytes. Later, proliferating VSM cells migrate into the lesion and a fibrous cap is laid down over the lipid deposit. Rupture of the cap can lead to platelet aggregation and thrombosis. Because the lesion involves the transendothelial passage of LDL and fibrinogen, and often platelet aggregation, endothelial dysfunction is thought to contribute to the pathogenesis. More specifically, impaired NO levels appear to be a contributory factor, as follows.

## Reduced nitric oxide levels facilitate atheroma formation

Endothelial NO is anti-atherogenic, because it inhibits VSM migration, platelet aggregation and endothelial expression of the monocyte glue, VCAM-1 (source of atheroma foam

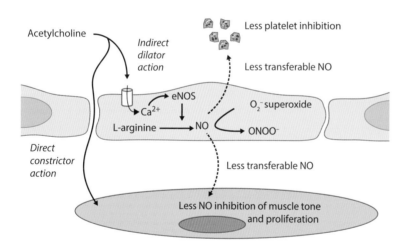

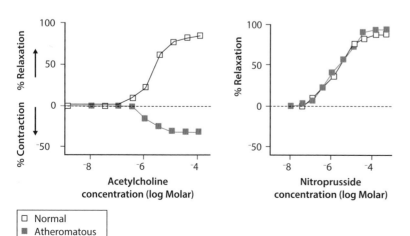

**Figure 9.13** Reduced nitric oxide (NO) availability in the atheromatous arteries of monkey. Response of normal (open squares) and atheromatous iliac artery (red filled squares) to acetylcholine (ACh; left panel) and to the NO donor nitroprusside (right panel). The NO-dependent vasodilator response to ACh becomes a constrictor response in atheromatous arteries. The sketch shows the proposed explanation: high levels of endothelial superoxide radicals in atheromatous vessels react with NO, reducing the amount of transferable NO. eNOS, endothelial nitric oxide synthase. (Redrawn from Freiman PC, Mitchell GC, Heistad DD, et al. *Circulation Research* 1986; 58(6): 783–9.)

cells) (Section 9.4). There is now considerable evidence that reduced NO levels contribute to atheroma formation. For example, atheroma formation in hypercholesterolaemic rabbits is reduced by L-arginine, which boosts NO production. Conversely, eNOS inhibitors increase the uptake of LDL and fibrinogen into the artery wall. Smokers and diabetics, who are especially prone to atheroma, have low NO levels and show impaired NO-dependent arterial vasodilatation. Diabetics have low insulin levels, or are insulin-resistant, and insulin is normally a significant tonic stimulus to NO production.

## Nitric oxide is depleted by increased superoxide production

Healthy arteries respond to ACh by endothelium-dependent vasodilatation, but atheromatous arteries show impaired dilatation or even constriction (Figure 9.13). This indicates that endothelial NO levels are low in atheromatous arteries. In early lesions, this is due to reduced endothelial NO generation, while in more advanced lesions, there is also increased inactivation of NO. Increased inactivation is caused by an overproduction of the superoxide radical $O_2^-$ by oxidases involved in oxidative metabolism and also generated by uncoupled NOS when cofactors such as $BH_4$ are scarce. Superoxide inactivates NO by reacting with it, to form peroxynitrite, $ONOO^-$. Superoxide generation is increased threefold in the aorta of cholesterol-fed rabbits, and is increased by smoking and diabetes. Moreover, superoxide dismutase, an enzyme that scavenges (removes) superoxide radicals, improves the endothelium-dependent vasodilatation of atheromatous vessels. Therefore, it appears that excessive superoxide production reduces NO concentration and hence the NO-based protection against atherogenesis.

Peroxynitrite is itself harmful because it undergoes further reactions that produce hydroxyl radicals, which damage cell membranes and oxidize LDL. Oxidized LDL reduces NO production further by displacing eNOS from its caveolar, cholesterol-rich binding site. By contrast, the 'good' HDL promotes eNOS localization in caveolae and boosts NO production.

## Oxidized low-density lipoprotein cholesterol and inflammation in atheromatous plaques

Oxidized LDL cholesterol is recognized by scavenger receptors on macrophages, triggering phagocytosis. Lipid-rich macrophages, or foam cells, ultimately die releasing their contents to form the lipid-rich core of the plaque. It is this stage of the atherosclerotic process for which the most effective treatments have been targeted. First, lowering plasma LDL cholesterol levels is known to reduce mortality in patients with atherosclerosis-related conditions.

Some benefit can be seen with improved diet, but inhibition of *de novo* synthesis of cholesterol in the liver by statins (3-hydroxy-3-methylglutaryl-coenzyme A reductase inhibitors) produces significant reductions in LDL cholesterol and are routinely prescribed to 'at risk' patients. Statins also have additional effects including reduced Ang II signalling, superoxide anion production and increased NO bioavailability, which help restore a healthy endothelium, as well as antiplatelet effects and plaque stabilization. Other primary prevention is aimed at reducing the prevalence of pro-oxidant species by stopping smoking and treating diabetes and hypertension.

If inflammation is resolved, atherosclerotic plaques may stabilize at this point, and can sometimes become calcified as they mature. A stable plaque will partially occlude the lumen of the artery and the extent and site of the occlusion (or 'stenosis') determine whether the patients suffers from symptoms.

## Plaque rupture and platelet activation

Plaques that remain inflamed can become unstable (prone to rupture). The mechanism that determines the stability of atherosclerotic plaques is not yet fully understood, but the consequences of plaque rupture can be devastating. If the fibrous cap is compromised, material from the core, which is highly thrombogenic, meets the blood leading to platelet adhesion, aggregation and activation of the coagulation cascade (see Section 9.11). The resulting thrombus can completely occlude the artery at the site of the plaque or become dislodged, forming an embolus that passes further down the arterial tree before occluding a smaller vessel.

## 9.11 ENDOTHELIUM, PLATELETS AND COAGULATION

Endothelial dysfunction, damage and exposure of collagen to the circulating blood leads to platelet activation and recruitment. Platelets are anucleate subcellular fragments whose function is to stop bleeding after injury. Platelet activation leads to the following interlinked processes:

1. Further platelet activation and recruitment (e.g. by ADP, thromboxane A2 [$TXA_2$] and 5-hydroxytryptamine release) to form a loose 'platelet plug' as a stopgap measure.
2. Local vasoconstriction to reduce blood flow to the affected area (via release of $TXA_2$, adrenaline and 5-hydroxytryptamine).
3. Activation of the coagulation cascade. Collagen and platelets stimulate the intrinsic pathway for blood coagulation, while tissue damage stimulates the extrinsic pathway. These pathways converge to convert prothrombin (so-called factor II) to thrombin (factor II-activated; IIa), which acts to convert fibrinogen to fibrin

and to further recruit platelets. Fibrin strands form a mesh around the platelet plug and trap other blood cells to generate a more permanent repair to the damaged vessel.

4. Recruitment of inflammatory cells to the site of injury to ward off any potential infection (e.g. through release of PDGF and PAF).

## Platelet activation

There are a range of different glycoprotein (GP) receptors on platelet membranes, which bind to a variety of ligands, including collagen and vWF, a factor secreted by the endothelium in response to injury as described in Section 9.6. Stimulation of these receptors results in an increase in intracellular $Ca^{2+}$, the trigger responsible for the following cellular effects (see Figure 9.14):

1. Increased surface area: pseudopodia emerge from the normal smooth discoid platelet surface, vastly increasing the surface area and, consequently, the adhesiveness of the platelets.

2. Degranulation: release of vasoconstrictor and PAFs to cause vasoconstriction and platelet recruitment, respectively.

3. Glycoprotein (GP) exposure: a change in the membrane leads to the exposure of the otherwise hidden glycoprotein, GPIIb/IIIa, which binds to fibrinogen to help stabilize the platelet plug.

## The coagulation cascade

Coagulation consists of two cascade pathways (see Figure 9.15) that converge to generate thrombin (factor IIa), which is responsible for the polymerization of soluble fibrinogen into fibrin strands. The cascade can be viewed as an amplification process whereby activation of a small amount of one factor generates large amounts of the next downstream factor. This results in the rapid formation of large amounts of fibrin in response to what may have been a weak initial signal. Each step in the cascade involves the activation of normally

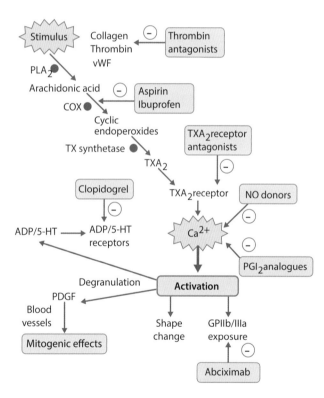

**Figure 9.14** Platelet activation pathways and therapeutic interventions. Platelet activation is triggered by stimuli, such as exposed collagen and thrombin, or the endothelial release of von Willebrand factor (vWF). These activate receptors that couple to phospholipase $A_2$ (PLA$_2$), which catalyses the production of cyclic endoperoxides from arachidonic acid via the enzyme cyclooxygenase (COX). Thromboxane (TX) synthetase then produces thromboxane $A_2$ (TXA$_2$), which acts at its receptor to raise intracellular $Ca^{2+}$ and activate the platelet. This results in platelet shape change, degranulation (releasing vasoconstrictors and platelet-activating factors, such as adenosine diphosphate [ADP], serotonin [5-hydroxytryptamine {5HT}], and platelet-derived growth factor [PDGF]), and exposure of glycoprotein (GP) IIb/IIIa, which binds to fibrinogen to help stabilize the platelet plug. The site of action of different antiplatelet agents (such as nitric oxide [NO], donors and prostacyclin [PGI$_2$] analogues) is highlighted. (Adapted from the *Oxford Handbook of Medical Sciences*, 2nd edn; 2011. Oxford: Oxford University Press. p. 465.)

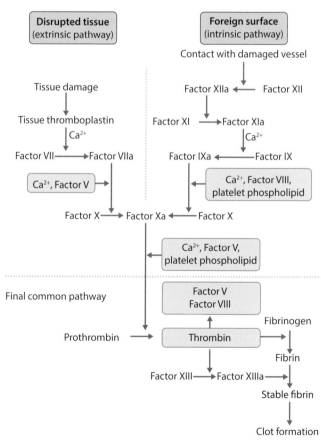

**Figure 9.15** The extrinsic and intrinsic pathways leading to the formation of a blood clot via a final common pathway. Note the central roles played by factor Xa and thrombin in the process of blood coagulation. (Adapted from *Human Physiology: The Basis of Medicine*, 3rd edn. Oxford: Oxford University Press; 2006. p. 240.)

inactive circulating enzymes known as 'clotting factors'. As each clotting factor becomes activated, it catalyses the activation of the subsequent factor in the cascade. Fibrin formed from soluble fibrinogen is finally stabilized by the action of factor XIIIa.

## Arterial versus venous thrombosis

The site (arterial or venous) of thrombus generation is important in determining the morphology of the thrombus. Arterial thrombi are predominantly composed of activated platelets (so-called 'white thrombus') with some fibrin. They can be caused by atherosclerotic plaque rupture, left atrial appendage blood stasis in atrial fibrillation or stasis surrounding a large myocardial infarction. They may remain at the initial site of thrombosis or be carried downstream as an embolus. Venous thrombi are mainly fibrin with few platelets and a large proportion of red blood cells that become trapped in the mesh (red thrombus). Venous thrombi tend to form in conditions where there is venous stasis, for example, deep vein thrombosis in the legs caused by extended physical inactivity. Venous thrombi are susceptible to distal embolization to the lungs as a life-threatening pulmonary embolism, or if a right-to-left intracardiac shunt exists (such as a patent foramen ovale, atrial or ventricular septal defect) as a paradoxical embolism into the systemic circulation. Drugs used to treat venous thrombosis are therefore targeted at the clotting cascade (such as low-molecular-weight heparin, warfarin or the novel oral anticoagulants: dabigatran, rivaroxaban, apixaban and edoxaban), while acute arterial ischaemic events tend to be treated with antiplatelet agents. When percutaneous coronary intervention is being undertaken to treat an acute coronary event, antiplatelet agents may be supplemented with the indirect factor Xa inhibitors low-molecular-weight heparin and fondaparinux, or the direct thrombin inhibitor bivalirudin (see Table 9.1).

**Table 9.1** Medications used as antithrombotic agents

| Drug class | Example (trial name)[a] | Mechanism of action | Side effects |
|---|---|---|---|
| Cyclooxygenase (COX) inhibitors | Aspirin (ISIS-2) | Inhibits COX1 and COX2 to prevent thromboxane action on platelet aggregation | Peptide/duodenal ulceration; bleeding; exacerbation of asthma; angio-oedema |
| Thienopyridine P2Y$_{12}$ receptor inhibitors | Clopidogrel (CURE) Prasugrel (TRITON-TIMI 38) | Platelet ADP receptor antagonists that prevent aggregation | Bleeding; neutropenia; TTP; bradycardia. Caution with prasugrel in those <60 kg or >75 years old |
| Non-thienopyridine P2Y$_{12}$ receptor inhibitors | Ticagrelor (PLATO) | Platelet ADP receptor antagonists that prevent aggregation | Bleeding; shortness of breath; bradycardia |
| Glycoprotein IIb/IIIa inhibitors | Abciximab (EPIC) | Platelet glycoprotein IIb/IIIa inhibitor to prevent aggregation | Bleeding; thrombocytopenia |
| Direct thrombin (II) inhibitors | Bivalent: bivalirudin (ACUITY/ HORIZONS-AMI) Univalent: dabigatran (RE-LY) | Thrombin inhibition | Bleeding |
| Direct Factor Xa inhibitors | Rivaroxaban (ROCKET AF) Apixaban (ARISTOTLE) Edoxaban (ENGAGE AF-TIMI 48) | Direct Factor Xa inhibition | Bleeding |
| Indirect Factor Xa inhibitors | Fondaparinux (OASIS5) Low-molecular-weight heparin (ESSENCE) | Potentiates antithrombin. Heparin also inactivates thrombin | Bleeding; heparin-induced thrombocytopenia (not fondaparinux) |
| Coumarins | Warfarin | Vitamin K antagonist inhibiting the production of clotting factors II, VII, IX and X | Bleeding; warfarin necrosis; osteoporosis |

[a] ACUITY, Acute Catheterization and Urgent Intervention Triage strategy; ARISTOTLE, Apixaban for Reduction in Stroke and Other Thromboembolic Events in Atrial Fibrillation; CURE, Clopidogrel in Unstable Angina to Prevent Recurrent Events; ENGAGE AF-TIMI 48, Effective Anticoagulation with Factor Xa Next Generation in Atrial Fibrillation–Thrombolysis in Myocardial Infarction 48; EPIC, A Phase III Double-Blind, Placebo-Controlled Multicenter Study of Abciximab In Patients Undergoing High Risk Coronary Angioplasty; ESSENCE, Efficacy and Safety of Subcutaneous Enoxaparin in Non–Q-Wave Coronary Events; HORIZONS-AMI, Harmonizing Outcomes with Revascularization and Stents in Acute Myocardial Infarction; ISIS-2, Second International Study of Infarct Survival; OASIS5, Fifth Organization to Assess Strategies in Acute Ischemic Syndromes; PLATO, Platelet Inhibition and Patient Outcomes; RE-LY, Randomized Evaluation of Long-Term Anticoagulation Therapy; ROCKET AF, Rivaroxaban Once Daily Oral Direct Factor Xa Inhibition Compared with Vitamin K Antagonism for Prevention of Stroke and Embolism Trial in Atrial Fibrillation; TRITON-TIMI 38, TRial to assess Improvement in Therapeutic Outcomes by optimizing platelet InhibitioN with prasugrel Thrombolysis In Myocardial Infarction 38. ADP, adenosine diphosphate; P2Y$_{12}$, P2Y purinoceptor 12; TTP, thrombotic thrombocytopenic purpura.

## SUMMARY

- The endothelium is a monolayer of flattened cells tethered to the basal lamina by integrins. The collagen IV-rich basal lamina prevents capillary rupture. Adjacent cells are joined by circumferential strands of junctional proteins, tethered internally to the actin cytoskeleton. Breaks in the junctional strands allow the intercellular passage of water and small solutes. Plasma proteins are prevented from entering the intercellular cleft by a semipermeable luminal coat, the glycocalyx. Some plasma protein is transported slowly across endothelium by a caveola/vesicle system.

- The endothelium has an intracellular potential very close to that of the adjacent VSM, approximately −30 to −60 mV, reflecting myoendothelial coupling via gap junctions. Receptors to inflammatory agonists (e.g. histamine, bradykinin) activate PLC, which leads to the activation of receptor-operated and store-operated $Ca^{2+}$ channels. The influx of extracellular $Ca^{2+}$ triggers endothelium-dependent vasodilatation and raises microvascular permeability. $Ca^{2+}$ also activates $SK_{Ca}$ and $IK_{Ca}$ channels, which hyperpolarizes the endothelial membrane potential to boost $Ca^{2+}$ entry.

- The endothelium regulates local vascular tone through the vasoconstrictor peptide endothelin and three vasodilator agents: NO, EDH/EDHF and $PGI_2$.

- Endothelin causes a long-lasting vasoconstriction. Circulating endothelin is elevated in hypoxia, pre-eclamptic toxaemia, heart failure and haemorrhagic strokes.

- NO is generated continuously from L-arginine by $Ca^{2+}$-calmodulin-dependent eNOS. eNOS activity can be increased by: (1) shear stress, leading to flow-induced vasodilatation in large arteries; and (2) agonists such as ACh, bradykinin and other inflammatory agents. The angina-relieving action of GTN is due to its NO-like vasodilatation of large veins and arteries.

- EDH dilates smaller arterial vessels. It mediates ascending (conducted) vasodilatation of feed arteries in exercising muscle. $PGI_2$, like NO, inhibits platelet aggregation; in some arteries, it causes vasodilatation.

- The endothelium also influences blood. ACE on the endothelial surface catalyses Ang II formation. vWF, released from the endothelial Weibel–Palade body, carries clotting factor VIII. NO and $PGI_2$ inhibit platelet aggregation to prevent/limit clotting.

- The venular endothelium contributes to the inflammatory response. Adhesive proteins (selectins, ICAM-1, VCAM-1) are inserted into the luminal membrane to capture circulating leukocytes. Also, the formation of wide intercellular gaps in venular endothelium speeds up the transfer of immunoglobulins and water, and leads to inflammatory swelling.

- Capillary permeability is regulated via changes in the organization of junctional proteins. Permeability is raised by flow and atrial natriuretic peptide, acting through cGMP. Conversely, agents that increase endothelial cAMP enhance the intercellular barrier.

- VEGF stimulates capillary sprouting (angiogenesis). Angiogenesis is necessary for tissue and tumour growth. Angiogenesis is inhibited by thrombospondin, angiostatin and anticancer angiostatic drugs.

- The trapping of plasma-derived LDL and fibrin under the arterial endothelium gives rise to atheroma, the biggest killer in westernized societies. Endothelial NO normally protects against atheroma by reducing LDL and fibrinogen uptake, VCAM-1 expression, smooth muscle proliferation and platelet aggregation. NO levels are low in atheromatous arteries, due in part to a reaction with superoxide.

- Endothelial dysfunction, damage and exposure of collagen to the circulating blood lead to platelet recruitment, activation of the coagulation cascade and thrombus formation. While this is a physiological response to prevent bleeding, inappropriate thrombus formation in arteries or veins can produce ischaemic events and organ damage if arterial blood flow is compromised.

## FURTHER READING

Garland CJ, Dora KA. EDH: endothelium-dependent hyperpolarization and microvascular signalling. *Acta Physiologica* 2017; **219**(1): 152–61.

Vanhoutte PM, Shimokawa H, Feletou M, et al. Endothelial dysfunction and vascular disease: a 30th anniversary update. *Acta Physiologica* 2017; **219**(1): 22–96.

Earley S, Brayden JE. Transient receptor potential channels in the vasculature. *Physiological Reviews* 2015; **95**: 645–90.

Longden, TA, Nelson, MT. Vascular inward rectifier K⁺ channels as external K⁺ sensors in the control of cerebral blood flow. *Microcirculation* 2015; **22**: 185–96.

Prakriya M, Lewis RS. Store-operated calcium channels. *Physiological Reviews* 2015; **95**: 1383–436.

Billaud M, Lohman AW, Johnstone SR, et al. Regulation of cellular signaling by microdomains in the blood vessel wall. *Pharmacological Reviews* 2014; **66**: 513–69.

Channon KM. Tetrahydrobiopterin: a vascular redox target to improve endothelial function. *Current Vascular Pharmacology* 2012; 10(6): 705–8.

Reitsma S, Slaaf DW, Vink H, et al. The endothelial glycocalyx: composition, functions, and visualization. *Pflügers Archiv: European Journal of Physiology* 2007; **454**: 345–59.

Tiruppathi C, Ahmmed GU, Vogel SM, et al. $Ca^{2+}$ signaling, TRP channels, and endothelial permeability. *Microcirculation* 2006; **13**(8): 693–708.

Carmeliet P. Angiogenesis in life, disease and medicine. *Nature* 2005; **438**(7070): 932–36.

Bazzoni G, Dejana E. Endothelial cell-to-cell junctions: molecular organization and role in vascular homeostasis. *Physiological Reviews* 2004; **84**(3): 869–901.

Cohen AW, Hnasko R, Schubert W, et al. Role of caveolae and caveolins in health and disease. *Physiological Reviews* 2004; **84**(4): 1341–79.

Shaul PW. Endothelial nitric oxide synthase, caveolae and the development of atherosclerosis. *The Journal of Physiology* 2003; **547**(Pt 1): 21–33.

Kvietys PR, Sandig M. Neutrophil diapedesis: paracellular or transcellular? *News in Physiological Sciences* 2001; **16**: 15–19.

Fisslthaler B, Dimmeler S, Hermann C, et al. Phosphorylation and activation of the endothelial nitric oxide synthase by fluid shear stress. *Acta Physiologica Scandinavica* 2000; **168**(1): 81–8.

Thurston G, Baluk P, McDonald DM. Determinants of endothelial cell phenotype in venules. *Microcirculation* 2000; **7**(1): 67–80.

Walzog B, Gaehtgens P. Adhesion molecules: the path to a new understanding of acute inflammation. *News in Physiological Sciences* 2000; **15**: 107–13.

Curry FE. Regulation of capillary permeability in single perfused microvessels. In: Reed RK, Rubin K, eds. *Connective Tissue Biology: Integration and Reductionism*. London: Portland Press; 1998. pp. 195–206.

Davies PF. Flow-mediated endothelial mechanotransduction. *Physiological Reviews* 1995; **75**(3): 519–60.

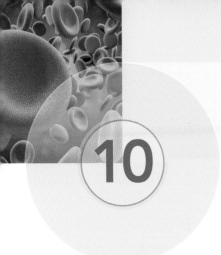

# The microcirculation and solute exchange

# 10

## LEARNING OBJECTIVES

*After reading this chapter you should be able to:*

- explain how terminal arterioles regulate capillary perfusion (10.1);
- sketch the key structural differences between three main types of capillary (10.2);
- distinguish between the laws governing solute exchange (diffusion) and water exchange (hydraulic flow) (10.3);
- list the factors governing the rate of diffusive transport (Fick's law) (10.3);
- define 'solute permeability' and explain how a porous membrane affects it (10.4);

- name three main categories of solute, based on capillary permeability (10.5–10.7);
- outline the special features of the blood–brain barrier (10.8);
- sketch the concentration profile of a metabolized solute (e.g. glucose) along a capillary and use the sketch to define 'Fick's principle' (cf. law), 'extraction' and 'plasma clearance' (10.9);
- explain the difference between flow-limited and diffusion-limited exchange (10.10);
- describe 'capillary recruitment', and list other factors that enhance solute exchange in exercising muscle (10.11).

A single, inescapable necessity has driven the evolution of the cardiovascular system – the need to deliver metabolic substrates, such as $O_2$ and glucose, rapidly to the cells of a large organism (Section 1.1). The delivery hatch, so to speak, is the capillary wall. The exchange of materials across the capillary wall is the payload for the entire, hugely complex system of pumps, valves, tubes and electrical potentials that we call the cardiovascular system – the primary reason for its existence.

## 10.1 ORGANIZATION AND PERFUSION OF EXCHANGE VESSELS

The term 'exchange vessel' embraces not only the capillaries but also, strictly speaking, the microvessels immediately upstream and downstream, since some $O_2$ transfer occurs

through the walls of terminal arterioles, and some fluid transfer across the walls of pericytic (postcapillary) venules. Nevertheless, capillaries account for the majority of solute and fluid exchange.

### Supply and drainage of a capillary bed

The smallest terminal arteries branch into first-order arterioles, and further divisions give rise to **terminal arterioles**, the last arterial vessels with smooth muscle in the wall. Each terminal arteriole divides into a cluster or **module of capillaries** (Figure 10.1). **Capillary** means 'hair-like', a typical capillary being 500–1000 μm long and 4–8 μm wide, hence invisible to the naked eye. The existence of capillaries was inferred by William Harvey, from his demonstration that blood flows from arteries into veins; it was not until the invention of the

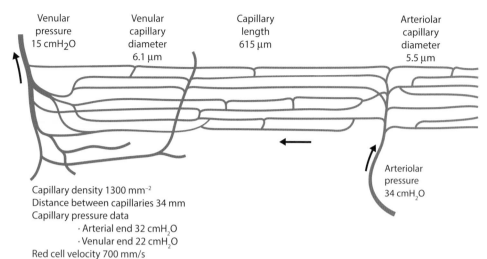

Figure 10.1 Capillary bed of relaxed cremaster muscle (rat), with a terminal arteriole feeding a module of ~14 capillaries. Numbers are means of observations. (From Smaje L, Zweifach BW, Intaglietta M. *Microvascular Research* 1970; 2(1): 96–110, with permission from Elsevier.)

Venular pressure 15 cmH$_2$O

Venular capillary diameter 6.1 μm

Capillary length 615 μm

Arteriolar capillary diameter 5.5 μm

Arteriolar pressure 34 cmH$_2$O

Capillary density 1300 mm$^{-2}$
Distance between capillaries 34 mm
Capillary pressure data
· Arterial end 32 cmH$_2$O
· Venular end 22 cmH$_2$O
Red cell velocity 700 mm/s

microscope that Malpighi, in 1661, first observed capillaries on the surface of the lung of the frog.

The venous ends of capillaries reunite to form **pericytic venules** (postcapillary venules). These are thin-walled vessels, ~15 μm wide, with pericytes but not smooth muscle surrounding the endothelium. Pericytic venules are highly permeable to water and play a major role in inflammation. Smooth muscle reappears in the walls of venules 30–50 μm wide.

**Arteriovenous anastomoses** are muscular microvessels, 20–130 μm wide, that link arterioles directly to venules, bypassing the capillary network. They are found chiefly in the skin of the extremities (fingers, nose, lips, earlobes), where they are important for temperature regulation (Section 15.3).

## Capillary density is adapted to tissue function

The number of capillaries packed into unit volume of tissue is called the capillary density, and is regulated by the hypoxia-inducible factor (HIF)-vascular endothelial growth factor (VEGF) pathway (Section 9.9). Skeletal muscle contains 300–1000 capillaries per mm$^2$ cross section, or 1–3 capillaries per muscle fibre. Endurance training stimulates angiogenesis and can raise the capillary-to-fibre ratio to 6–8. In the myocardium and brain, where the metabolic rate is both high and sustained, capillary density is correspondingly high, ~3000 per mm$^2$. This has two advantages:

- A high capillary density increases the endothelial surface area available for gas and nutrient exchange. Capillary surface area increases from ~100 cm$^2$ per gram in skeletal muscle to ~500 cm$^2$ per gram in myocardium or brain.
- A high capillary density reduces the distance between the bloodstream and tissue cells. This is important because distance profoundly affects the time needed for diffusive transport (see Section 1.1).

The lungs provide the most extreme example of capillary packing; here, the capillary surface area is a staggering 3500 cm$^2$ per gram, for obvious functional reasons.

## Terminal arterioles regulate the number of perfused capillaries

The contractile state of the terminal arterioles controls the number of capillaries that are well perfused with blood at any one moment. The relaxation of an individual arteriole allows a brisk perfusion of the associated capillary module, and such capillaries are referred to as 'open'. The contraction of a terminal arteriole slows or halts the blood flow through its associated capillary module, and such capillaries are referred to as 'closed'. In skeletal muscle at rest, some arterioles are relaxed and others are contracted at any one moment. As a result, a substantial fraction of the capillaries is 'closed' at any one instant, and the distribution of flow is uneven. This **heterogeneity of tissue perfusion** is characteristic of many resting tissues. When arteriolar tone decreases, capillary perfusion becomes more uniform; in other words, vasodilatation improves the homogeneity of tissue perfusion.

The regulation of the number of perfused capillaries used to be ascribed to a largely mythical beast, the 'precapillary sphincter'. In reality, **there is no discrete sphincteric ring of muscle at the capillary entrance** in most tissues. It is the terminal arteriole that regulates the numbers of open and closed capillaries in general.

## Capillary blood flow varies with time because of vasomotion

An individual arteriole does not usually remain relaxed or contracted for long; its muscle tone changes constantly. This is called **vasomotion**. In some tissues, such as resting skeletal muscle, vasomotion has a regular rhythm, with a cycle time of ~15 s; in other tissues, such as skin, vasomotion is

less regular. Because of arteriolar vasomotion, blood flow in an individual capillary tends to fluctuate; it may wax and wane every 15 s or so, and can stop for a while in 'closed' capillaries.

## Capillary transit time governs the time available for exchange

The time that it takes a red cell to pass through the capillary bed, from entrance to exit, is called the **transit time**. Transit time represents the time available for each unit of blood to unload $O_2$ and glucose, and load up with $CO_2$ and urea. Vasomotion causes transit times to vary, but a typical transit time in a well-perfused capillary is 0.5–2 s (blood velocity is 300–1000 µm/s). The transit time can fall to around 0.25 s during exercise because the arterioles dilate and blood velocity increases. During extreme human exercise, when cardiac output is very high, the transit time through the lung capillaries can become so short that the blood emerges without having had time to achieve full $O_2$ saturation (see section 10.10).

## 10.2 THREE TYPES OF CAPILLARY

Electron microscopy has revealed three basic types of capillary. They are, in order of increasing permeability to water, the continuous, fenestrated and discontinuous capillary.

## The continuous capillary

Continuous capillaries occur in skeletal muscle, myocardium, skin, lung, connective tissue and fat. A specialized form, the tight capillary, occurs in the central nervous system and testes. The circumference comprises a ring of 1–3 endothelial cells surrounded by a continuous basement membrane (Figure 10.2a). Due to the thinness of the cells, the transcapillary diffusion distance is only ~0.3 µm. **Pericytes**, formerly called Rouget's cells, partly envelop the outside of the capillary. Recent genetic knockout studies in mice have indicated that the pericytes regulate capillary diameter and structure. Pericytes are unusually well developed around retinal capillaries, and seem to be contractile in this tissue.

The structural features of continuous capillaries that influence solute exchange are primarily the following:

- The **intercellular cleft** transmits water and small lipid-insoluble solutes, for example, glucose. These small molecules weave their way through the breaks in the junctional strands (Figures 9.2, 9.4 and 10.3).
- The luminal **glycocalyx** excludes plasma proteins from access to the cleft, but is permeable to water and small solute (Figure 9.3).
- The **caveola/vesicle** system transfers large molecules slowly across the wall (Figure 9.6).

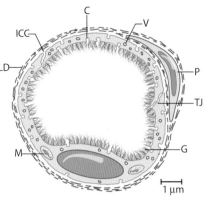

(a) Continuous capillary

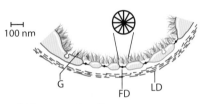

(b) Fenestrated capillary

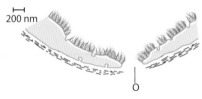

(c) Discontinuous capillary

**Figure 10.2** Sketches of capillary wall in transverse section, based on electron micrographs. **(a)** Continuous capillary. **(b)** Fenestrated capillary. **(c)** Discontinuous capillary. C, caveola (open surface vesicle); FD, fenestral diaphragm; inset shows diaphragm viewed face-on; G, glycocalyx; ICC, intercellular cleft; LD, lamina densa of basal lamina; M, mitochondrion; O, open gap; P, pericyte; TJ, tight part of intercellular junction; V, vesicle.

## Fenestrated capillaries are specialized for rapid fluid filtration

Fenestrated capillaries are at least an order of magnitude more permeable to water and small lipid-insoluble solutes than are continuous capillaries. They are found in tissues that specialize in fluid exchange (kidneys, exocrine glands, intestinal mucosa, synovial lining of joints, choroid plexus, ciliary body of the eye) and in endocrine glands. The endothelium is perforated by clusters of small, circular windows, or fenestrae, with a diameter of 50–60 nm (Figure 10.2b). Each fenestra is bridged by an extremely thin membrane, the diaphragm, which is 4–5 nm thick, except in renal glomerular capillaries, where the diaphragm is absent. The diaphragm resembles a cartwheel, with wedge-shaped apertures between the spokes, through which water, nutrients and hormones can pass very rapidly to reach the surrounding tissue. The only currently known diaphragmatic constituent is a glycoprotein, plasma-lemmal vesicle associated protein (PV-1).

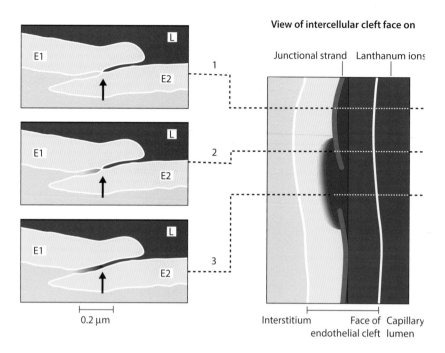

**View of intercellular cleft face on**

Junctional strand    Lanthanum ions

1

2

3

0.2 μm

Interstitium    Face of    Capillary
endothelial cleft    lumen

**Figure 10.3** Three sections of the same intercellular cleft (left). The capillary was perfused with a solution of lanthanum ions (black) for 10 s before fixation. The cleft is depicted face-on on the right. The tight junction (red lines on the right, arrows on the left) blocks the cleft in Section 1, but a break in the junctional strands creates an open pathway in Section 3. The intermediate Section 2 gives the false impression that the tight junction is permeable. L, lumen; E1 and E2, endothelial cells. (Redrawn from Adamson RH, Michel CC. *The Journal of Physiology* 1993; 466: 303–27, with permission from Wiley-Blackwell.)

Fenestrae appear to form when VEGF from neighbouring cells causes a local removal of the endothelial F-actin cytoskeleton. This closely approximates the luminal and abluminal membranes. Renal glomerular capillaries have an exceptionally high density of fenestrae and the surrounding cells (podocytes) express very high levels of VEGF. Conversely, in heterozygous knockout mice with low VEGF levels, fenestrae fail to develop.

## Discontinuous capillaries allow blood cell turnover

Discontinuous or sinusoidal capillaries have endothelial gaps over 100 nm wide, with a corresponding discontinuity in the basal lamina, so these capillaries are highly permeable, even to plasma proteins. Discontinuous capillaries occur in organs where red cells or white cells need to migrate between the blood and tissue, namely in the bone marrow, spleen and liver.

## 10.3 DIFFUSION, CONVECTION AND REFLECTION ACROSS A POROUS MEMBRANE

Before dealing with solute permeation through the capillary wall, a brief overview of passive transport through porous membranes may be helpful.

## Solutes diffuse, whereas water flows

Water and solutes (e.g. glucose) cross the capillary wall by **passive** transport; that is, without any energy expenditure by the endothelium being involved. However, solutes cross the wall by an entirely different physical process from water. Water **flows** across the wall down a **pressure gradient**, whereas a metabolized solute, such as glucose or $O_2$, **diffuses** across the wall down its **concentration gradient** (Figure 10.4). As long ago as 1919, the Danish physiologist August Krogh established that passive diffusion accounts for $O_2$ transfer from blood to muscle.

It is true that solutes such as glucose are also swept along in the water that is continuously flowing out through the capillary wall in a process called **convective transport**. However, the flow of water is so slow that it generally contributes little to the transport of a metabolite or drug; diffusion is much faster over capillary-to-cell distances. (For proof, see the footnote to Table 10.2) A further source of confusion is the common textbook statement that water molecules can cross the wall very quickly by diffusion. While this is true, it is a red herring because water diffusion is bidirectional and achieves no net transport.

Thus, to understand the transcapillary movement of glucose, amino acids, drugs and other lipid-insoluble metabolites in most tissues (except brain; see Section 10.8), we need to focus on passive, non-carrier-mediated diffusion through a porous membrane.

## Fick's law describes free diffusive transport in a fluid

The basic physics of diffusive transport was worked out by Adolf Fick, Professor of Physiology at the University of Würzburg in Germany. **Fick's first law of diffusion** (1855) states that the mass of solute transferred by diffusion per unit time, $J_s$, across a body of liquid depends on four factors (Figure 10.5a):

1. $J_s$ is directly proportional to the **concentration difference**, $C_1 - C_2$ or $\Delta C$ (delta means 'a difference in').

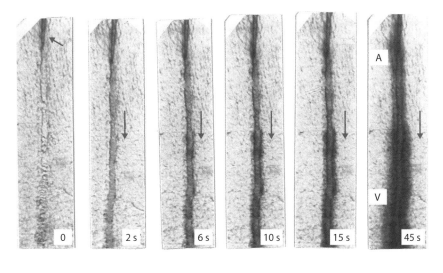

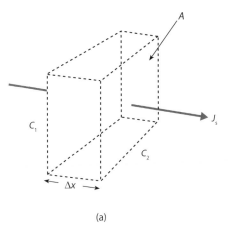

**Figure 10.4** Timed sequence showing diffusion of Evans blue (small, lipid-insoluble solute, radius ~1 nm) out of a perfused frog mesenteric capillary. Dye-filled micropipette (arrow) is visible at the arterial end of the capillary in the first frame; other arrows show the direction of flow. The arteriovenous (A, V) gradient of permeability is obvious; venous capillaries are normally more permeable than arterial capillaries. (From Levick JR. Doctoral thesis, Oxford.)

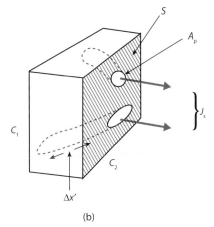

**Figure 10.5 (a)** Free diffusion in bulk solution. The solute diffuses through an unimpeded layer of fluid of thickness $\Delta x$ and surface area $A$, driven by concentration difference $(C_1 - C_2)$. $J_s$ is the diffusion rate (mole/s). **(b)** A porous membrane reduces $J_s$ by confining the solute to pores of total area $A_p$. The pore pathlength $\Delta x'$ is usually greater than the membrane thickness $\Delta x$.

2. $J_s$ is inversely proportional to the **diffusion distance**, $\Delta x$. The ratio $\Delta C/\Delta x$ is called the concentration gradient.

3. $J_s$ is directly proportional to the **surface area**, $A$.

4. $J_s$ is directly proportional to the solute **diffusion coefficient** or diffusivity, $D$.

Fick's law can thus be written:

$$J_s = -DA\Delta C/\Delta x \qquad (10.1)$$

The negative sign, which often puzzles students, is a mathematical convention to show that transport is 'downhill', that is, down the concentration gradient. The **diffusion coefficient** is a measure of the ease with which a given molecular species slips through the solvent. Since big molecules encounter more friction than little ones, $D$ is inversely related to solute size; small molecules, such as glucose, have a large $D$ and diffuse faster than big molecules, such as albumin.

## Pores impede diffusive transport

When a solute diffuses through a large body of solvent, the distant walls of the container do not affect the solute and the process is called free diffusion. By contrast, when a solute diffuses through very narrow pores in a membrane, as in the capillary wall, diffusion is slowed down by three distinct factors.

## Reduction of area available for diffusion

When a solute is confined to water-filled pores, the maximum area available for diffusion is the total pore area $A_p$, which is usually a very small percentage of the total surface area of the membrane $S$ (Figure 10.5b). This reduces the transport rate by the factor $A_p/S$. A further effect, **steric exclusion**, can reduce the available area to less than $A_p/S$ (Figure 10.6a). For a solute molecule of radius '$a$', the closest the centre of the molecule can get to the pore wall is $a$. Consequently, in a cylindrical pore of radius $r$ the diffusive movements are confined to the central column of fluid, of radius $r - a$. The area available for diffusion is now only a fraction of the total pore area $A_p$.

## Restricted diffusion inside a pore

When the solute radius is >1/10th of the pore radius, the proximity of the pore wall impedes diffusion by a hydrodynamic mechanism. For the solute molecule to advance along

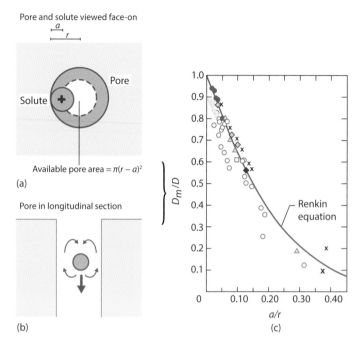

Pore and solute viewed face-on

Available pore area = $\pi(r - a)^2$

(a)

Pore in longitudinal section

(b)

(c)

**Figure 10.6** Difficulties encountered by a spherical molecule of radius '$a$' (grey) diffusing through a water-filled cylindrical pore of radius $r$. **(a)** End-on, bird's eye view of pore, showing steric exclusion of solute centre from an annulus of fluid (pink). The solute can only move around in the central clear area, reducing the available pore area to $\pi(r - a)^2$. **(b)** Longitudinal section through the pore. As the solute molecule diffuses down the pore (thick arrow), water molecules must squeeze past it, through the narrow gap between wall and solute. This increases the hydrodynamic drag on the solute (restricted diffusion). **(c)** Plot of reduced diffusion across a membrane, $D_m$, as fraction of free diffusion coefficient $D$, against ratio of solute to pore size, $a/r$. The Renkin equation predicts $D_m/D$ from the steric exclusion and restricted diffusion phenomena. (From Beck RE, Schultz JS. *Biochimica et Biophysica Acta* 1972; 255(1): 273–303, with permission from Elsevier.)

the pore, water molecules ahead of it must slip back through the narrow gap between the pore wall and solute, to make space for the advancing solute particle (Figure 10.6b). The narrower the gap between the solute and the pore wall, the less easily the water slips past; in biophysical terms, the hydrodynamic drag of water on the solute increases as the solute size approaches the pore diameter. As a result, the solute diffusion coefficient inside a narrow pore, $D_{res}$, is smaller than the free diffusion coefficient in bulk solution, $D$. This is called **restricted diffusion**, and can be a substantial reduction. For example, $D_{res}$ is half $D_{free}$ when the solute radius $a$ is 15% of pore radius $r$.

## Increased pathlength

Most endothelial junctions pass obliquely through the capillary wall (Figures 9.4 and 10.3). Consequently, the true diffusion distance, $\Delta x'$, is greater than the membrane thickness $\Delta x$ (Figure 10.5b).

Because of these three effects, the transcapillary diffusion of lipid-insoluble solutes, such as glucose, lactate, amino acids, peptides, hormones and drugs, is slowed down by more than two orders of magnitude. **Membrane permeability** is an index of this depression of diffusion (Section 10.4).

## Narrow pores cause molecular reflection: the reflection coefficient

In the previous account, there was no solvent flow across the membrane, so solute transport was purely diffusive. If there is also pressure-driven fluid filtration across the membrane, solute transport is partly by filtration and

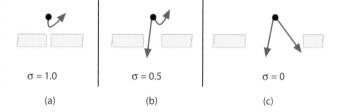

$\sigma = 1.0$  (a)

$\sigma = 0.5$  (b)

$\sigma = 0$  (c)

**Figure 10.7** The osmotic reflection coefficient $\sigma$ is a measure of the molecular selectivity of a pore **(a–c)**. It depends on the solute width-to-pore width ratio.

partly by diffusion, and we need a new membrane parameter to deal with this, namely the reflection coefficient, $\sigma$ (sigma). The reflection coefficient is the fraction of solute molecules reflected by the membrane during filtration at a high rate; it is an index of the difficulty a solute experiences in passing through a pore, relative to water. When a small solute (radius $a$) is washed into a large pore (radius $r$), steric exclusion is negligible, so the solute passes through the pore as freely as water. Its reflection is zero ($\sigma = 0$; Figure 10.7c) and the solute exerts no osmotic pressure across the membrane. At the other extreme, if the solute is wider than the pore ($a > r$), steric exclusion is total, so all the solute molecules are reflected ($\sigma = 1.0$) and the ultrafiltrate contains no solute (Figure 10.7a). The solute exerts its full osmotic potential in these circumstances. In the intermediate state, where $a/r$ is >0.1 but <1, the solute is partially excluded from the pore (Figure 10.6a), so a fraction is reflected ($\sigma$ is >0 but <1) and the ultrafiltrate has a reduced solute concentration, $1 - \sigma$ (Figure 10.7b). The solution exerts a fraction of its osmotic pressure in these circumstances (Section 11.1).

Because the reflection coefficient depends simply on $a/r$, it has been measured in capillaries using solutes of known radius $a$, to estimate the equivalent radius $r$ of the transendothelial channels at their narrowest point. The result was 4–5 nm. The capillary wall is perforated by water-filled channels with similar properties to cylindrical channels of radius 4–5 nm. The channels are not cylindrical in reality; they are the interfibre spaces of the glycocalyx (Figure 9.3).

The reflection coefficient and permeability, though related, are distinct; permeability depends on the number and length of pores, as well as their width, whereas reflection depends solely on pore width.

## 10.4 THE CONCEPT OF 'PERMEABILITY'

### Definition of permeability

Because a membrane impedes diffusion by multiple, hard-to-measure effects (steric exclusion, restricted diffusion, porous area and pathlength), it is convenient to encapsulate them in one catch-all parameter, namely permeability. The permeability of a membrane $P$ is the rate of diffusion of solute ($J_s$) across unit area of membrane per unit concentration difference across the membrane $\Delta C$, in the absence of fluid filtration. If we write the definition out in symbols, using $S$ for capillary surface area, we have the permeability equation:

$$P = J_s/S\Delta C \qquad (10.2)$$

Rearranging the permeability equation, we see that it is a simplified version of Fick's first law of diffusion (equation 10.1);

$$J_s = PS\Delta C \qquad (10.3)$$

Permeability has the units of velocity, cm/s. The product $PS$ is called the capillary diffusion capacity of a tissue and has the units of $cm^3/s$.

### Permeability and local concentration gradient determine solute flux

The rearranged permeability equation 10.3 tells us that the amount of solute transported across a segment of capillary in a given time depends on three factors (Figure 10.11):

- endothelial permeability;
- surface area;
- the transcapillary concentration difference for that segment.

It is necessary to consider each segment separately, rather than the whole capillary, because solute concentration changes non-linearly as blood passes along the capillary, due to diffusion (Figure 10.11). Consequently, $\Delta C$ is different in each successive segment along the capillary (see Section 10.9).

## Permeability depends on the properties of both membrane and solute

If we compare Fick's free diffusion equation 10.1 with the transcapillary diffusion equation 10.3, we see that endothelial permeability $P$ to a lipid-insoluble solute depends on both **pore geometry** and **solute properties**, namely:

- the restriction to diffusivity $D$ caused by the solute/pore width ratio, $a/r$;
- the pore area $A_p$ per unit endothelial area $S$, which is determined by the extent of the breaks in the junctional strands;
- the non-excluded fraction of the pore area, which is again determined by $a/r$;
- the path length $\Delta x$, which is governed by the length of the intercellular cleft.

For example, when the number of junctional strands is increased by cyclic adenosine monophosphate (Section 9.7), fractional pore area $A_p/S$ falls, so permeability falls.

The key solute properties are **size**, which influences exclusion and restricted diffusion, and **lipid solubility**. Lipid-soluble solutes, such as $O_2$, diffuse through the entire lipid cell membrane, and therefore have a vastly greater area for diffusion than lipid-insoluble solutes, such as glucose, which are confined to the aqueous pores. Therefore, solutes fall into three main permeability categories, namely **lipid-soluble molecules** (e.g. $O_2$), **small lipid-insoluble molecules** ($a \ll r$, little restriction or exclusion, e.g. glucose, electrolytes) and **large lipid-insoluble molecules** ($a \geq r$, major restriction and exclusion, e.g. plasma proteins). Capillaries are many thousand times more permeable to lipid-soluble $O_2$ than to lipid-insoluble glucose, and nearly 1000 times more permeable to glucose (180 Da) than albumin (69 000 Da; Table 10.1). Therefore, we need to consider each class of solute separately.

## 10.5 LIPID-SOLUBLE MOLECULES DIFFUSE EXTREMELY RAPIDLY ACROSS THE ENDOTHELIUM

The permeability of the endothelium to lipophilic ('fat-loving') molecules increases in proportion to their oil-to-water partition coefficient. Since virtually the entire capillary surface is available for diffusion, the permeability is extremely high. Respiratory gases, general anaesthetics and the blood flow tracer xenon are examples of lipophilic solutes. The oil-to-water partition coefficient is ~5 for $O_2$ and 1.6 for $CO_2$. The permeability to $O_2$ is so high that there is a significant diffusion of $O_2$ out of arterioles, reducing the haemoglobin saturation to ~80% by the time blood enters the capillary. However, only part of the deoxygenation is due to $O_2$ transfer into the tissue. The rest is caused by **diffusive, countercurrent**

**Table 10.1** Capillary permeability to different types of solute

| Solute | $M^a$ (Dalton) | Diffusivity $D^b$ (×10⁻⁵ cm²/s) | Radius $a^c$ (nm) | Membrane | Permeability (×10⁻⁶ cm/s) |
|---|---|---|---|---|---|
| $O_2$ | 32 | 2.11 | 0.16 | Continuous capillary | ~100 000 |
| Urea | 60 | 1.90 | 0.26 | Continuous capillary | 26–28 |
| Glucose | 180 | 0.91 | 0.36 | Continuous capillary | 9–13 |
| Sucrose | 342 | 0.72 | 0.47 | Continuous capillary | 6–9 |
| | | | | Cerebral capillary | 0.1 |
| | | | | Fenestrated capillary | >270 |
| Albumin | 69 000 | 0.085 | 3.55 | Continuous capillary | 0.03–0.01 |
| | | | | Fenestrated capillary | 0.04 |

*Source:* After Renkin EM. *Circulation Research* 1977; 41: 735–43; Clough GE, Smaje LH. *The Journal of Physiology* 1984; 354: 445–55; Landis EM, Pappenheimer JR. In: Hamilton WF, Dow P, eds. *Handbook of Physiology: Circulation*, Section 2. Washington, DC: American Physiological Society; 1963. pp. 961–1034.

ª $M$, molecular mass.

ᵇ $D$, free diffusion coefficient in water at 37°C.

ᶜ $a$, Stokes–Einstein diffusion radius.

**shunting** of $O_2$ from the supplying arterioles into the draining venules, which commonly run alongside the arterioles.

## 10.6 SMALL LIPID-INSOLUBLE MOLECULES PERMEATE THE SMALL PORE SYSTEM

Lipophobic (fat-hating), hydrophilic (water-loving) solutes include the plasma electrolytes, glucose, lactate, amino acids, vitamins such as $B_{12}$, hormones such as adrenaline and insulin and many drugs. These solutes cannot diffuse through the lipid endothelial membrane; they are confined to the water-filled pathways through the intercellular junctions and fenestrae. The intercellular clefts occupy only 0.2–0.4% of the capillary surface, so the permeability of a continuous capillary to small lipophobic solutes is a fraction of its permeability to lipophilic solutes, though still high.

## Restricted diffusion provided the first clue to capillary pore size

In 1951 Pappenheimer, Renkin and Borrero proposed the seminal 'small pore theory' of capillary permeability. Their measurements of lipophobic solute permeation indicated that the capillary wall is perforated by narrow, aqueous channels that occupy only 0.01%–0.04% of the capillary surface (about one tenth of the cleft area), of width equivalent to 3–5 nm radius pores. The estimate of pore size was based on their discovery that, as lipophobic solute radius increases, capillary permeability falls faster than the free diffusion coefficient (Figure 10.8). Pappenheimer and colleagues realized that this must be due to steric exclusion and restricted diffusion in narrow pores (Figure 10.6), and from the degree of restriction they calculated the equivalent pore size to be 3–5 nm. As noted in Section 10.3, pore size

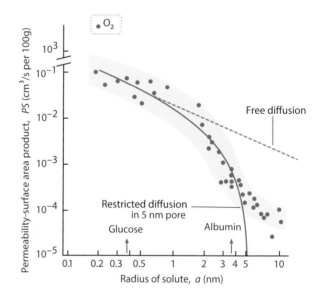

**Figure 10.8** Effect of Stokes–Einstein radius of solute molecule on capillary permeability. Except for $O_2$, the points denote lipophobic solutes. The dashed line of slope −1 shows the effect of the fall in free diffusion coefficient with increasing molecular size. The red line shows the decline in permeability for the cylindrical pores with a radius of 5 nm, as discovered by Pappenheimer, Renkin and Borrero in 1951. A small but persistent permeability to solutes larger than albumin reveals the existence of a small number of larger pores. Data from mammalian skeletal muscle and skin, except for $O_2$ (lung). (After Renkin EM, Curry FE. In: Giebisch G, Tosteson DC, Ussing HH, eds. *Membrane Transport in Biology*, Vol. IV. Berlin: Springer-Verlag; 1978. pp. 1–45. With kind permission of Springer Science and Business Media.)

has also been calculated from capillary reflection coefficients. Taking a broad average, the transcapillary channels in the myocardium, skeletal muscle and intestine have similar restrictive and reflective properties to cylindrical, water-filled pores with a radius of 4–5 nm. However, it must be emphasized that nobody believes that the small pores are cylindrical tubes, only that some of their properties resemble those of narrow tubes.

## Differences in permeability between capillaries often result from differences in pore numbers, not size

The permeability of capillaries in the different tissues of the body to a given lipophobic solute or water spans a very wide, ~100-fold range. Fenestrated capillaries are 10–100 times more permeable than continuous capillaries, because each fenestra contains a collection of small pores of very short path length, namely the gaps between the cartwheel spokes (Figure 10.2). However, there are up to tenfold differences in permeability even among continuous capillaries (e.g. muscle versus mesenteric capillaries) with no immediately obvious anatomical cause. An important clue to the cause is that the solute permeability and the hydraulic conductance of the capillary wall correlate linearly; that is, if one is ten times higher, so is the other. This indicates that permeability differences are not caused by differences in pore radius since hydraulic flow is proportional to $r^4$ (Poiseuille's law, equation 8.7), whereas diffusion is proportional to pore area and hence $\pi r^2$ (Fick's law). Therefore, physiological differences in permeability must be caused by differences in **pore numbers**. It appears that the proportion of the intercellular cleft that is 'open for business', due to breaks in the junctional strands, varies from tissue to tissue (Figures 9.2, 9.4 and 10.3). The open fraction is typically ~10%. A vessel with more extensive breaks in the junctional strands (equivalent to more pores) has a higher permeability, as in the postcapillary venule. Conversely, less extensive breaks produce a vessel of lower permeability, such as the arterial capillary. Ultrastructural investigations with markers such as ferrocyanide ions, lanthanum ions and microperoxidase have confirmed that small lipophobic solutes do indeed permeate the intercellular cleft through breaks in the junctional strands (Figure 10.3).

## The glycocalyx is the site of the size-selective small pores

Although the intercellular cleft is undoubtedly the pathway through which water and small solutes cross the capillary wall, the cleft itself is unlikely to be the size-limiting structure, that is, the small pore of radius 4–5 nm, because it is ~20 nm wide. Moreover, discrepancies between the estimates of small pore size from hydraulic data versus diffusion data indicate that the small pore is unlikely to have a continuous, solid wall. In 1980, this led Curry and Michel to suggest that the size-limiting pores are in the glycocalyx, the luminal coat of biopolymers that spans the entrance to the intercellular cleft (Figures 9.3 and 9.5). This is the **fibre matrix theory of capillary permeability**.

The fibre matrix theory (Figure 10.9) proposes that the glycocalyx biopolymers form a fine network that acts as a size-selective sieve, that is, the small pore system. There is now considerable evidence supporting this view. For example, the glycocalyx excludes fluorescent macromolecules perfused through a capillary. Also, enzymatic digestion of the glycocalyx increases endothelial permeability. Conversely, the binding of albumin to the glycocalyx greatly reduces endothelial permeability (the **protein effect**), as does cationized ferritin (Figure 9.5), whereas macromolecules that do not bind to the glycocalyx do not reduce capillary permeability. It is thought that bound albumin regulates the pore size within the network (Figure 10.9b). The highly anionic plasma protein orosomucoid likewise binds to the glycocalyx, increasing the negative charge density and the exclusion of negatively charged plasma proteins.

The modern view is that **two different structures, the glycocalyx and the breaks in junctional strands, together determine the permeability** of continuous endothelium to solutes and water. The **area** available for the passage of water and small solutes, and hence the permeability, depends on the extent of the breaks in the junctional strands. However, the **size and charge selectivity** of the pathway is determined by the spacing and charges within the glycocalyx polymer network covering the entrance to the clefts. The uniform coating of the intercellular junctions and fenestrae by glycocalyx (Figure 10.10b) also explains the remarkable constancy of the reflection coefficient to plasma proteins (0.8–0.95) across different capillary beds with a 400-fold range in hydraulic permeability.

The concepts of John Pappenheimer and Gene Renkin, the originators of pore theory, and Charles Michel and Roy Curry, the originators of the fibre matrix theory, might be summarized as follows:

*The Pappenheimer pore's so small*
*You cannot make it out at all,*
*Though many sanguine doctors hope*
*To see one through the microscope –*
*Rectangular or round in shape*
*With many nanometres gape.*
*Some say the pore is made of fluff,*
*A glycocalyxacious stuff,*
*Whose fibres subdivide the space*
*Constructing there a random lace*
*Till albumin, a protein, lands*
*And tidies up those tangled strands,*
*Through which there flows dilute saline.*
*All this has never yet been seen,*
*But Scientists, who ought to know,*
*Assure us that it must be so.*
*Oh let us never, never doubt*
*What nobody is sure about.*

(With apologies to Hilaire Belloc's *The Microbe*)

In addition to its role as a semipermeable, size-selective ultrafilter, the glycocalyx has **haemodynamic effects** in microvessels, and contributes to **endothelial mechanosensitivity** in larger vessels (Section 9.2).

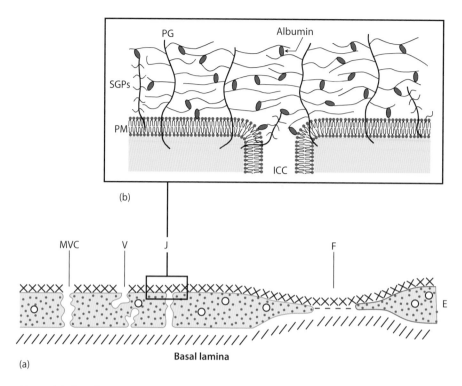

**Figure 10.9** Fibre matrix model of capillary permeability. **(a)** The glycocalyx covers the endothelium (E) and fenestrae (F) and intercellular junction (J) and sieves out plasma proteins. The number of open junctions and fenestrae determines net permeability to smaller lipophobic solutes and water. The multivesicular transcellular channel (MVC) or vesicles (V) may represent the large pore system. Large pores are few. (Adapted from Michel CC. *The Journal of Physiology* 1980; 309: 341–55; by permission.) **(b)** The inset outlines key features of the glycocalyx. Negatively charged proteoglycan fibres (PG) and sialoglycoproteins (SGPs) bind to the positively charged arginine groups of albumin (red ellipsoids). This creates a three-dimensional sieve that reflects plasma proteins. Reflection is governed primarily by the glycocalyx mesh size, and secondarily by its net negative charge. PM, plasmalemma membrane; ICC, intercellular cleft. (After Curry FE. *Circulation Research* 1986; 59(4): 367–80.)

## Specific transporters generally contribute little to transcapillary exchange

In most tissues, carrier-mediated solute transport by integral membrane proteins and water transport through membrane aquaporins (water channels) contribute negligibly to transcapillary transport, because their transport capacities are orders of magnitude lower than that of the intercellular cleft. However, there are important exceptions. The brain endothelium has a very low intercellular permeability, and therefore relies on integral membrane proteins to transport solutes such as glucose (Section 10.8). Also, carrier-mediated urea transport is important in the descending vasa recta of the kidney (medullary capillaries).

## 10.7 LARGE LIPID-INSOLUBLE MOLECULES PASS THROUGH A LARGE PORE SYSTEM

The permeability of the continuous and fenestrated endothelium to plasma proteins is around one millionth of their permeability to $O_2$. Nevertheless, there is a small but important flux of plasma proteins into the tissues, as demonstrated by their presence in lymph at 20%–70% of the plasma concentration. This flux is needed for immunoglobulins to exercise their defence role, and for the transfer of protein-bound substances, such as iron, copper, vitamin A, thyroxine, testosterone, oestradiol, lipids and short-chain fatty acids.

## The permeability versus molecular size plot reveals a large-diameter transport system

As solute radius approaches 3.6 nm (albumin), which is approximately the size of the small pores (glycocalyx mesh size), solute permeation falls off steeply (Figure 10.9). Indeed, one might expect zero permeability to solutes bigger than the small pores, namely the plasma proteins. However, there is still a finite, albeit low permeability to plasma protein of radius >4 nm. This led Grotte to propose, in 1956, the existence of a second transport pathway, with properties equivalent to a small number of large pores, with a radius of 20–30 nm. Reflection coefficient measurements support this view; macromolecule reflection coefficients are <1, even for fibrinogen (radius: 10 nm). Nevertheless, the permeability to

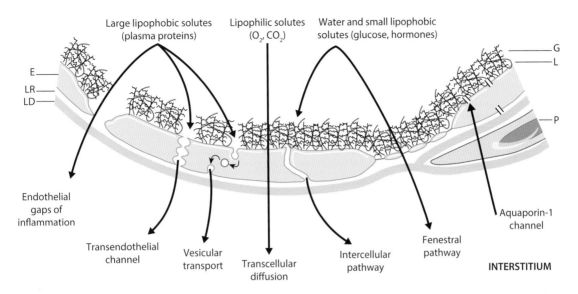

**Figure 10.10** Main transport pathways across the capillary wall. Water flows mainly through the small pore system, that is, the glycocalyx overlying the intercellular clefts and fenestrae. Only a little passes through membrane aquaporin-1 channels or the scanty large pore system. Note the large gap and break in glycocalyx in inflammation. E, endothelium; G, glycocalyx; L, lipid plasma membrane; LR, lamina rara of basement membrane; LD, lamina densa of basement membrane; P, pericyte.

macromolecules is very low, showing that the large pores are few in number – around one large pore per 4000 small pores in continuous capillaries – and essentially none in cerebral and renal glomerular capillaries.

## Macromolecular permeation depends on charge as well as size

Large plasma proteins such as fibrinogen cross the endothelial layer less readily than smaller proteins such as albumin. Moreover, negatively charged macromolecules, such as albumin, permeate the endothelial barrier less readily than neutral or positively charged ones of similar size. This is due to electrical repulsion by the fixed negative charges of the glycocalyx.

## The identity of large pores: continuous channels and/or vesicular transport?

The large pore system is a functional concept, inferred from permeability data (Figure 10.9). There is controversy as to whether the system consists of true pores, that is, hydraulically continuous channels, in the form of multivesicular channels (Figures 9.6b and 10.10) or glycocalyx gaps, or whether it is really the caveola/vesicle transport system.

'True pore' protagonists point out that the rate of transport of macromolecules across the capillary wall is proportional to the pressure driving fluid across the wall, as expected for a hydraulically continuous large pore. Moreover, tissue cooling, which should inhibit active vesicular transport, has only a small effect on macromolecular permeation. Also, caveolin knockout mice lack endothelial caveolae, yet show no impairment of transendothelial protein permeation.

Nevertheless, vesicular transport may contribute significantly to macromolecular transfer at low filtration rates. Macromolecules such as gold-labelled albumin and ferritin (radius: 5.5 nm) undoubtedly enter the luminal caveolae and appear soon afterwards in the abluminal caveolae (Figures 9.5 and 9.6). However, it remains unclear how much this contributes to total protein transport. It is possible that, at normal, low capillary filtration rates, conductive channels and vesicular transport both contribute to protein permeation.

The current understanding of the various parallel pathways for solute movement across the capillary wall is summarized in Figure 10.10.

## 10.8 THE BLOOD–BRAIN BARRIER AND CARRIER-MEDIATED TRANSPORT

### Cerebral capillaries form a tight blood–brain barrier

Brain capillaries, like all capillaries, are highly permeable to lipophilic solutes ($O_2$, $CO_2$, general anaesthetics), but are exceptionally impermeable to lipophobic solutes, such as L-glucose, catecholamines and plasma proteins. This is called the blood–brain barrier. The function of the barrier is to protect the neurons from circulating stimulants, such as catecholamines, and to prevent the washout of neurotransmitters from the brain parenchyma by the bloodstream. The blood–brain barrier is formed by complex, multiple junctional strands between the endothelial cells, with no breaks; the strands form a continuous, unbroken seal around the cell perimeter. The caveola/vesicle system is also very scanty. Breakdown of the barrier is common in pathological conditions such as local cerebral ischaemia (strokes), cerebral haemorrhage and cerebral inflammation, and leads to cerebral oedema.

## Specific endothelial carriers transport solutes into the brain parenchyma

In stark contrast to most capillaries, cerebral capillaries rely on specific carrier proteins in the endothelial cell membrane to transport essential, lipid-insoluble solutes between the blood and brain parenchyma. There are specific carrier proteins for D-glucose, the natural, dextrose form of glucose (carrier glucose transporter 1, GLUT-1), lactate, pyruvate, amino acids and adenosine. This form of transport is **transcellular**, as opposed to paracellular. The transport is not active, but is brought about by the diffusion of the carrier-bound solute down its concentration gradient (facilitated diffusion). In addition, the cerebral endothelium can regulate the $K^+$ concentration of cerebral interstitial fluid by active transport, via $Na^+/K^+$-ATPase in the abluminal membrane (Section 15.4).

## 10.9 EXTRACTION AND CLEARANCE IN CAPILLARIES

The concentration of a consumed solute, such as $O_2$, glucose or a drug, falls along the capillary (Figure 10.11), and this decay is crucial to understanding the effect of blood flow on solute transfer. This section describes the concentration profile along a capillary and the related concepts of extraction and clearance; Sections 10.10 and 10.11 build on this to explain the effects of blood flow and exercise on solute exchange. To illustrate the capillary concentration profile, let us consider glucose transfer into active muscle. The interstitial glucose concentration is lower than the arterial concentration because the muscle is consuming glucose; for simplicity, we will assume that the interstitial glucose concentration is uniform.

## Concentration decays non-linearly along a capillary

At the start of the capillary, plasma glucose concentration is close to arterial level and the difference in concentration across the capillary wall is high (point A, Figure 10.11). Consequently, glucose diffuses rapidly out of the first part of the capillary, as dictated by Fick's law of diffusion (arrow $J_{sA}$, Figure 10.11). Due to this solute efflux, the plasma concentration falls off steeply at first, for example, from A to B in Figure 10.11. Further along the capillary, the concentration difference across the wall is smaller (point C, Figure 10.11), so the solute efflux is slower (flux $J_{sC}$). As a result, the plasma concentration falls off less steeply, as from C to D. In the case of lactate or $CO_2$, where the concentration is higher in the tissue than the capillary, the concentration increases rather than decays along the capillary axis, but again in a curvilinear fashion. The capillary concentration profile is thus a curve, and mean capillary concentration is less than the average of the arterial and venous concentrations. If the curvature is pronounced, with a steep initial decay, almost all the solute exchange happens near the start of the capillary, with little downstream. The degree of curvature depends on the permeability and blood flow (Section 10.10).

## Fick's principle (cf. Fick's law) describes the exchange across the whole capillary bed

The net solute exchange across an entire capillary bed is easily worked out using Fick's *principle* (Section 7.1), which should not be confused with Fick's law of diffusion! Fick's principle states that the solute exchange rate equals the arteriovenous concentration difference $C_a - C_v$ multiplied by the blood flow $\dot{Q}$:

$$J_s = \dot{Q}(C_a - C_v) \qquad (10.4)$$

For example, the glucose flux into a muscle can be evaluated by measuring the blood flow, the arterial glucose concentration and the local venous concentrations. Conversely, Fick's principle can be used to work out the concentration drop $C_a - C_v$ that will be produced by any combination of solute consumption and blood flow (Figure 10.11).

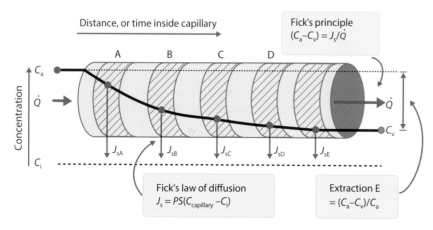

**Figure 10.11** The concentration of a rapidly diffusing solute falls non-linearly along a capillary, from arterial concentration $C_a$ to venous concentration $C_v$. Black arrows indicate the size of diffusional fluxes $J_s$. $PS$, permeability-surface area product; $Q$, blood flow. The concentration profile is exponential, if the interstitial concentration $C_i$ is zero or uniform.

## Extraction (E) is the fraction of solute removed from plasma during one capillary transit

Let us suppose that glucose enters a capillary bed at an arterial concentration of 5 mM and leaves at a venous concentration of 4.5 mM. Clearly, 0.5 mM has been removed by diffusion into the tissues. This is 10% of the amount delivered in the arterial blood (0.5/5.0), so the 'extraction' is 10%. Extraction is defined as the arteriovenous concentration difference, $C_a - C_v$, as a fraction of the arterial concentration $C_a$: $E = (C_a - C_v)/C_a$ (Figure 10.11). $O_2$ extraction in many tissues is ~25% at rest, rising to 80%–90% in heavily exercising muscle.

Solute extraction following an intra-arterial injection is illustrated in Figure 10.12. The solute was vitamin $B_{12}$ in this case, and the injected solution also contained a non-exchanging or 'reference' solute, namely radiolabelled albumin. Samples of the venous effluent showed that the diffusible solute concentration fell below the reference solute concentration, due to diffusion out of the capillaries. The reference solute concentration shows what the test solute concentration would have been if no exchange had taken place. The extraction of vitamin $B_{12}$, calculated from the difference between the test and reference solute concentrations, was initially ~40% (Figure 10.12b). Extraction then declined because the interstitial concentration increased, reducing the concentration gradient across the capillary wall. This pattern of extraction shows that solute exchange is a diffusive process that obeys Fick's law of diffusion.

## Clearance (Cl) is the volume of plasma cleared of solute per unit time

The plasma clearance is the volume of plasma that has been emptied of a specified solute per minute, due to the extraction of that solute. The clearance equals the plasma flow multiplied by extraction $E$:

$$Cl = \text{plasma flow} \times E \qquad (10.5a)$$

For example, if the plasma flow through an exercising muscle is 100 mL/min and the glucose extraction is 10%, then 10 mL of plasma is cleared of glucose per minute.

Note that the units of clearance are plasma volume/time, not solute mass/time; the mass of solute removed per unit time is called the solute flux ($J_s$, equation 10.1). Solute flux equals plasma clearance × arterial concentration; $J_s = Cl \cdot C_a$. Therefore, clearance can also be defined as solute flux per unit arterial concentration ($Cl = J_s/C_a$), which again has the units of volume/time. The relationships between clearance, extraction and solute flux may thus be summarized as:

$$Cl = \text{Plasma flow} \times E = \\ \text{Plasma flow} \times (C_a - C_v)/C_a = J_s/C_a \qquad (10.5b)$$

The concept of plasma clearance is used a great deal in renal physiology. For example, the renal clearance of the waste product creatinine from plasma is ~140 mL/min in young humans and declines in renal failure. The concept of

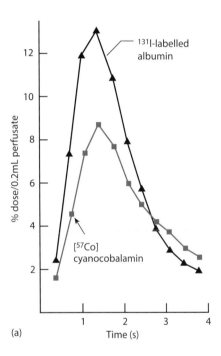

(a)

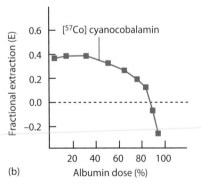

(b)

**Figure 10.12** Diffusion of vitamin $B_{12}$ (cyanocobalamin, radius 0.8 nm) out of the fenestrated microcirculation of the cat salivary gland, following a bolus arterial injection. Albumin (radius 3.6 nm) served as a non-extracted reference solute (see text). **(a)** Amount of vitamin $B_{12}$ and albumin in successive venous samples as a percentage of the initial arterial dose. The lines cross after 3 s because the interstitial concentration of $B_{12}$ is now higher than the falling level in the blood, causing a net back-diffusion into the blood. **(b)** Extraction of $B_{12}$ is high at first, then falls as interstitial concentration rises. Permeability can be calculated from the extraction and blood flow, using the Renkin–Crone relation, equation 10.6. (From Mann GE, Smaje LH, Yudilevich DL. *The Journal of Physiology* 1979; 297(0): 335–54, with permission from Wiley-Blackwell.)

'clearance' can also be applied to any other organ or solute. For example, the pulmonary clearance of $CO_2$ is ~370 mL/min in a resting human.

## 10.10 HOW BLOOD FLOW AFFECTS SOLUTE TRANSFER

Raising the blood flow through a tissue can boost solute exchange, or have virtually no effect at all! This is because there are two basic exchange states, called flow-limited and diffusion-limited exchange. Each state has a different, distinctive capillary concentration profile. In **flow-limited exchange**, the solute concentration decays very steeply in the first part of the capillary (Figure 10.13, red curves), and the transcapillary solute flux is limited by the rate at which blood delivers

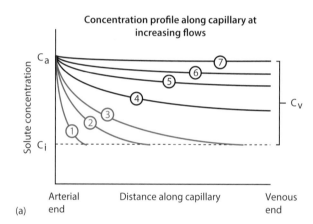

**Concentration profile along capillary at increasing flows**

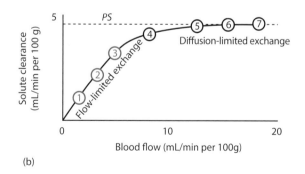

**Effect of flow on solute exchange rate**

**Figure 10.13** Effect of blood flow on diffusive transport across the capillary wall. **(a)** Decay of plasma concentration along the capillary at low-to-high blood flows (curves 1–7), for a constant or zero pericapillary concentration $C_i$. $C_a$, $C_v$, arterial and venous concentrations. Slow transits allow time for equilibration ($C_v = C_i$) before the end of the capillary (curves 1–3). This is flow-limited exchange. With fast transits, there is not enough time for equilibration across the diffusion barrier; $C_v$ is $>C_i$ (curves 5–7). This is diffusion-limited exchange. **(b)** Resulting effect of blood flow on transcapillary exchange, expressed as plasma clearance (solute flux/$C_a$, equation 10.5b). The plateau clearance value equals the capillary diffusion capacity $PS$. Data are for urea in muscle capillaries. (Data of Renkin EM. In: Marchetti G, Taccardi B, eds. *Coronary Circulation and Energetics of the Myocardium*. Basel: Karger; 1967. pp. 18–30.)

solute to the capillary (see next section). In **diffusion-limited exchange**, the solute concentration profile is relatively flat (Figure 10.13, black curves) and the transcapillary solute flux is limited by the rate at which the solute can permeate the capillary wall.

### In flow-limited exchange, solute transfer rate is proportional to blood flow

If capillary permeability to the solute is very high (e.g. $CO_2$ in lung capillaries), the solute crosses the wall so quickly that its plasma concentration equilibrates with the concentration outside the capillary (pericapillary interstitial fluid or alveolar gas) long before the blood reaches the end of the capillary (Figure 10.13a, curve 1). This is usually the case for lipophilic solutes such as $O_2$ and $CO_2$, and for small lipophobic solutes in fenestrated capillaries. It can also be true for small lipophobic solutes such as urea and glucose in continuous capillaries if blood flow is slow. Since the plasma concentration quickly falls to that of the surrounding interstitial fluid, only the initial part of the capillary contributes to exchange. When the blood flow is raised, the time available for exchange shortens but equilibration may still occur before the capillary exit, albeit further downstream (curves 2 and 3). Since the arteriovenous difference ($C_a - C_v$) is unchanged yet blood flow has increased, transcapillary solute flux $J_s$ has increased (Fick's principle, equation 10.4; $J_s$ = blood flow $\times [C_a - C_v]$). In fact the solute flux increases in direct proportion to the blood flow, as shown by points 1–3 in panel (b) of Figure 10.13.

**Gas exchange in the lungs** is a prime example of flow-limited exchange of major physiological importance. The $CO_2$ and $O_2$ in the pulmonary capillary blood equilibrate with the alveolar gas long before the end of the capillary is reached. Consequently, an increase in pulmonary blood flow, that is, cardiac output, causes a directly proportional increase in capillary $O_2$ uptake and $CO_2$ removal.

In flow-limited exchange, the solute clearance rate is a measure of blood flow, not capillary permeability. This is the basis of the Kety xenon clearance method (Figure 8.6). It is not possible to measure capillary permeability $P$ when exchange is flow-limited because the fraction of the capillary wall that is contributing to exchange is unknown; that is, $S$ is unknown.

### In diffusion-limited exchange, solute transfer rate is little affected by blood flow

Diffusion-limited exchange is at the opposite end of the spectrum to flow-limited exchange. In diffusion-limited exchange the solute transfer is limited by endothelial permeability rather than by solute delivery rate, that is, blood flow. The plasma solute concentration has not equilibrated with the pericapillary space by the time the end of the capillary is reached, and the concentration profile is relatively flat, as in curve 5 of Figure 10.13a. Medium-to-large lipophobic solutes, such as inulin and cyanocobalamin (vitamin $B_{12}$), behave in this way. So too do small solutes, such as urea and glucose, when the transit time is shortened by high blood flows; diffusion-limited exchange occurs with big molecules at normal flow and with small molecules at high flows.

In diffusion-limited exchange, raising the blood flow causes relatively little increase in solute exchange because the blood is already spending too little time in the capillary to unload its solute fully. If the transit time is shortened further by raising blood flow, the extraction fraction falls and the venous concentration rises (curves 6 and 7 of Figure 10.13a). Therefore, the arteriovenous concentration difference ($C_a - C_v$) declines. Applying Fick's principle (equation 10.4), we find that solute exchange $J_s$ increases relatively little; the effect of the rise in $\dot{Q}$ is largely offset by the fall in ($C_a - C_v$). Thus, points 5–7 in Figure 10.13b show little increase in solute clearance with increasing blood flow.

## Ratio of diffusion capacity to blood flow, $PS/\dot{Q}$, determines whether exchange is flow-limited or diffusion-limited

The nature of the exchange process – whether diffusion-limited or flow-limited – is determined by the ratio of the permeability-surface area product of the capillary bed, $PS$ (the diffusion capacity), to blood flow $\dot{Q}$. Both factors have the same units, $cm^3/s$, so the ratio is dimensionless. If the diffusion capacity substantially exceeds the blood flow ($PS/\dot{Q} > 5$), equilibration is reached before the end of the capillary and the exchange is flow-limited. If blood flow exceeds the diffusion capacity ($PS/\dot{Q} < 1$), equilibration is not achieved and the exchange is diffusion-limited. This follows from the nonlinear relationship between extraction $E$ and blood flow, the **Renkin–Crone relation**:

$$E = 1 - \exp(-PS/\dot{Q}) \qquad (10.6)$$

Renkin and Crone pointed out that at $PS/\dot{Q} = 5$ the solute extraction $E$ is >99%, so there is almost complete equilibration and exchange is flow-limited. By contrast, when $PS/\dot{Q}$ is ≤1, the extraction is ≤63%, so equilibration is not achieved and exchange is diffusion-limited. Typical values for glucose in skeletal muscle capillaries are ~5 at rest, because blood flow is low in resting muscle, and <1 during exercise, because blood flow is raised.

It is clear from the Renkin–Crone equation and Figure 10.13b that flow-limited exchange and diffusion-limited exchange are just the extremes of a continuous spectrum. There are many **intermediate states** (Figure 10.13b, region between points 3 and 5) where raising the blood flow increases the solute flux, via an increase in mean capillary concentration (Fick's law of diffusion), but fails to increase it proportionately (as in purely flow-limited exchange), because $C_v$ rises. This is illustrated by the increase in solute flux between point 4 and point 5 in Figure 10.13b (intermediate regime).

## An increase in blood flow can also trigger an increase in permeability

The preceding section describes the purely passive, biophysical effect of blood flow on solute exchange. However, recent work indicates that blood flow can also induce active increases in endothelial permeability to lipophobic solutes. This is described in the next section because it is one of several ways in which the body adjusts the rate of solute transfer to meet increased demand during exercise.

## 10.11 PHYSIOLOGICAL REGULATION OF SOLUTE TRANSFER

The transfer of $O_2$ and nutrients across the capillary wall should, ideally, match tissue demand; when demand increases, as in exercising muscle or myocardium, transfer needs to increase too. However, if the supply artery is narrowed by atheroma, solute delivery is restricted and transfer may lag behind the increased demand. In patients with coronary artery disease, this results in exercise-induced angina, while in patients with femoral artery disease it results in calf pain during exercise (intermittent claudication).

The $O_2$ consumption of skeletal muscle can increase up to 20–40-fold during exercise, and a matching increase in the transcapillary flux of $O_2$ is normally brought about by three mechanisms:

1. more uniform perfusion of the capillary bed, due to capillary recruitment;
2. an increase in the concentration gradient from plasma to tissue;
3. an increase in local blood flow.

Additional factors include an increase in the $O_2$ diffusion velocity through muscle myoglobin as intracellular $O_2$ partial pressure falls, and in the case of small lipophobic solutes such as glucose, probably an increase in capillary permeability with flow.

## Capillary recruitment improves solute exchange in exercising muscle

In skeletal muscle, each capillary supplies a cylindrical envelope of surrounding muscle fibres, called a Krogh muscle cylinder (Figure 10.14). The number of muscle fibres supplied by one capillary, and hence the radius of the Krogh cylinder, depends on the anatomical capillary density and the fraction that is well perfused at any moment in time. The injection of visible particles or dyes has shown that, in resting skeletal muscle, half to three quarters of the capillaries are not perfused, or are perfused only sluggishly, at any one moment because the terminal arterioles supplying them are in the constricted phase of their vasomotion cycle (Section 10.1). Since a

185

**REST**

Terminal arteriole 1, dilated.
VSM relaxed.
Capillary module perfused.

Oxygen flux

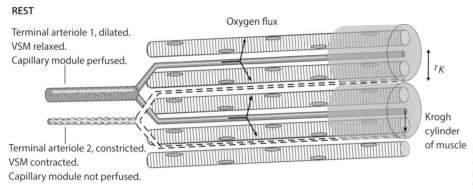

$r_K$

Krogh
cylinder
of muscle

Terminal arteriole 2, constricted.
VSM contracted.
Capillary module not perfused.

**EXERCISE - metabolic hyperaemia**

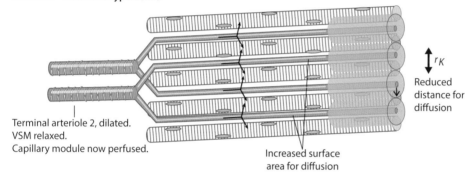

$r_K$

Reduced
distance for
diffusion

Terminal arteriole 2, dilated.
VSM relaxed.
Capillary module now perfused.

Increased surface
area for diffusion

**Figure 10.14** The Krogh muscle cylinder and capillary recruitment. In resting skeletal muscle (top), contraction of terminal arteriole 2 arrests the perfusion of one capillary module (dashed lines). Each perfused capillary must therefore supply a broad cylinder of muscle (Krogh cylinder). The radius of the Krogh cylinder $r_K$ is the maximum diffusion distance. When exercise commences (bottom), metabolic vasodilatation dilates terminal arteriole 2, leading to perfusion of the previously closed-off capillaries. This improves the homogeneity of $O_2$ supply, increases the perfused capillary surface area, reduces the radius of each Krogh cylinder and thus reduces the maximum diffusion distance $r_K$. VSM, vascular smooth muscle.

relatively small number of capillaries is well perfused at rest, each capillary must supply a large zone of surrounding muscle fibres. Therefore, in resting muscle the Krogh cylinder radius is large.

During exercise the terminal arterioles are dilated by metabolites released by the contracting muscle fibres (Section 13.7, 'Metabolic hyperaemia'). This increases the number of well-perfused capillaries, a process termed **capillary recruitment**. Capillary recruitment increases the **surface area** of the endothelium available for exchange ($S$) and at the same time reduces the Krogh cylinder radius and hence the solute **diffusion distance**, $\Delta x$ (Figure 10.14). These changes improve the uniformity of the $O_2$ supply; that is, they reduce the heterogeneity present in resting muscle (Section 10.1). The increase in $S/\Delta x$ greatly increases the rate of diffusive transport, as dictated by Fick's law (equation 10.1).

## Increased metabolic consumption steepens the concentration gradient

The increased metabolic rate of an active tissue lowers the tissue concentration of glucose and $O_2$, and therefore increases the concentration difference between the capillary blood and the tissue. For example, the mean concentration difference for glucose across the capillary wall is estimated to increase from ~0.3 mM in resting muscle to ~3 mM during heavy exercise (Table 10.2). The increased concentration difference, coupled with the shortening of diffusion distance by capillary

recruitment, can increase the concentration gradient $\Delta C/\Delta x$ by more than an order of magnitude.

## Blood flow increases with increased metabolic activity

Blood flow increases in direct proportion to metabolic rate in most organs, including skeletal muscle (Figure 10.15), myocardium (Figure 15.4) and brain (Figure 15.15). The metabolic hyperaemia increases the rate of delivery of $O_2$ and glucose and prevents the transcapillary exchange from becoming flow-limited. Metabolites such as glucose are diffusion-limited at the high flows that occur during exercise, so solute transfer is not limited by solute delivery rate.

## Endothelial permeability increases in response to flow

Recent measurements of $K^+$, $Na^+$, urea and fluorescein exchange show that an increase in blood flow not only increases the delivery of solute to the capillaries but also triggers a rapid rise in capillary permeability. The flow-mediated rise in permeability involves an active endothelial response mediated by nitric oxide. The raised permeability helps to explain the large increase in transcapillary glucose flux into exercising muscle.

To draw together the various concepts introduced in this chapter, let us finish with two specific examples of how solute flux is increased to meet an increase in demand.

**Table 10.2** Transport of glucose from blood to 100 g skeletal muscle *in vivo*

| | Notation | Units | Rest | Heavy exercise | Fractional change (exercise/rest) |
|---|---|---|---|---|---|
| Glucose consumption rate[a] | $J_s$ | µmol/min | 1.4 | 60 | 43× |
| Arterial concentration | $C_a$ | mM | 5.0 | 5.0 | – |
| Venous concentration | $C_v$ | mM | 4.44 | 4.0 | 0.9× |
| Extraction | $E$ | % | 11.2% | 20% | 1.8× |
| Blood flow | $\dot{Q}$ | mL/min | 2.5 | 60 | 24× |
| Perfused capillary density | | number/mm² | 250 | 1000 | 4× |
| Diffusion capacity[b] | $PS$ | cm³/min | 5 | 20 | 4× |
| Mean concentration difference across capillary wall | $\Delta C$[c] | mM | 0.3 | 3 | 10× |
| Mean pericapillary concentration | $C_i$ | mM | 4.7 | 2 | 0.4× |
| Krogh cylinder radius | $r_K$ | µm | 36 | 18 | 0.5× |

*Source:* After Crone C, Levitt DG. In: Renkin EM, Michel CC, eds. *Handbook of Physiology: the Cardiovascular System*, Section 2, Vol. IV, Microcirculation. Bethesda, MD: American Physiological Society; 1984. p. 431.

[a] Diffusion, not fluid filtration, accounts for most of the transcapillary transport of glucose and other small metabolites. Proof: resting skeletal muscle consumes 1.4 µmol glucose/min (100 g)⁻1. Net transcapillary filtration rate is 0.005 mL/min (100 g)⁻1 and glucose concentration is 5 µmol/mL, so convective glucose transport is 0.025 µmol/min. This is only 2% of the total glucose flux.

[b] Recent evidence shows that some of the increase in $PS$ (the capillary diffusion capacity of a tissue) may be due to increased capillary permeability as flow increases (see text), as well as recruitment.

[c] $\Delta C$ is calculated as $J_s/PS$ (see equation 10.3).

## How glucose transfer is increased in exercising muscle

Human muscle contains ~400 g of glycogen (1%–2% by weight), providing an internal source of glucose in the early stages of exercise. As exercise proceeds, muscle glycogen levels fall and glucose transport from blood to muscle increases (Figure 10.15). During 25 min of cycling, the glucose consumption of leg muscles is proportional to the exercise intensity. Arterial plasma glucose itself is kept constant through increased glucose production by the liver and other tissues. The factors that increase the transfer of blood glucose to the exercising muscle fibres are brought together in Table 10.2 and Figure 10.15. **Capillary recruitment** reduces the radius of the Krogh cylinder and hence the **diffusion distance** $\Delta x$. Recruitment also enhances the **surface area** for diffusion, $S$, and the effect of flow on capillary permeability $P$ may further raise the net capillary diffusion capacity, $PS$. A fall in tissue glucose concentration raises the concentration gradient across the capillary wall, and the resulting increase in diffusive flux raises the fractional extraction and arteriovenous concentration difference $(C_a - C_v)$ (Figure 10.15). Increased **blood flow** delivers glucose faster to the capillary and prevents a major fall in the mean intracapillary plasma concentration, thereby avoiding flow limitation of exchange. Fick's principle (Figure 10.11) tells us that the new transcapillary glucose flux equals the increased blood flow multiplied by the increased $(C_a - C_v)$ (Figure 10.15).

## How oxygen transfer is increased in exercising muscle

$O_2$ diffuses through endothelial cells so rapidly that the capillary wall offers no significant resistance to its transport. The main factor impeding $O_2$ transport into a muscle fibre is the length of the extravascular pathway, ~20 µm, which is over 60 times longer than the transcapillary pathway,

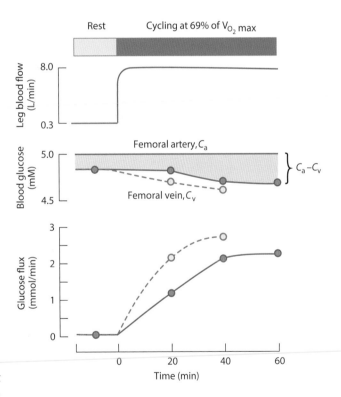

**Figure 10.15** Increase in glucose flux from blood to leg muscles during cycling, calculated by Fick's principle (solute flux = blood flow × arteriovenous concentration difference). At first, the muscle uses both stored glycogen and extracted glucose. As the glycogen store is depleted, blood glucose extraction $(C_a - C_v)/C_a$ increases. When muscle glycogen is depleted prior to exercise, glucose extraction is increased (dashed lines with blue circles). $V_{O_2max}$ is the individual's maximum $O_2$ consumption rate. (Data from Blomstrand E, Saltin B. *The Journal of Physiology* 1999; 514(Pt 1): 293–302.)

0.3 µm. Therefore, the main $O_2$ concentration gradient is from pericapillary space to muscle mitochondria, rather than from plasma to pericapillary space (Figure 10.16, top). Net

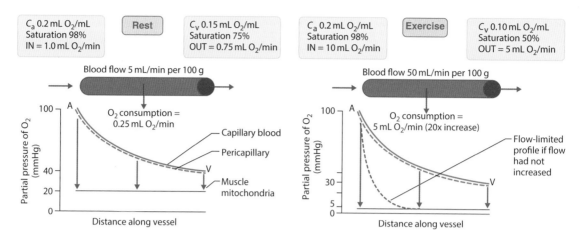

**Figure 10.16** $O_2$ exchange along a capillary in resting versus exercising skeletal muscle. Mitochondrial $P_{O2}$ is estimated from myoglobin saturation data. Note that the $O_2$ demand of the exercising muscle, 5 mL $O_2$/min, exceeds the total resting arterial supply, 1 mL $O_2$/min. If blood flow did not increase, the $O_2$ content of the blood would approach zero soon after it entered the capillary (dotted-dashed line). A, arterial end of exchange microvessels (strictly, the terminal arteriole); V, venous end of exchange system.

transfer is intermediate between flow- and diffusion-limited exchange, as in curve 4 of Figure 10.13a; the end-capillary $P_{O2}$ of 40 mmHg ($O_2$ partial pressure, resting muscle) is lower than arterial $P_{O2}$, 100 mmHg, but has not equilibrated to mitochondrial $P_{O2}$, namely ~20 mmHg in resting muscle (Figure 10.16, top).

During exercise, **capillary recruitment** occurs, as described previously for glucose. This raises the **surface area** available for exchange and reduces the **diffusion distance**. Mitochondrial $P_{O2}$ is estimated to fall to ~5 mmHg, due to increased $O_2$ consumption, and this **raises the concentration gradient** from arterial blood to muscle. Consequently, $O_2$ extraction increases and the end-capillary $P_{O2}$ can fall as low as ~15 mmHg. **Increased blood flow**, and hence increased $O_2$ delivery, prevents the end-capillary $P_{O2}$ from falling lower

(Figure 10.16, bottom). If flow did not increase, $O_2$ exchange would become severely flow-limited, since a moderately exercising muscle consumes more $O_2$ per minute than its total resting arterial supply.

An additional factor that speeds up $O_2$ transport in exercising muscle is the partial deoxygenation of the **myoglobin** that is present at up to 7 g/kg in the sarcoplasm of red muscle. Although there is a large $O_2$ gradient from the blood to a point just inside the sarcoplasm, the $P_{O2}$ is surprisingly uniform across the muscle fibre itself, despite the considerable transport distance, and this is due to the transport-enhancing effect of myoglobin. Partially deoxygenated myoglobin greatly speeds up the rate of $O_2$ diffusion through the sarcoplasm, because the $O_2$ molecules can 'hop' from one unoccupied myoglobin binding site to the next. This is called **facilitated diffusion**.

## SUMMARY

- A dense network of fine, thin-walled capillaries subserves nutrient and water exchange between blood and tissue.
- Solutes such as $O_2$ and glucose **diffuse rapidly** across the capillary wall down **concentration gradients**. Water, by contrast, **flows slowly** across the wall down a **pressure gradient** across the intercellular cleft and fenestrae.
- **Fick's law of diffusion** states that the amount of solute transferred per unit time by diffusion is proportional to the concentration gradient (concentration difference/distance), the area available for diffusion and the solute diffusion coefficient.
- A **porous membrane**, such as the capillary wall, limits the area available for diffusion and restricts the intrapore diffusivity. These effects are lumped together in the parameter '**membrane permeability**'. Diffusive transport rate $J_s$ equals permeability $P$ × membrane area $S$ × concentration drop across the membrane $\Delta C$; $J_s = PS\Delta C$.
- Capillary permeability depends on both ultrastructure and solute properties. Three types of capillary – continuous,

fenestrated and discontinuous – form a hierarchy of increasing permeability to lipid-insoluble solutes. Solutes fall into three classes:

- **Lipid-soluble molecules**, such as $O_2$, $CO_2$ and general anaesthetics, diffuse across the entire endothelial cell membrane; so, they permeate capillaries extremely rapidly.
- **Small, lipid-insoluble molecules**, such as salts, glucose, amino acids and many drugs, diffuse through an aqueous pathway, namely the intercellular cleft and fenestrae. The intercellular space is small, so permeation is much slower than for lipid-soluble molecules. The entrance to the intercellular pathway is guarded by small pores (equivalent radius: 4–5 nm) that exclude and reflect the plasma proteins. The pores are the tiny spaces between the polymers of the endocapillary coat, the glycocalyx. Blood–brain barrier capillaries have exceptionally tight intercellular junctions, so glucose and amino acid transfer is mediated by specific carrier proteins, through facilitated diffusion.

- **Large, lipid-insoluble molecules**, such as plasma proteins (radius: >4 nm), cross the endothelium slowly through a limited large pore system, the identity of which is controversial. Both vesicular transport and porous channels may contribute.

- **Solute extraction** $E$ is the fraction of the arterial solute that is extracted by the tissue during capillary transit. $E = (C_a - C_v)/C_a$, where $C_a$ and $C_v$ are the arterial and venous plasma concentrations. For $O_2$, $E$ averages ~25% in a resting human. **Plasma clearance** (mL/min) = plasma flow × $E$. **Solute transfer rate** $J_s$ can be determined by applying **Fick's principle**; $J_s$ = plasma flow × $(C_a - C_v)$.

- **Solute transfer rate** can be increased hugely, for example, in exercising muscle, through a combination of: (1) **an increase in the blood-to-tissue concentration difference** $\Delta C$,

due to increased metabolic consumption by the tissue; (2) **recruitment** of underperfused capillaries by arteriolar dilation, which raises $S$, reduces diffusion distance $\Delta x$ across the Krogh cylinder and improves perfusion homogeneity; and (3) **increased capillary blood flow**.

- The **effect of increased blood flow** depends on whether solute exchange is **flow-limited**, **diffusion-limited** or **intermediate**. If capillary diffusion capacity $PS$ is ≥5 times blood flow, blood equilibrates with pericapillary fluid before the capillary exit is reached. Such exchange is flow-limited; raising the blood flow increases the exchange rate proportionately, as with $O_2$ uptake by pulmonary capillaries. If $PS/\dot{Q}$ is <1, equilibration is not achieved before the end of the capillary and exchange is diffusion-limited (e.g. glucose in exercising muscle); transfer is not limited by solute delivery rate.

## FURTHER READING

Komarova YA, Kruse K, Mehta D, et al. Protein interactions at endothelial junctions and signaling mechanisms regulating endothelial permeability. *Circulation Research* 2017; **120**(1): 179–206.

Pittman RN. Oxygen transport in the microcirculation and its regulation. *Microcirculation* 2013; **20**(2): 117–37.

Poole DC, Copp SW, Ferguson SK, et al. Skeletal muscle capillary function: contemporary observations and novel hypotheses. *Experimental Physiology* 2013; **98**(12): 1645–58.

Michel CC. Microvascular permeability, ultrafiltration, and restricted diffusion. *American Journal of Physiology. Heart and Circulatory Physiology* 2004; **287**(5): H1887–8.

Tuma P, Hubbard AL. Transcytosis: crossing cellular barriers. *Physiological Reviews* 2003; **83**(3): 871–932.

Wittenberg JB, Wittenberg BA. Myoglobin function reassessed. *Journal of Experimental Biology* 2003; **206**(Pt 12): 2011–20.

Firth JA. Endothelial barriers: from hypothetical pores to membrane proteins. *Journal of Anatomy* 2002; **200**(6): 541–8.

Wolf MB. A three-pathway pore model describes extensive transport data from mammalian microvascular beds and frog microvessels. *Microcirculation* 2002; **9**(6): 497–511.

Duelli R, Kuschinsky W. Brain glucose transporters: relationship to local energy demand. *News in Physiological Sciences* 2001; **16**: 71–6.

Abbott NJ. Inflammatory mediators and modulation of blood–brain barrier permeability. *Cellular and Molecular Neurobiology* 2000; **20**(2): 131–47.

Jürgens KD, Papadopoulos S, Peters T, et al. Myoglobin: just an oxygen store or also an oxygen transporter? *News in Physiological Sciences* 2000; **15**: 269–74.

Intaglietta M, Johnson PC. Functional capillary density: active and passive determinants. *International Journal of Microcirculation* 1995; **15**: 213–76.

Ellsworth ML, Ellis CG, Popel AS, et al. Role of microvessels in oxygen supply to tissue. *News in Physiological Sciences* 1994; **9**(3): 119–23.

Hudlicka O, Egginton S, Brown MD. Capillary diffusion distances: their importance for cardiac and skeletal muscle performance. *News in Physiological Sciences* 1988; **3**(4): 134–8.

Curry FE, Michel CC. A fiber matrix model of capillary permeability. *Microvascular Research* 1980; **20**(1): 96–9.

Pappenheimer JR, Renkin EM, Borrero LM. Filtration, diffusion and molecular sieving through peripheral capillary membranes; a contribution to the pore theory of capillary permeability. *American Journal of Physiology* 1951; **167**(1): 13–46.

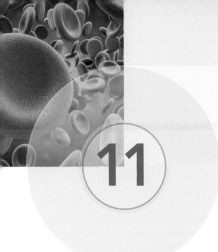

# 11

# Circulation of fluid between plasma, interstitium and lymph

## LEARNING OBJECTIVES

*After reading this chapter you should be able to:*

- name the factors determining capillary fluid exchange and relate them using the Starling equation (11.1);
- define 'osmotic reflection coefficient' and explain its importance (11.1, 11.3, 11.11);
- outline the factors determining capillary pressure (11.2);
- give typical values for human capillary pressure and plasma colloid osmotic pressure (11.2, 11.3);
- sketch how extravascular protein concentration alters with filtration rate, and explain its importance (11.4);
- outline how Starling pressures and fluid flux change along the capillary axis (11.6);

- state the circumstances under which capillaries absorb interstitial fluid (11.6);
- explain why normal tissue does not 'pit' but oedematous tissue does (11.7);
- draw an interstitial pressure–volume relation, marking the normal and oedematous zones (11.7);
- list the functions of the lymphatic system and outline how lymph is moved (11.8);
- categorize the causes of oedema and explain the 'safety margin' (11.10);
- list the changes that bring about inflammatory swelling (11.11).

Capillary blood pressure causes fluid to filter slowly across the capillary wall into the interstitial space. From here, the fluid drains into the lymphatic system, which returns it to the bloodstream. Although this fluid turnover is usually very slow, the cumulative turnover over many hours is substantial; in fact, **the entire plasma volume completes an extravascular circulation in under one day**, except for the plasma proteins. Consequently, the distribution of fluid between the plasma and interstitial compartment can be distorted relatively quickly by changes in capillary or lymphatic function. For example, increased capillary filtration during prolonged standing or exercise reduces the plasma volume by up to 20%, and increased capillary filtration during cardiac failure drives

an excess of water in the tissues (oedema). To understand such fluid shifts, we must first identify the forces that determine fluid exchange.

## 11.1 THE STARLING PRINCIPLE OF FLUID EXCHANGE

Transcapillary fluid movement is a process of **plasma ultrafiltration across a semipermeable membrane**. Water and electrolytes pass through the wall more easily than plasma proteins, producing an ultrafiltrate with a substantially reduced protein content – the interstitial fluid. The ultrafilter is the endocapillary coating of biopolymers, the glycoca-lyx (Figures 9.3, 9.5 and 10.10). The glycocalyx interpolymer spaces function as a system of small pores (radius 4–5 nm), that are permeable to water and small solutes but are too nar-row to transmit plasma proteins readily. The glycocalyx is thus a semipermeable membrane; it covers the entrance to the intercellular cleft, through which the plasma ultrafiltrate flows to reach the pericapillary, interstitial space (Figure 11.1b). In fenestrated capillaries, the fenestrae provide an additional, subglycocalyx pathway permeable to water (Figures 10.10 and 10.11). In discontinuous capillaries, the gaps further enhance permeability (Figure 10.2).

## Blood pressure drives filtration whereas plasma colloid osmotic pressure opposes it

The primary force driving plasma ultrafiltration is the **capil-lary blood pressure**, as Carl Ludwig recognized in 1850. The primary force opposing ultrafiltration is the **osmotic pres-sure of the plasma proteins**, which tends to suck fluid into the capillary, as shown by Ernest Starling in 1896. Starling injected isotonic saline or serum into the tissues of a dog hindlimb and found that the saline was absorbed into the bloodstream, as revealed by haemodilution, whereas serum was not. He con-cluded that the capillary wall is a semipermeable membrane,

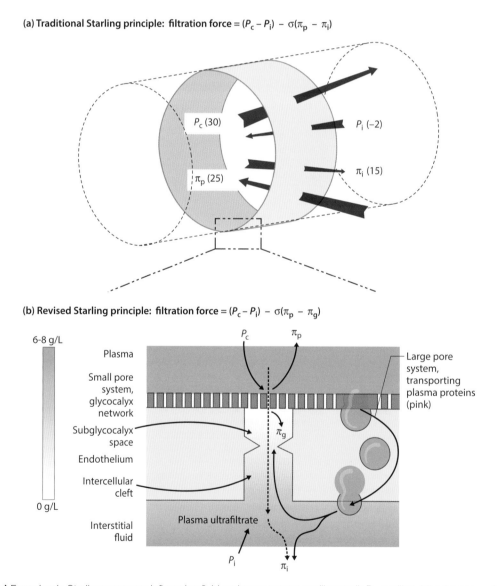

**Figure 11.1 (a)** Four classic Starling pressures influencing fluid exchange across capillary wall: $P_c$, capillary blood pressure (mmHg, human skin, heart level); $P_i$, interstitial fluid pressure; $\pi_p$, plasma colloid osmotic pressure (COP); and $\pi_i$, interstitial fluid COP. Pressures are relative to atmospheric pressure (760 mmHg), so $P_i = -2$ mmHg means an absolute pressure of 758 mmHg, hence the direction of the arrow. **(b)** Cross section of intercellular cleft to show the gradient of the extravascular plasma protein extending into the subglycocalyx space (COP = $\pi_g$); concentration indicated by shade of pink. The gradient is the result of the battle between upstream diffusion of extravascular plasma protein (solid curves) and its washout by plasma ultrafiltrate emerging from the glycocalyx small pore system (dashed line). At a fenestration, the dif-ference between $\pi_g$ and $\pi_i$ is less extreme, because the small pore outlets are less confined. (a: Data from Levick JR, Michel CC. *The Journal of Physiology* 1978; 274: 97–109; Bates DO, Levick JR, Mortimer PS. *The Journal of Physiology* 1994; 477(Pt 2): 355–63. b: Adapted from Levick JR. *The Journal of Physiology* 2004; 557(Pt 3): 704. Data from Levick JR. Microvascular Research 1994; 47(1): 90–125.)

across which the plasma proteins ('colloids') exert an absorptive force, the **colloid osmotic pressure (COP)**. This is the **Starling principle of fluid exchange**.

COP and oncotic pressure are synonyms for the osmotic pressure of the plasma proteins. Students unfamiliar with osmosis should note that osmotic pressure is a **suction** force, not a pushing force (Section 11.3). Plasma COP is of major importance because **plasma COP is the sole force retaining water within the plasma compartment**. Starling's discovery led to the use of solutions of artificial colloids to replace lost plasma in wounded soldiers during World War I, and more recently to the development of plasma substitutes such as urea-linked gelatin solution, a nice example of practical benefit arising from 'pure' research.

## Rate and direction of fluid exchange are governed by four pressures

The Starling principle of fluid exchange (not to be confused with Frank–Starling's law, Section 6.4) states that the transcapillary filtration rate is proportional to the hydraulic pressure difference across the wall minus the opposing COP difference (Figure 11.1a). In other words:

Capillary filtration rate ∝ [ hydraulic push – osmotic suction]

When hydraulic push exceeds osmotic suction, fluid filters from the bloodstream into the interstitium. This is normal. However, if osmotic suction exceeds hydraulic push, the filtration rate becomes negative; that is, fluid is absorbed from the interstitial compartment into the plasma, as happens after a haemorrhage.

We can easily convert this statement into an equation that predicts the volume filtered per unit time, $J_v$. The net hydraulic push equals capillary blood pressure $P_c$ minus interstitial fluid pressure $P_i$. The net osmotic suction equals plasma COP, $\pi_p$, minus the COP of fluid on the downstream side of the semipermeable membrane, the glycocalyx, $\pi_g$. So, replacing words with symbols:

$$J_v \propto [(P_c - P_i) - (\pi_p - \pi_g)] \tag{11.1a}$$

$P_c$, $P_i$ and $\pi_p$ have all been measured. Unfortunately, $\pi_g$ cannot be measured at present, only computed. However, interstitial fluid COP ($\pi_i$) can be measured, and the interstitial fluid is connected to the subglycocalyx fluid via the intercellular cleft (and fenestrae, when present) (Figure 11.1b). Therefore, $\pi_i$ has traditionally been substituted for $\pi_g$ (for caveats, see Section 11.6). This gives us the traditional formula:

$$J_v \propto [(P_c - P_i) - (\pi_p - \pi_i)] \tag{11.1b}$$

The proportionality factor depends on capillary surface area $S$ and the hydraulic conductance of the wall, $L_p$, so we can write:

$$J_v \cong L_p S[(P_c - P_i) - (\pi_p - \pi_i)] \tag{11.1c}$$

However, this equation still lacks one crucial term; it neglects the fact that endothelium is as an **imperfect** semipermeable membrane; that is, it is slightly leaky to plasma proteins. This is dealt with by introducing the reflection coefficient, as follows.

## The reflection coefficient quantifies imperfect semipermeability

When a membrane is leaky to a solute, the solute's potential osmotic pressure is not exerted fully (Figure 10.7). The ratio of the effective osmotic pressure across a leaky membrane ($\Delta\pi_{effective}$) to the full osmotic pressure across a perfect semipermeable membrane ($\Delta\pi_{ideal}$) is called the osmotic reflection coefficient $\sigma$:

$$\sigma = \frac{\Delta\pi_{effective}}{\Delta\pi_{ideal}} \tag{11.2}$$

Endothelial $\sigma$ for plasma proteins is 0.80–0.95, so 80%–95% of the plasma COP is exerted at the capillary wall. (NB: The reduction is not caused by protein outside the membrane. The effective osmotic pressure of extravascular protein is likewise reduced by factor $\sigma$.) Thus, the osmotic pressures in equation 11.1 must be reduced by fraction $\sigma$, giving us the **classic Starling equation for fluid filtration**.

$$J_V = L_p S[(P_c - P_i) - \sigma(\pi_p - \pi_i)] \tag{11.3}$$

As we shall see, the Starling equation is central to understanding disorders such as oedema, inflammatory swelling and posthaemorrhagic fluid absorption. However, it must be remembered that $\pi_i$ is a rough substitute for the true factor $\pi_g$, and in some circumstances the distinction is important (Section 11.6).

## Key features of the starling principle have been proved in single capillaries

Transcapillary fluid movement was first measured in an individual capillary by an American medical student, Eugene Landis, in 1926. The capillary is cannulated with a micropipette and blocked downstream by a glass rod (Figure 11.2a). If ultrafiltration occurs out of the blocked segment, the lost fluid is replaced from the pipette, sweeping the trapped red cells towards the blocker. Conversely, if interstitial fluid is absorbed into the capillary, the red cells are pushed back towards the pipette. The flow is calculated from the red cell velocity, and the capillary pressure is measured through the micropipette.

The Landis red cell method established that the capillary filtration rate increases linearly with pressure $P_c$, as the Starling equation predicts (Figure 11.2b). The slope equals endothelial hydraulic conductance, $L_p$. The results also prove that the capillary wall is a semipermeable membrane, because the filtration rate is zero when capillary pressure is close to the plasma COP $\pi_p$, and reverses direction to

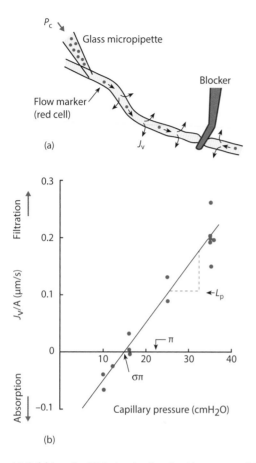

(a)

(b)

**Figure 11.2 (a)** Landis–Michel red cell method to measure fluid exchange in a single capillary. Filtration rate in the blocked vessel ($J_v$) equals axial shift in red cell per unit time × vessel cross-sectional area. Measurements are made at several capillary pressures. **(b)** Initial filtration rate per unit wall area ($J_v/A$) increases with capillary pressure. The 'plasma' here was an infused albumin solution of colloid osmotic pressure ($\pi_p$) 22 cmH$_2$O. The pressure intercept at zero filtration, 15 cmH$_2$O, is the effective osmotic pressure of the albumin *in vivo*, $\sigma\pi_p$. $P_i$ and $\pi_i$ were probably close to zero, because the tissue was continuously washed with saline. The slope is the endothelial hydraulic conductance, $L_p$. (From Michel CC. *The Journal of Physiology* 1980; 309: 341–55, with permission from Wiley-Blackwell.)

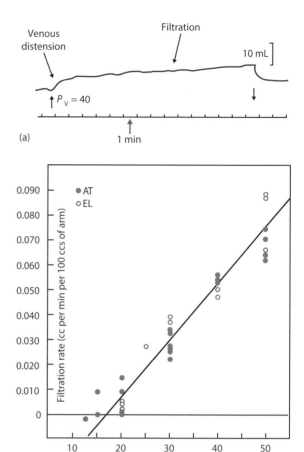

(a)

(b)

**Figure 11.3** Capillary filtration in the human forearm. **(a)** Forearm volume was measured by plethysmography (Figure 8.5). The arrows mark the inflation of the venous congesting cuff around the upper arm to 40 cmH$_2$O and deflation after 15 min. After the initial phase of venous distension (<2 min), the slow swelling is caused by capillary filtration. **(b)** Capillary filtration rate at a series of venous pressures. The slope, 0.003 mL min$^{-1}$ mmHg$^{-1}$ per 100 mL forearm, is called the capillary filtration capacity. (From the classic study of Krogh A, Landis EM, Turner AH. *The Journal of Clinical Investigation* 1932; 11(1): 63–95.)

absorption when capillary pressure is lowered below $\pi_p$. The transient nature of fluid absorption is considered later in the chapter (Section 11.6).

## Filtration rate increases with venous pressure in human limbs

Capillary filtration rate can be measured in human limbs and isolated perfused organs using the slow rise in volume or weight that occurs when capillary pressure is raised. Capillary pressure can be raised in a human limb by inflating a proximal sphygmomanometer cuff to ~40 mmHg, thereby raising distal venous pressure. After the vascular volume has stabilized, the limb swells slowly because of increased capillary filtration (Figure 11.3a). A **deep vein thrombosis** of the leg causes leg oedema in this way. The swelling rate increases linearly with

venous pressure (Figure 11.3b), and the slope of the relation, the **capillary filtration capacity**, equals the sum of the capillary area × wall conductance values, $\Sigma(L_pS)$, in a given volume of tissue.

The effect of venous pressure on capillary filtration raises the question 'What determines capillary pressure?' The next section addresses this issue.

## 11.2 CAPILLARY BLOOD PRESSURE ($P_C$) AND ITS REGULATION

Capillary blood pressure is the most variable of the four Starling pressures and is the only factor under nervous control. It is affected by arterial and venous pressures, vascular resistance, gravity and distance along the capillary axis.

## The pre- to postcapillary resistance ratio (R_A/R_V) regulates capillary pressure

Capillary pressure lies between arterial pressure and venous pressure, and is usually closer to venous than arterial pressure. How close capillary pressure is to arterial or venous pressure depends on the ratio of precapillary, arteriolar resistance $R_A$ to postcapillary, venular resistance $R_V$ (Figure 11.4). If $R_A/R_V$ is high, the pressure drop across the arterioles is large, so the pressure reaching the capillary is much attenuated, as in the 'vasoconstriction' curve of Figure 8.16. As a result, capillary pressure is close to venular pressure. Conversely, if $R_A/R_V$ is low, as it is during inflammation, capillary pressure is high (Figure 8.16, vasodilatation curve). $R_A/R_V$ is normally quite large, ~4, so capillary pressure is normally low and four times more sensitive to venous pressure than to arterial pressure. Therefore, venous hypertension causes oedema, but arterial hypertension does not.

Since capillary pressure is regulated by $R_A/R_V$, **the sympathetic vasomotor nerves can influence fluid exchange**. After a haemorrhage, sympathetic-mediated arteriolar vasoconstriction raises $R_A/R_V$, which reduces capillary pressure. Plasma COP now predominates over capillary pressure, so interstitial fluid is absorbed into the

capillary bloodstream, topping up the depleted circulation (Section 18.2). The active regulation of capillary pressure by $R_A/R_V$ is a daily occurrence in the human leg during standing, as described next.

## The rise in capillary pressure below heart level is attenuated by precapillary vasoconstriction

Due to gravity, arterial and venous pressures increase with vertical distance below heart level, to ~180 mmHg and ~90 mmHg, respectively, in the feet of a standing human (Figure 8.2). Capillary pressure also increases, to ~95 mmHg in the foot. Therefore, oedema is common in the feet and ankles, or over the sacrum if bedridden. However, capillary pressure does not increase as steeply as the arterial and venous pressures (Figure 11.5). This is because a local, arteriolar vasoconstriction, the **veni-arteriolar response**, raises $R_A/R_V$ to 20–30 (Figure 11.5, top right). The large rise in precapillary resistance shifts the capillary pressure towards the lower, venous limit of its range. In this way, the veni-arteriolar response attenuates the fluid filtration rate and helps minimize postural oedema.

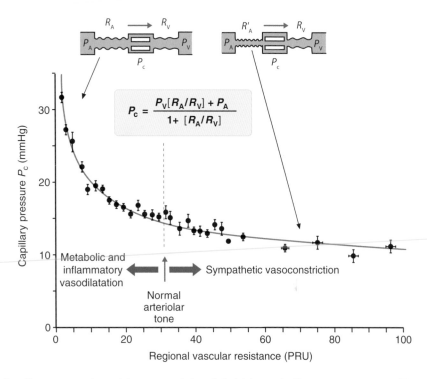

**Figure 11.4** Control of capillary pressure by resistance vessels in cat skeletal muscle. Pressure was measured towards the venous end of the capillary bed; the venous pressure $P_V$ was 7 mmHg, the arterial pressure $P_A$ 100 mmHg. Peripheral resistance (unit, PRU) is generated mainly by precapillary, arteriolar resistance. The inset shows how the ratio of precapillary resistance $R_A$ to postcapillary resistance $R_V$ regulates capillary pressure $P_c$. Blood flow from artery to mid-capillary equals $(P_A - P_c)/R_A$. Flow from mid-capillary to vein equals $(P_c - P_V)/R_A$. Since the two flows are virtually equal, $(P_A - P_c)/R_A = (P_c - P_V)/R_V$. Rearranging, we get the Pappenheimer–Soto-Rivera equation for capillary pressure in the box. (Data from Maspers M, Björnberg J, Mellander S. *Acta Physiologica Scandinavica* 1990; 140(1): 73–83, by permission.)

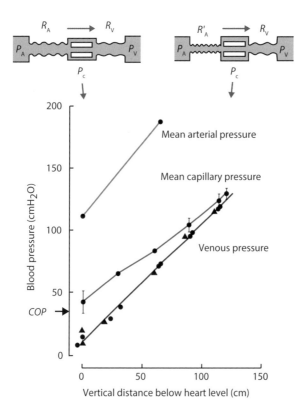

**Figure 11.5** Capillary blood pressure in nail-fold skin of the human foot, measured by micropuncture, with the foot at various distances below heart level. Popliteal artery pressure and dorsal foot vein pressure increase with distance below heart level in the simple way predicted by physics (effect of gravity), but capillary pressure increases less than expected. The top insets show how the rise in capillary pressure is attenuated by a vasoconstrictor response. This 'veni-arteriolar response' may be mediated by the myogenic response (Bayliss effect), but also requires an intact sympathetic innervation. (From Levick JR, Michel CC. *The Journal of Physiology* 1978; 274: 97–109, by permission.)

## Blood pressure decays along a capillary

Due to the capillary's hydraulic resistance, blood pressure falls along a capillary, from ~32–36 mmHg at the arterial end to 12–25 mmHg at the venous end of human skin capillaries at heart level. Capillary pressure is considerably lower in the lungs (~10 mmHg) and portal circulations (renal tubular capillaries ~14 mmHg, hepatic sinusoids ~6–7 mmHg).

Next, we must consider the main force opposing capillary filtration, the plasma COP.

## 11.3 OSMOSIS ACROSS CAPILLARIES: PLASMA COLLOID OSMOTIC PRESSURE ($\pi_P$)

Capillaries can absorb interstitial fluid by osmosis under certain circumstances (Figure 11.2), so let us consider next the process of osmosis.

## Osmosis is the flow of water molecules across a semipermeable membrane from a dilute to a stronger solution

The total pressure acting on the entrance to a pore in a semipermeable membrane is the result of the bombardment of the pore entrance by both solvent molecules and solute molecules, which are in a state of continuous, thermodynamic motion (Figure 11.6). If the solution is at, say, atmospheric pressure, the sum of the solvent and solute bombardments equals 1 atm. Therefore, the solvent itself must exert <1 atm of pressure, just as, in a mixture of gases at 1 atm, each gas has a partial pressure of <1 atm. The solute thus reduces the solvent free energy (Figure 11.6, red line). If the opposite side of the membrane is exposed to pure solvent or a less concentrated solution at atmospheric pressure, there is now a difference in solvent energy level across the pore. This drives a hydraulic flow of solvent through the pore into the more concentrated solution – osmotic flow. The osmotic flow can be halted by applying pressure to the concentrated solution, to raise its solvent free energy to the same level as on the opposite side. **The hydrostatic pressure that halts the osmotic flow from pure solvent into a solution is called the 'osmotic pressure' of the solution**. This way of measuring osmotic pressure accounts for the fact that a suction effect is referred to as a 'pressure'.

Note that, during osmosis, the solvent flows hydraulically through the pore. Contrary to a popular belief, perpetuated in some textbooks, the net water movement is **not by diffusion**. Experiments half a century ago proved that osmotic flow through pores of known radius $r$ obeys Poiseuille's law of hydraulic flow (flow $\propto r^4$, Section 8.7), not Fick's law of diffusion (flux $\propto$ area $\propto r^2$, Section 10.3).

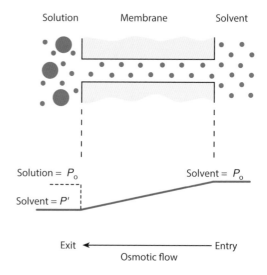

**Figure 11.6** Osmotic flow from solvent (right) to solution (left), both at atmospheric pressure, $P_o$. The solute lowers the 'partial pressure' $P'$ of the solvent in the solution (i.e. its free energy), so $P'$ is less than $P_o$. The resulting pressure gradient across the pore drives the osmotic flow of solvent into the solution. Osmosis is a process of hydraulic flow, not water diffusion. (After Mauro A. In: Ussing HH. *Water Transport Across Epithelia: Barriers, Gradients, and Mechanisms*. Copenhagen: Munksgaard, 1981: 107–10, with permission from Wiley-Blackwell.)

Osmotic pressure is a 'colligative' property, like freezing point depression; that is, it depends primarily on solute concentration, not chemical identity. The osmotic pressure ($\pi$) of an ideal solution is described by van't Hoff's law, namely

$$\pi = RTC$$

($R$, gas constant; $T$, absolute temperature; $C$, molal concentration).

## Albumin contributes disproportionately to colloid osmotic pressure $\pi_p$

As a rough rule, in different vertebrates, the plasma COP equals mid-capillary blood pressure; both are high in humans and low in amphibia. Human plasma contains 65–80 g protein per litre, and its COP is 21–29 mmHg (Figure 11.7). Albumin, which accounts for half the plasma protein mass, generates about two thirds of the COP. Albumin's osmotic pressure greatly exceeds the 'ideal' osmotic pressure predicted by van't Hoff's law, partly because the albumin molecule has 17 negative charges at physiological pH. These attract extra $Na^+$ ions into the solution (**Gibbs–Donnan effect**), which contribute about one third of albumin's osmotic pressure.

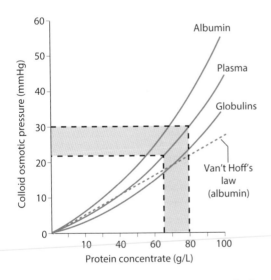

**Figure 11.7** Osmotic pressure of human plasma proteins in isotonic saline (pH 7.4; 37 °C). The pink region shows the normal human range. The dashed line is van't Hoff law prediction for albumin. Colloid osmotic pressure is bigger than predicted and is described (in mmHg) by polynomial equations:

albumin $\pi = 0.28C + 1.8 \times 10^{-3}C^2 + 1.2 \times 10^{-5}C^3$;
plasma $\pi = 0.21C + 1.6 \times 10^{-3}C^2 + 0.9 \times 10^{-5}C^3$;
globulins $\pi = 0.16C + 1.5 \times 10^{-3}C^2 + 0.6 \times 10^{-5}C^3$;

where $C$ is g/L. (From Scatchard G et al., summarized by Landis EM, Pappenheimer JR. In: Hamilton WF, Dow P, eds. *Handbook of Physiology 2, Circulation III*. Washington: American Physiological Society, 1963: 961–1034, by permission.)

## Colloid osmotic pressure differs massively from crystalloid osmotic pressure

The total osmotic pressure of plasma is extremely high, ~5800 mmHg, but 99.6% is due to the 300 millimoles of 'crystalloids' per litre, chiefly sodium chloride ($Na^+Cl^-$). The crystalloid osmotic pressure, though massive, does not affect capillary fluid exchange under most circumstances, because the salt concentration in interstitial fluid and plasma is almost identical and the endothelial reflection coefficient for crystalloids is only ~0.1. Plasma protein concentration is only ~1 mM, but plasma proteins exert a sustained osmotic pressure of ~25 mmHg, due to their high reflection coefficient. The plasma proteins are thus responsible for retaining fluid in the circulation. However, there are a few circumstances in which crystalloid osmotic pressure influences transcapillary fluid exchange, as follows.

## Aquaporins provide a water-only, transcellular pathway of low conductance

The endothelial glycocalyx–intercellular cleft pathway provides a high-conductance pathway for both water and crystalloids. Continuous capillaries also have low-conductance channels in the endothelial cell membrane, formed by the transmembrane glycoprotein aquaporin-1. Aquaporin channels conduct water but not crystalloids and their discovery by Peter Agre led to him receiving the Nobel Prize in Chemistry in 2003. Their main role is cell volume regulation. Aquaporins normally contribute little to transcapillary flow, due to their low hydraulic conductance and the absence of a significant transcapillary crystalloid gradient. However, if interstitial crystalloid concentration increases, flow through the aquaporin pathway can become significant because crystalloids exert their full osmotic pressure on the water-only aquaporin channels ($\sigma = 1$). Interstitial crystalloid concentration increases in the following situations:

- **Exercising muscle fibres** release lactate and $K^+$ ions into the interstitial fluid, raising the local crystalloid osmotic pressure. This draws water from the plasma compartment through the aquaporin-1 channels. Consequently, muscles swell during exercise, and plasma volume falls (Section 11.9).
- The **renal outer medulla** has long capillaries (descending vasa recta) with abundant aquaporin-1 channels. A gradient of $Na^+Cl^-$ created by the renal tubules draws water through these channels.
- In **peritoneal dialysis**, a concentrated glucose solution is infused into the peritoneal cavity of renal failure patients. The glucose, a crystalloid, sucks fluid osmotically from the plasma into the peritoneal cavity, enabling the physician to control the plasma volume. Mercuric chloride, which blocks aquaporin-1 channels, blocks this fluid transfer.

## 11.4 MAGNITUDE AND DYNAMICS OF EXTRAVASCULAR COP ($\pi_i$, $\pi_g$)

Having considered plasma COP, we must next consider the smaller but by no means insignificant extravascular COP. As noted earlier, the underside of the semipermeable glycocalyx is exposed to the subglycocalyx fluid of the intercellular cleft and fenestrations, which connects with the interstitial fluid compartment (Figures 10.10 and 11.1b). If the filtration rate is slow, interstitial albumin and other escaped plasma proteins can diffuse upstream in the intercellular cleft to influence the COP $\pi_g$ at the outer face of the semipermeable membrane (Section 11.6). We must therefore consider the interstitial fluid plasma protein concentration and the factors that change it.

### Interstitial plasma protein concentration and COP are *not* insignificant

There is widespread, time-hallowed misconception that the plasma protein content and COP of interstitial fluid are insignificant. This is simply not true for most tissues. Mean interstitial plasma protein concentration is ~20–30 g/L, and because interstitial fluid is 16% of the body weight, over half of the entire plasma protein mass is extravascular. Interstitial fluid composition has been determined by collecting fluid from prenodal lymphatics and implanted wicks. Human leg lymph contains 15–35 g/L plasma protein, intestinal lymph 30–40 g/L and lung lymph 40–50 g/L, representing 23% (leg) to 70% (lung) of the plasma concentration. Since the interstitial plasma proteins can diffuse into the subglycocalyx space, they can affect the COP gradient across the semipermeable glycocalyx, and hence fluid exchange (Section 11.6). So, what determines the interstitial plasma protein concentration?

### Interstitial protein concentration and COP are a dynamic function of filtration rate

Plasma protein concentration in the bulk interstitial fluid is not a fixed quantity; it varies with fluid exchange rate, due to the following simple relation. Plasma proteins pass slowly from plasma to interstitium through the large pore system, which is spatially separate from the main filtration pathway (intercellular clefts, fenestrae; Figures 10.11 and 11.1b). If the large pores transmit a plasma protein mass $m$ into the interstitium in time $t$ (flux $J_s$), and the small pores transmit a water volume $V$ over the same period (flow $J_v$), the interstitial protein concentration $C_i$ is given by the **interstitial dilution relation**:

$$C_i = \frac{m/t}{V/t} = \frac{J_s}{J_v} \tag{11.4}$$

In other words, interstitial protein concentration equals the rate of arrival of protein divided by the rate of arrival of water, in the steady state (Figure 11.8a). Interstitial protein concentration is thus a **dynamic variable**, governed by two continuous influxes,

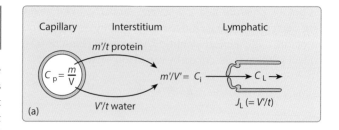

(a)

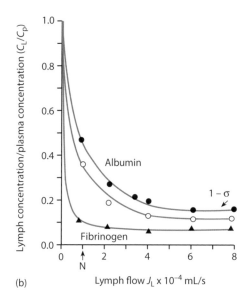

(b)

**Figure 11.8** Effect of capillary filtration rate on interstitial protein concentration. **(a)** Mass of protein entering the interstitium in a given time ($m'/t$ or $J_s$) is diluted by the volume of filtrate produced over the same time interval ($V'/t$ or $J_v$); so interstitial protein concentration $C_i = J_s/J_v$. This drains away as lymph ($C_i = C_L$). **(b)** Effect of the filtration rate on the lymph/plasma concentration ratio, $C_L/C_p$, in dog paw. The filtration rate was measured as lymph flow $J_L$ and was varied by venous congestion. $N$ is the normal value. Curves are for albumin (●, radius 3.55 nm), γ-globulin (○, radius 5.6 nm) and fibrinogen (▲, radius 10 nm). At high flows, $C_L/C_p$ falls to a limit, the transmitted fraction $1 - \sigma$. (From Renkin EM, et al. 1977, plotted by Curry FE. In: Renkin EM, Michel CC, eds. *Handbook of Physiology, Cardiovascular System*, Vol. IV, Part II, Microcirculation. Bethesda, MD: American Physiological Society, 1984: 309–74, by permission.)

one of which ($J_v$) varies with capillary pressure. When capillary pressure is raised, the water transfer rate increases more than the protein transfer rate, since small pores sieve out the plasma proteins. Consequently, **interstitial protein concentration varies inversely with capillary filtration rate** (Figure 11.8b). This is sometimes called the 'protein washdown' effect. Conversely, if the water filtration rate were reduced to zero, the interstitial protein concentration would eventually equilibrate with the plasma level, due to protein permeation through the large pores.

In Section 11.1, we saw that the pericapillary COP (COP just outside the membrane) can be a **determinant** of filtration rate (equation 11.3), while here we have seen that pericapillary COP is also **dependent** on filtration rate (equation 11.4). The interdependence of filtration rate and pericapillary COP has important consequences (Section 11.6), but before tackling these we must review the fourth Starling pressure, the interstitial fluid pressure.

## 11.5 INTERSTITIAL MATRIX AND INTERSTITIAL FLUID PRESSURE ($P_i$)

### Interstitium is a biphasic, porous material composed of fluid and biopolymers

The interstitium, or extracellular matrix, is the complex substance between the parenchymal cells of a tissue; it is not just a pool of liquid bathing the cells (Figure 11.9). **Collagen fibrils** provide tensile strength, and in skin and large arteries **elastin** confers elasticity (Figure 1.11). The interfibrillar spaces contain **glycosaminoglycan (GAG) chains**, which are long-chain polymers of amino sugars, up to 40 nm long, mostly rich in negative sulphate groups (chondroitin, keratan, dermatan and heparan sulphates). Multiple sulphated GAG chains are anchored to a linear core protein, forming a large, brush-shaped molecule, the **proteoglycan**. Multiple proteoglycans are anchored to an enormously long chain of non-sulphated GAG, **hyaluronan** (length ~5000 nm, size 2–3 million dalton). All GAG chains have fixed negative charges in the form of carboxyl groups ($-COO^-$) and most also have sulphate groups ($-SO_4^-$). **Glycoproteins**, such as the cell-attachment 'glue' fibronectin, add further to the structural complexity. The interstitium thus comprises a three-dimensional network of negatively charged biopolymer fibres, the solid phase, and a space-filling solution of electrolytes and escaped plasma proteins, the fluid phase.

### GAG chains reduce interstitial permeability; interstitial fluid is not easily displaced

GAG chains have two major roles: they are **water-attracting, expansion elements**, and they determine **interstitial permeability**. Regarding the latter role, interstitial water and solutes occupy the minute spaces within the GAG matrix. The effective radius of these spaces, or mean hydraulic radius, ranges from a mere 3 nm in cartilage, which has a very high GAG concentration, to 300 nm in the vitreous body of the eye, which has a very low GAG concentration. Because the spaces are tiny, their resistance to flow is high. As a result, the interstitium has a gel-like consistency, as exemplified by Wharton's jelly (mean hydraulic radius 30 nm) in the umbilical cord. The low mobility of interstitial water stabilizes tissue shape, prevents interstitial fluid displacement by gravity and impedes bacterial spread.

### GAG chains expand the interstitial compartment

GAG chains are responsible for the large volume of the interstitial compartment, because they attract water and swell. If a slice of connective tissue, or Wharton's jelly from the umbilical cord (almost pure interstitium), is placed in saline, the interstitial matrix imbibes the saline and swells. The swelling can be halted by lowering the saline pressure to a sufficiently subatmospheric value. The subatmospheric pressure that exactly counteracts the suction effect of the GAG is called the **gel swelling pressure**. As with osmosis, this kind of 'pressure' is really a suction force, not a pushing force. The gel swelling pressure is caused by the osmotic activity of the GAG chains, which is due chiefly to $Na^+$ ions attracted by their fixed negative charges (the **Gibbs–Donnan effect**). *In vivo*, the interstitial matrix is under-saturated; that is, it still has a swelling tendency, despite the continuous input of plasma ultrafiltrate by capillaries. The unsaturated state is due to the operation of the lymphatic system, which pumps water away from the interstitium, leaving the interstitial fluid at a subatmospheric pressure.

In some tissues, such as skin, the swelling tendency of the interstitial matrix is partly counteracted by fibroblasts. The fibroblasts exert tension on the collagen fibrils through $\alpha_2\beta_1$-integrins at their membrane focal contact points, and the tensed collagen fibrils help to limit the matrix swelling.

### Interstitial fluid pressure $P_i$ is often subatmospheric

Interstitial fluid pressure is difficult to measure, due to the low mobility of fluid in the interstitium. This problem was first overcome in the 1960s by the American physiologist Arthur Guyton, who implanted a hollow perforated capsule under the skin of dogs (Figure 11.10). Over several weeks, the **Guyton capsule** filled with interstitial fluid, and the fluid pressure was subatmospheric, around −5 mmHg. This caused considerable controversy, since interstitial fluid pressure was previously thought to be positive. Subsequently, acute techniques, such as the **wick-in-needle** and **servo-null micropipette** methods (Figure 11.10), confirmed that interstitial fluid pressure is slightly subatmospheric in the skin, subcutis (Table 11.1), relaxed muscle, joint spaces and epidural space (−1 to −3 mmHg). Interstitial pressure is above atmospheric in

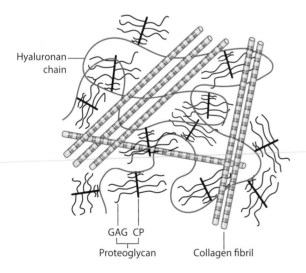

**Figure 11.9** The interstitial matrix is a network of fibrous biopolymers with interstitial fluid in the tiny spaces between the chains. The hyaluronan chain acts as the 'string' to which proteoglycan 'pearls' are anchored (string-of-pearls model). Cutting the string with hyaluronidase raises interstitial hydraulic permeability about fivefold. GAG, sulphated glycosaminoglycan chain (long, chondroitin sulphate; short, keratan sulphate); CP, core protein (of proteoglycan). Microfibrils and glycoproteins, such as fibronectin, are not shown.

Hyaluronan chain

GAG CP
Proteoglycan        Collagen fibril

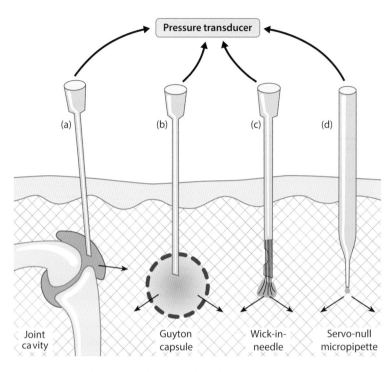

**Figure 11.10** Measurement of interstitial fluid pressure. **(a)** Cannulation of a free fluid space in contact with the interstitium, for example, joint cavity, epidural space. **(b)** Guyton's chronic capsule method. **(c)** Acute wick method of Fadnes, Reed and Aukland; fine cotton filaments conduct interstitial pressure into a hypodermic needle. **(d)** Acute micropipette method; micropipette filled with 1 M Na⁺Cl⁻, a good electrical conductor, is connected to a motorized pump that varies the intrapipette pressure until fluid neither enters nor leaves the tip (null flow), as indicated by its electrical resistance. All four methods rely on equilibrating a small volume of free fluid (blue) to interstitial fluid pressure. The arrows show how the linking fluid is absorbed by the interstitial matrix until its subatmospheric pressure equals that in the matrix.

**Table 11.1** Starling pressures in human subcutaneous tissue (mmHg)

|  | Normal | Congestive cardiac failure |
|---|---|---|
| **Chest** | | |
| Plasma COP | 26.8 | 23.3 |
| Interstitial fluid COP | 15.6 | 10.5 |
| Interstitial fluid pressure | −1.5 | −1.4 |
| | | |
| **Ankle** | | |
| Plasma COP (arterial) | 26.8 | 23.3 |
| Interstitial fluid COP | 10.7 | 3.4 (mild oedema) |
| Interstitial fluid pressure | 0.1 | 0.4 (mild oedema) |

*Source:* Interstitial fluid colloid osmotic pressure (COP) measured in soaked wick fluid. Interstitial fluid pressure measured by wick-in-needle. (From Noddeland H, Omvik P, Lund-Johansen P, et al. *Clinical Physiology* 1984; 4(4): 283–97.)

the kidney (+1 to +10 mmHg), myocardium, resting salivary gland, bone marrow, tooth pulp and flexed joints.

Like interstitial COP, **interstitial fluid pressure is not a fixed quantity**, but varies with fluid exchange. In the small intestine, for example, water absorption from the gut lumen raises mucosal $P_i$ from 1 mmHg to 5 mmHg, which promotes water transfer into the fenestrated mucosal capillaries. Conversely, in salivary glands, secretion reduces $P_i$ from 3 mmHg to −0.8 mmHg, which boosts capillary filtration and thus supplies the extra water needed for saliva formation. Interstitial fluid pressure is also influenced by fibroblasts, which exert a mild compressive effect on the interstitial matrix via integrin bonding to collagen fibres, a point we will return to when considering inflammation (Section 11.11).

## 11.6 TISSUE FLUID BALANCE: FILTRATION VERSUS ABSORPTION

Having covered the forces affecting fluid exchange, we can now address the problem of volume homeostasis; that is, how does the interstitium avoid accumulating plasma ultrafiltrate? The most important factor is the drainage of interstitial fluid by the lymphatic system. A second possibility, long believed and still taught tenaciously in most textbooks, yet clearly disproved by a large body of evidence over the past 20 years, is that venous capillaries continuously reabsorb the filtrate generated by arterial capillaries.

### Lymphatics drain away the capillary filtrate

Almost all tissues form lymph; indeed, the lungs generate lymph even though pulmonary capillary pressure is less than plasma COP (see later). Lymph formation shows that there is normally a net filtration of fluid from the microcirculation into the interstitium, from where the fluid drains into the lymphatics. The ratio of lymph-to-plasma flow tells us the fraction of the plasma water that escapes during one transit through the capillary – the **filtration fraction**. The filtration fraction is tiny, ~0.1%–0.3% in most tissues. However, over a day some 4000 L of plasma pass through the human microcirculation, so the tiny filtration fraction generates a substantial volume of lymph, ~4–8 L/day. In some microcirculations, such as the fenestrated vessels of the renal glomerulus and salivary glands, or the capillaries of the foot during standing, the filtration fraction can be a hundred times higher, for example, 20% in glomerular capillaries.

## Filtration rate decays along the capillary axis

Blood pressure falls as the blood passes along a capillary, so the filtration rate dwindles along the capillary (Figure 11.11). Arterial capillary pressure (~35 mmHg in human skin at heart level) exceeds plasma COP (25 mmHg), whereas venous capillary pressure (~15 mmHg) is below plasma COP (Figure 11.11, top left). This led to the traditional view that arterial capillaries are in a filtration state, while venous capillaries continuously reabsorb most of the filtrate, thus preventing tissue swelling. However, this line of reasoning ignores the by no means negligible interstitial force. The Starling equation (11.3) tells us that, at the balance point for zero filtration, filtration pressure $P_c$ equals the sum of the opposing pressures $\sigma(\pi_p - \pi_i) + P_i$. (We can temporarily ignore differences between interstitial and subglycocalyx protein concentrations, because at zero filtration rate they will equilibrate by diffusion.) Measurements in human skin, muscle and mesentery show that the factor $\sigma(\pi_p - \pi_i) + P_i$ is ~12.5 mmHg. This is lower than venous capillary pressure, ~15 mmHg. There is thus a small net filtration pressure in venous capillaries, and even in venules (Figure 11.11, bottom left). Figure 11.12 summarizes similar data for 12 tissues. In all cases, the venular blood pressure exceeds the opposing force $\sigma(\pi_p - \pi_i) + P_i$. The Starling forces thus indicate that a **well-perfused capillary is normally in a state of filtration along its entire length** in most tissues.

## Venous capillaries absorb fluid transiently when pressure falls

Although venous capillaries do not normally have a net absorptive force, they can absorb interstitial fluid for a while if the Starling pressures are changed. This was demonstrated in Starling's seminal experiment (Section 11.1) and in the studies of Figures 11.2 and 11.13. In a clinical setting, a fall in blood pressure coupled with precapillary vasoconstriction, as during haemorrhage and other form of **hypovolaemic shock**, can reduce the capillary pressure sufficiently for osmotic absorption to occur transiently (Figure 11.11b). However, absorption gradually tails off because (1) ultrafiltration of the absorbed interstitial fluid at the underside of the glycocalyx raises subglycocalyx plasma protein concentration, $\pi_g$ and $\pi_i$, and (2) interstitial pressure $P_i$ falls as fluid is removed from the interstitium. The changes in $\pi_g$ and $P_i$ gradually abolish the net absorptive force, so the absorption rate decays, until finally a steady state of slight filtration is restored (Figure 11.11c).

Proof that **absorption is not sustained at capillary pressures below the plasma COP** was provided by the seminal study of Figure 11.13. Capillary pressure was lowered to venular levels and held there. At first, there was a transient absorption of fluid, in agreement with the Starling principle. However, within a few minutes absorption ceased, as predicted by modern exchange theory (see the glycocalyx–cleft model).

## Fluid exchange in the lung

As pointed out earlier, the lung generates lymph (i.e. capillary filtrate) even though pulmonary capillary pressure, ~10 mmHg, is much lower than plasma COP, 25 mmHg. Pulmonary capillaries are in a filtration state because pulmonary interstitial protein concentration is high, ~70% of plasma level, creating an interstitial COP of 16–20 mmHg. As a result, the difference

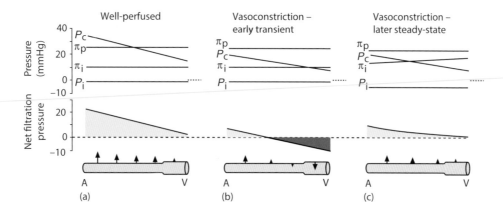

**Figure 11.11** Pressure gradients from the arterial end of the capillary (A) to the venule (V). The yellow region shows the sum of four classic Starling pressures, $(P_c - P_i) - \sigma(\pi_p - \pi_i)$, as measured in skin, muscle and mesentery at heart level. The arrows show fluid flux inferred from the Starling forces. A broadly similar pattern is predicted when differences between $\pi_i$ and $\pi_g$ are considered. **(a)** Net filtration along the entire length of a well-perfused capillary. Note that neglect of measured $\pi_i$ and $P_i$ would lead to the spurious prediction of absorption in the downstream half of the capillary. (Data from Levick JR. *Experimental Physiology* 1991; 76(6): 825–57.) **(b)** Transient absorptive force (red region) immediately after a haemorrhage or arteriolar constriction, which lower $P_c$. **(c)** Loss of absorptive force with time, due to progressive rise in $\pi_i$ and $\pi_g$ and fall in $P_i$. See text for symbols.

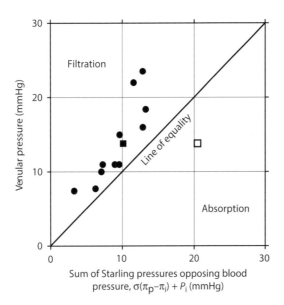

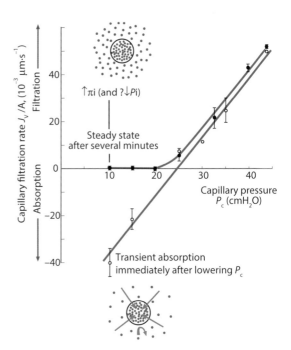

**Figure 11.12** Comparison of venular blood pressure and the net pro-absorption Starling pressures in 12 tissues, showing a moderate net filtration force in venules. When the differences between $\pi_i$ and $\pi_g$ are considered, the net filtration force is smaller. Tissues include muscle, skin, joints, lung (lowest left point) and mesentery (highest right point) (filled circles). The filled square shows fasting rat intestinal mucosa. The unfilled square shows the switch to absorption into mucosal capillaries after the rat drank water, mediated by a fall in $\pi_i$ and rise in $P_i$. These changes illustrate the importance of interstitial forces in determining the direction of fluid movement (Data from many laboratories, reviewed in Levick JR, Mortimer PS. Fluid 'balance' between microcirculation and interstitium in skin and other tissues; revision of classical filtration-reabsorption scheme. In: Messmer K, ed. Microcirculation in Chronic Venous Insufficiency. *Progress in Applied Microcirculation*. Basel: Karger; 1999. Vol. 23. pp. 42–62.)

**Figure 11.13** Demonstration that lowering capillary pressure below plasma colloid osmotic pressure (32 cmH$_2$O here) causes transient but not sustained fluid absorption. Method as for Figure 11.2. On lowering capillary pressure to venular levels, there was transient fluid absorption (open circles); however, after several minutes of perfusion at low pressure, the absorption ceased (closed circles). The lower inset shows extravascular plasma protein (red dots) reflected by capillary wall during water absorption (long arrows). This raises extravascular protein concentration (upper sketch). (Adapted from Michel CC, Phillips ME. *The Journal of Physiology* 1987; 388: 421–35, with permission from Wiley-Blackwell.)

in COP across the capillary wall is smaller than the hydraulic pressure difference. Fluid exchange in the lung thus falls on the flat part of the steady-state line of Figure 11.13.

## Venous capillaries are not normally in a state of sustained absorption

The antiquated view that venous capillaries are normally in a state of sustained absorption is still widely taught as an established fact, based usually on inaccurate interstitial force values derived from differing tissues. This view has now been disproved by:

- measurement of all four Starling forces in the same tissue (Figure 11.12);
- direct measurement of fluid exchange at venous capillary pressures (Figure 11.13);
- experimental and theoretical proof that extravascular COP is inversely related to filtration rate (Figure 11.8).

Therefore, the traditional dogma must be abandoned for most tissues. Its dogged persistence, despite extensive contrary evidence, is characteristic of the antisocial behaviour of factoids! As William Harvey aptly put it in his seminal work *De Motu Cordis*: "I tremble lest I have mankind at large for my enemies, so much doth wont and custom become a second

nature. Doctrine once sown strikes deep its root, and respect for antiquity influences all men."

## Michel–Weinbaum glycocalyx–cleft theory of fluid exchange

The modern form of the Starling principle recognizes that the capillary wall is a two-layer membrane, comprising a thin semipermeable membrane, the glycocalyx, over a more coarsely porous sheet, the endothelial intercellular cleft ± fenestrae. Many commercial semipermeable membranes are constructed similarly. The Michel–Weinbaum theory (Figures 11.1b and 11.14) states that (1) since the endocapillary glycocalyx is the semipermeable membrane, the Starling equation must incorporate the subglycocalyx COP, $\pi_g$:

$$J_V = L_p S[(P_c - P_i) + \sigma(\pi_p - \pi_g)] \qquad (11.5)$$

(2) the low subglycocalyx protein concentration, and hence the osmotic absorption gradient $(\pi_p - \pi_g)$, depends on the continuous, outward ultrafiltration of plasma. If filtration declines or ceases, plasma proteins entering the interstitium via the large pore system accumulate there, raising the interstitial protein concentration (Figure 11.8). When the filtration stream in the intercellular cleft is slow, zero or reversed, the interstitial protein can

diffuse more easily up the cleft into the subglycocalyx space, raising $\pi_g$ and reducing the absorption force ($\pi_p - \pi_g$) (Figure 11.14, dashed line). The glycocalyx–cleft model thus predicts that absorption at low capillary pressure should dwindle and cease with time, as demonstrated experimentally in Figure 11.13.

## How is net filtration rate kept so low?

Continuous capillaries generate lymph very slowly, indicating a low net filtration rate. For example, the foot of a supine human produces only 0.22 mL lymph per 100 g per hour overnight. To explain the low filtration rates, the Starling pressure imbalance must be very small, ~1 mmHg or less. This has been attributed to two factors, pore exit gradients and vasomotion.

## Pore exit gradients: differences between $\pi_g$ and $\pi_i$

The glycocalyx small pore system transmits essentially protein-free plasma ultrafiltrate into the subglycocalyx space,

upstream of the intercellular junctional strands. From the subglycocalyx space, the ultrafiltrate must converge and pass through narrow breaks in the strands, creating a rapid local current, like a lake draining through a narrow gorge. Interstitial plasma proteins diffuse up the filtration stream, against the current, to act osmotically on the underside of the glycocalyx (Figure 11.14). This 'race' between upstream diffusion and downstream washout results in a subglycocalyx protein concentration that is lower than the interstitial concentration. Consequently, the true transmembrane osmotic difference, $\pi_p - \pi_g$, is greater than the classical one, $\pi_p - \pi_i$. This helps explain the low rate of filtration and lymph production.

In support of the cleft gradient model, recent studies showed that raising $\pi_i$ around rapidly filtering capillaries has much less effect on filtration rate than predicted by the classic Starling equation, because $\pi_g$ is ~10% of $\pi_i$ in such capillaries. At normal capillary pressure and filtration rate, $\pi_g$ may be 70%–90% of $\pi_i$, because diffusion makes better progress against a slow current of filtrate. Under these conditions $\pi_g$ mirrors $\pi_i$ more closely.

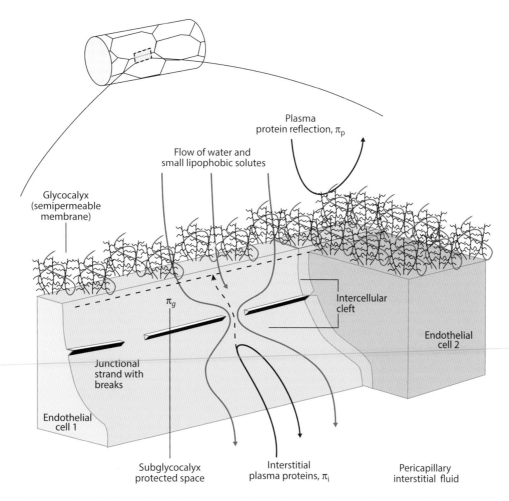

**Figure 11.14** Michel–Weinbaum glycocalyx–junctional break model of fluid exchange in a continuous capillary. The colloid osmotic pressure acting on the underside of the semipermeable glycocalyx, $\pi_g$, can differ from that in the interstitium, $\pi_i$, because the diffusion of interstitial plasma proteins up the cleft is opposed by the outward stream of ultrafiltrate, particularly where it converges in the narrow break between junctional strands ($\pi_g < \pi_i$). Conversely, during interstitial fluid absorption, the reversed intercellular flow causes reflected protein to accumulate in the subglycocalyx space ($\pi_g > \pi_i$). EC (1,2), endothelial cell. (Based on Adamson, Lenz JF, Zhang X, et al. *The Journal of Physiology* 2004; 557(Pt 3): 889–907, with permission from Wiley-Blackwell.)

## Vasomotion

Vasomotion is the cycling of arterioles between dilatation and constriction. In some tissues, such as skeletal muscle, vasomotion occurs rhythmically, several times per minute. Because capillary pressure depends partly on precapillary resistance (Figure 11.4), each contraction phase reduces capillary pressure, allowing a transient absorption of interstitial fluid. Under these conditions the microcirculation alternates between states (**a**) and (**b**) in Figure 11.11, reducing the rate of lymph formation.

## Tissues with an independent fluid input can sustain fluid absorption

Fluid absorption is sustained (cf. transient) in **intestinal mucosa fenestrated capillaries** after drinking water (Figure 11.12, unfilled square). It is also sustained in **renal peritubular fenestrated capillaries** and in **lymph node continuous capillaries**. Sustained absorption becomes possible when the interstitial compartment receives an independent fluid input, that is, fluid from a source other than capillary filtration, such as water absorbed by the gut lumen or renal tubules or supplied by afferent lymphatics. Much of the fluid is absorbed, while the remainder flushes the interstitial space, washing away the interstitial plasma proteins so that they do not accumulate and abolish the absorption gradient. In the intestinal mucosa, 80% of the water absorbed from the gut lumen is absorbed by the microcirculation. The remaining 20% acts as the flushing solution, lowering $\pi_i$ and raising

$P_i$ to maintain a net transendothelial absorption force. This abolishes the inverse link between interstitial protein concentration and capillary filtration rate, which halts absorption in other tissues (Figure 11.8).

The human interstitial compartment contains 10–12 L of fluid and serves as a reservoir for the plasma compartment (3 L). If the plasma volume is reduced by a haemorrhage, a transient absorption of fluid from the interstitial compartment helps top up the depleted plasma compartment. Conversely, if the plasma compartment is overexpanded, due to renal fluid retention or overtransfusion, some of the excess fluid spills over into the interstitium, raising the interstitial volume. The relationship between interstitial fluid volume and pressure – the interstitial compliance curve – is as follows.

## Interstitial compliance is normally low, but is raised in oedema

### Normal hydration

In the subcutaneous interstitium, where clinical oedema commonly accumulates, the interstitial volume–pressure relation is sigmoidal (Figure 11.15). At normal interstitial hydration, the interstitial fluid pressure $P_i$ is subatmospheric and is very sensitive to fluid addition or removal. The normal compliance

### CONCEPT BOX 11.1

#### THE STARLING PRINCIPLE OF FLUID EXCHANGE

- Capillary filtration rate depends on four classic Starling pressures, namely capillary blood pressure minus interstitial fluid pressure, and the opposing plasma COP minus extravascular COP (or more accurately, subglycocalyx COP).

- The filtration rate also depends on the hydraulic conductance and osmotic reflection coefficient of the endothelial layer.

- In most tissues the Starling pressures add up to a net filtration force, even in venous capillaries and lungs. This generates interstitial fluid, which drains away as lymph.

- Osmotic absorption occurs transiently when capillary pressure is reduced by hypovolaemia or precapillary vasoconstriction. Absorption is transient because it raises extravascular COP and lowers interstitial pressure.

- Oedema is caused by increased capillary pressure (e.g. heart failure), or reduced plasma COP (e.g. malnutrition), or increased endothelial conductance and reduced reflection coefficient (inflammation), or reduced lymphatic drainage (e.g. postmastectomy arm oedema).

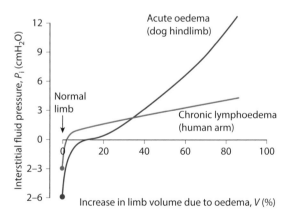

**Figure 11.15** The interstitial compliance curve of limb subcutis. The steeper relation was observed in dog hindlimbs made acutely oedematous by intravenous saline infusion; pressure was recorded in subcutaneous capsules. Pressure gradually declines with time, for a given degree of swelling ('creep'). Consequently, in the chronically swollen human arm (lymphoedema caused by breast cancer surgery) the interstitial compliance curve is flatter. Human subcutis interstitial pressure was measured with the wick-in-needle technique. (Data from Bates DO, Levick JR, Mortimer PS. *International Journal of Microcirculation, Clinical and Experimental* 1992; 11(4): 359–73, and Guyton AC, Taylor, Granger. *Circulation Physiology: Dynamics and Control of Body Fluid*. Philadelphia: WB Saunders; 1975.)

(volume change required for unit pressure change) is small because a change in interstitial water content alters the GAG concentration, and hence the gel swelling pressure (Section 11.5).

## Oedematous tissue

When excess fluid is added, acutely, to the interstitium, GAG dilution reduces the swelling pressure to essentially zero, eliminating this influence on the compliance curve. Interstitial pressure $P_i$ is close to atmospheric pressure at this point (Table 11.1). In an acutely oedematous limb, ~98% of the excess fluid is in the subcutis, stretching the overlying skin. Since skin is very stretchy, $P_i$ increases relatively little with further volume expansion; the oedema pressure–volume relation is relatively flat, and interstitial compliance is ~20-fold normal. By contrast, in tissues bounded by an inelastic fibrous capsule, such as the muscle compartments of the limbs, the pressure–volume curve is steeper and $P_i$ can reach high levels.

## The pitting test for increased interstitial conductivity in oedema

Depending on the tissue, water makes up to 65%–99% of normally hydrated interstitial matrix by weight. Interstitial water is not easily displaced because the GAG chains massively reduce interstitial hydraulic conductivity (Section 11.5 and Figure 11.9). Interstitial hydraulic conductivity depends on the fraction of the interstitial matrix that is water (the 'porosity' $\varepsilon$) relative to the surface area of the fixed biopolymers ($S$), which create hydraulic resistance. The ratio $\varepsilon/S$ is called the **mean hydraulic radius** and ranges from 3 nm in articular cartilage to 300 nm in the vitreous body of the eye. When the mean hydraulic radius is raised by increased tissue hydration, as in clinical oedema, interstitial conductivity increases dramatically. This is the basis of the clinical **pitting test** for subcutaneous oedema. When finger pressure is applied to normal skin for 1 min, then removed, little to no indentation remains, because interstitial fluid mobility is normally low and little fluid is displaced. In oedema, by contrast, interstitial conductivity is high and fluid is rapidly displaced by the applied pressure, leaving a distinct pit in the tissue (Figure 11.16).

## Solute transport and exclusion in the interstitium

Small solutes, such as $O_2$ and glucose, diffuse freely through the spaces between the negatively charged interstitial proteoglycans. Macromolecules, such as albumin, experience restricted diffusion and partial exclusion in the interstitial matrix. (See Section 10.3 for an explanation of these terms.) Albumin is excluded from 20%–50% of the water in subcutaneous and muscle interstitium, due to its size (steric exclusion) and net negative charge (electrical exclusion). Consequently, the effective interstitial protein concentration, that is, protein

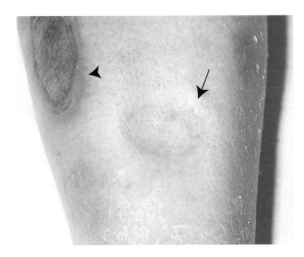

**Figure 11.16** Human calf showing pitting oedema (arrow) in a patient with cardiac failure. The oedema was exacerbated by dependency. Note the skin damage (arrowhead, top left) caused by an oedema blister. The ankle is off the lower edge of the picture. (Courtesy of Professor P Mortimer, Department of Dermatology, St. George's Hospital, London.)

mass divided by available water volume, is higher than the apparent concentration (protein mass/total water volume). Protein is transported through the interstitium to the lymphatic system by convection; that is, it is washed along by the stream of capillary filtrate.

## 11.8 LYMPH AND THE LYMPHATIC SYSTEM

Parts of the lymphatic system were recognized in the early 17th century by Aselli, Pecquet, Rudbeck and Bartholin, but it was not until the 18th century that William Hunter concluded "lymphatic vessels are the absorbing vessels all over the body … they constitute one great and general system dispersed throughout the whole body for absorption." The three main functions are as follows.

### Preservation of fluid balance

Lymph vessels return the capillary ultrafiltrate and escaped plasma proteins to the bloodstream, by draining into the neck veins (Figure 1.8). This completes the extravascular circulation of fluid and protein and maintains tissue volume homeostasis (Figure 11.17). If lymphatic function is impaired, the tissue develops a severe, intractable form of oedema called **lymphoedema**.

### Nutritional function

Intestinal lymph vessels, or 'lacteals', take up and transport tiny globules of digested fat (chylomicra) that have been absorbed by the mucosa, as Aselli noted in 1627 (Figure 11.18).

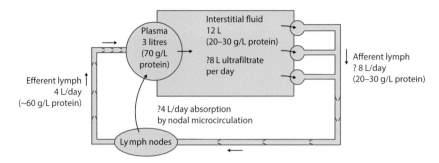

**Figure 11.17** Estimate of extravascular circulation of fluid and plasma protein in a 65-kg human. (After Renkin EM. *The American Journal of Physiology* 1986; 250(5 Pt 2): H706–10, with permission from the American Physiological Society.)

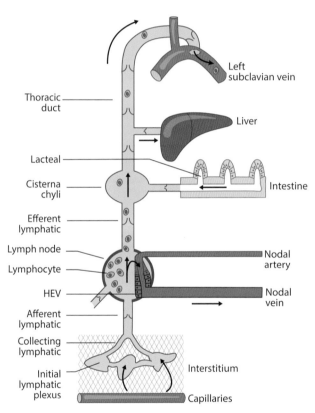

**Figure 11.18** The lymphatic system. The curved arrow within the node indicates absorption of some of the fluid by the nodal capillaries. HEV, high endothelial venule, where circulating lymphocytes re-enter the node.

## Defence function

As interstitial fluid drains into the lymphatic system, it carries foreign materials, such as antigens, viruses, bacteria and inhaled carbon particles, to the lymph nodes. This is an effective, economical method of immunosurveillance (Figure 11.18). The lymph nodes phagocytose particulate matter, which accounts for the blackened nodes in the lungs of smokers and coal miners. Bacterial and viral antigens activate nodal lymphocytes, which are released into the efferent (postnodal) lymph for transport to the bloodstream. Efferent lymph thus has a higher white cell count than afferent (prenodal) lymph.

## Genetic disorders can impair lymphatic development

During embryogenesis, the lymphatics sprout from the venous system and join up with a superficial lymphatic plexus (network) formed by mesenchymal lymphangioblasts. This is why lymph drains, ultimately, into the large veins of the neck (Figure 11.18). Lymphatic growth is driven by an isoform of vascular endothelial growth factor C (VEGFC), and by the transcription factors forkhead box protein C2 (FOXC2) and prospero homeobox protein 1 (PROX1). Inherited defects in the VEGFC receptor or FOXC2 cause different forms of hereditary lymphoedema.

- **VEGFC** is crucial for lymphatic growth and acts on the lymphatic endothelial receptor, vascular endothelial growth factor receptor 3 (VEGFR-3), a receptor tyrosine kinase. **Milroy's disease** is an autosomal dominant form of human hereditary lymphoedema, caused by heterozygous mutation of VEGFR-3. This results in a severely hypoplastic (underdeveloped) peripheral lymphatic plexus and leg lymphoedema.
- **FOXC2** is a transcription factor promoting the maturation of primary lymphatics into lymphatics with valves. FOXC2 −/− knockout mice still develop a lymphatic system, but the main lymphatics lack valves; also, the finest lymphatics, normally simple endothelial tubes, acquire smooth muscle. **Lymphoedema-distichiasis syndrome** is an autosomal dominant form of human hereditary lymphoedema caused by heterozygous, loss-of-function point mutations of the *forkhead box C2 (FOXC2)* gene. This results in leaky lymphatic valves, leg lymphoedema and a double row of eyelashes (distichiasis). Leg venous valves are leaky too, emphasizing the common ancestry of lymphatics and veins.
- **PROX1** is a transcription factor whose deletion in mice results in a total aplasia (absence) of the lymphatic system and perinatal death.

## Structure of the lymphatic vessels

### Lymphatic capillaries

The initial lymphatic vessels are microscopic lymphatic capillaries (diameter 10–50 µm), which form a network of anastomosing tubes in most tissues, and blind-ended sacs in the intestinal villi (Figure 11.18). The wall is a single layer of endothelial cells with an incomplete basement membrane. Some of the endothelial intercellular clefts are ≥14 nm wide, so interstitial proteins and fine particles readily enter lymphatic capillaries. Due to its oblique orientation, the intercellular cleft is thought to act as a flap valve, allowing fluid into the lumen when lymph pressure is low, but closing when lymph pressure is raised above interstitial pressure by local tissue movements (Figure 11.19). The outer surface of the wall is tethered to the surrounding tissues by radiating microfibrils, the **anchoring filaments**, composed of the protein fibrillin. In swollen, oedematous tissue, tension in the anchoring filaments helps to dilate the initial lymphatics.

### Collecting and afferent lymphatics

The initial lymphatic network drains into collecting vessels, which feed into afferent lymph trunks running beside major blood vessels. **Semilunar valves** direct the lymph centrally. From the collecting vessel onwards, the lymphatic wall acquires a coat of smooth muscle and is actively contractile. Lymphatic smooth muscle is abundant in man and ruminants, but scanty in dogs and rabbits. The contractile segment between successive pairs of valves is called a **lymphangion**.

### Lymph nodes

The lower vertebrates have a lymphatic system but no lymph nodes; nodes evolved in mammals, marsupials and some aquatic birds. Lymph enters the node at its hilum through multiple afferent vessels. The node is a mass of lymphocytes and phagocytic cells, permeated by a network of sinuses carrying the lymph flow. The sinuses are endothelial tubes, with gaps to allow lymphocytes to join the lymph. Nodal blood vessels supply $O_2$ and nutrients, and the blood capillaries drain into **high-endothelial venules** involved in lymphocyte trafficking. High-endothelial venules express a receptor for L-selectin on circulating lymphocytes. The captured lymphocytes penetrate the venule intercellular junctions to re-enter the node, thus completing their own unique circulation; that is, efferent lymph → blood → node.

### Efferent lymphatics and the thoracic duct

Lymphocyte-rich efferent lymph from the legs and viscera is actively pumped into a large lymphatic vessel on the posterior abdominal wall. A saccular dilatation of the vessel, the **cisterna chyli**, receives chyle, the fatty lymph formed in intestinal lacteals after a fatty meal. The ultimate lymphatic trunk, the thoracic duct, carries about three quarters of the total efferent lymph and drains into the left subclavian vein, near its junction with the jugular vein. Smaller cervical and right lymphatic trunks carry lymph from the head, neck and upper right quadrant, and drain into the neck veins. There may also be minor, small lymphovenous communications at more peripheral sites. The brain, uniquely, has no lymphatic system, but has a specialized fluid drainage system (Section 15.4).

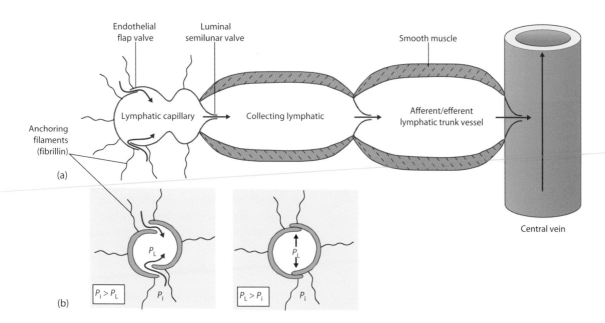

**Figure 11.19** Lymphatic transport mechanisms. **(a)** Interstitial fluid enters the initial lymphatic through the intercellular cleft flap valves down a pressure gradient. Each muscular segment then pumps lymph into the next segment and ultimately into the venous system. **(b)** Proposed operation of initial lymphatic endothelial junctions as flap valves (see text). $P_i$, interstitial pressure; $P_L$, lymph pressure.

## Initial lymphatics may fill by a squeeze–recoil mechanism

The composition of prenodal lymph (water, salts, diluted plasma proteins) shows that it is simply interstitial fluid that has drained into the lymphatic capillaries. The filling mechanism is not certain, but probably resembles that of a Pasteur (rubber teat) pipette. To fill the pipette, one first squeezes the rubber bulb empty (phase 1), then one allows its elastic recoil to suck up fluid (phase 2). Similarly, it is thought that tissue movements compress the initial lymphatic plexus, driving fluid proximally; the intercellular flap valves prevent backflow into the interstitium (phase 1). Then, when the tissue compression ceases, the elastic recoil of the tissue and tethering filaments reduce the intralymphatic pressure below the interstitial fluid pressure. This opens the intercellular flap valves and draws interstitial fluid into the initial lymphatics, re-expanding them (phase 2) (Figure 11.20).

## Lymph flow is coupled to capillary filtration rate

The rate of lymph formation depends on interstitial fluid pressure and volume; the higher they are, the greater the lymph flow, up to a limit (Figure 11.21). Since interstitial fluid

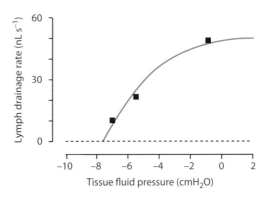

**Figure 11.21** Effect of raising tissue fluid pressure on lymphatic drainage rate from pleural and peritoneal spaces in rabbit. The coupling of lymph drainage to interstitial pressure is essential to prevent fluid accumulation in the extravascular compartment. (Based on data from Miserocchi G, Negrini D, Mukenge P, et al. *Journal of Applied Physiology* 1989; 66(4): 1579–85; and Miserocchi G, Negrini D. In: Crystal RG, et al., eds. *The Lung: Scientific Foundations*. Philadelphia, PA: Lippincott-Raven, 1997, with permission of the American Physiological Society.)

pressure and volume depend on capillary filtration rate, these interstitial parameters couple lymph flow to capillary filtration rate. This coupling is essential, because lymph drainage rate must match capillary filtration rate if oedema is to be avoided.

## Extrinsic and intrinsic mechanisms contribute to lymph flow

Lymph cannot drain passively along the lymphatic system, because the pressure at the venous outlet is higher (~3 mmHg) than in the initial lymphatics (~0). Lymph is therefore pumped. Collecting lymphatics and the more proximal vessels have smooth muscle to pump the lymph along – the intrinsic pump. Initial lymphatics lack smooth muscle in most tissues, so extrinsic pumping is needed here. Because the initial lymphatics are in series with the muscular lymphatics, both intrinsic and extrinsic propulsion are necessary overall.

### Extrinsic propulsion

Flow in the non-contractile lymph vessels is induced by tissue movements, which intermittently compress the lymphatics, for example, skeletal muscle contractions, intestinal peristalsis, pulsation of adjacent arteries. Extrinsic propulsion accounts for the large increase in lymph flow from the leg of an anaesthetized animal when the leg is cycled passively.

### Intrinsic propulsion

Lymphatic contraction was first described by Arnold Ludwig Gotthilf Heller in 1869. Lymphatic vessels with abundant encircling smooth muscle, such as those in the human leg, exhibit spontaneous, rhythmic contractions at ~8–15 cycles per minute (Figure 11.22a). Successive regions, comprising one or more lymphangia, behave like mini-hearts linked in

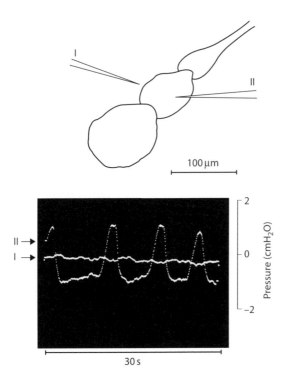

**Figure 11.20** Suction of interstitial fluid into initial lymphatics of bat wing. (**Top**) Micropipettes were inserted into the interstitium and into a contractile lymphatic to record the interstitium-to-lymph pressure gradient. (**Bottom**) Interstitial pressure (I) exceeded lymph pressure (II) for 43% of the time because lymph pressure fell to subatmospheric levels during lymphatic relaxation. (From Hogan RD. In: Hargens AR, ed. *Tissue Fluid Pressure and Composition*. Baltimore, MD: Williams & Wilkins, 1981: 155–63.)

series, and the pumping cycle of each region bears a striking resemblance to the cardiac cycle. Each region has longitudinally running **pacemaker cells**, that trigger local action potentials in the circumferentially orientated smooth muscle, leading to rhythmic contractions. As in the heart, the pacemaker cells express the 'funny' pacemaking current $i_f$ and T-type $Ca^{2+}$ channels. The smooth muscle action potentials are generated by L-type $Ca^{2+}$ channels and fast $Na^+$ channels. As in the cardiac ventricle, a diastolic filling phase, with the distal valve open and the proximal valve closed, is followed by an isovolumetric contraction phase (all valves closed), then an ejection phase (proximal valve open; ejection fraction ~25%) and an isovolumetric relaxation phase (all valves closed). Thus, each contractile segment traces out a pressure–volume loop analogous to that of the ventricle (Figure 11.22b). Human limb lymphatics can pump to 40–50 mmHg against a resistance, an important point when dealing with **envenomation** by a snake or spider bite. To prevent venom transmission by

active lymphatic pumping, the tourniquet pressure needs to be >40–50 mmHg.

## Lymphatic contraction is regulated by filling pressure, sympathetic nerves and vasoactive agents

Lymphatic contractile frequency, and to a lesser degree stroke volume, are increased by **distension**. In this way, a lymphatic segment can increase its output in response to an increased input from a more distal segment. Maximal output occurs at a diastolic filling pressure of ~4–8 $cmH_2O$ in isolated lymphatics; at higher pressures the stroke volume and output begin to fall.

Large lymphatics are innervated by an outer plexus of **sympathetic noradrenergic fibres** and an inner plexus of peptidergic fibres. Sympathetic activity and circulating adrenaline both increase contractile frequency. Following a haemorrhage,

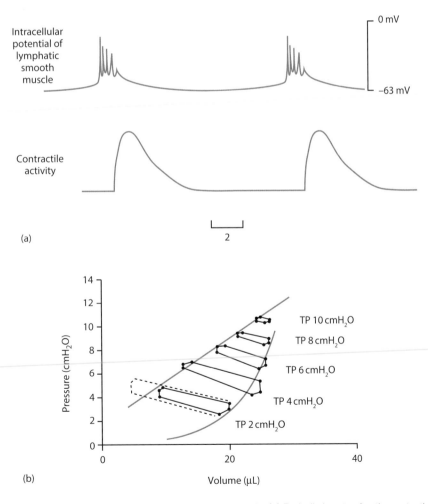

**Figure 11.22** Electrical and contractile properties of lymphatic smooth muscle. **(a)** Periodic bursts of action potentials and contraction in isolated bovine lymphatic trunk. **(b)** Pressure–volume cycle of contracting sheep mesenteric lymphatic vessels at various diastolic distensions. The dashed loop shows increased contractility and ejection fraction after a haemorrhage. Note the analogy with cardiac pressure–volume loops of Figure 6.11b. TP, transmural pressure. (a: From McHale N and colleagues. *Journal of Physiology* 1977; 272: 33P–4P; and *The Journal of Physiology* 1991; 438: 168P, with permission from Wiley-Blackwell. b: From Li B, Silver I, Szalai JP, et al. *Microvascular Research* 1998; 56(2): 127–38, with permission from Elsevier.)

lymphatic contractile frequency rises and ejection fraction increases to ~40%, boosting the transfer of interstitial fluid into the depleted circulation (Figure 11.22b, dashed loop). Substance P, a chemical mediator of inflammation, stimulates lymphatic contraction, whereas nitric oxide (NO) inhibits lymphatic contraction.

## Lymph nodes absorb some lymph: postnodal versus prenodal lymph

The concentration of plasma proteins in postnodal lymph from the legs of dogs and sheep is up to twice that in the prenodal lymph, due mainly to the absorption of water by nodal blood capillaries. Therefore, postnodal lymph composition is unrepresentative of interstitial fluid composition, and postnodal lymph flow underestimates capillary filtration rate. Considering this, our estimate of fluid turnover in humans, based on thoracic duct lymph flow, has been revised upwards (Figure 11.17). However, the exact proportion of afferent lymph that is absorbed in human lymph nodes is unknown, and probably depends on posture, since capillary pressure in the nodes must increase with dependency.

## Lymph flow and composition differs from tissue to tissue

Postnodal lymph flow in the human thoracic duct averages 1–3 L per day, of which the **liver** contributes 30%–50% (Table 11.2). Hepatic lymph is particularly rich in plasma protein, due to the discontinuities in the hepatic capillary endothelium. The **intestine** makes the second greatest contribution to total lymph flow, especially after a meal. **Lung** and **renal** lymph flows are substantial too. The **limbs** contribute a variable quantity of lymph, depending on exercise intensity. The concentration of plasma protein in lymph varies from tissue to tissue; it depends on protein size and charge, capillary permeability, reflection coefficient and capillary filtration rate (Figures 11.8 and 11.23).

The **brain**, unusually, lacks a lymphatic system. Cerebral interstitial fluid is in contact with the cerebrospinal fluid (CSF), which drains into the cerebral venous sinuses through specialized structures called arachnoid granulations. Some

CSF also drains along perineural sheaths around the olfactory nerve, passing through the long cribriform plate to reach lymphatics in the nasal submucosa.

## 11.9 CHALLENGES TO TISSUE FLUID BALANCE: ORTHOSTASIS AND EXERCISE

Two physiological events can increase the capillary filtration rate so much that plasma volume falls. They are orthostasis (upright posture) and physical exercise.

## Orthostasis causes dependent swelling and a fall in plasma volume

During standing/sitting, blood pressure is raised in all the capillaries below heart level (Figure 11.5). This increases their filtration rate, especially in the most dependent (lowermost) tissues. The foot, for example, swells at a rate of ~30 mL/h, driving people to unlace their shoes during long-haul flights or long films. During a 15–40 min period of standing, the increased plasma ultrafiltration into dependent tissues reduces plasma volume by 6%–20%, with a concomitant haemoconcentration and rise in plasma COP. The latter increased from 25 mmHg to 29 mmHg in university students over an 8-h period of sitting in lectures, reading, etc. These changes would be considerably worse, were it not for the following attenuating mechanisms.

### Postural vasoconstriction

Strong precapillary vasoconstriction in dependent tissues raises $R_A/R_V$, which attenuates the increase in capillary pressure (Figure 11.5). Dependent vasoconstriction is a local reaction, mediated by the myogenic response (Section 13.2) and veni-arteriolar response (Section 15.3).

### Local haemoconcentration

Postural vasoconstriction reduces blood flow through the dependent tissues (Figure 8.6), while the increased capillary pressure raises the filtration rate. Together, these changes can greatly increase the filtration fraction, from ~0.1%–0.3% at heart level to 20%–27% in the foot during standing. The resulting local haemoconcentration raises the plasma COP in the venous capillaries to 35–44 mmHg. This attenuates filtration in these vessels, which have a higher $L_p$ than arterial capillaries.

### Reduced capillary filtration capacity

The contraction of some terminal arterioles may stop flow completely through capillary modules for short periods, thereby reducing the capillary filtration capacity. However, the evidence for this in human limbs is conflicting.

**Table 11.2** Postnodal lymph flow and composition in man

|  | Flow (%)[a] | L/P[b] |
|---|---|---|
| Thoracic duct | 1–3 L/day | 0.66–0.69 |
| Liver | 30%–49% | 0.66–0.89 |
| Gastrointestinal | ~37% | 0.50–0.62 |
| Kidneys | 6%–11% | 0.47 |
| Lungs | 3%–15% | 0.66–0.69 |
| Limbs and cervical trunks | <10% | 0.23–0.58 |

*Source:* From Joffey JM, Courtice FC. *Lymphatics, Lymph and the Lymphomyeloid Complex.* London: Academic Press, 1970.
[a] Expressed as percentage of total thoracic duct flow.
[b] Protein concentration in postnodal lymph (L) relative to plasma (P).

## The skeletal muscle pump

Dynamic exercise in the upright position reduces venous pressure in the active limbs (Figure 8.27), which in turn reduces capillary pressure and hence filtration rate. Movement also enhances **lymph transport**.

## Exercise causes muscle swelling and a fall in plasma volume

People working out at the gym notice that intensively exercised skeletal muscles becomes swollen and tense. Likewise, rock-climbers, for reasons not unconnected with their well-being, become keenly aware of swollen, pumped forearm muscles during steep, fingery climbs. A temporary 20% increase in muscle volume is not uncommon. The causes are as follows:

- **Increased interstitial osmolarity** is the main cause of the acute swelling. The contracting muscle fibres release small solutes, such as lactate and $K^+$ ions, which raise the local interstitial fluid osmolarity by 7%–10% (20–30 mmol/L), corresponding to a rise in crystalloid osmotic pressure of 380–580 mmHg (van't Hoff's law). The increased crystalloid osmotic pressure is exerted across endothelial **aquaporin channels**, which are strongly expressed in the continuous capillaries of muscle. Although aquaporin conductance is low, the increase in interstitial osmotic suction is large, so capillary filtration rate increases substantially. Since aquaporins are water-only channels, the $Na^+Cl^-$ concentration rises in the venous blood of active muscle. In addition, muscle sarcoplasm osmolarity increases during exercise, due to phosphocreatine breakdown and lactate formation. Consequently, **intracellular swelling** contributes to the muscle swelling.
- **Vasodilatation** of the resistance vessels in exercising skeletal muscle not only increases blood flow but also reduces $R_A/R_V$. This raises capillary pressure, which contributes to the increased filtration rate (Figure 11.4).
- **Capillary recruitment** in the exercising muscle not only boosts $O_2$ transport but also raises the capillary filtration capacity. This contributes to the increased filtration rate (Figure 10.14).

During prolonged heavy exercise involving multiple, large muscle groups, such as strenuous cycling, net muscle volume can increase by up to 1100 mL and plasma volume falls by ~600 mL (20%). The relative preservation of plasma volume is brought about by a compensatory absorption of interstitial fluid from the non-exercising tissues into the plasma compartment.

Oedema is an excess of interstitial fluid. Clinical oedema can develop in the subcutis (peripheral oedema), lungs (pulmonary oedema), abdominal cavity (ascites) or other body cavities (synovial, pleural and pericardial effusions). Inflammation can cause oedema in almost any tissue.

In **subcutaneous oedema**, the tissue has reached the flat part of the interstitial compliance curve (Figure 11.15); consequently, the addition of more fluid causes little further rise in interstitial fluid pressure to oppose ongoing capillary filtration and volume expansion. The oedema is not usually detected until interstitial volume has doubled, which corresponds to ~10% limb swelling. Peripheral oedema causes discomfort, impaired limb mobility, impaired cell nutrition (due to increased diffusion distance), and may lead to cellulitis, ulceration or blistering (Figure 11.16).

**Pulmonary oedema** is often secondary to left ventricular failure, which raises left ventricular filling pressure and hence pulmonary venous pressure (Section 18.5). The congested, oedematous lungs are difficult to inflate, causing **dyspnoea** (difficulty in breathing). In the most severe cases the interstitial oedema spills over into the alveolar spaces, impairing $O_2$ exchange, with potentially fatal consequences.

## Causes of oedema

Oedema develops when capillary filtration rate exceeds lymphatic drainage rate for a sufficient period. The key relation is:

$$\text{Tissue swelling rate} = \text{Capillary filtration rate} - \text{Lymphatic drainage rate}$$

From this relation we see that oedema can result from a raised capillary filtration rate and/or a low lymph drainage rate. Since capillary filtration is governed by the Starling principle (equation 11.3), the Starling factors allow a logical classification of oedema, as follows.

## Raised capillary pressure, $P_c$

Capillary pressure is elevated when venous pressure is chronically raised, as in the oedema of:

- cardiac failure;
- overtransfusion;
- deep vein thrombosis (DVT);
- dependent tissues, such as the ankles, or the sacral area during recumbency.

Pressures of 20–40 mmHg have been recorded in the venous limbs of skin capillaries at heart level during right ventricular failure (cf. normal 12–15 mmHg). The resulting oedema fluid has a low protein concentration, 1–10 g/L, due to the interstitial dilution relation (Figure 11.8).

## Reduced plasma COP, $\pi_p$

Clinical oedema develops when the plasma protein concentration falls below ~30 g/L, because the fall in plasma COP raises the capillary filtration rate. The oedema fluid again has a low protein

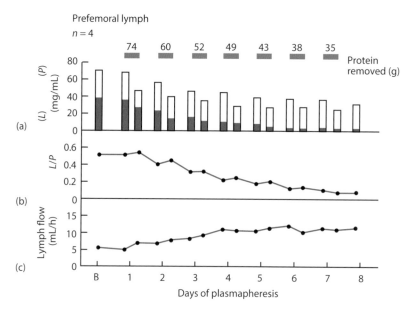

**Figure 11.23** Effect of hypoproteinaemia on fluid exchange. **(a)** Protein was removed from sheep by daily plasmapheresis (removal of blood, reinjection of cells, water and electrolytes). This progressively lowered the plasma protein concentration *P* (top of white bars). **(b)** The protein concentration fell relatively more in postnodal leg lymph (*L*, red bars) than plasma, so the *L/P* ratio declined. **(c)** Lymph flow, a measure of capillary filtration rate in the steady state, more than doubled. Two of the safety factors against oedema are seen operating here: the dilution of interstitial protein (reducing extravascular colloid osmotic pressure, π$_i$); and increased lymphatic drainage rate. (From Kramer G, et al. In: Renkin EM. *American Journal of Physiology* 1986; 250: H706–10, with permission from the American Physiological Society.)

concentration, 1–6 g/L, lowering the interstitial COP. This, along with an increased lymph flow (Figure 11.23), helps to limit the severity of the oedema. The hypoproteinaemia can be caused by:

- malnutrition (inadequate protein intake);
- intestinal disease (malabsorption and protein loss);
- nephrotic syndrome (albumin leakage into urine, >20 g/day, due to a breakdown of the glomerular ultrafilter);
- hepatic failure (failure to synthesize albumin, fibrinogen, α- and β-globulins). Hepatic failure is often caused by alcoholic cirrhosis. The attendant fibrosis raises portal vein pressure, and hence intra-abdominal capillary pressures. As a result, the oedema is predominantly peritoneal (**ascites**).

## Increased capillary permeability ($\uparrow L_p$, $\downarrow \sigma$, $\uparrow P_{protein}$)

In **inflammation**, there is a major breakdown of the capillary barrier, due to the formation of wide gaps and glycocalyx disruption (Figure 10.11). The hydraulic conductance $L_p$ and protein permeability $P_{protein}$ increase and the protein reflection coefficient σ falls. These changes cause severe oedema with a raised protein content, >30 g/L. Section 11.11 describes the signal pathways involved.

## Lymphatic insufficiency

Lymph is the only way of returning escaped plasma proteins to the circulation, so an impairment of lymphatic drainage causes both water and plasma proteins to accumulate in the

interstitium. Lymphoedema is thus characterized by a protein content of >30 g/L. Chronic lymphoedema provokes the gradual deposition of a fibrous, adipose tissue in the interstitium, as a result of which long-standing lymphoedema may not pit easily ('brawny' non-pitting oedema). In Western countries, the most common cause of lymphatic insufficiency is damage to the lymph nodes during **cancer** surgery and radiotherapy (Figure 11.24). The rarer **hereditary lymphoedemas** are due to inadequate limb lymphatic development, as in **Milroy's disease** and **lymphoedema-distichiasis** (see earlier). The most common cause of lymphoedema worldwide is **filariasis**, a nematode worm infestation transmitted by mosquitoes. The nematodes impair lymphatic function in the limbs and scrotum, causing a gross lymphoedema associated with hyperkeratotic, elephant-like skin (**elephantiasis**).

## Oedema only develops when a 'safety margin' is exceeded

Clinicians have long recognized that oedema does not appear until the plasma COP or venous pressure has changed adversely by ~15 mmHg. There is thus a 15 mmHg margin of safety against oedema. The safety margin is attributed to three factors that 'buffer' the capillary filtration rate, namely, a fall in extravascular COP, rise in interstitial fluid pressure and rise in lymph flow as filtration rate increases (Figure 11.25).

## Fall in extravascular colloid osmotic pressure

A rise in capillary filtration rate reduces the extravascular plasma protein concentration (Figures 11.8 and 11.23) and

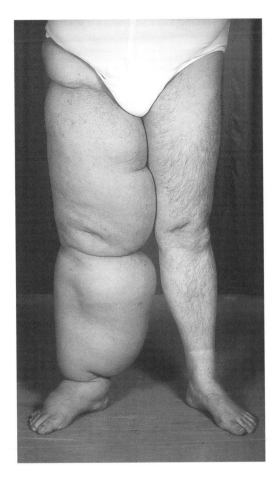

**Figure 11.24** Lymphoedema caused by surgery to treat testicular cancer. (Courtesy of Professor P Mortimer, Department of Dermatology, St. George's Hospital, London.)

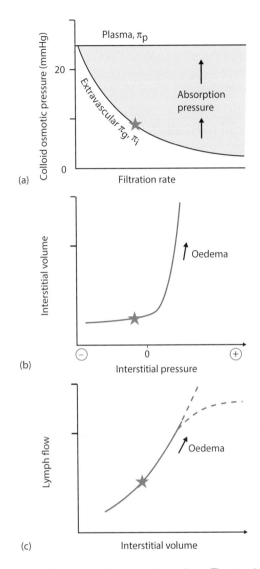

**Figure 11.25** Three safety factors against oedema. The stars indicate normal state. **(a)** When capillary filtration rate increases, the colloid osmotic pressure difference opposing filtration, $(\pi_p - \pi_g)$, increases because extravascular plasma protein concentration falls in the interstitial and subglycocalyx compartments. **(b)** Interstitial fluid pressure changes markedly with hydration in normal subcutis. However, once oedema develops, interstitial compliance becomes very large, so there is little further rise in the supra-atmospheric pressure. (NB: This is Figure 11.15 turned on its side.) **(c)** Lymphatic drainage rate increases with increasing interstitial hydration, thereby opposing oedema formation. The dashed lines indicate that lymph flow reaches a limit in stationary tissue, but perhaps not in moved limbs. (After Taylor AE, Townsley MI. *News in Physiological Science* 1987; 2: 48–52, with permission from the American Physiological Society.)

opposes the diffusion of extravascular plasma protein up the intercellular cleft into the subglycocalyx space (Figure 11.14). Consequently, the subglycocalyx COP $\pi_g$ falls and the absorptive force $\pi_p - \pi_g$ rises (Figure 11.25a). This attenuates the capillary filtration rate. This buffering mechanism is most effective in tissues with normally high extravascular protein concentrations, such as the lung ($\pi_i \geq 18$ mmHg).

## Rise in interstitial fluid pressure

In normally hydrated tissue, a small rise in interstitial volume causes a relatively large rise in interstitial pressure (Figures 11.15 and 11.25b). This reduces the pressure drop across the capillary wall, $P_c - P_i$. If $P_i$ is normally −2 mmHg and clinical oedema becomes apparent at around +1 mmHg, the change in $P_i$ provides a safety margin of 3 mmHg. In oedematous interstitium, by contrast, large volumes of capillary filtrate can accumulate with little further rise in the opposing pressure $P_i$.

## Rise in lymph flow

Lymphatic drainage rate increases as interstitial pressure and volume increase, helping prevent oedema formation (Figures 11.21, 11.23 and 11.25c). For example, lymph flow increases 20-fold in response to a 30-mmHg elevation of

venous pressure in the cat intestine. However, there comes a point at which lymph flow cannot keep pace with capillary filtration, and oedema then develops.

## 11.11 THE SWELLING OF INFLAMMATION

The six definitive characteristics of inflammation are tissue swelling, redness, heat, pain, loss of function and leukocyte migration. The swelling is caused by a protein-rich

213

oedema, which can form very rapidly. Examples include blisters, rashes, swollen joints, pleural, pericardial and peritoneal effusions and cerebral oedema. The key change precipitating the swelling is the formation of gaps in the endothelial barrier, as follows.

## Chemical mediators initiate gap formation in venules

When a tissue is damaged, whether by trauma, infection, ischaemia or allergy, numerous pro-inflammatory chemicals are released by the tissue cells. These agents include histamine, bradykinin, prostaglandins, serotonin, thrombin, substance P, platelet-activating factor (PAF), superoxide radicals, leukotrienes and cytokines. The cytokines interleukin-1β (IL-1β) and tumour necrosis factor α (TNFα) are pro-inflammatory agents secreted by monocytes/macrophages, fibroblasts and endothelial cells, and they induce leukocyte adhesion and migration (Figure 9.12).

Most chemical mediators of inflammation act primarily on receptors expressed by the **postcapillary venule** to cause **endothelial gap formation** (Figures 11.26 and 11.27). The endothelial gaps create holes in the normally continuous glycocalyx, disrupting the semipermeable barrier. Consequently, water and plasma proteins leak out rapidly into the tissue (Figure 11.28). The greater the inflammatory stimulus, the greater the number of the leakage spots. In ischaemia–reperfusion injury (Section 6.12), glycocalyx damage may possibly raise permeability without gap formation. A common pharmacological test for inflammation, the **skin blueing test**, is based on the raised protein permeability. The dye Evans blue is injected into the plasma of a rat. Little escapes into normal skin because the dye binds to circulating plasma albumin; however, if an inflammatory

agent is injected into the skin, the dye-albumin complex leaks out, producing a blue skin patch.

The inflammatory response to an agonist often shows two phases. Over the first 10–30 min there is a large but transient rise in permeability, which then decays (Figures 11.26 and 11.28). This is followed by a second, more sustained increase lasting hours. Histamine, serotonin and bradykinin cause only a transient rise in permeability, whereas thrombin and VEGF cause more prolonged rises.

## The extravasated fluid has a high fibrinogen content

Due to the barrier breakdown, inflammatory oedema has a high plasma protein concentration (≥30 g/L). This is termed an **exudate**, to distinguish it from the low-protein oedema, or **transudate**, of cardiac failure, venous thrombosis, etc. (≤15 g/L). One of the exuded proteins is **fibrinogen**. The formation of extravascular, insoluble fibrin clots can lead to serious complications, such as intestinal adhesions following peritonitis or abdominal surgery.

## Net filtration force and permeability both increase

Exudation is rapid and severe because the chemical agonists alter almost every factor in the Starling principle (equations 11.3 and 11.5).

### Capillary pressure, $P_c$

Many inflammatory agonists cause arteriolar vasodilatation, leading to the characteristic **redness** and **heat** of inflamed tissue. The vasodilatation reduces $R_A/R_V$, which raises capillary filtration pressure (Figure 11.4).

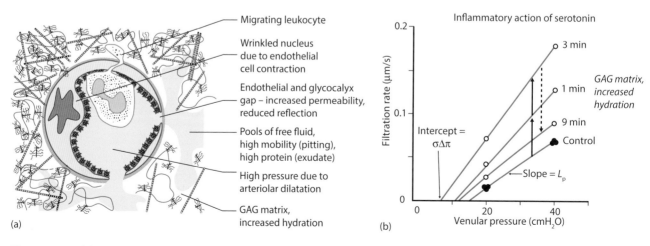

**Figure 11.26 (a)** Gap formation, oedema and leukocyte migration in an acutely inflamed, postcapillary venule. **(b)** Effect of an inflammatory agonist, serotonin, on permeability of a single venule (rat). Hydraulic permeability increases (slope, $L_p$) and osmotic reflection coefficient decreases (intercept at zero filtration, $\sigma\Delta\pi$). Although serotonin was infused continuously, the hyperpermeability was transient and returned towards baseline by 9 min. GAG, glycosaminoglycan. (Adapted from Michel CC, Kendall S. *The Journal of Physiology* 1997; 501(Pt 3): 657–62, with permission from Wiley-Blackwell.)

## Interstitial fluid pressure, $P_i$

In established swelling, $P_i$ is increased to ~2 mmHg, and serves as a minor check on filtration. However, at the onset of the inflammation in skin and submucosa, $P_i$ falls transiently to a more subatmospheric level, before rising as oedema accumulates. This curious effect is mediated by fibroblasts. Normally, fibroblasts slightly tense the surrounding collagen fibrils, to which they adhere through transmembrane $\alpha_2\beta_1$-integrins. The collagen tension slightly compresses the interstitial matrix, reducing its swelling tendency (Section 11.5). Release of the fibroblast's gel-compressing bonds at the onset of inflammation lowers $P_i$ by several mmHg, which in turn enhances the initial swelling rate. In **burns**, $P_i$ can fall more dramatically, to −30 mmHg transiently, so plasma extravasation is very rapid in burn injuries. The large suction force is attributed to the denaturation of collagen by heat to gelatin, which is water-soluble and has a large swelling pressure.

## Extravascular osmotic pressure, $\pi_i$, $\pi_g$

Interstitial protein concentration increases as plasma proteins leak out through the endothelial gaps. This reduces the difference in COP across the capillary wall and thus increases the filtration rate.

## Osmotic reflection coefficient, $\sigma$

The residual difference in COP across the endothelium itself becomes less effective, because $\sigma$ is reduced to ~0.4 by the impairment of the glycocalyx barrier. The fall in $\sigma$ is evident from the leftward shift of the intercept in the filtration rate versus pressure plot (Figure 11.26), and from the outpouring of plasma macromolecules (Figure 11.28).

## Hydraulic conductance of the wall, $L_p$

The changes in $P_c$, $P_i$, $\pi_i$ and $\sigma$ greatly increase the net filtration force across the venules (term inside the square brackets in equations 11.3 and 11.5). The effect of the increased filtration force is amplified many times by the increase in wall hydraulic conductance caused by gap formation. $L_p$ can increase around sevenfold. The increase in $L_p$ is evident from the increase in slope of the filtration rate versus pressure plot (Figure 11.26).

The net effect of these five changes is a 50–100-fold rise in fluid extravasation rate. This rapid leakage, along with flow obstruction by marginating leukocytes (Section 9.8), can lead to plugging of the microvessels by packed columns of red cells (**stasis**).

## Endothelial gaps can be intercellular or transcellular

During inflammation, gaps up to 1 μm wide form in the endothelial lining of the postcapillary venules, with accompanying breaks in the glycocalyx layer. The venular gaps can be **intercellular**, resulting from a separation of the junction between two endothelial cells, or **transcellular**, resulting from the formation of a hole directly through the endothelial cell, close to but not through the intercellular junction (Figure 11.27). Histamine, serotonin, substance P and PAF induce mainly intercellular gaps, whereas VEGF, heat injury, pressure overload, psoriasis and encephalomyelitis induce relatively more transendothelial gaps.

## A biochemical cascade leads to gap formation

Inflammatory mediators, such as histamine, bradykinin, serotonin and thrombin, trigger multiple signalling pathways that lead to cytoskeletal reorganization and gap formation. Different mediators may trigger different pathways. Many mediators, such as histamine, act via an NO pathway; however, bradykinin may act via reactive $O_2$ species. The signal pathway leads to loosening of the intercellular junctions and endothelial cell contraction, as described next.

## Increased cytosolic $Ca^{2+}$ is an early step in the signal cascade

Agonists, such as histamine, activate their cognate endothelial receptor, which is coupled by Gq-protein to phospholipase C. The latter generates two chemical messengers, inositol 1,4,5 trisphosphate ($IP_3$) and diacylglycerol (DAG). $IP_3$ releases the endothelial $Ca^{2+}$ store and triggers **store-operated $Ca^{2+}$ channels** (SOCs) (Figure 9.7). DAG activates **receptor-operated $Ca^{2+}$ channels** (ROCs). Consequently, extracellular $Ca^{2+}$ passes into the cell, raising its cytosolic $Ca^{2+}$ concentration four- to tenfold within a minute (Figure 11.29). DAG also activates **protein kinase C**, which activates a mitogen-activated protein kinase cascade implicated in some inflammatory responses (Figure 11.30). The **extracellular $Ca^{2+}$ influx is obligatory for the inflammatory response**; if it is reduced, the change in hydraulic conductance is likewise reduced (Figure 11.29). But the rise in $Ca^{2+}$ does not directly initiate

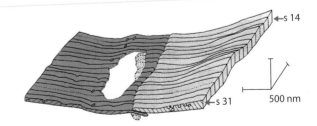

**Figure 11.27** Three-dimensional reconstruction of an inflammatory gap in frog endothelium, induced by mild heat injury. The gap is transcellular; it passes through the cell on the left, close to but separate from the intercellular junction. Part of an underlying third cell is visible through the gap (stippled grey). (Based on 18 serial electron micrograph sections by Neale CR, Michel CC, with permission from Wiley-Blackwell.)

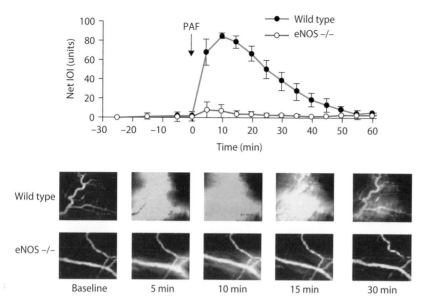

Figure 11.28 Hyperpermeability of venules in cremaster muscle induced by inflammatory agonist platelet-activating factor (PAF), applied for 3 min in wild-type mice. Intravenous fluorescein-labelled dextran (77 000 Da) leaked out rapidly following inflammation, as shown by the integrated optical intensity (IOI) of the images. In endothelial nitric oxide synthase (eNOS –/–) knockout mice, the hyperpermeability response was greatly reduced, demonstrating the obligatory role of NO in the inflammation signalling pathway. (From Hatakeyama T, Pappas PJ, Hobson RW 2nd, et al. *The Journal of Physiology* 2006; 574(Pt 1): 275–81, with permission from Wiley-Blackwell.)

gap formation, since $Ca^{2+}$ still increases when NO production is blocked, yet permeability hardly changes (Figure 11.28). Therefore, $Ca^{2+}$ must act by stimulating NO formation.

## Nitric oxide, cGMP and cAMP continue the signal cascade

The increased cytosolic $Ca^{2+}$ raises the $Ca^{2+}$-calmodulin level, which stimulates endothelial NO synthase activity (Section 9.4). Although small amounts of NO can lower permeability (by scavenging toxic $O_2$ radicals), **high levels of NO are pro-inflammatory** (Figure 11.28). NO activates soluble guanylyl cyclase, which produces cyclic guanosine monophosphate (cGMP). **cGMP is a permeability-raising messenger** that activates phosphodiesterase 2 (PDE2) (Figure 11.30). Because PDE2 is more abundant in venular than arterial endothelium, this helps localize the inflammatory response to venules. PDE2 degrades cyclic adenosine monophosphate **(cAMP), an anti-inflammatory, barrier-enhancing messenger**, so a fall in cAMP raises permeability. Conversely, cAMP-raising agonists, such as the β adrenergic receptor agonists isoprenaline and terbutaline, attenuate gap formation and inflammation. The anti-inflammatory action of cAMP is mediated by two pathways: (1) cAMP activates protein kinase A (PKA), which inhibits myosin contraction (Section 9.7); (2) cAMP activates the factor exchange protein directly activated by cAMP 1 (EPAC1), which activates pathways that stabilize the junctional strands and actin cytoskeleton. A fall in cAMP therefore favours gap formation by **loosening the intercellular junction** and by **endothelial contraction** (retraction). In intact venules, junction loosening seems the more important factor because inhibitors of myosin light chain kinase, a key initiator of contraction, do not block the inflammatory response. By contrast, active contraction is important in cultured endothelial cells, a much used but potentially misleading research 'model'.

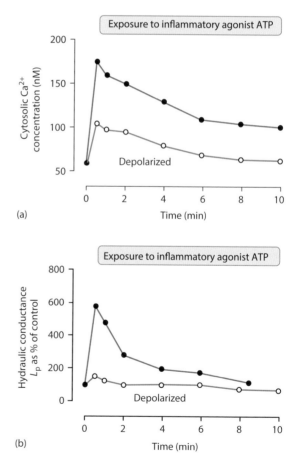

(a)

(b)

Figure 11.29 Parallel changes in free cytosolic $Ca^{2+}$ **(a)** and hydraulic permeability **(b)** during the inflammatory response of frog venule to inflammatory agonist adenosine triphosphate (ATP). ATP was used because frogs do not respond to mammalian agonists such as histamine. Endothelial depolarization by a high $K^+$ solution (open symbols) reduced the $Ca^{2+}$ transient and conductance changes in parallel (see text). (Redrawn from work of He P, Zhang X, Curry FE. *American Journal of Physiology* 1996; 271(6 Pt 2): H2377–87 with permission from the American Physiological Society.)

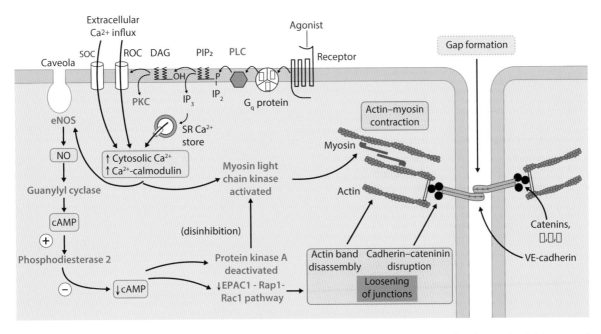

**Figure 11.30** Simplified summary of signal transduction cascade leading to endothelial gap formation in inflammation. Major second messengers are in the grey boxes, enzymes in red. cAMP, cyclic adenosine monophosphate; cGMP, cyclic guanosine monophosphate; DAG, diacylglycerol; eNOS, endothelial nitric oxide synthase; EPAC1, exchange protein directly activated by cAMP 1; $IP_3$, inositol trisphosphate; NO, nitric oxide; $PIP_2$, phosphatidylinositol bisphosphate; PKC, protein kinase C (this activates a mitogen-activated protein kinase cascade [not shown] implicated in some inflammatory responses); PLC, phospholipase C; Ras-related protein Rap-1A (Rap1) and Ras-related C3 botulinum toxin substrate 1 (Rac1) are small GTPases that promote cortical actin stability; ROC, receptor-operated $Ca^{2+}$ channel; SR, sarcoplasmic reticulum; SOC, store-operated $Ca^{2+}$ channel.

## Intercellular junctions are loosened by junctional protein redistribution

Intercellular gaps form when the key transmembrane protein, vascular endothelial cadherin (**VE-cadherin**), diffuses away from the junction (Figure 9.3). The duration of a VE-cadherin bond is only about half a second, so cadherins can dissipate quickly by lateral diffusion in the cell membrane. This is normally prevented by their attachment to catenins, which in turn are held in place by the actin cytoskeleton. During inflammation **fragmentation of the anchoring peripheral F-actin band**, along with **altered phosphorylation of VE-cadherin and β-catenin**, weakens the junction, facilitating its separation. A fall in cAMP and EPAC1 activity appears to mediate the changes in F-actin and junctional proteins.

## Endothelial cell contraction may contribute to gap formation

Endothelial contraction was originally inferred from the nuclear wrinkling seen in inflamed venules, and it certainly occurs in inflamed, cultured endothelial cells. The contractile process is unlike that in the heart, and resembles that in smooth muscle (Chapter 12). The rise in endothelial $Ca^{2+}$-calmodulin activates **myosin light chain kinase** (MLCK), which activates actin-myosin contraction. Since MLCK is inhibited by cAMP-activated PKA, the fall in cAMP during inflammation may increase the tension on the weakened junction (Figure 11.30).

**Transcellular gaps** are thought to arise from a thinning of the cell, brought about by actin-myosin contraction. As the cell thins, vacuoles and vesicles fuse across the cell to form fenestrations, transcellular gaps and breaks in the glycocalyx.

## Cytokines, VEGF and leukocytes mediate longer-lasting hyperpermeability

The preceding account describes acute inflammation. In chronically inflamed tissue, such as rheumatoid arthritis, psoriasis and cancer, microvascular permeability is raised for months or years, sustained by continuous **cytokine** production. Chronic hyperpermeability is mediated partly by **VEGF**, which used to be called 'vascular permeability factor'. **Leukocytes** also contribute to chronic inflammation. Leukocyte migration through the endothelium (Section 9.8) does not in itself raise permeability because the endothelium reseals quickly behind the migrating leukocyte; however, activated leukocytes raise permeability by releasing pro-inflammatory agents, such as the potent leukotrienes and PAF (Section 13.5). Other leukocyte products, such as superoxide anions, hydrogen peroxide and elastase (a potent protease), damage the endothelium directly and increase its permeability.

**Steroids** (glucocorticoids) are often used to suppress chronic inflammatory states, such as rheumatoid arthritis. Steroids suppress leukocyte migration, cytokine production, gap formation and vasodilatation.

## SUMMARY

- The transcapillary filtration of ~4–8 L/day (humans) affects plasma and interstitial fluid volumes, and washes escaped plasma proteins and antigens into the lymphatic system. The filtration fraction is low in continuous capillaries (0.1%–0.3%) but high in fenestrated capillaries (renal glomerulus 20%).

- The capillary wall is coated internally by a **semipermeable membrane, the glycocalyx**, which overlies the intercellular clefts and fenestrae. The glycocalyx reflects the plasma proteins, which therefore exert a COP. The **Starling principle** states that the filtration rate, per unit surface area, equals the hydraulic conductance of the wall, $L_p$, multiplied by the sum of the pressures acting on the wall, namely the hydraulic pressure drop across the wall [capillary blood pressure $P_c$ – interstitial fluid pressure $P_i$], minus the effective COP difference, $\sigma \times$ [plasma COP $\pi_p$ – interstitial COP $\pi_i$ (or more accurately subglycocalyx COP, $\pi_g$)]. The protein reflection coefficient $\sigma$ is 0.8–0.95.

- **Human capillary pressure** $P_c$ is ~35 mmHg at the inlet, falling to ~12 mmHg at the outlet (heart level). $P_c$ depends on arterial pressure, venous pressure and precapillary, arteriolar resistance, which is under sympathetic nervous control. Gravity increases capillary pressure greatly in dependent tissues (ankles, sacral region), which are therefore prone to oedema.

- **Human plasma COP** $\pi_p$ is 21–29 mmHg. Albumin contributes disproportionately, due to $Na^+$ ions attracted by its net negative charge (Gibbs–Donnan distribution).

- **Interstitial COP** $\pi_i$ is typically about one third of plasma COP, due to escaped plasma proteins. Interstitial protein concentration and $\pi_i$ are not fixed quantities. They fall as filtration rate increases, thereby attenuating the filtration rate. Conversely, when interstitial fluid is absorbed by capillaries after a haemorrhage, $\pi_i$ and subglycocalyx $\pi_g$ rise and eventually halt the absorption process.

- **Interstitial fluid pressure** $P_i$ is slightly subatmospheric in many tissues. $P_i$ increases to ~2 mmHg in oedema. Interstitial fluid mobility is normally low, due to interstitial GAG chains. In oedema, GAG dilution results in a high mobility (clinical pitting test). The $P_i$ versus hydration curve (compliance curve) is steep at physiological hydrations, but flat in the oedema range.

- The Starling pressures generally cause **filtration**, even in postcapillary venules, contrary to traditional teaching. If capillary pressure is reduced, by hypovolaemia or precapillary vasoconstriction, capillaries **absorb** interstitial fluid transiently; however, absorption tails off as $\pi_i$ and $\pi_g$ rise and $P_i$ falls.

- Absorption is only sustained in tissues where the interstitium is flushed by an independent stream of liquid (intestinal mucosa during water absorption; renal peritubular capillaries; lymph nodes).

- In **orthostasis**, capillary pressure is high in the dependent tissues, so filtration rate increases and plasma volume falls. **Exercise** also reduces plasma volume because interstitial crystalloids released by the active muscle fibres (lactate, $K^+$) exert osmotic pressure across endothelial, water-only aquaporin channels, promoting filtration into the active muscle.

- **The lymphatic system** preserves tissue volume homeostasis by returning escaped plasma proteins and fluid to the circulation. Flow in the non-contractile initial lymphatics is driven by extrinsic compression, whereas the contractile main lymphatic vessels pump lymph actively. Pumping is enhanced by distension and sympathetic activity. Some lymph can be reabsorbed by blood capillaries in the lymph nodes. The rest drains via efferent lymph trunks (chiefly the thoracic duct) into neck veins. Impaired lymph transport, whether hereditary, post-surgical or infective (filariasis), results in high-protein **lymphoedema**.

- **Clinical oedema** develops when the capillary filtration rate exceeds the lymphatic drainage rate. Increased capillary filtration can cause a low-protein oedema (transudate, <15 g/L) following capillary pressure elevation (dependent oedema, cardiac failure, DVT); or plasma COP reductions (malnutrition, intestinal disease, hepatic failure, nephrotic syndrome); or a high-protein oedema (exudates, >30 g/L) following inflammation.

- **Inflammatory swelling** is caused by increases in venular permeability to water and plasma proteins ($\uparrow L_p$, $\downarrow \sigma$). Also, net filtration force is increased by vasodilatation ($\uparrow P_c$), an initial dip in interstitial pressure ($\downarrow P_i$, especially in burns) and plasma protein leakage ($\uparrow \pi_i$, $\pi_g$).

- The inflammatory hyperpermeability is due to the formation of intercellular and transcellular **gaps** in the venular endothelium and glycocalyx. Inflammatory mediators, such as histamine, bradykinin and thrombin, raise endothelial **cytosolic $Ca^{2+}$**, which activates a pathway involving NO, cGMP and cAMP. This leads to gap formation by loosening intercellular junctions, possibly aided by endothelial cell contraction. Also, the cytokines IL-1β and TNFα initiate **leukocyte** margination and emigration. The activated leukocytes release endothelium- and glycocalyx-damaging agents, such as free $O_2$ radicals and proteases.

## FURTHER READING

Jacob M, Chappell D, Becker BF. Regulation of blood flow and volume exchange across the microcirculation. *Critical Care* 2016; **20**(1): 319.

Tarbell JM, Cancel LM. The glycocalyx and its significance in human medicine. *Journal of Internal Medicine* 2016; **280**(1): 97–113.

Levick JR, Michel CC. Microvascular fluid exchange and the revised Starling principle. *Cardiovascular Research* 2010; **87**(2): 198–210.

Reed RK, Rubin K. Transcapillary exchange: role and importance of the interstitial fluid pressure and the extracellular matrix. *Cardiovascular Research* 2010; **87**(2): 211–17.

Alitalo K, Tammela T, Petrova T. Lymphangiogenesis in development and human disease. *Nature* 2005; **438**(7070): 946–53.

Aukland K. Arnold Heller and the lymph pump. *Acta Physiologica Scandinavica* 2005; **185**(3): 171–80.

Curry FR. Microvascular solute and water transport. *Microcirculation* 2005; **12**(1): 17–31.

Zawieja D. Lymphatic biology and the microcirculation: past, present and future. *Microcirculation* 2005; **12**(1): 141–50.

Wiig H, Rubin K, Reed RK. New and active role of the interstitium in control of interstitial fluid pressure: potential therapeutic consequences. *Acta Anaesthesiologica Scandinavica* 2003; **47**(2): 111–21.

Michel CC. Starling: the formulation of his hypothesis of microvascular fluid exchange and its significance after 100 years. *Experimental Physiology* 1997; **82**(1): 1–30.

Sabolic I, Brown D. Water channels in renal and nonrenal tissues. *News in Physiological Sciences* 1995; **10**(1): 12–17.

Aukland K. Why don't our feet swell in the upright position? *News in Physiological Sciences* 1994; **9**(5): 214–19.

Varani J, Ward PA. Mechanisms of neutrophil-dependent and neutrophil-independent endothelial cell injury. *Biological Signals* 1994; **3**(1): 1–14.

Aukland K, Reed RK. Interstitial-lymphatic mechanisms in the control of extracellular volume. *Physiological Reviews* 1993; **73**(1): 1–78.

Levick JR. Flow through interstitium and other fibrous matrices. *Quarterly Journal of Experimental Physiology* 1987; **72**(4): 409–37.

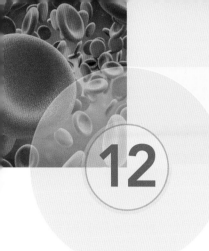

# 12

# Vascular smooth muscle: excitation, contraction and relaxation

## LEARNING OBJECTIVES

*After reading this chapter you should be able to:*

- outline the ultrastructural basis of vascular contraction (12.2);
- contrast contraction in vascular and cardiac myocytes (12.1, 12.3);
- outline the roles of $Ca^{2+}$, $K^+$ and $Cl^-$ channels in vascular tone regulation (12.4);
- state the roles of myosin light-chain kinase (MLCK), myosin light-chain phosphatase (MLCP), phospholipase C (PLC),

inositol 1,4,5 trisphosphate ($IP_3$) and diacylglycerol (DAG) in excitation-contraction coupling (12.3, 12.5);
- explain the difference between depolarization-dependent and depolarization-independent contraction (12.5);
- state the role and mechanism of $Ca^{2+}$-sensitization during tonic contraction (12.5);
- explain how sympathetic nerve activity evokes vasoconstriction (12.5);
- outline four mechanisms mediating vasodilatation (12.7).

## 12.1 OVERVIEW

The tunica media (middle coat) of arteries, arterioles, venules and veins consists mainly of vascular smooth muscle (VSM) cells (vascular myocytes). These are small, spindle-shaped cells, varying in length from ~70–200 μm long by ~4 μm wide at the centre and wrapped helically around the vessel (Figure 1.11). Changes in their contractile tension (tone) cause the vessel to constrict or dilate as required. There are substantial differences in the way contraction is regulated in different blood vessels, making this a tricky subject for teacher and student alike. Nevertheless, two principles apply to nearly all vessels: (1) **contractile tension is governed primarily by cytosolic $Ca^{2+}$ concentration**; and (2) **contractile tension is also regulated by changes in sensitivity to $Ca^{2+}$**. Other key features, often contrasting sharply with cardiac contraction, are as follows.

## Membrane depolarization may or may not initiate VSM contraction

Most blood vessels do not normally generate action or spike potentials, due to powerful membrane stabilization by myocyte $K^+$ channel activity (cf. heart and skeletal muscle). Depending on the vessel, three types of activation can be discerned:

1. Most commonly, vascular myocytes may show a graded, sustained depolarization on activation, but no action potential generation. This causes a graded, sustained contraction (Figure 12.1).
2. In some vessels, vascular myocytes fire action potentials on top of the underlying depolarized state. This evokes transient increments of the underlying contractile tension (Figures 12.2a,b).

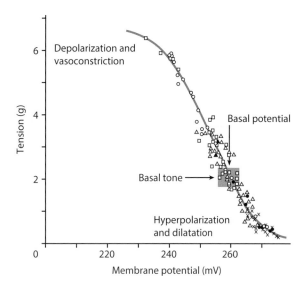

**Figure 12.1** Dependence of contractile tone on membrane potential in isolated canine carotid artery. Membrane potential was altered by extracellular $H^+$ ($\triangle$), extracellular $K^+$ ($\square$), extracellular $Ca^{2+}$ ($\bullet$), noradrenaline ($\bigcirc$) and hypoxia ($\times$). The highlighted box indicates the membrane potential and tone in the 'resting', basal state. (Data from Siegel G, et al. *Journal of Vascular Medicine and Biology* 1991; 3: 140–9.)

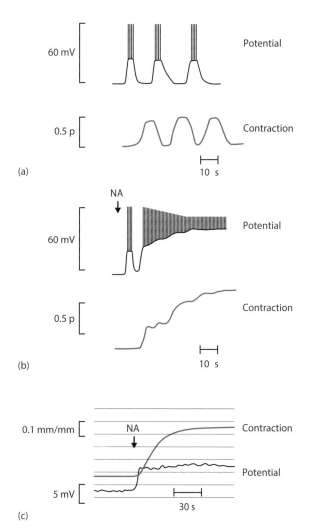

3. In large vessels, contraction is often induced by intracellular, biochemical signalling, with little change in membrane potential; any associated change in membrane potential is secondary, and not the cause of myocyte contraction (Figure 12.2c).

Patterns (1) and (2) have been called **electromechanical coupling**, while pattern (3) is **pharmacomechanical coupling**.

## Myosin activation causes contraction

Cardiac contraction occurs when $Ca^{2+}$ binds to troponin on the actin filament. VSM lacks troponin and contraction is brought about primarily by the activation of the myosin filament. The VSM myosin isoform is activated by a phosphorylating enzyme, **myosin light chain kinase (MLCK)**, which is itself activated when cytosolic $Ca^{2+}$ rises.

## Active tension (tone) is regulated not only by $Ca^{2+}$ concentration but also by $Ca^{2+}$ sensitivity

In the heart, an agonist such as adrenaline increases contractile force by increasing the cytosolic $Ca^{2+}$ concentration. In VSM, agonists can increase contractile force by increasing $[Ca^{2+}]$ and by increasing the sensitivity of the contractile apparatus to $Ca^{2+}$.

## Contraction duration can be very long

A cardiac contraction lasts ~300 ms, whereas many blood vessels are in a partially contracted state, called **basal tone** throughout life. In the smallest arteries, basal tone is spontaneous and referred to as **myogenic tone**. Vascular dilatation results from a reduction in the tone, vascular constriction from an increase in the tone.

To understand these features, we must consider the structure of VSM and its varied expression of ion channels and signal pathways. To avoid undue repetition, it is assumed that the reader is familiar with the electrophysiology basics introduced in Chapter 3.

**Figure 12.2** Diverse characteristics of vascular smooth muscle. **(a)** (Upper trace) Membrane potential in spontaneously active portal vein of guinea pig, showing automaticity. Regular, slow depolarizations trigger bursts of action potentials. (Lower trace) Contractions followed the membrane depolarization (p is tension). **(b)** Response of portal vein to noradrenaline (NA), showing further depolarization-dependent contraction. **(c)** Contrasting response of sheep carotid artery to noradrenaline. There are no action potentials and the sustained contraction is not dependent on the slight accompanying depolarization (depolarization-independent contraction). (a, b: From Golenhofen K, Hermstein N, Lammel E. *Microvascular Research* 1973; 5(1): 73–80, with permission from Elsevier; c: From Keatinge WR, Harman MC. *Local Mechanisms Controlling Blood Vessels*. London: Academic Press, 1980, by permission.)

## 12.2 STRUCTURE OF A VASCULAR MYOCYTE

### Actin and myosin filaments form the contractile machinery

As in the heart, contraction depends on crossbridge formation between thick myosin filaments (2.2 μm × 0.315 μm) and overlapping, parallel thin actin filaments (1.5 μm × 0.037 μm) (Figure 12.3). However, the similarities end here. The smooth muscle thin filament is longer than in cardiac muscle, allowing greater shortening, and it lacks troponin, the cardiac $Ca^{2+}$-dependent regulatory protein. Troponin is replaced by the proteins caldesmon and calponin on VSM thin filaments. The myosin also differs from that in the heart, and only participates in contraction when **phosphorylated**, that is, when phosphate groups are added to it, by the enzyme **MLCK**. Therefore, VSM contraction depends primarily on thick-filament rather than thin-filament activation.

VSM lacks the Z lines that align the filaments in a cardiac myocyte. Instead, the actin filaments are rooted in **dense bands** on the inner cell membrane and in **dense bodies** in the cytoplasm. These structures are composed of α-actinin, the protein forming the cardiac Z lines. The dense bodies are not aligned across the cell, so VSM lacks the striated appearance of cardiac and skeletal muscle. A third kind of filament, the intermediate filament (meaning intermediate in thickness) acts as a cytoskeletal element; it links the various dense bodies and dense bands, so that the entire cell contracts as a single unit. Vascular intermediate filaments are composed mainly of the proteins desmin and vimentin.

### The VSM sarcoplasmic reticulum is a $Ca^{2+}$ store with two kinds of $Ca^{2+}$ release channel

The VSM smooth endoplasmic reticulum, or sarcoplasmic reticulum (SR), contains a releasable store of $Ca^{2+}$ ions. In VSM, the SR is relatively poorly developed (1%–4% of the cell volume), and the $Ca^{2+}$ store is not very big, especially in small resistance vessels. The proximity of the SR to the cell membrane (sarcolemma), ~15 nm in places, and the presence of multiple invaginations or caveolae favours the formation of signalling clusters or domains. These factors facilitate store release of $Ca^{2+}$ by agonists such as noradrenaline. The limited store in resistance vessels means that tonic vasoconstriction requires extracellular $Ca^{2+}$ influx, as well as store release, and this is mainly due to influx through voltage-dependent $Ca^{2+}$ channels (VDCC) associated with caveolae, and present in larger numbers in VSM of resistance vessels compared with larger vessels. This explains why $Ca^{2+}$ channel blockers, such as nifedipine, are good resistance vessel dilators. Release from the SR $Ca^{2+}$ store is due to a soluble factor, inositol 1,4,5 trisphosphate ($IP_3$), formed when vasoconstrictor agonists like noradrenaline bind to their membrane receptors. SR $IP_3$ receptors are linked to $Ca^{2+}$ release channels (**$IP_3$-$Ca^{2+}$ release channels**) that form part of their structure. Release is enhanced by $IP_3$ in a random, 'all or nothing' (stochastic) manner and referred to as a $Ca^{2+}$ blip or puff. Enhancement may be sufficient to raise cytosolic $Ca^{2+}$ 'globally' (i.e. throughout the cell) and if so, vascular tone increases.

Unlike the adjacent endothelial cells, the VSM SR membrane also has a second type of $Ca^{2+}$ release channel, the **ryanodine receptor** (RyR), as in cardiac myocytes. In the basal state,

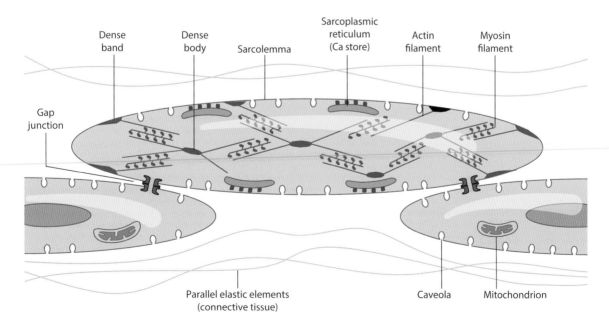

**Figure 12.3** Structure of the vascular myocyte. Fine, periodic, dark-staining elements, thought to be $Ca^{2+}$ release channels, extend from the subsarcolemmal sarcoplasmic reticulum towards the sarcolemma. The local, subsarcolemmal region may therefore experience higher $Ca^{2+}$ concentrations than the cytosol. The general organization of the tunica media and myoendothelial gap junctions is shown in Figure 1.11. (Based partly on Gabella G. *Physiological Reviews* 1984; 64(2): 455–77, with permission of the American Physiological Society.)

RyRs spontaneously release brief bursts of $Ca^{2+}$, called $Ca^{2+}$ sparks. RyRs are often aligned with sarcolemmal $Ca^{2+}$-dependent $K^+$ channels. Because a $Ca^{2+}$ spark only raises the $Ca^{2+}$ concentrations locally (cf. globally), in the subsarcolemmal region, this can activate the $Ca^{2+}$-dependent $K^+$ channels, leading to an outward hyperpolarizing current, first described as a spontaneous transient outward current (STOC), serving to limit vasoconstriction (Section 12.4).

## Gap junctions transmit ionic currents

Vascular myocytes are connected to each other by ion-permeable, electrically conductive gap junctions (**homocellular gap junctions**) (Figure 12.3). The gap junction, or nexus, is composed of the protein connexin, as in the heart. Six connexin molecules form a hemichannel (connexon), and the hemichannels of adjacent cells join end-to-end, connecting the cytoplasm of the two cells. This allows ionic currents to transmit depolarization from cell to cell. The spread of current is electrotonic, so it decays with distance and usually only extends ~1 mm along the vessel longitudinally.

The innermost myocytes of the tunica media also form gap junctions with the endothelial cells. These **heterocellular** or **myoendothelial gap junctions** transmit hyperpolarizing signals from the lining endothelium to the vascular myocytes, as described under 'Endothelium-derived hyperpolarizing factors' (Section 9.5).

## Caveolae

The cell surface of VSM is heavily invaginated with tiny flask-shaped pits, called caveolae ('little caves'). The caveolae are so numerous that they increase the total membrane area by up to 75%. The cytoplasmic surface of each caveola has a striated coat of protein, caveolin-1, and the membrane of the caveolae is enriched in cholesterol and sphingomyelin, so they are a type of lipid raft. They function as signalling microdomains, because they contain high concentrations of G-protein-coupled receptors such as β adrenergic receptors, and G proteins, L-type $Ca^{2+}$ channels, $K_{ATP}$ channels and signal pathway proteins such as adenylyl cyclase and protein kinase Cα. So, caveolae operate as 'signalosomes' where cell signalling pathways are integrated.

## 12.3 CONTRACTILE PROPERTIES AND ROLE OF $Ca^{2+}$

Resistance vessels and large arteries are normally in a state of partial contraction called **basal tone**. In the smaller resistance arteries, VSM contraction is spontaneous and referred to as myogenic tone (see Chapter 13). Whether spontaneous or evoked, regulatory mechanisms exist to increase the tone (**vasoconstriction**) or reduce it (**vasodilatation;** see Section 12.7). Vasoconstriction can be induced by depolarizing

the cell, for example, by isotonic $K^+Cl^-$ in the laboratory (Figure 12.4), or more physiologically by:

- sympathetic vasomotor fibres releasing noradrenaline;
- circulating hormones, such as adrenaline (acting on α adrenergic receptors), angiotensin II (Ang II) (acting on AT1 receptors) and vasopressin;
- paracrine agents, such as endothelin (ET; $ET_A$ and $ET_B$ receptors), histamine ($H_1$ receptors) and 5-hydroxytryptamine (5HT, serotonin) ($5HT_{2A}$ receptor) and thromboxane released by activated blood platelets.

The receptor type is specified here because agonists can have an opposite effect when bound to a different receptor type, by linking to a different signalling pathway within the cell. For example, adrenaline bound to α adrenergic receptors causes vasoconstriction, but when bound to $β_1$ or $β_2$ adrenergic receptors causes vasodilatation (NB: there is now increasing

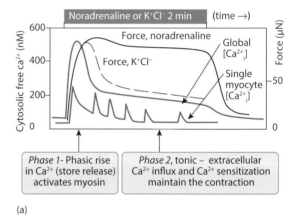

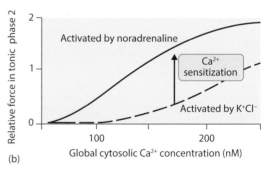

**Figure 12.4** Contraction and cytosolic free $Ca^{2+}$ concentration in the rabbit mesenteric artery. **(a)** Contraction in response to noradrenaline was well sustained (upper black line). The effect of a depolarizing concentration of extracellular $K^+Cl^-$ was less sustained (lower, dashed black line). The 'global' cytosolic $Ca^{2+}$ concentration over the whole tunica media (upper red line) is the average of hundreds of asynchronous $Ca^{2+}$ waves in individual myocytes (lower red line). After the initial, transient phase of store release, $Ca^{2+}$ wave frequency and magnitude decline, reducing the global average $[Ca^{2+}]$; yet, the noradrenaline-induced contraction is maintained (tonic phase). This shows that the noradrenaline-triggered pathway raises the sensitivity to $Ca^{2+}$. **(b)** Dependence of contractile force on mean cytosolic free $[Ca^{2+}]$ in phase 2. Noradrenaline steepens the relation, demonstrating $Ca^{2+}$ sensitization. (Based on Itoh T, Kajikuri J, Kurigama H. *The Journal of Physiology* 1992; 457: 297–314, with permission from Wiley-Blackwell; and Wier WG, Morgan KG. *Reviews of Physiology, Biochemistry and Pharmacology* 2003; 150: 91–139.)

evidence that $\beta_1$ adrenergic receptors are as important for vasodilatation as $\beta_2$ adrenergic receptors). Likewise, $H_1$ receptors elicit vasoconstriction, whereas $H_2$ receptors elicit vasodilatation. Vasoconstriction is illustrated in Figures 12.2, 12.4 and 12.9, and has the following characteristics.

## Vascular contraction is slow but sustained

### Speed of contraction

The vascular myocyte has evolved for slow, sustained contraction (Figure 12.4a), unlike the brief twitch of a cardiac myocyte. The shortening velocity is about one tenth that of striated muscle, because the myosin crossbridges form and break much more slowly in VSM than in striated muscle.

### Degree of shortening

The vascular myocyte can shorten by a half or more, whereas striated muscle fibres shorten by only about one third. The enhanced shortening of VSM is due to the greater actin filament length and a difference in myosin filament structure. The myosin heads on one side of the filament all face the same direction, and those on the opposite side face the opposite direction (Figure 12.3), unlike the arrangement in cardiac myosin filaments (Figures 3.3 and 6.3).

### Contractile force

This is regulated by agonists, as listed earlier.

### Duration of contraction

The sustained nature of vascular contraction is remarkable; many arterioles and arteries maintain tone throughout life. This is vitally important to support arterial blood pressure (BP), and is a prerequisite for vasodilatation, which is simply a reduction in tone. In vessels with a high tone, each myocyte is tonically contracted, and excessive adenosine triphosphate (ATP) consumption is avoided by means of a special 'latch state'. In vessels with low tone, individual myocytes show asynchronous, recurring contraction-relaxation cycles, associated with Ca²⁺ waves (Figure 12.4a).

## Contraction is mediated by Ca²⁺-calmodulin, leading to myosin phosphorylation

As noted earlier, vascular contraction depends primarily on global cytosolic Ca²⁺ ion concentration (Figure 12.4), which triggers myosin filament activation as follows.

### Myosin light-chain kinase activates the myosin motor

A rise in cytosolic Ca²⁺ concentration causes the formation of Ca²⁺-calmodulin complex; calmodulin is a cytoplasmic protein, related to troponin C, that binds four Ca²⁺ ions. The Ca²⁺-calmodulin

complex activates the enzyme MLCK. The light chain is a component of the myosin head involved in crossbridge formation with actin, and vascular myosin only forms crossbridges when the light chain is phosphorylated (unlike striated muscle myosin). MLCK transfers a phosphate group from ATP to the myosin light chain, enabling the myosin head to form a crossbridge with actin. The myosin head then rotates to generate tension, as in striated muscle. However, instead of quickly detaching as it would in cardiac muscle, the crossbridge remains attached in the tense, flexed state for a prolonged period (see 'latch state').

## Myosin light-chain phosphatase inactivates the myosin motor, causing relaxation

The phosphate group can be removed by the enzyme myosin light chain phosphatase (MLCP) (Figure 12.7). When intracellular Ca²⁺ concentration falls, MLCK activity declines and the competing myosin phosphatase dominates, dephosphorylating the myosin. Since dephosphorylated myosin cannot form new crossbridges, the phosphatase in effect turns off the myosin motor. As existing crossbridges detach, new ones cannot form, so the myocytes relax, leading to vasodilatation. Increased myosin phosphatase activation may explain cases of vascular relaxation with little fall in cytosolic Ca²⁺ concentration, for example hypoxic vasodilatation (Figure 13.5). Phosphatase inhibition is promoted by the activation of RhoA kinase (see Figure 12.7).

## Slow crossbridge cycling (the latch state) maintains vascular tension economically

The energy cost of maintaining vascular tone throughout the body would be substantial, were it not for the ability of VSM to maintain tension with just 1/300th of the energy expenditure of striated muscle. This is due to a difference in crossbridge duration. In a skeletal muscle fibre, crossbridge duration is very short, so tension can only be maintained by the continuous, rapid making and breaking of crossbridges, consuming one ATP molecule per crossbridge cycle. In smooth muscle, a crossbridge lasts much longer, so tension maintenance consumes much less ATP. This is called the **latch state**. The muscle is in effect locked into the crossbridged state, in a similar way to the latch muscle of a bivalve shell. VSM can thus maintain tension for a long period with little ATP consumption and without fatiguing.

## Cytosolic free Ca²⁺ depends on rate of influx versus removal

The cytosolic free Ca²⁺ concentration regulating VSM tone is typically in the range 100–350 nM (Figure 12.4), and is determined by three factors (Figure 12.5):

1. **Extracellular Ca²⁺** enters the myocyte through Ca²⁺-conducting channels in the sarcolemma. These fall into three functional classes: **Voltage-dependent Ca²⁺ channels (VDCCs), receptor-operated channels (ROCs)** and **store-operated channels (SOCs)**;

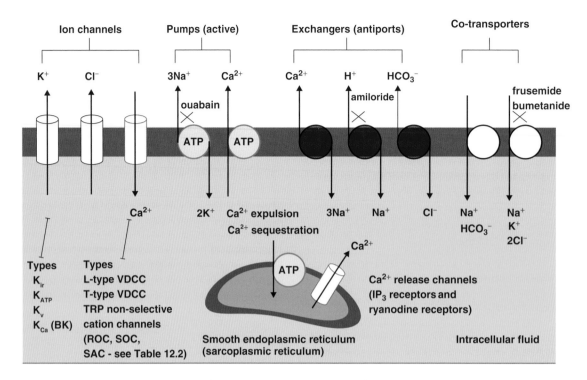

**Figure 12.5** Ion channels, pumps, exchangers and co-transporters in sarcolemma of vascular myocyte. For channel abbreviations, see text. Crosses denote transport blockers. The $Na^+/HCO_3^-$ co-transporter and $Na^+/H^+$ exchanger combat intracellular acidosis during a sustained contraction. The $Na^+K^+2Cl^-$ co-transporter and $HCO_3^-/Cl^-$ exchanger generate a high intracellular $Cl^-$ concentration, which affects the $Cl^-$ electrochemical gradient (see text). ATP, adenosine triphosphate; $IP_3$, inositol 1,4,5 trisphosphate; $K_{ATP}$, ATP-dependent $K^+$ channel; $K_{Ca}$, $Ca^{2+}$-activated $K^+$ channel; $K_{ir}$, inwardly rectifying $K^+$ channel; $K_v$, voltage-dependent (delayed rectifying) $K^+$ channel; ROC, receptor-operated channel; SAC, stretch-activated channel; SOC, store-operated channel; TRP, transient receptor potential; VDCC, voltage-dependent $Ca^{2+}$ channel.

see the next section. The VDCCs have a low but finite open-state probability under basal conditions, allowing a small extracellular $Ca^{2+}$ influx that contributes to **basal tone**.

2. **Stored $Ca^{2+}$** is released from the SR store through the $IP_3$-dependent $Ca^{2+}$ release channels, when the myocyte is stimulated by noradrenaline. The released $Ca^{2+}$ can spread across the cell as a $Ca^{2+}$ wave, reflecting the activation of both IP3 receptors and RyRs. At the same time, the activation of sarcolemmal SOCs increases extracellular $Ca^{2+}$ entry.

3. **$Ca^{2+}$ ATPase pumps** in the sarcolemma and SR membrane continuously pump $Ca^{2+}$ out of the cytoplasm. SR uptake is called **$Ca^{2+}$ sequestration** and extracellular transfer is called **$Ca^{2+}$ expulsion**. A sarcolemmal $Na^+/Ca^{2+}$ exchanger also contributes to $Ca^{2+}$ expulsion (Figure 12.5). Due to the relatively small but continuous influx of $Ca^{2+}$ through $Ca^{2+}$ channels in the basal state, the sarcolemmal $Ca^{2+}$ pumps must expel $Ca^{2+}$ continuously, otherwise $Ca^{2+}$ would accumulate in the cell.

Because $Ca^{2+}$ channels and membrane potential are major factors influencing VSM contraction, we must next consider the mix of ion channels in the VSM membrane.

## 12.4 VASCULAR ION CHANNELS

This section introduces the players in the game. In a pressurized artery, the VSM membrane potential will vary depending on the intraluminal pressure within a range of approximately −60 mV to −30 mV (Figure 12.1). This is a more depolarized state than the cardiac myocyte, owing to differences in the ion channel population. The VSM sarcolemma has, rather dauntingly, four types of $K^+$-conducting channel, four types of $Ca^{2+}$-conducting channel and one $Cl^-$ conducting channel (Figures 12.5 and 12.6a). These channels are expressed to different degrees in different vessels and tissues, so VSM shows very diverse electrical behaviour (Figure 12.2). Voltage-operated $Na^+$ channels, which are of major importance in cardiac electrophysiology, generally play no role in VSM. The key channels are as follows.

### $K^+$ channels generate the negative membrane potential

Like all cells, the vascular myocyte has a high intracellular $K^+$ concentration (Figure 12.5) maintained by the $Na^+/K^+$ pump. The sarcolemma also has ~50 000 $K^+$ channels, a substantial fraction of which is open at any one moment, transmitting a

**Table 12.1** Ionic composition of vascular smooth muscle (VSM)

| Ion | Intracellular fluid (mM) | Extracellular fluid (mM) | Nernst equilibrium potential (mV)[a] |
|---|---|---|---|
| $K^+$ | 165 | 5 | −89 |
| $Na^+$ | 9 | 137 | +69 |
| $Ca^{2+}$ | 0.0001[b] | 1.2[c] | +124 |
| $Cl^{-}$[d] | 54 | 134 | −23 |
| $HCO_3^-$ | 7.3 | 15.5 | −19 |
| $H^+$ | $8.7 \times 10^{-8}$ (pH 7.06) | $4.0 \times 10^{-8}$ (pH 7.40) | −20 |

[a] See Section 3.6.
[b] Relaxed state.
[c] Total plasma $Ca^{2+}$ is ~2.5 mM, but only 1.2 mM is in unbound, ionic form.
[d] $Cl^-$ concentration is unusually high in VSM.

small outward current of $K^+$ ions down their electrochemical gradient (Table 12.1). The negative charges left behind create the negative basal membrane potential. Also, the $Na^+/K^+$ pump, by expelling three $Na^+$ ions in exchange for two $K^+$ ions, contributes around ~11 mV to the membrane potential.

Since the Nernst equilibrium potential for $K^+$, $E_K$, is approximately −90 mV, whereas the membrane potential is less than −60 mV, the sarcolemma clearly has a significant basal conductance to other ions also, notably $Na^+$ ions (due to transient receptor potential (TRP) channel constitutive activity) and $Cl^-$ ions (due to $Cl_{Ca}$ channels). The chemical gradient and equilibrium potential for these ions are listed in Table 12.1. The influx of $Na^+$ and slight efflux of $Cl^-$ down their electrochemical gradients contribute to the low membrane potential (by convention, $Cl^-$ efflux is referred to as an inward current).

$K^+$ channel status (open/closed) is important because it determines the membrane potential, which in turn controls VDCCs and hence vascular tone. For example, **hypoxia** increases the fraction of open $K^+$ channels, leading to hyperpolarization (a more negative potential) and therefore closure of the VDCCs. This reduces $Ca^{2+}$ influx, which contributes to hypoxic vascular relaxation (Figure 12.1, crosses).

The four main types of $K^+$ channel expressed by VSM are the inwardly rectifying $K^+$ channel ($K_{ir}$), its structural relative the ATP-dependent $K^+$ channel ($K_{ATP}$), the voltage-dependent $K^+$ (delayed rectifying) channel ($K_V$) and its relative the $Ca^{2+}$-activated $K^+$ channel ($K_{Ca}$) (Table 12.2). Their properties differ markedly, and each makes a specific contribution to vascular behaviour, as follows.

## Inwardly rectifying channel $K_{ir}$ senses extracellular $K^+$ and contributes to vasodilatation in exercising muscle, myocardium and brain

The structure of $K_{ir}$ is shown in Figure 3.12 (top left). The channel serves as a sensor of external $K^+$ concentration, being the only $K^+$ channel whose conductance **is increased by a rise in extracellular [$K^+$]**, in the range 5–20 mM. The conductance is raised by driving $Mg^{2+}$ and polyamines from the channel pore. The increased $K^+$ conductance shifts the membrane potential

towards $E_K$, causing hyperpolarization and hence vasodilatation. This is important in exercising muscle, myocardium and active areas of the brain (Figure 15.15), where increased metabolic activity raises the local interstitial [$K^+$]. The resulting vascular hyperpolarization and vasodilatation help raise blood flow, to match demand ('metabolic hyperaemia', Section 13.4). By contrast, a very high, non-physiological extracellular $K^+$ concentration depolarizes the myocyte, because it abolishes the [$K^+$] gradient responsible for the membrane potential. The depolarization activates $Ca^{2+}$ channels, leading to contraction (Figure 12.4).

## ATP-dependent channel $K_{ATP}$ senses ischaemia and contributes to hypoxic vasodilatation

The ATP-dependent $K^+$ channel comprises four α subunits of $K_{ir}$ protein, each surrounded by a sulphonylurea receptor unit that confers sensitivity to ATP and sulphonylurea-related drugs (Figure 3.12, top right). The channel open probability is increased by a fall in intracellular ATP, as in severe ischaemia, and by a rise in adenosine diphosphate (ADP), guanosine diphosphate (GDP), adenosine and $H^+$ concentration, which occurs during moderate hypoxia. The $K_{ATP}$ channel thus helps link vascular tone to tissue $O_2$ status; ischaemia and hypoxia increase the $K_{ATP}$ open probability, leading to vascular hyperpolarization, vasodilatation and increased $O_2$ delivery (Figure 12.1, crosses). An alternative name sometimes used for this channel, emphasizing its ADP sensitivity, is 'nucleotide diphosphate-dependent channel', $K_{NDP}$.

Even under normal, non-hypoxic conditions, some $K_{ATP}$ channels are open, due to phosphorylation by background levels of active protein kinase A (PKA) (Section 12.7). Consequently, the $K_{ATP}$-blocker **glibenclamide** causes partial depolarization and vasoconstriction. Conversely, the $K_{ATP}$-activating drug **nicorandil** causes vasodilatation; it is also a nitrovasodilator, and is used to treat angina.

## Voltage-dependent K+ channel $K_v$ and $Ca^{2+}$-dependent K+ channels $K_{Ca}$ (BK) contribute to resting potential and prevent vasospasm

The **voltage-dependent $K^+$ channel** $K_v$ is a heterotetramer (Figure 3.12). $K_v$ is activated by depolarization, and thus brings about repolarization after an action potential. It also contributes to the basal membrane potential.

The large or big conductance **$Ca^{2+}$-dependent $K^+$ channel** $BK_{Ca}$ is a specialized form of $K_v$ that is expressed by VSM but not native endothelial cells. Unlike the endothelial isoforms of $Ca^{2+}$-dependent $K^+$ channels, namely small and intermediate conductance $K_{Ca}$ ($SK_{Ca}$, $IK_{Ca}$), that are only sensitive to cytoplasmic $Ca^{2+}$, $BK_{Ca}$ is activated by depolarization as well as $Ca^{2+}$. Increases in cytoplasmic $Ca^{2+}$ shift the level at which membrane depolarization activates the channel to more negative potentials. Normally, the $BK_{Ca}$ channels are

**Table 12.2** Ion channels in sarcolemma (plasma membrane) of vascular smooth muscle (VSM)

| Channel | Properties | Roles |
|---|---|---|
| **K⁺-conducting channels** | | |
| *Inwardly rectifying K⁺ channel, $K_{ir}$ (2T)[a]* | Expressed in arterioles. Open at basal membrane potential. Open state increased by $K_o^+$. Blocked by $Ba^{2+}$. | Supplies part of outward current for basal membrane potential. Mediates vasodilatation by interstitial K⁺ in exercising muscle, myocardium, brain. |
| *ATP-dependent K⁺ channel, $K_{ATP}$ ($K_{NDP}$) (2T, specialized form of $K_{ir}$)[b]* | Opened by low ATP, raised ADP, GDP, adenosine $A_1$ receptors and [H⁺]. Inhibited by α2 adrenergic receptors. Blocked by glibenclamide → contraction. Activated by diazoxide, pinacidil, cromakalim, nicorandil, CGRP, VIP → dilatation. | Links vascular tone to metabolic state in exercise and hypoxia. Low, basal open state due to basal PKA activity. Open state raised in cAMP/PKA-mediated vasodilatation. |
| *Voltage-dependent (delayed rectifying) K⁺ channel, $K_v$ (6T)[c]* | Opens slowly on depolarization beyond −30 mV. Blocked by 4-aminopyridine. | Part of outward current for basal potential in resistance vessels. Action potential repolarization. |
| *$Ca^{2+}$-activated K⁺ channel, $K_{Ca}$ (BK) (6T, specialized form of $K_v$)* | Open state promoted by $Ca^{2+}$ and depolarization. Big conductance type (BK) strongly expressed in large artery VSM (cf. small and intermediate conductance isoforms, SK, IK, in endothelium). Blocked by tetramethylammonium, iberiotoxin, charybdotoxin, ethanol. | Contributes to basal membrane potential and repolarization. If abundantly expressed, BK suppresses action potentials. Provides a 'brake', e.g. on myogenic contraction. Implicated in action of nitric oxide. |
| **Selective $Ca^{2+}$-conducting channels** | | |
| *Voltage-dependent $Ca^{2+}$ channel (VDCC)* | Mainly L-type, meaning Large conductance, Long opening. Abundant in resistance vessels. Blocked by dihydropyridines, e.g. nifedipine. | Supplies inward current for action potentials, graded electromechanical coupling and Bayliss myogenic response. |
| **Non-selective, cation-conducting TRP channels ($Ca^{2+}$ channels)** | | |
| *Receptor-operated channel (ROC), (TRPC proteins, e.g. TRPC3, TRPC6)* | Poorly selective between $Ca^{2+}$, Na⁺, K⁺. Activated by diacylglycerol when α1 adrenergic receptor and other $G_q$-protein-coupled receptors activated. Insensitive to nifedipine. | Mediates pharmacomechanical coupling by NAd (noradrenaline), angiotensin, vasopressin, 5HT, histamine. Related channel contributes depolarizing current $i_{cat}$ of slow excitatory junction potential (EJP). |
| *Store-operated channel (SOC) (cation-conducting TRP channels of low selectivity, cat-SOC, TRPC1 protein)* | Activated when $IP_3$ discharges the SR $Ca^{2+}$ store. | Conducts extracellular $Ca^{2+}$ into VSM when $Ca^{2+}$ store released. |
| *Stretch-activated channel (SAC) (?TRPC6, ?TRPV2, ?TRPV4, ?TRPM4 proteins)* | Activated by stretch. Inward Na⁺ and $Ca^{2+}$ currents → depolarization → VDCC activation. | Contractile response of VSM to stretch (myogenic response). Autoregulation of blood flow. |
| **Cl⁻-conducting channels** | | |
| *$Ca^{2+}$-activated Cl⁻ channel, $Cl_{Ca}$* | Open state promoted by $Ca_i^{2+}$ at >200 μM. | Contributes 'inward' current $i_{Cl(Ca)}$ (efflux of negative ions) for slow EJP. Modulates membrane potential. Contributes to vasomotion. |

*Note:* 5HT, 5-hydroxytryptamine; ADP, adenosine diphosphate; ATP, adenosine triphosphate; cAMP, cyclic adenosine monophosphate; CGRP, calcitonin gene-related peptide; GDP, guanosine diphosphate; IK, intermediate conductance; $IP_3$, inositol 1,4,5 trisphosphate; NAD, nicotinamide adenine dinucleotide; PKA, protein kinase A; SK, small conductance; SR, sarcoplasmic reticulum; TRP, transient receptor potential; TRPC, transient receptor potential channel; VIP, vasoactive intestinal peptide.

[a] 2T, Two transmembrane helices per α subunit; four α subunits make up one conducting channel.

[b] An octamer. Four $K_{ir}$ 6.1 α subunits form the pore, and four sulphonylurea receptor subunits (SUR2B) surround them, conferring sensitivity to ATP and drugs.

[c] 6T, Six transmembrane helices per α subunit; each α unit is a $K_v$ protein produced by the *KCNA* gene. Four α subunits make up the conducting channel. The channel is a heterotetramer, that is, a mix of different $K_v$ α isoforms, for example, $K_v$ 1.2/1.5 (rat cerebral artery), $K_v$ 1.3/1.6 (mouse cerebral artery), $K_v$ 1.5/1.6 (rabbit pial artery).

activated intermittently by the spontaneous SR $Ca^{2+}$ sparks (from RyRs, see earlier), generating hyperpolarizing STOCs. Thus, $BK_{Ca}$ channels reduce vascular excitability and prevent vasospasm because, as $Ca^{2+}$ enters VSM, $BK_{Ca}$ activation suppresses membrane depolarization, which reduces the VDCC open probability. For the same reason, vessels with a high $BK_{Ca}$ density do not generate action potentials, except after treatment with the $BK_{Ca}$ blockers iberiotoxin or charybdotoxin (each a component of scorpion venom). In mice, knockout of the accessory b1 regulatory subunit of the $BK_{Ca}$ channel raises vascular tone and arterial BP. Conversely, gain-of-function mutations in the human $BK_{Ca}$ subunit protect against diastolic hypertension, indicating these channels influence our susceptibility to hypertension. The alignment between $BK_{Ca}$ channels and $Ca^{2+}$ sparks requires the caveolar protein caveolin-1, and is lost when this protein is knocked out.

## Voltage-dependent $Ca^{2+}$ channels mediate depolarization-dependent contraction

The VDCC (also known as voltage-operated, voltage-gated or voltage-sensitive $Ca^{2+}$ channel) is highly selective for divalent cations ($Ca^{2+}$ and $Ba^{2+}$), and its open probability is increased by depolarization. As a result, **vascular tone is a graded function of membrane depolarization in most vessels** (Figure 12.1). The predominant VDCC is the L-type $Ca^{2+}$ channel ($Ca_v1.2$, Figure 4.3). Since the open probability is a continuous, graded function of membrane potential, there is a very low, but finite, open-state probability at resting potentials (around −50 mV to −40 mV). This, along with some constitutive TRP channel activity, allows a small flux of extracellular $Ca^{2+}$ into the myocyte under basal conditions. The resulting cytosolic $Ca^{2+}$ concentration, though low, may be enough to activate sufficient myosin heads to generate **basal, myogenic vascular tone**.

L-type $Ca^{2+}$ channels are expressed more abundantly in arterioles and terminal arteries (up to ~5000 per myocyte) than in large arteries, so their contribution to vasoconstriction is most pronounced in small resistance vessels. Many arterioles and small arteries express L-type $Ca^{2+}$ channels so abundantly that they may fire $Ca^{2+}$-based **action potentials** following sympathetic stimulation (Figure 12.6a). The inward $Ca^{2+}$ current, $i_{Ca-L}$, generates the upstroke of the action potential. The dihydropyridine **nifedipine** inhibits L-type $Ca^{2+}$ channels, leading to vasodilatation of resistance vessels; therefore, nifedipine is used to treat clinical hypertension.

## $Ca^{2+}$-conducting TRP channels mediate depolarization-independent contraction and contribute to agonist-induced electrical excitation

If the VSM membrane potential of an artery is abolished by extracellular isotonic $K^+Cl^-$ solution, noradrenaline can still evoke a contraction when VDCCs are blocked, provided that $Ca^{2+}$ ions are added to the extracellular solution. This finding showed that VSM expresses channels that are permeable to extracellular $Ca^{2+}$, but are not classic voltage-operated channels; rather, they are activated by the agonist-receptor interaction. These channels were initially called receptor-operated channels (ROCs); they are now thought to be composed of mainly TRP proteins.

The **TRP protein** was discovered in mutant *Drosophila* fruit flies with photoreceptors that responded with a transient depolarization to light. The mammalian TRP channel comprises a ring of four TRP proteins, each with six transmembrane helices, like $K_v$ (Figure 3.12, middle) but lacking the S4 arginine charges that confer voltage sensitivity. There are 28 different mammalian TRP proteins, and they can form homo- or heterotetrameric channels (a mix of TRP species). Thus, TRP channels are very diverse, and include ROCs, SOCs and stretch-activated channels (SACs) (see Table 12.2). In total, 13 different TRP proteins have been identified in VSM.

**ROCs** are cation-conducting channels that are about three- to fivefold more permeable to $Ca^{2+}$ than $Na^+$. A lag of ~0.1–1.0 s between agonist application and channel activation indicates that a relatively slow, biochemical pathway leads to channel activation (Figure 12.6a). When an agonist binds to its G-protein-coupled receptor, for example, noradrenaline to the $\alpha_1$ adrenergic receptor, the activated receptor splits trimeric $G_q$ protein into $G_q\alpha$ and $G_q\beta\gamma$ components, and the former activates the membrane-bound enzyme phospholipase C$\beta$ (PLC$\beta$). PLC$\beta$ catalyses the breakdown of a membrane lipid, phosphatidylinositol 4,5-bisphosphate ($PIP_2$), into cytosolic $IP_3$ and lipophilic DAG (Figure 12.6b). DAG activates the ROCs directly, leading to extracellular $Ca^{2+}$ influx and VSM contraction. Available evidence supports the involvement of short TRP channels 3, 6 and 7 (TRPC3, TRPC6 and TRPC7) as VSM ROCs, but as TRPs can form heteromultimeric channels this is almost certainly a simplified view. It also seems that $IP_3$, like DAG, may activate TRPs directly (independently of $Ca^{2+}$), certainly in the case of TRPC3. Note that the 'pharmacomechanical' contraction due to ROCs does not require an initial membrane depolarization, although the ROC-conducted current can cause a small, incidental depolarization (Figure 12.2c). **Depolarization-independent contraction is typical of large arteries.** It also appears that TRPC3 displays **constitutive activity,** which provides a low, background permeability in unstimulated vessels, resulting from background levels of DAG. The consequent small, inward cation current contributes to the resting potential in some arteries, and can be enhanced by vasoconstrictor agonists like noradrenaline to increase VDCC open probability.

**SOCs** in contractile VSM are cation-conducting TRP channels of low selectivity (cat-SOCs), unlike the highly $Ca^{2+}$-selective $Ca^{2+}$ release-activated channel (CRAC)/SOC in non-contractile cultured VSM cells. The cat-SOC is activated when $IP_3$, generated by the receptor/$G_q$/PLC$\beta$ pathway, releases the ER store. This results in the translocation of the stromal interaction molecule 1 from the SR to the surface membrane where it associates with TRPC1. This complex then associates with and activates PLC$\beta$1 generating DAG that causes channel opening through protein kinase C (PKC) phosphorylation of TRPC1. Receptor activation thus leads to contraction through both ROC and cat-SOC activation.

**SACs** are mechano-dependent TRP channels that are activated by stretch of the vessel wall. They contribute to a contractile response of blood vessels to stretch, called the myogenic response, which is the basis of autoregulation (Sections 13.2 and 13.6). A variety of TRP channels have been implicated including TRPC6, TRP cation channel subfamily V member 2 and 4 and TRP cation channel subfamily M member 4.

**Depolarization-dependent contraction**

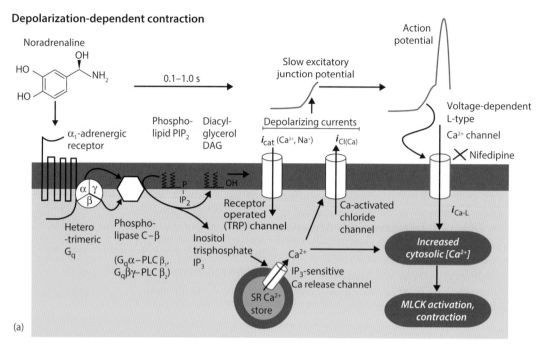

(a)

**Depolarization-independent contraction**

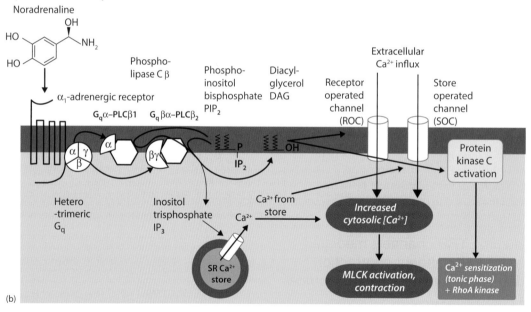

(b)

**Figure 12.6** Pathways by which noradrenaline $\alpha_1$ adrenergic receptors evoke depolarization-dependent and depolarization-independent contraction. Histamine $H_1$ receptors, serotonin, angiotensin II and vasopressin receptors are coupled similarly to evoke contraction. **(a)** Small arterial resistance vessels and the portal vein express abundant L-type $Ca^{2+}$ channels. Electrical depolarization via a slow excitatory junction potential activates the L-type $Ca^{2+}$ channels, leading to contraction. **(b)** In large arteries, contraction is often independent of membrane potential; it is mediated by receptor-operated and store operated channels and by $Ca^{2+}$ release from the sarcoplasmic reticulum store (SR), followed by $Ca^{2+}$ sensitization. DAG, diacylglycerol; $IP_3$, inositol 1,4,5 trisphosphate; $PIP_2$, phosphatidylinositol 4,5-bisphosphate; MLCK, myosin light-chain kinase; PLC, phospholipase C; RhoA, Ras homolog gene family, member A; ROC, receptor-operated channel; SR, sarcoplasmic reticulum; TRP; transient receptor potential.

## Chloride channels contribute to agonist-induced electrical excitation

Electrically excitable myocytes express ROCs and also $Cl^-$-conducting channels activated by cytosolic $Ca^{2+}$ ($Cl_{Ca}$, Figure 12.6a). VSM intracellular $Cl^-$ concentration is unusually high, ~54 mM (Table 12.1), due to the activity of $Na^+K^+2Cl^-$ co-transporters and $Cl^-/HCO_3^-$ exchangers (Figure 12.5). The resulting $Cl^-$ equilibrium potential is $-23$ mV (Table 12.1). Consequently, when the $Cl^-$ channels open, the basal membrane potential of approximately $-55$ mV drives $Cl^-$ ions out of the cell (cf. $Cl^-$ influx in neurons), depolarizing it towards the Cl⁻ equilibrium potential. The Cl⁻ current, along with a current from ROCs $i_{cat}$, also generates the agonist-evoked **excitatory junction potential** (EJP). A few Cl⁻ channels may also be open in the basal state, contributing to the relatively depolarized basal potential.

Vascular myocytes thus express a bewildering armoury of diversely activated ion-conducting channels. The next section draws the threads together to show how receptor activation leads, via ion channel activation, to myocyte contraction.

## 12.5 FROM SYMPATHETIC STIMULATION TO CONTRACTILE RESPONSE

Most arteries and arterioles are innervated by the sympathetic vasoconstrictor system, which continuously stimulates a basal level of vasoconstriction by releasing **noradrenaline** (Section 14.1) to activate VSM $\alpha_1$ adrenergic receptors (synonym, $\alpha_1$ adrenoreceptor). Many other vasoconstrictor agonists, such as angiotensin II, vasopressin, serotonin (5HT), thromboxane A₂ and endothelin activate G protein-coupled receptors that trigger broadly similar pathways to the $\alpha$ adrenergic receptor. The importance of this basal activity is clear from the drop in BP observed with drugs that block autonomic ganglia.

### Sympathetic junctional varicosities release noradrenaline and ATP

The terminal part of a sympathetic axon runs along the adventitia-media border of arteries and develops a string of swellings, ~1000 per fibre, called **junctional varicosities** (Figures 1.11 and 14.2). There can be up to six varicosities per myocyte, and the distance from varicosity to nearest myocyte is ~75 nm. Each varicosity contains ~500 small, dense-cored vesicles grouped near the membrane and a smaller number of large vesicles. The vesicles contain a variable mixture of noradrenaline and ATP, and release is promoted when an action potential arrives.

### Transmitter release is quantal

When a sympathetic action potential reaches a varicosity, the depolarization activates N-type Ca²⁺ channels in the varicosity membrane, raising neuronal [Ca²⁺]. The Ca²⁺ triggers the discharge of a single vesicle into the junctional cleft. Neurotransmitter is thus released as a discrete, standard-size packet or **quantum**. However, only ~1 in every 100 action potentials succeeds in releasing a quantum from a given varicosity. The released noradrenaline diffuses rapidly across the short neuromuscular gap and binds to adrenergic receptors on the vascular myocyte, while ATP binds to vascular P2X purinergic receptors, which contain an ion channel within their structure.

## Adrenergic receptors differ in type, agonist affinity, coupling and effect

Adrenergic receptors are not linked directly to the ion channels that they regulate, but activate intracellular secondary messenger signalling, so they are termed '**metabotropic**'. There are two main classes, $\alpha$ and $\beta$ adrenergic receptors. Both are G protein-coupled receptors, but they are linked to different intracellular pathways, so that $\alpha$ adrenergic receptors elicit vasoconstriction and $\beta$ adrenergic receptors elicit vasodilatation. In most, but not all, tissues, $\alpha$ adrenergic receptors predominate. The $\alpha$ and $\beta$ adrenergic receptors are further subdivided as follows:

- **$\alpha_1$ receptors** are abundant in most systemic blood vessels, and noradrenaline and adrenaline have similar potency when evoking vasoconstriction. The activated receptor triggers the $G_q$–PLCβ–IP₃–DAG cascade (Figures 12.6 and 12.7), which increases sarcolemmal conductance to cations and Cl⁻. The resulting depolarization leads to vasoconstriction, as described more fully below.
- **$\alpha_2$ receptors** are abundant in cutaneous blood vessels and junctional varicosities, the latter providing negative feedback against the release of noradrenaline (Figure 14.2). The $\alpha_2$ receptor has a similar affinity for adrenaline and noradrenaline. The receptor is coupled to a different G-protein from the $\alpha_1$ adrenergic receptor, namely $G_i$. Therefore, it acts through a different intracellular pathway. $G_i$ activity inhibits the adenylyl cyclase–cyclic adenosine monophosphate (cAMP) pathway, which is a vasodilator pathway in VSM (Section 12.7). The net effect is a fall in $K_{ATP}$ channel conductance leading to depolarization. This can reinforce $\alpha_1$ adrenergic receptor-mediated vasoconstriction.
- **$\beta_1$ receptors** are found in the cardiac pacemaker and myocardium. The $\beta_1$ adrenergic receptor has a slightly greater affinity for adrenaline than noradrenaline. It is coupled to $G_s$-protein, which stimulates the adenylyl cyclase–cAMP pathway, leading to an increase in heart rate and contractility (Figure 4.9). Generally, $\beta_1$ adrenergic receptors have not been thought to have a role in vasodilatation, but recent evidence from resistance arteries has indicated that they contribute as much as $\beta_2$ adrenergic receptors.
- **$\beta_2$ receptors** are abundant in the arterial vessels of the myocardium, skeletal muscle and liver, while in other blood vessels they are outnumbered by $\alpha_1$ adrenergic receptors. The $\beta_2$ adrenergic receptor has a far greater affinity for adrenaline than noradrenaline. Like $\beta_1$, $\beta_2$ adrenergic receptors are coupled to $G_s$-protein, which stimulates the adenylyl cyclase–cAMP pathway. This leads to vasodilatation (Section 12.7).

To summarize, noradrenaline has similar potency to adrenaline in activating $\alpha$ and $\beta_1$ adrenergic receptors, but adrenaline is more potent than noradrenaline in activating

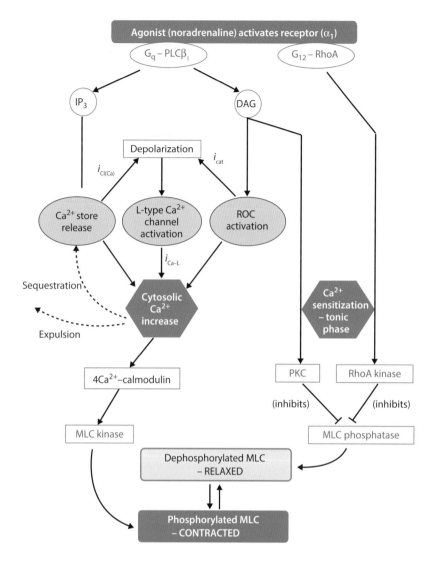

**Figure 12.7** Pathways mediating noradrenaline-induced vasoconstriction. Relative importance of various pathways varies with vessel type, tissue and agonist. DAG, diacylglycerol; $IP_3$, inositol 1,4,5 trisphosphate; MLC, myosin light-chain; PKC, protein kinase C; PLC, phospholipase C; RhoA, Ras homolog gene family, member A; ROC, receptor-operated channel; $i_{cat}$, current generated by opening of receptor operated channels (ROCs).

$\beta_2$ adrenergic receptors. The rest of this section concentrates on the pathways activated by the ubiquitous, physiologically most important receptor, the $\alpha_1$ adrenergic receptor.

## $\alpha_1$-adrenergic receptors activate the PLC–IP$_3$–DAG pathway

The $\alpha_1$ adrenergic receptor is coupled to the trimeric membrane GTPase, **$G_q$ protein**. The activated receptor splits the trimer into its component subunits, $G_q\alpha$ and $G_q\beta\gamma$. These activate the membrane-bound enzymes **PLCβ1** and **β2**, respectively (Figures 12.6 and 12.7). PLC splits a membrane phospholipid, $PIP_2$, into two messenger molecules, $IP_3$ and DAG.

**IP$_3$** activates Ca$^{2+}$ release channels on the SR, releasing the Ca$^{2+}$ store. The consequences depend on SR distribution. If the SR is scanty and close to the sarcolemma, the increase in free Ca$^{2+}$ may be confined largely to the subsarcolemmal space, activating Ca$^{2+}$-activated Cl$^-$ channels. With nerve-released noradrenaline, the resulting depolarizing current, $i_{Cl(Ca)}$, contributes to a slow-rising excitatory junction potential (EJP), described in the next section. If the SR is extensive, as

in large artery myocytes, store discharge contributes to a rise in global cytosolic Ca$^{2+}$ concentration, leading to contraction.

**DAG**, the other messenger product, activates $i_{cat}$ TRP channels. The depolarizing current $i_{cat}$, along with $i_{Cl(Ca)}$, creates a slow-rising EJP. DAG and Ca$^{2+}$ also activate PKC, which contributes to Ca$^{2+}$ sensitization.

## $\alpha_1$-adrenergic receptors can evoke membrane depolarization

The release of both noradrenaline and ATP by sympathetic fibres evokes a complex electrical and mechanical response. To simplify matters, let us consider first the effect of a pulse of noradrenaline alone, delivered by a micropipette to an isolated vascular myocyte (Figure 12.8). The $\alpha_1$ adrenergic receptor activation is followed by a 0.1–1.0 s delay, as the $G_q$–PLCβ–DAG/IP$_3$–Ca$^{2+}$ pathway grinds into action. Then, a slow depolarization develops, the **slow EJP**. The slow EJP is generated by $i_{cat}$ (DAG-activated TRP channels) and $i_{Cl(Ca)}$ (Ca$^{2+}$-activated Cl$^-$ channels) (Figure 12.6a). If the EJP is big enough and the myocyte has abundant VDCCs (e.g. arteriolar VSM), an action

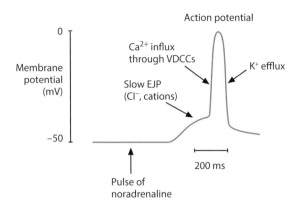

**Figure 12.8** Response of an action potential-generating vascular myocyte to a brief pulse of noradrenaline from a micropipette (cf. sympathetic vesicle, Figure 12.9). EJP, excitatory junction potential; VDCC, voltage-dependent $Ca^{2+}$ channel. (Courtesy of Professor WA Large, Department of Pharmacology, St. George's Hospital Medical School, London.)

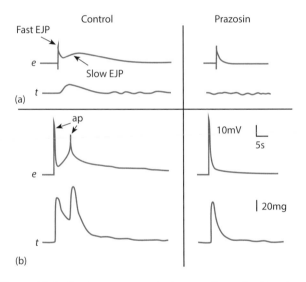

**Figure 12.9** Simultaneous records of contractile tension (*t*) and membrane potential (*e*) recorded by an intracellular microelectrode in a rat tail artery. The perivascular nerves were stimulated with a single external pulse in each frame in the absence (left) or presence (right) of an α adrenergic receptor blocker, prazosin. **(a)** Medium-intensity stimulation produced a fast, ATP-mediated excitatory junction potential (EJP) and a slow, noradrenaline-mediated EJP. Contraction preceded the slow EJP and was blocked by prazosin (depolarization-independent contraction). **(b)** Stimulation at higher intensity evoked larger fast and slow EJPs, each of which triggered an action potential (ap), with associated twitch contractions (depolarization-dependent contractions). Only the slower potentials and contraction were blocked by prazosin. (From Cheung DW. *Pflügers Archiv: European Journal of Physiology* 1984; 400(3): 335–7, with kind permission from Springer Science and Business Media.)

potential ensues; VDCCs activated by the EJP cause more depolarization, activating more VDCCs, and so on (positive feedback). The rapidly increasing inward current $i_{Ca-L}$ generates the upstroke of the action potential (Figure 12.8). The action potential is of variable amplitude, but does not overshoot 0 mV, and lasts 10–100 ms. The attendant transient increase in cytosolic $[Ca^{2+}]$ causes a brief twitch contraction.

Repolarization is brought about by a $K^+$ efflux through $K_v$, $K_{Ca}$ and $K_{ir}$ channels.

## Contraction may or may not depend on membrane depolarization

Although $\alpha_1$ adrenergic receptor activation can trigger contraction through action potentials, as described earlier, it can also cause contraction without action potentials via depolarization-independent pathways. Depending on the mix of ion channels in a vessel, contraction can be triggered in three ways:

- **Contraction induced by action potentials** (Figure 12.2a,b). In some arterioles, small arteries and certain veins, VDCCs are so abundant that strong sympathetic stimulation triggers VDCC-based action potentials. Extracellular $Ca^{2+}$ influx during the action potential raises intracellular $Ca^{2+}$, causing a twitch contraction. This has been called electromechanical coupling.
- **Contraction induced by graded, sustained depolarization** (Figure 12.1). In many blood vessels, noradrenaline evokes a graded, sustained depolarization, but no action potentials. The depolarization is brought about by $i_{cat}$ and $i_{Cl(Ca)}$, which are activated via the $G_q$–PLCβ–$IP_3$/DAG pathway (Figure 12.6a). The depolarization activates VDCCs, leading to a sustained contraction. This is again electromechanical coupling.
- **Contraction unrelated to membrane potential** (Figures 12.2c and 12.6b). In large arteries, the myocytes often have abundant ROCs but few VDCCs. Noradrenaline raises the cytosolic $Ca^{2+}$ partly through DAG-activated ROCs and partly through $IP_3$-mediated stored release and cat-SOCs. The contraction is not evoked by membrane depolarization, though the ROC current may cause a small, coincidental depolarization. This type of activation has been called pharmacomechanical coupling.

## Sympathetic stimulation can evoke fast and slow EJPs, and both depolarization-dependent and depolarization-independent contraction

Having considered how noradrenaline alone affects vascular myocytes, we can return to the more complex case of sympathetic stimulation, which releases both noradrenaline and ATP. Sympathetic stimulation can evoke both depolarization-independent and depolarization-dependent contraction in the same myocyte. This is illustrated by the response of a small arterial vessel to moderate sympathetic stimulation (Figure 12.9a). When the local sympathetic fibres are stimulated briefly, the myocyte electrical response has two components. After a very short latency, ~15 ms, there is a small, rapidly rising depolarization of ~10 mV that is short-lived (1 s) – the **fast EJP**. This is followed by a slow-rising, longer-lasting depolarization, like the **slow EJP** evoked by noradrenaline (Figure 12.8). What causes the two electrical responses?

The **fast EJP** is abolished by inhibitors of the purinergic (ATP) receptor, P2X, so it must be triggered by sympathetic ATP (for proof, see Figure 14.3). Unlike the metabotropic adrenoceptor, the P2X receptor is an '**ionotropic**' receptor; that is, the receptor is directly linked to a cation-conducting channel, which is part of the same macromolecule (a **ligand-gated** channel). Channel activation is therefore very fast. The activated channel conducts a small depolarizing current of $Ca^{2+}$ and $Na^+$ into the myocyte. The **slow EJP** is abolished by $\alpha_1$ adrenergic receptor blockers, such as prazosin, so it is clearly triggered by noradrenaline (Figure 12.9a, top right). It is generated by $i_{cat}$ and $i_{Cl(Ca)}$, as described earlier (Figure 12.6a).

The **mechanical response** in Figure 12.9a, a slow contraction, is puzzling on close inspection. It cannot be caused by the slow EJP because the contraction starts before the slow EJP. Nor can the contraction be caused by the fast EJP because prazosin abolishes the contraction but not the fast EJP (Figure 12.9a, top right). The slow contraction is in fact an example of **depolarization-independent contraction**, due to ROC and SOC activation by $\alpha_1$ adrenergic receptors.

At a higher intensity of sympathetic stimulation, the fast EJP becomes larger and activates sufficient VDCCs to trigger an action potential and twitch contraction (Figure 12.9b). The slow depolarization becomes larger too, triggering another action potential, which produces a twitch superimposed on the underlying slow contraction. The twitches are examples of **depolarization-dependent contraction**, while the underlying slow contraction reflects depolarization-independent contraction. Both processes can occur in the same myocyte. However, the electrical response to sympathetic stimulation varies greatly from vessel to vessel; not all vessels respond as described here, although the pattern is a common one.

## Intracellular free $Ca^{2+}$ shows two phases during a vasoconstriction

If the vessel wall is loaded with a $Ca^{2+}$-dependent fluorescent dye, it is found that the cytosolic free $Ca^{2+}$ concentration exhibits two distinct phases following stimulation. In the **initial, transient phase**, there is a rapid increase in cytosolic $Ca^{2+}$ concentration, from ~0.1 $\mu$M to ~1 $\mu$M. This occurs synchronously in all the myocytes throughout the vessel wall, and is followed almost immediately by a rise in tension (Figure 12.4a). In the **second, tonic phase**, starting 30–60 s later, the average cytosolic $[Ca^{2+}]$ in the vessel wall retreats to a lower but still suprabasal level; yet, the force of contraction is well maintained. During the second phase, individual myocytes may exhibit intermittent, asynchronous $Ca^{2+}$ waves (Figure 12.4a), especially in small artery myocytes with a low contractile tone; the second-phase $Ca^{2+}$ tend to be more stable

in vessels with a high basal tone. The pathways responsible for the two phases are as follows.

## The initial phase is due to $Ca^{2+}$ store release and extracellular $Ca^{2+}$ influx

The initial large increase in myocyte free $Ca^{2+}$ results from the release of stored $Ca^{2+}$ from the SR, particularly in large arteries, aided by an influx of extracellular $Ca^{2+}$, particularly in small arteries and arterioles (Figure 12.7). In large arteries, $Ca^{2+}$ store release accounts for most of the initial cytosolic $Ca^{2+}$ transient, because the SR is well developed. Store discharge is triggered chiefly by receptor-induced $IP_3$ production. Store replenishment is brought about by an influx of extracellular $Ca^{2+}$ ions through the store-operated TRP channels in the adjacent sarcolemma (capacitative $Ca^{2+}$ entry). In smaller, resistance arteries/arterioles, extracellular $Ca^{2+}$ influx is more important because small resistance vessels tend to have scanty SR but abundant VDCCs. The VDCCs are activated by depolarization, which is brought about by $i_{cat}$ and $i_{Cl(Ca)}$. Extracellular $Ca^{2+}$ influx through the activated VDCCs, and through ROCs, raises the cytosolic $Ca^{2+}$ concentration.

**To summarize the initial 30–60s phase of vasoconstriction**, the agonist-receptor complex activates the PLC$\beta$–$IP_3$–DAG pathway. $IP_3$ releases stored $Ca^{2+}$, which raises cytosolic $Ca^{2+}$ and activates depolarizing current $i_{Cl(Ca)}$. The DAG activates depolarizing current $i_{cat}$. The depolarization by $i_{cat}$ and $i_{Cl(Ca)}$ increases the open-state probability of sarcolemmal VDCCs, admitting extracellular $Ca^{2+}$. DAG also activates sarcolemmal ROCs that admit extracellular $Ca^{2+}$. A $4Ca^{2+}$-calmodulin complex then activates MLCK, which phosphorylates the myosin light chains, enabling the myosin heads to form crossbridges with the actin filament. Crossbridge flexion then generates shortening and tension.

## The second phase is sustained by extracellular $Ca^{2+}$ influx and $Ca^{2+}$ sensitization

During the tonic phase, the mean cytosolic $Ca^{2+}$ concentration, averaged across the whole tunica media, drops below the transient peak value; in some vessels, the individual myocytes develop intermittent $Ca^{2+}$ waves (Figure 12.4a). Each $Ca^{2+}$ wave is generated by SR store discharge by $IP_3$. Since the sarcolemmal pumps expel some $Ca^{2+}$ during each wave, extracellular $Ca^{2+}$ influx through VDCCs and cat-SOCs is needed to recharge the stores. The importance of extracellular $Ca^{2+}$ influx during tonic contraction is demonstrated by the relaxation induced by nifedipine and cat-SOC blockers.

During the tonic phase, vasoconstriction is well maintained despite a fall in mean cytosolic $[Ca^{2+}]$ (Figure 12.4a). Therefore, some additional mechanism must come into play. This mechanism is **Ca$^{2+}$ sensitization**; that is, a given level of Ca$^{2+}$ has an increased contractile effect during the tonic phase.

## Tonic Ca$^{2+}$ sensitization is mediated by RhoA kinase and PKC

Ca$^{2+}$ sensitization is brought about by kinases that are activated by the G protein-coupled receptors (Figure 12.7). Kinases are a large family of enzymes that phosphorylate other proteins to change their activity. The kinase chiefly responsible for Ca$^{2+}$ sensitization is **RhoA kinase**. Agonist-receptor complexes coupled to G$_{12/13}$ protein activate **RhoA**, a monomeric GTPase that activates RhoA kinase. RhoA kinase inhibits MLCP, the enzyme responsible for dephosphorylating the myosin head and turning off the myosin motor. This shifts the dynamic balance between MLCK and MLCP in favour of phosphorylation, despite a fall in Ca$^{2+}$-calmodulin.

Ca$^{2+}$ sensitization is also promoted in some vessels by PKCα, which is activated by DAG and cytosolic Ca$^{2+}$ (Figure 12.6b). PKCα activates the CPI-17 protein, which,

---

### CONCEPT BOX 12.1

#### REGULATION OF VASCULAR MYOCYTE TONE

- Active vascular tension (tone) is sustained. Tone is regulated by the sympathetic neuroeffector noradrenaline, circulating hormones (adrenaline, angiotensin II, vasopressin) and local factors (e.g. nitric oxide, endothelium-derived hyperpolarization (EDH), endothelin, hypoxia, histamine and other autacoids).

- Tone depends primarily on cytosolic [Ca$^{2+}$]. The Ca$^{2+}$-calmodulin complex activates myosin light chain kinase (MLCK), which phosphorylates myosin heads to cause crossbridge formation. Conversely, if [Ca$^{2+}$] falls, dephosphorylation by constitutively active myosin light chain phosphatase (MLCP) causes relaxation.

- Agonists (e.g. noradrenaline) that activate G$_q$-protein-coupled receptors (e.g. α$_1$ adrenergic receptor) can raise cytosolic [Ca$^{2+}$] in three ways:
  - G$_q$-activated PLCβ generates IP$_3$, which releases the Ca$^{2+}$ store and activates cat-SOCs;
  - PLCβ generates DAG, which activates ROCs;
  - IP$_3$ and DAG trigger depolarizing currents that activate L-type voltage-dependent Ca$^{2+}$ channels (VDCCs).

- Tone is also regulated by RhoA kinase and PKC, which sensitize the cell to Ca$^{2+}$ by inhibiting MLCP.

- Vascular relaxation is brought about by reducing the free cytosolic [Ca$^{2+}$] or Ca$^{2+}$ desensitization. Free [Ca$^{2+}$] can be reduced by hyperpolarization-induced closure of VDCCs (e.g. metabolic hyperaemia, EDH), or by cAMP-activated PKA (e.g. adrenaline-activated β$_2$ adrenergic receptors), or by cyclic guanosine monophosphate (cGMP)-activated protein kinase G (PKG; e.g. NO, penile erection).

---

like RhoA kinase, inhibits MLCP. PKCα also triggers a mitogen-activated protein kinase pathway that phosphorylates **caldesmon**, a regulatory protein on the actin filament, facilitating crossbridge formation. This may explain why adrenergic-stimulated tone is maintained in some vessels despite a fall in myosin light chain phosphorylation.

### 12.6 VASOMOTION (RHYTHMIC CONTRACTIONS)

Most arteries and veins exhibit a stable vascular tone, but many arterioles (e.g. skeletal muscle, skin; Figure 15.10c), along with terminal pial arteries and the portal vein (Figure 12.2a), exhibit rhythmic contractions called vasomotion. Arteriolar vasomotion may help reduce net capillary filtration rate (Section 11.6) and optimize tissue O$_2$ delivery. Vasomotion occurs several times per minute and is brought about by co-ordinated, synchronous oscillations in cytosolic [Ca$^{2+}$] throughout the tunica media (cf. asynchronous oscillations in the myocytes of tonically contracted vessels). The oscillations are due primarily to the cyclical release of the SR Ca$^{2+}$ store by IP$_3$, boosted by VDCCs that are activated as $i_{Cl(Ca)}$ depolarizes the myocyte. The relaxation phase is due to Ca$^{2+}$ sequestration by the SR pumps and repolarization by the Ca$^{2+}$-activated BK current. Synchronization between the myocytes is probably mediated by the homocellular gap junctions, and in some cases the myoendothelial gap junctions, since vasomotion is endothelium-dependent in some vessels. In the portal vein, a different mechanism seems to operate; spontaneous myocyte depolarization triggers action potentials, which open VDCCs and cause the Ca$^{2+}$ oscillation.

### 12.7 PHYSIOLOGICAL VASODILATOR MECHANISMS

The account so far has concentrated on vascular contraction. But a major function of blood vessels, especially resistance vessels, is to dilate, to raise blood flow to exercising muscle, myocardium, and so on. Vasodilatation is not an active process; it is simply a reduction of tonic contractile tension, that is, a relaxation, and it can be brought about by four mechanisms:

- hyperpolarization;
- the adenylyl cyclase–cAMP–PKA pathway;
- the guanylyl cyclase–cGMP–PKG pathway;
- desensitization to Ca$^{2+}$.

The first three mechanisms produce vasodilatation by **reducing the cytosolic Ca$^{2+}$ concentration**, which reduces MLCK activity. This allows the constitutive background MLCP activity to predominate and turn off the myosin motor. The fourth vasodilator mechanism, **desensitization to Ca$^{2+}$**, produces vascular relaxation despite little fall in cytosolic Ca$^{2+}$ concentration.

# Hyperpolarization mediates vasodilatation by extracellular K+, endothelium-derived hyperpolarization, hypoxia and neuropeptides

Hyperpolarization closes VDCCs, leading to a fall in cytosolic free [Ca²⁺] and vasodilatation (Figure 12.1). Examples are as follows:

- **Skeletal muscle contraction, myocardial contraction and brain activity** raise the K⁺ concentration in the local interstitial fluid, due to K⁺ efflux during action potential repolarization. Extravascular K⁺ increases vascular $K_{ir}$ activity (Section 12.4), leading to hyperpolarization and vasodilatation. This is one of several mechanisms that match blood flow to tissue metabolic activity (metabolic hyperaemia, Section 13.4).
- **Endothelium-derived hyperpolarization** (EDH) elicits vasodilatation by VSM hyperpolarization. EDH is the spread of hyperpolarization from the endothelium to VSM via myoendothelial gap junctions and the diffusion of endothelium-derived hyperpolarizing factors (EDHFs), such as K⁺, epoxyeicosatrienoic acid (EET) as reviewed in Section 9.5. In feed arteries, conducted vasodilatation is due to the conduction of endothelial hyperpolarization into myocytes through myoendothelial gap junctions (Section 13.7).

- **Hypoxia**, if severe, can activate myocyte $K_{ATP}$ channels (Section 12.4), leading to hyperpolarization, reduced cytosolic [Ca²⁺] and hypoxic vasodilatation. However, in many arteries Ca²⁺ desensitization is the main mechanism underlying hypoxic vasodilatation, and there is little reduction in cytosolic [Ca²⁺].
- **Sensory nerve neuropeptides**, such as calcitonin gene-related peptide (CGRP) and vasoactive intestinal polypeptide (VIP), are released during inflammation, and contribute to the vasodilatation of inflammation by causing hyperpolarization (Section 14.4).
- **$K_{ATP}$-activating drugs**, such as diazoxide, pinacidil and cromakalim, elicit vasodilatation through myocyte hyperpolarization.

## cAMP-PKA-mediated vasodilatation is triggered by β adrenergic receptors

Circulating adrenaline dilates the resistance vessels of skeletal muscle, myocardium and liver because vascular β adrenergic receptors are strongly expressed in these tissues. (In most other tissues, $\alpha_1$ density exceeds β density, so adrenaline causes vasoconstriction.) The β adrenergic receptor is coupled to the trimeric membrane GTPase $G_s$, which activates membrane-bound adenylyl cyclase (Figure 12.10). Although β adrenergic receptor-mediated vasodilation was ascribed to $\beta_2$ adrenergic receptors, recent evidence indicates

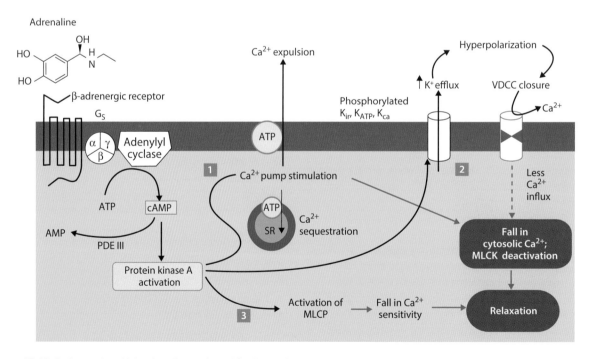

**Figure 12.10** Pathways by which adrenaline-activated β adrenergic receptors bring about vasodilatation. Adenosine $A_{2A}$ receptors, histamine $H_2$ receptors, VIP and CGRP receptors are likewise coupled to adenylyl (adenylate) cyclase, leading to vasodilatation. Adenylyl cyclase can be activated directly by the drug forskolin. AMP, adenosine monophosphate; ATP, adenosine triphosphate; cAMP, cyclic adenosine monophosphate; CGRP; calcitonin gene-related peptide; $K_{ATP}$, ATP-dependent K⁺ channel; $K_{Ca}$, Ca²⁺-activated K⁺ channel; $K_{ir}$, inwardly rectifying K⁺ channel; MLCP, myosin light chain phosphatase PDE3, phosphodiesterase 3; SR, sarcoplasmic reticulum; VIP, vasoactive intestinal peptide; VDCC, voltage-dependent Ca²⁺ channel. (After Ushio-Fukai M, Abe S, Kobayashi S, et al. *The Journal of Physiology* 1993; 462: 679–96, with permission from Wiley-Blackwell.)

an important role for $\beta_1$ adrenergic receptors also. Many other physiological vasodilators also activate $G_s$-coupled receptors, including **adenosine** ($A_{2A}$ receptor), **prostacyclin** ($EP_4$ receptor), **histamine** ($H_2$ receptor), **VIP** and **CGRP**. The activation of adenylyl (or adenylate) cyclase by any of these $G_s$-coupled receptors catalyses the conversion of ATP to cAMP; cAMP activates the phosphorylating enzyme **protein kinase A (PKA)**. PKA induces vascular relaxation by multiple actions (Figure 12.10):

- PKA phosphorylates **phospholamban**, a protein that normally acts as a brake on the $Ca^{2+}$ ATPase pump. Phosphorylation reduces this braking effect. PKA therefore stimulates SR and sarcolemma **$Ca^{2+}$ pump activity**, leading to a fall in cytosolic free $Ca^{2+}$.
- PKA also phosphorylates **$K_{ir}$, $K_{ATP}$ and $K_{Ca}$ channels**, increasing their open-state probability. The resulting hyperpolarization closes VDCCs and thus reduces extracellular $Ca^{2+}$ influx.
- PKA phosphorylates **MLCP,** increasing activity and relaxing VSM.

The PKA activator, cAMP, is continuously degraded by the enzyme **phosphodiesterase 3** (PDE3; Figure 12.10). Drugs that inhibit PDE3, such as milrinone and cilostazol, raise intracellular cAMP, leading to vasodilatation.

## cGMP/PKG-mediated vasodilatation is induced by nitric oxide

NO, nitrovasodilator drugs such as glyceryl trinitrate (commonly used to relieve angina), and the hormone atrial natriuretic peptide (ANP) cause vasodilatation by raising the intracellular concentration of **cGMP**. NO activates soluble guanylyl (guanylate) cyclase, which catalyses the production of cGMP from guanosine trisphosphate (Section 9.4; Figure 9.10). The cGMP activates **protein kinase G (PKG)**, which has similar actions to PKA; it phosphorylates phospholamban to disinhibit the $Ca^{2+}$ ATPase pumps, leading to $Ca^{2+}$ sequestration and $Ca^{2+}$ expulsion; it also reduces $Ca^{2+}$ sensitization. In this way, NO contributes to flow-induced vasodilatation, inflammatory vasodilatation, endotoxin shock and sexual erection (Chapter 13). The treatment of erectile dysfunction by the cGMP-boosting drug **sildenafil** (**Viagra**) is covered in Section 13.3.

## Desensitization to $Ca^{2+}$ occurs in hypoxic arteries

In many arteries, hypoxia causes vasodilatation despite little fall in cytosolic free $Ca^{2+}$ concentration (Figure 13.5). The vasodilatation is brought about by reduced myosin phosphorylation, possibly through the inhibition of RhoA kinase (Figure 12.7).

## SUMMARY

- VSM comprises circumferential, spindle-shaped myocytes. Gap junctions provide an electrical connection between the myocytes, and between myocyte and endothelium. The contractile machinery comprises interdigitating thick myosin filaments and thin actin filaments. The latter are anchored to cytoplasmic dense bodies and sarcolemmal dense bands.
- Contraction is driven primarily by cytosolic $[Ca^{2+}]$, which forms a $Ca^{2+}$-calmodulin complex that activates **MLCK**. MLCK phosphorylates myosin heads, which then form myosin–actin crossbridges, causing contraction. The long duration of the crossbridges (latch state) maintains vascular tone with relatively little energy expenditure. When MLCK activity is reduced, dephosphorylation by **MLCP** leads to relaxation.
- Sarcolemmal **$K^+$ channels** conduct an outward current that generates a basal potential of about −50 mV. Inwardly rectifying $K_{ir}$, ATP-dependent $K_{ATP}$, voltage-dependent (delayed rectifying) $K_V$ and $Ca^{2+}$-activated $K_{Ca}$ (BK) channels all contribute. An inward cation current through constitutively active TRP channels contributes to the relatively depolarized basal potential.
- Sarcolemmal **L-type VDCCs** exhibit an increase in open probability with membrane depolarization, leading to extracellular $Ca^{2+}$ influx and contraction. **Depolarization-dependent contraction** is prominent in small, arterial resistance vessels because they strongly express VDCCs.
- **Sympathetic fibre activity** causes resistance vessel contraction. Fibre varicosities release ATP and noradrenaline,

which evoke VSM **fast and slow EJPs** (depolarizations), respectively. Noradrenaline $\alpha_1$ adrenergic receptors are $G_q$-coupled to $PLC\beta$, which generates $IP_3$ and DAG. DAG activates cation-conducting receptor-operated channels (ROCs), which can generate a small current ($i_{cat}$); $IP_3$ releases stored $Ca^{2+}$ to activate $Cl^-$ channels (current $i_{Cl(Ca)}$). Depolarization by $i_{cat}$ and $i_{Cl(Ca)}$ creates the slow EJP. If the EJPs are large and VDCCs are abundant, as in arterioles, VDCC activation generates a **$Ca^{2+}$-mediated action potential** and twitch.

- **Depolarization-independent contraction** can occur in large arteries. When a $G_q$-protein-coupled receptor, such as $\alpha_1$ or $H_1$, activates the $PLC\beta$–$IP_3$–DAG pathway, the $IP_3$ releases the SR **$Ca^{2+}$ store** (substantial in large arteries), which can open sarcolemmal store-operated channels (**SOCs**), while DAG activates **ROCs** that conduct extracellular $Ca^{2+}$ into the cell.
- During prolonged vasoconstriction, an initial, transient phase of high cytosolic $[Ca^{2+}]$ due to store release is followed by a sustained phase of lower but still elevated $[Ca^{2+}]$. The contraction is maintained by (1) continuing **$Ca^{2+}$ influx** through VDCCs, ROCs and SOCs; and (2) increased sensitivity to $Ca^{2+}$. **$Ca^{2+}$ sensitization** is brought about by the inhibition of MLCP by RhoA kinase and PKC.
- Some arterioles undergo rhythmic contractions (**vasomotion**), caused by regular, spontaneous waves of $Ca^{2+}$ discharge from the SR store.

- **Vasodilatation** is usually brought about by a **fall in cytosolic [Ca²⁺]**, which deactivates MLCK, allowing myosin phosphatase to predominate and turn off the myosin motor. In addition, **desensitization to Ca²⁺** can contribute to vasodilatation. Cytosolic [Ca²⁺] can be reduced by the following three mechanisms:

  - **Hyperpolarization** reduces VDCC open probability, leading to vasodilatation. In active skeletal muscle, myocardium and brain, increased interstitial [K⁺] raises the $K_{ir}$ channel open probability, leading to hyperpolarization. This contributes to metabolic hyperaemia. EDHFs (K⁺, EET) likewise cause myocyte hyperpolarization and vasodilatation, as do some neuropeptides. Severe hypoxia activates $K_{ATP}$ channels, leading to hyperpolarization and vasodilatation.

  - **cAMP–PKA.** $G_s$-coupled receptors, such as $\beta_{1/2}$ adrenergic receptors, adenosine $A_{2A}$ and histamine $H_2$ receptors, activate the adenylate cyclase–cAMP–PKA pathway. PKA stimulates Ca²⁺ ATPase pumps to reduce cytosolic [Ca²⁺]; it phosphorylates K⁺ channels to cause hyperpolarization, leading to VDCC closure, and activates MLCP. This is how adrenaline causes vasodilatation in the myocardium and skeletal muscle.

  - **cGMP–PKG.** NO, nitrovasodilator drugs and ANP activate the guanylate cyclase–cGMP–PKG pathway. PKG has similar effects to PKA. NO mediates flow-induced dilatation, the vasodilatation of inflammation and sexual erection.

## FURTHER READING

Garland CJ, Dora KA. EDH: endothelium-dependent hyperpolarization and microvascular signalling. *Acta Physiologica* 2017; **219**(1): 152–61.

Schinzari F, Tesauro M, Cardillo C. Vascular hyperpolarization in human physiology and cardiovascular risk conditions and disease. *Acta Physiologica* 2017; **219**(1): 124–37.

Tykocki NR, Boerman EM, Jackson WF. Smooth muscle ion channels and regulation of vascular tone in resistance arteries and arterioles. *Comprehensive Physiology* 2017; **7**(2): 485–581.

Brozovich FV, Nicholson CJ, Degen CV, et al. Mechanisms of vascular smooth muscle contraction and the basis for pharmacologic treatment of smooth muscle disorders. *Pharmacological Reviews* 2016; **68**(2): 476–532.

Dora KA. Endothelial-smooth muscle cell interactions in the regulation of vascular tone in skeletal muscle. *Microcirculation* 2016; **23**(8): 626–30.

Shimokawa H, Sunamura S, Satoh K. RhoA/Rho-kinase in the cardiovascular system. *Circulation Research* 2016; **118**(2): 352–66.

Earley S, Brayden JE. Transient receptor potential channels in the vasculature. *Physiological Reviews* 2015; **95**(2):645–90.

Westcott EB, Segal SS. Perivascular innervation: a multiplicity of roles in vasomotor control and myoendothelial signaling. *Microcirculation* 2013; **20**(3): 217–38.

Aalkjær C, Boedtkjer D, Matchkov V. Vasomotion: what is currently thought? *Acta Physiologica* 2011; **202**(3): 253–69.

Albert AP, Large WA. Signal transduction pathways and gating mechanisms of native TRP-like cation channels in vascular myocytes. *The Journal of Physiology* 2006; **570**(Pt 1): 45–51.

Ledoux J, Werner ME, Brayden JE, et al. Calcium-activated potassium channels and the regulation of vascular tone. *Physiology* 2006; **21**: 69–78.

Cohen AW, Hnasko R, Schubert W, et al. Role of caveolae and caveolins in health and disease. *Physiological Reviews* 2004; **84**(4): 1341–79.

Somlyo AP, Somlyo AV. Ca²⁺ sensitivity of smooth muscle and nonmuscle myosin II: modulated by G proteins, kinases, and myosin phosphatase. *Physiological Reviews* 2003; **83**(4): 1325–58.

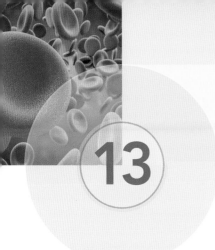

# Control of blood vessels: intrinsic control

# 13

## LEARNING OBJECTIVES

*After reading this chapter, you should be able to:*

- sketch the myogenic response of arterioles to a pressure change and explain its importance (13.2);
- list the chief roles of nitric oxide in the circulation (13.3);
- state the role of metabolic hyperaemia and name the putative mediators (13.4);
- give thumbnail sketches of the autacoids histamine, bradykinin, serotonin, platelet-activating factor, prostacyclin and thromboxane (13.5);

- illustrate 'autoregulation' by drawing a plot of blood flow versus perfusion pressure, and draw a second curve to show how autoregulation is affected by metabolic hyperaemia (13.6);
- explain how dilatation is co-ordinated along the arterial tree during exercise (13.7);
- outline how post-ischaemic hyperaemia arises (13.8);
- explain the basis of ischaemia-reperfusion injury (13.9).

## 13.1 OVERVIEW OF VASCULAR CONTROL AND ITS ROLES

The tension exerted by vascular smooth muscle is called the vascular 'tone'. Vascular tone regulates the calibre of the resistance vessel, and hence the blood flow through it. An increase in tone causes vasoconstriction and reduces local flow. Conversely, a fall in tone causes vasodilatation, by allowing the blood pressure (BP) to distend the relaxed vessel. Vascular tone is thus an essential prerequisite for vasodilatation (loss of tone), and basal vascular tone is high in tissues capable of substantially increasing their blood flow (hyperaemia), for example, skeletal muscle.

Arterial vessels maintain some vascular tone even when the tonic sympathetic vasoconstrictor nerve activity is blocked. This is called **basal tone**. Basal tone is generally low in veins. Basal tone is the result of tonic vasoconstrictor influences – constitutively active myocyte transient receptor potential channels (TRPCs), myogenic response, endothelin (ET), partially offset by tonic

vasodilator influences – nitric oxide (NO), endothelium-derived hyperpolarization (EDH). Vascular tone *in vivo* is generally suprabasal due to the tonic vasoconstrictor activity of sympathetic fibres.

Before we delve further into the processes that regulate vascular tone, let us first summarize its many roles, drawing together key points from earlier chapters.

## Vascular tone regulates regional blood flow, arterial blood pressure, capillary filtration rate and central venous pressure

**Regional blood flow** through a tissue is altered through changes in resistance vessel radius, $r$. A small change in $r$ has a huge effect on resistance to flow, due to the $r^4$ term in Poiseuille's law (Section 8.7). This allows tissues to alter their blood flow over a huge range. In skin, skeletal muscle and exocrine glands, the **flow can be increased 20-fold** by vasodilatation to meet the demands of temperature regulation, exercise

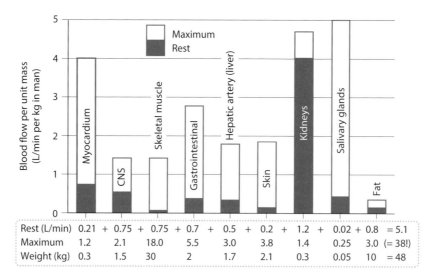

**Figure 13.1** Wide range of blood flow, from rest to maximal, in tissues of a 70-kg human. Maximal flow through all organs simultaneously can never be achieved because at 38 L/min it exceeds maximum cardiac output. CNS, central nervous system. (Data from Mellander S, Johansson B. *Pharmacological Reviews* 1968; 20(3): 117–96, with permission.)

and liquid secretion, respectively (Figure 13.1). Indeed, the maximal tissue blood flows are so huge that they could never be achieved simultaneously, because the total flow would then exceed the maximum output of the heart.

**Arterial BP** is the product of total peripheral resistance and cardiac output (Section 8.5). The continual adjustment of resistance vessel tone helps control arterial pressure during normal activities, such as standing up. During hypovolaemic emergencies such as haemorrhage, vasoconstriction helps to maintain BP.

**Capillary recruitment** and **capillary pressure** are regulated by local arteriolar tone. Vasodilatation in exercising muscle improves perfusion homogeneity and perfused capillary surface area, boosting solute exchange (Figure 10.14). Arteriolar tone also regulates capillary pressure, and therefore fluid exchange and plasma volume (Figure 11.4).

**Central venous pressure** (CVP) is regulated by the tone of the peripheral veins and venules. Peripheral venoconstriction displaces blood into the central veins, thus raising the cardiac filling pressure and stroke volume (Frank–Starling's law of the heart, Section 6.4).

From this summary, we see that changes in vascular tone act both at a **local** level to regulate tissue perfusion, nutrient and water exchange; and at the level of the **whole animal** to regulate arterial BP, plasma volume, CVP and stroke volume.

## Vascular tone is controlled by intrinsic and extrinsic mechanisms

The processes that regulate vascular tone fall into two classes: intrinsic and extrinsic (Figure 13.2). Intrinsic regulation is regulation by factors located entirely within an organ or tissue.

Extrinsic regulation is regulation by factors from outside the organ. **Intrinsic regulatory mechanisms** include:

- the **Bayliss myogenic response** (Bayliss effect) to arterial pressure;
- **endothelial secretions** (NO, EDH, prostacyclin ($PGI_2$), ET);
- **vasoactive metabolites** generated by active tissues, for example, adenosine;
- **autacoids** (vasoactive paracrine secretions such as histamine); and
- **temperature**, which is chiefly important in the skin (Chapter 15).

Many major responses are mediated purely by intrinsic regulation, notably **flow autoregulation, functional and reactive hyperaemia, inflammatory vasodilatation** and **arterial vasospasm**.

**Extrinsic regulation** is brought about by:

- **vasomotor nerves**, mainly sympathetic; and
- **vasoactive hormones** such as adrenaline, angiotensin II and vasopressin.

## The control hierarchy

Vascular regulation involves a hierarchy of control processes. The lowest level is intrinsic regulation by the Bayliss myogenic response (Bayliss effect). The middle level is the modulation of the myogenic response by endothelial secretions, vasoactive metabolites and autacoids. These two levels of control provide for local tissue needs, for example, constancy of renal perfusion (myogenic response), hyperaemia of exercising muscles (vasoactive metabolites). The highest level of control is exercised by the extrinsic factors (Chapter 14), which modify or override the intrinsic controls to meet the needs of the whole animal, as in the sympathetic-mediated peripheral vasoconstriction during a haemorrhage.

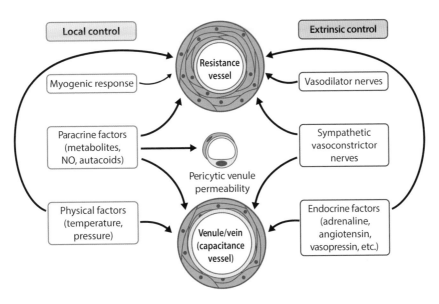

**Figure 13.2** Overview of local and extrinsic vascular control. NO, nitric oxide.

## 13.2 MYOGENIC RESPONSE TO BLOOD PRESSURE CHANGES

Arterial vessels respond actively to changes in transmural pressure, as follows.

### Arterial vessels contract when blood pressure is raised: the Bayliss myogenic response

The myogenic response was first described by Sir William Bayliss, brother-in-law of Ernest Starling, in 1902. When BP is raised acutely in an artery or arteriole, the pressure at first distends the vessel. However, within seconds most systemic arterioles and arteries react and undergo a well-sustained contraction – the myogenic response (Figure 13.3). Conversely, a fall in BP triggers a fall in vascular tone and vasodilatation. The myogenic response is important because (1) it contributes to basal tone and (2) it stabilizes tissue blood flow and capillary filtration pressure if arterial pressure changes (autoregulation; Section 13.6). The myogenic response is well developed in the brain, kidney and myocardium, but not in the skin.

### The myogenic response is mediated by depolarization and $Ca^{2+}$

When an arterial myocyte is stretched, it depolarizes to around −40 mV. This activates L-type $Ca^{2+}$ channels, leading to a rise in cytosolic free $[Ca^{2+}]$ and contraction. The depolarization is attributed to stretch-activated channels, namely TRP cation channels, volume-regulated $Cl^-$ channels and epithelial $Na^+$

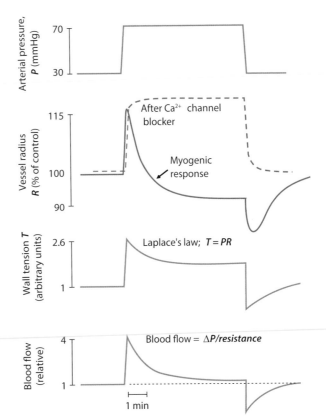

**Figure 13.3** Change in diameter of isolated rat cerebral artery on raising luminal pressure $P$. Initial passive stretch is followed by active contraction – the Bayliss myogenic response. This is abolished by the L-type $Ca^{2+}$ channel blocker, nimodipine. Wall tension $T$, calculated from Laplace's law (equation 8.8), is increased and provides a sustained stimulus. (Based on McCarron JG, Crichton CA, Langton PD, et al. *The Journal of Physiology* 1997; 498(Pt 2): 371–9, with permission from Wiley-Blackwell; and Carlson BE, Secomb TW. *Microcirculation* 2005; 12(4): 327–38, with permission from Taylor & Francis Group.)

channels (ENaCs), because the myogenic response is impaired by gadolinium (TRP channel blocker), Cl⁻ channel blockers and amiloride (ENaC blocker), as well as $Ca^{2+}$ channel blockers (Figure 13.3).

This pathway drives the initial myogenic vasoconstriction. Over longer periods, $Ca^{2+}$ sensitization by protein kinase C and Ras homolog gene family, member A (RhoA) kinase helps maintain the response (Figure 12.7). The depolarization is sustained by reduced $K_{Ca}$ channel activity, elicited by the vasoconstrictor 20-hydroxyeicosatetraenoic acid (20-HETE). 20-HETE is produced from arachidonic acid by the enzyme cytochrome P450 ω-hydroxylase.

When a vessel narrows due to the myogenic response, the endothelial shear stress increases, stimulating the endothelium to produce more NO and EDH. These vasodilators help prevent excessive myogenic constriction.

## Wall tension sustains the myogenic response

A puzzling feature of the myogenic response is that the vessel wall is only stretched temporarily, at the start. During the tonic contraction, the vessel circumference and myocyte lengths are smaller than at the outset, yet the response is well maintained (Figure 13.3). However, the wall **tension** is increased, due to the rise in pressure (Laplace's law, Section 8.7). Therefore, the response is probably mediated by tension, acting on the membrane ion channels and on membrane integrins linked to protein kinases.

## External pressure impairs flow and can cause pressure ulcers

When pressure is applied to the outside of a blood vessel, the vessel is compressed and blood flow falls. This happens to the intramural coronary arteries during systole, temporarily impairing myocardial perfusion (Figure 15.5). Similarly, blood flow to skeletal muscle is impaired during a contraction because intramuscle pressure can reach 270–570 mmHg (Figure 13.8). Sitting, kneeling and lying compresses blood vessels in the skin. If this is prolonged, as in older bedridden or paralysed patients, the resulting impairment of skin nutrition can cause horrific ulcers over the buttocks and heels, called **pressure ulcers (bed sores)**. These can be avoided by good nursing care, namely regularly turning the patient to relieve the cutaneous compression.

## 13.3 REGULATION BY ENDOTHELIUM

Endothelium produces the vasoconstrictor ET and the vasodilators NO, EDH and $PGI_2$. These are paracrine agents, acting locally on neighbouring myocytes. Their production and roles were covered in Sections 9.4 and 9.5; here, we concentrate on vascular regulation by NO and ET.

The chief roles of NO in vascular control are:

- continuous modulation of **basal tone**;
- reduction of basal tone in **pregnancy**;
- **flow-induced vasodilatation** of conduit arteries to muscle during exercise;
- vasodilatation mediated by **cholinergic parasympathetic fibres**;
- vasodilatation of **sexual erection**;
- vasodilatation during **inflammation** and **endotoxic shock**.

## Shear-stimulated nitric oxide production modulates basal vascular tone

The chief, normal stimulus for endothelial NO production is the **shear stress** exerted by the bloodstream, which drives ~60%–80% of tonic NO formation. Other stimuli include circulating **insulin** and **oestrogen**. Shear stress, not flow, is clearly the stimulus because raising the blood viscosity (and hence shear stress) evokes vasodilatation when flow is held constant. Shear stress is sensed by the endothelial glycocalyx, which activates the phosphatidyl inositol-3 kinase–protein kinase B ($PI_3$–PKB) pathway (Figure 9.10). This increases the activity of endothelial NO synthase (**eNOS**). Since NO causes local vasodilatation, it reduces shear stress. Thus, shear-dependent NO production results in a negative feedback loop that helps to stabilize endothelial shear stress.

NO is evidently produced continuously and influences human peripheral resistance, since the synthesis inhibitor L-N$^G$-monomethylarginine reduces blood flow in the forearm (Figure 13.4). NOS inhibitors also approximately halve renal blood flow, a greater effect than in most other tissues. Human vascular tone is thus the result of a balance between tonic relaxation mediated by NO (also EDH and $PGI_2$) and tonic vasoconstriction mediated by constitutive TRP channel activity, the myogenic response, ET, sympathetic vasomotor activity and circulating hormones.

During **pregnancy**, high oestrogen levels stimulate NO production, leading to a generalized vasorelaxation. Along with the expansion of the uterine and placental vascular beds by angiogenesis, this greatly reduces peripheral resistance. Consequently, BP falls, despite a 50% increase in cardiac output.

## Shear-stimulated nitric oxide production causes large-artery dilatation during exercise

When fluid is pumped through an isolated, large artery, raising the flow causes vasodilatation. This flow-induced dilatation is mediated by shear stress, and can be blocked by inhibitors of NO secretion. Flow-induced dilatation occurs in small arteries also, where EDH may contribute to the response. Flow-induced vasodilatation can be demonstrated in human

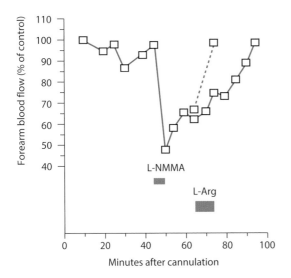

**Figure 13.4** Role of nitric oxide (NO) in regulating vascular resistance of the human forearm. An inhibitor of NO production, L-N^G-monomethylarginine (L-NMMA), was infused into the brachial artery. The 50% reduction in flow indicates that there is normally a tonic production of the vasodilator NO. Inhibition was reversed by the NO substrate, L-arginine (L-Arg, broken line). (After Vallance P, Collier J, Moncada S. *Lancet* 1989; 2(8670): 997–1000, with permission from Elsevier.)

arteries *in vivo* during exercise. For example, the diameter of the human brachial artery increases by >10% during forearm exercise. At the onset of the exercise, the small resistance vessels inside the active muscle dilate first (metabolic vasodilatation, Sections 13.4 and 13.7), lowering the vascular resistance. This raises the blood flow through the conduit artery supplying the muscle. The resulting rise in artery shear stress stimulates NO secretion. Thus, the conduit artery dilates, even though it is a considerable distance from the intra-muscle vasodilator metabolites.

The pressure profiles in Figures 1.10 and 8.16 show that conduit artery resistance is only a tiny fraction of the resting vascular resistance. So, is the dilatation of a large artery of any real value during exercise? The answer is 'yes', for two reasons. First, dilatation attenuates the rise in endothelial shear stress in the big vessels. Second, once resistance vessel dilatation in the exercising muscle has reduced the downstream resistance to a low level, the upstream conduit artery resistance becomes a significant fraction of the total vascular resistance. This would limit the increase in blood flow, were it not for the flow-induced artery vasodilatation. Thus, endothelial NO **couples conduit artery resistance to arteriolar resistance**.

## Neural nitric oxide mediates the vasodilatation of sexual erection

Penile erection is brought about by the dilatation of helicine arteries and smooth muscle in the corpus cavernosum; clitoral erection has a similar basis. The dilatation is triggered

by nitridergic parasympathetic nerves; that is, nerve fibres that contain a neural isoform of NOS, **nNOS**, and generate NO (Section 14.2). NO produces vasodilatation through the guanylyl cyclase–cyclic guanosine monophosphate (cGMP)–protein kinase G pathway (Figure 9.10). Male impotence can be treated by inhibitors of the cGMP-degrading enzyme **phosphodiesterase type 5**, such as sildenafil (Viagra), which raise vascular cGMP and thereby amplify the erectile effect of nitridergic fibre activity.

## Endothelial nitric oxide contributes to the vasodilatation of inflammation

The familiar redness and heat of an inflamed tissue are caused by vasodilatation. The vasodilatation is due partly to an increase in NO production. Several inflammatory autacoids, including bradykinin, thrombin and substance P, produce vasodilatation by activating **eNOS**. In addition, inflammatory cytokines induce the synthesis of a third isoform, inducible NOS, **iNOS**.

## Inducible nitric oxide synthase contributes to endotoxin shock

Endotoxin shock is a severe, intractable form of hypotension caused by bacterial infection. Endotoxin is a bacterial lipopolysaccharide that stimulates circulating monocytes and tissue macrophages to secrete cytokines, such as interferon-γ. Over several hours, the cytokines induce the transcription-translation of an isoform of NOS called **iNOS** (NOS-II). iNOS differs from constitutively expressed eNOS in that it is a cytosolic enzyme (cf. caveolin-bound eNOS); it does not require activation by $Ca^{2+}$-calmodulin, and it produces NO at a much faster rate than eNOS. The induction of iNOS in vascular myocytes, macrophages and endothelial cells (ECs) contributes to a generalized vasodilatation and hypotension. Disappointingly, to date, the treatment of endotoxin shock with iNOS inhibitors has not significantly improved survival rates.

## Nitrate drugs act through nitric oxide release

The drugs glyceryl trinitrate, sodium nitroprusside and isosorbide dinitrate have long been used as vasodilators to treat cardiac angina. It is now appreciated that these drugs act by mimicking endothelial NO. They are very effective as venodilators and large-artery dilators. Their therapeutic benefit is due partly to the reduction of CVP by peripheral venodilatation, and partly to the reduction of systolic BP through arterial relaxation (increased compliance) and reduced wave reflection (Section 8.4). Both changes reduce the cardiac stroke work and hence $O_2$ demand.

## Endothelin contributes to basal tone and pathological conditions

The endothelium also constitutively secretes a vasoconstrictor peptide, ET. $ET_A$ and $ET_B$ receptors on arterial and venous myocytes activate the phospholipase C (PLC)–diacylglycerol pathway, which activates non-selective cation TRPCs and thereby raises the cytosolic free $[Ca^{2+}]$ (Figure 12.6b). Due to the prolonged binding of ET, vasoconstriction and venoconstriction last 2–3 h.

### Physiological role

Although plasma ET levels are low, the $ET_{A/B}$-receptor antagonist **bosentan** causes a small fall in BP. Similarly, phosphoramidon, an inhibitor of ET production, causes dilatation in the human forearm and rat coronary artery. These observations show that ET makes a small contribution to the basal tone of resistance vessels.

### Pathological roles

Hypoxia stimulates ET production, so plasma levels increase with altitude and may contribute to **high-altitude pulmonary hypertension**. Plasma ET is also raised in **pre-eclamptic toxaemia**, the acute hypertension of pregnancy. ET makes a small contribution to essential hypertension (Chapter 18). In **heart failure**, a raised plasma ET also contributes to the characteristic renal and peripheral vasoconstriction. Consequently, bosentan significantly increases peripheral blood flow, dilates veins and reduces BP in heart failure patients. **Subarachnoid haemorrhage, ischaemic strokes** and **brain trauma** raise the ET content of cerebrospinal fluid, contributing to the **cerebral vasospasm** associated with these conditions. Cerebral vasospasm is ameliorated by bosentan.

## 13.4 REGULATION BY METABOLIC VASOACTIVE FACTORS

As the celebrated 18th century anatomist John Hunter pointed out, blood flow goes where it is needed. When the metabolic activity of the **myocardium, skeletal muscle** or **cerebral neurons** increases, the blood flow to the active region increases substantially, within seconds (Figures 13.1, 13.7 and 13.8). This metabolism-driven increase in blood flow is called **functional hyperaemia** or **metabolic hyperaemia** or **metabolic vasodilatation**. Metabolic hyperaemia is graded, so $O_2$ delivery increases in proportion to $O_2$ demand (Figure 15.4). The hyperaemia is caused by vasodilator substances released from the active cells, as indicated by experiments in which the fluid bathing stimulated cardiac myocytes acquires a vasodilator capacity, in proportion to stimulation intensity. The metabolic vasodilators act locally on the resistance vessels within the active tissue, with the more distal, smallest resistance vessels showing greater sensitivity than the more

proximal, larger vessels (Figure 13.9). However, despite a century of research we still do not know for certain which agents account for metabolic hyperaemia. $K^+$, $H^+$ (acidosis), hypoxia, adenosine, adenosine triphosphate (ATP), phosphate ions, hyperosmolarity and hydrogen peroxide ($H_2O_2$) all increase in the interstitium with increased tissue activity, and each has a vasodilator effect. Their relative importance seems to depend on the time point and the tissue. $K^+$ and $CO_2$, for example, are particularly important regulators of cerebral vessels, while $K^+$ and adenosine seem important in striated muscle.

### Interstitial $K^+$

When muscles contract or cerebral neuron activity increases, the outward, repolarizing current of the action potential ($I_K$) transfers intracellular $K^+$ into the extracellular space. In the early stage of exercise, interstitial $[K^+]$ can more than double in an active skeletal muscle, from 4 to 9 mM because of an incomplete reuptake of $K^+$ by the $Na^+/K^+$ pump. This stimulates the hyperpolarizing $3Na^+/2K^+$ pumps of vascular myocytes and increases their $K_{ir}$ channel activity (Section 12.4). The resulting hyperpolarization leads to vasodilatation (Section 12.7). Rises in interstitial $[K^+]$ are most pronounced at early time points, then decay as the tissue approaches a new steady state, especially in the brain. Therefore, interstitial $[K^+]$ may contribute more to the rapid-onset initial phase of metabolic hyperaemia (first few seconds) than the later, sustained phase. While physiological increases (up to ~10 mM) cause vasodilatation, pharmacological concentrations >20 mM cause vasoconstriction. A plot of vascular tone versus extracellular $K^+$ is thus U-shaped. Pharmacological $K^+$ levels depolarize the myocyte; see the Nernst equation, Section 3.3.

### Acidosis

A decrease in pH can be brought about by metabolic acid (e.g. lactic acid or inorganic acid – $H^+Cl^-$) or respiratory acidosis – high partial pressure of $CO_2$ in arterial blood ($PaCO_2$). Inorganic acids can also cause hyperkalaemia. As a rule of thumb, for every 0.1 pH unit decrease caused by an inorganic acid, $[K^+]_o$ increases by 0.7 mM. A similar decrease in pH caused by hypercapnia causes a more modest (0.3 mM) increase in $[K^+]_o$. These two ions interact synergistically to bring about the contractile state of cardiac (negative inotropic) and smooth muscle (vasodilatation). Metabolic activity causes local tissue acidosis, due to the generation of more $CO_2$ (forming carbonic acid in solution) and lactic acid that is produced during exercise or grand mal seizure. Acidosis causes vasodilatation (Figure 12.1), as discovered by WH Gaskell in 1880. **Cerebral blood vessels** are particularly sensitive to the partial pressure of $CO_2$ in arterial blood ($PaCO_2$), so $PaCO_2$ is an important regulator of cerebral blood flow (Figure 15.13). However, vessels in skeletal muscle and myocardium respond only weakly, so acidosis probably contributes relatively little to exercise hyperaemia. Indeed, patients who cannot make lactic acid during exercise (McArdle's disease) still vasodilate. In healthy individuals, acidosis causes vasorelaxation by multiple mechanisms:

1. Intracellular acidosis hyperpolarizes the vascular myocytes, probably because $K_{ATP}$ channels respond to pH. Hyperpolarization closes voltage-sensitive $Ca^{2+}$ channels, leading to vasodilatation.
2. If vascular myocytes are depolarized by raised external $K^+$, acidosis still reduces cytosolic $Ca^{2+}$ because acidosis reduces the open probability of $Ca^{2+}$ channels.
3. $CO_2$ causes endothelium to release NO in the mesentery, but less certainly in the brain. Lactate by contrast has a non-endothelium-dependent action.

## Hypoxia

Hypoxia can affect blood vessels locally or via reflexes. This section describes the local effect; hypoxia-induced reflexes are covered in Chapter 18. Hypoxia affects systemic and pulmonary vessels differently, as follows.

### Hypoxia dilates systemic resistance vessels

$PaO_2$ is normally 100 mmHg or 13 kPa. When blood with a $PaO_2$ of ~40 mmHg (5 kPa) is perfused through skeletal muscles, myocardium or the brain, the arterioles dilate (Figure 13.5). Thus, hypoxia has a local vasodilator effect, and the increase

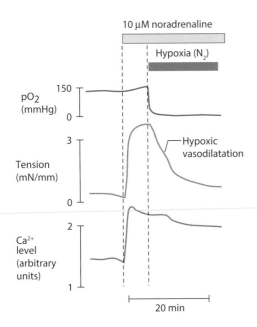

**Figure 13.5** Vasodilator response of isolated rat mesenteric artery to acute hypoxia. Because vasodilatation is a loss of tone, tone was first established with noradrenaline. Hypoxic vasodilatation of this vessel involves little to no fall in $Ca^{2+}$, and is due to a fall in sensitivity to $Ca^{2+}$. In some arteries, hypoxia reduces intracellular free $Ca^{2+}$, due to a hyperpolarization-mediated closure of L-type $Ca^{2+}$ channels. (Adapted from Bruce J, Taggart M, Austin C. *Microvascular Research* 2004; 68(3): 303–12, with permission from Elsevier.)

in blood flow helps offset the low $O_2$ content. Even isolated vascular myocytes exhibit hypoxic relaxation, so it is not endothelium- or NO-dependent. Hypoxic vasodilatation is mediated by multiple mechanisms, which differ between vessels. In some vessels, hypoxia activates $K_{ATP}$ and possibly $K_{ir}$ channels, leading to a hyperpolarization-mediated fall in $[Ca^{2+}]$ and relaxation (Figure 12.1). In other vessels, $[Ca^{2+}]$ remains almost unchanged; instead, $Ca^{2+}$ sensitivity falls (Figure 13.5). Desensitization is probably due to hypoxic inhibition of RhoA kinase, leading to reduced myosin light chain phosphorylation (Figure 12.7).

Although hypoxia causes vasodilatation, the arterioles are perfused with blood of normal $O_2$ content in exercising muscle or myocardium. Since $O_2$ permeates the arteriole wall freely, the vascular myocytes are unlikely to be hypoxic, except during a sustained muscle contraction (which impairs perfusion). The skeletal muscle fibres, by contrast, become hypoxic as their $O_2$ consumption rises, leading to the formation of the vasodilator **adenosine**.

### Hypoxia constricts pulmonary vessels and large systemic arteries

Although hypoxia dilates systemic arterioles, it constricts pulmonary blood vessels. Hypoxic pulmonary vasoconstriction is a normal, physiologically beneficial response (Section 15.5), though it can cause problems at high altitude. Hypoxia can also trigger vasospasm in large systemic arteries, such as coronary arteries, due partly to the release of noradrenaline (NAd) from the hypoxic sympathetic fibres and the local release of autacoid vasoconstrictors, such as PAF.

## Adenosine

The vasodilator adenosine may account for ~20%–40% of the sustained phase of metabolic hyperaemia in exercising skeletal muscle, and contributes to myocardial hyperaemia. Adenosine is formed in active myocardium and skeletal muscles by the dephosphorylation of extracellular adenosine monophosphate (AMP) by AMP 5′-nucleotidase, an ectoenzyme (outward facing enzyme). AMP, a breakdown product of ATP, is released into the extracellular fluid in increasing amounts during exercise or systemic hypoxia. Adenosine causes vasodilatation through multiple pathways:

1. $A_{2A}$ receptors on vascular myocytes activate the adenylate (or adenylyl) cyclase–cAMP–protein kinase cascade (Figure 12.10).
2. $A_1$ receptors are coupled to $K_{ATP}$ channels, leading to hyperpolarization-mediated relaxation.
3. Adenosine binds to receptors on sympathetic varicosities to reduce NAd release (Figure 14.2).

A good correlation has been reported between myocardial metabolic rate, coronary blood flow and coronary venous adenosine content. Experimental degradation of myocardial adenosine, by infusing adenosine deaminase, approximately halves metabolic hyperaemia. Similarly, metabolic hyperaemia of skeletal muscle or brain is substantially attenuated by perfusion with the adenosine receptor blocker 8-phenyltheophylline. However, considerable hyperaemia always persists, so adenosine is clearly not the sole factor mediating metabolic hyperaemia.

By contrast, adenosine $A_1$ receptors in the kidney are coupled to $G_i$ protein, so adenosine triggers vasoconstriction in renal afferent arterioles. This is part of a feedback system to stabilize glomerular filtration rate (tubuloglomerular feedback).

## Phosphate ions and hyperosmolarity

A rise in interstitial phosphate or osmolarity elicits vasodilatation, and both changes occur during exercise. **Inorganic phosphate ions** are released into the interstitial fluid of active muscle following the breakdown of creatine phosphate and ATP. This change, in combination with the accumulating $K^+$ ions and lactate (30 mM lactate during intense exercise, cf. 0.6 mM normally), raises the **osmolarity** of the interstitial fluid during the early stages of exercise. As a result, the osmolarity of the venous blood from active muscle increases by 4–40 milliosmoles/L.

## Hydrogen peroxide

$H_2O_2$ is a freely permeable, hyperpolarizing vasodilator. It is generated by mitochondrial superoxide dismutase from superoxide, $O_2^-$. Mitochondrial production of $O_2^-$ increases as $O_2$ consumption increases. A good correlation between $H_2O_2$ production and the degree of metabolic hyperaemia has been reported in myocardium and skeletal muscle.

**To summarize**, no one metabolic vasodilator can explain the rapid onset and sustained nature of metabolic hyperaemia. Many factors seem to contribute, and a full 'accountancy' still eludes us, despite more than a century of research.

## 13.5 REGULATION BY AUTACOIDS

Autacoids (auto + *akos*, remedy) are organic, paracrine vasoactive chemicals; they are agents produced locally, released locally and acting locally on nearby vascular myocytes. Autacoids are involved mainly in pathological events, such as inflammation and bleeding. They include histamine, bradykinin, serotonin (5-hydroxytryptamine [5HT]), prostaglandins, thromboxane $A_2$ (TXA$_2$), leukotrienes and platelet-activating factor (PAF). The following 'thumbnail sketches' describe the principal autacoids.

## Histamine

Histamine is formed by the decarboxylation of the amino acid histidine. It is stored in granules in basophilic leukocytes and tissue mast cells, particularly in tissues that interface with the environment, that is, skin, lungs and gut. Histamine is one of the chemical mediators of **inflammation**, being released in response to trauma and allergic reactions (urticaria, anaphylaxis, asthma). Histamine $H_1$ receptors on postcapillary venules are coupled to the $G_q$–PLC pathway, leading to increased venular permeability (Figure 11.30). $H_2$ receptors on arteriolar myocytes are coupled to the $G_s$–adenylate cyclase pathway, leading to vasodilatation (Figure 12.10). Thus, histamine dilates arterioles and increases venular permeability, the characteristic features of inflammation. Cutaneous histamine elicits the itchy, prickling sensation of mild inflammation, and the triple response of Lewis (Section 14.4). The culprits, the $H_1$ receptors, can be blocked by the 'antihistamine' mepyramine.

## Bradykinin

Bradykinin is a nonapeptide, cleaved from its parent plasma protein, kininogen, by the enzyme kallikrein. Kallikrein is activated during **inflammation**. Bradykinin, like histamine, elicits vasodilatation and venular hyperpermeability, thereby contributing to the hyperaemia and swelling of inflammation. Bradykinin is also the most potent **pain-producing** autacoid. The endothelium constitutively expresses bradykinin $B_2$ receptors, which are $G_q$- or $G_i$-coupled; $B_1$ receptors are induced by inflammation. Receptor activation stimulates the endothelium to produce NO in some tissues, PGI$_2$ in others, and possibly EDH in human skin. These agents then act locally to cause vasodilatation.

## Serotonin

Serotonin (5HT) is synthesized by tryptophan hydroxylase from the amino acid tryptophan in intestinal enterochromaffin cells, endothelium, some central neurons and stinging nettles. Circulating serotonin also accumulates inside platelets at a high concentration. There are at least seven types of serotonin HT receptor. The principle effects are vasoconstriction, venular hyperpermeability and pain.

## Platelet serotonin

When the circulation is breached, platelets encounter collagen, which causes the platelets to release their serotonin into the serum (hence the name serotonin). Arterial myocyte 5HT$_{2A}$ receptors are coupled to the PLC–IP$_3$ pathway (Figure 12.7), so an intense vasospasm ensues, slowing or arresting the bleeding. However, this beneficial mechanism can cause harm in atheromatous coronary arteries. If the surface of the atheromatous plaque splits, exposing collagen, platelets are activated inappropriately, and the released serotonin, along with TXA$_2$ and PAF cause **coronary vasospasm** and angina.

## Enterochromaffin (argentaffin) cells

Enterochromaffin (argentaffin) cells in the intestinal mucosa contain ~90% of all serotonin. Here serotonin helps regulate intestinal motility. Argentaffin cells occasionally give rise to a **carcinoid tumour**, which releases large quantities of serotonin into the circulation. This causes attacks of hypertension and diarrhoea.

## Central neuron serotonin

Serotonin is a central neurotransmitter, and the serotonin antagonist, lysergic acid diamine, is hallucinogenic. Serotonin is also found in neurons close to large intracranial blood vessels and in perivascular nerve fibres. Its release following a cerebral haemorrhage activates $5HT_{1D}$ receptors on the cerebral blood vessels, leading to **cerebral artery vasospasm** and hence cerebral infarction (haemorrhagic stroke). Conversely, excessive cerebral vasodilatation, which can cause vascular headaches and migraine (Section 15.4), can be treated with the selective $5HT_{1D}$ agonist **sumatriptan**.

## Pulmonary hypertension

Pulmonary arterial hypertension is a chronic, little-understood condition that leads to right ventricular failure. There is growing evidence that some forms of this condition are due to the proliferation of pulmonary arterial myocytes under the influences of serotonin.

## Prostaglandins and thromboxane (eicosanoids, prostanoids)

**Prostaglandins** and $TXA_2$ are vasoactive agents synthesized from a 20-carbon unsaturated fatty acid in the cell membrane, **arachidonic acid** (AA). Since AA is an eicosatetraenoic acid (eicosa-, 20 carbon chain; tetra-, four double bonds), these agents are called 'eicosanoids'. The rate-limiting step in eicosanoid production is usually the formation of AA from membrane phospholipids by phospholipase $A_2$ ($PLA_2$). The downstream pathway from AA to both prostaglandins and $TXA_2$ involves the constitutively expressed enzyme **cyclooxygenase 1** (COX1) and, in inflamed tissues, COX2. Anti-inflammatory **steroids** inhibit COX production. **Nonsteroidal anti-inflammatory drugs** (NSAIDs; aspirin, ibuprofen, indomethacin) are COX1/2 inhibitors.

**Prostaglandins** are synthesized by the vascular endothelium, fibroblasts, macrophages and leukocytes. The F series, PGFs, are mainly vasoconstrictors. The important E series (e.g. $PGE_2$) and $PGI_2$ are **vasodilators** (Figure 9.8). They contribute to **reactive hyperaemia** (see later), **sweating-related cutaneous vasodilatation** and to the **vasodilatation and oedema of inflammation**, for example, in arthritis. Although not inflammatory by themselves, $PGE_2$ and $PGI_2$ potentiate the inflammatory action of histamine and bradykinin and sensitize the nociceptive C fibres ('pain' receptors), hence the effectiveness of NSAIDs in reducing the inflammatory swelling and pain of arthritis. $PGI_2$, which is produced continuously by the endothelium, also inhibits platelet aggregation and is thus **antithrombotic** (Section 9.5).

$TXA_2$ is synthesized by COX in platelets. It is a powerful vasoconstrictor and thrombotic agent. Following a bleed, the shed platelets release both $TXA_2$ and serotonin, and the ensuing vasoconstriction helps stop the bleeding. Since coronary atheroma sometimes activates platelets inappropriately (see 'Serotonin' subsection), the resulting shower of $TXA_2$ and serotonin can cause **coronary artery vasospasm** and angina at rest. $TXA_2$ also has a key role in **thrombosis**, the formation of an organized blood clot inside a vessel; released $TXA_2$ mediates the aggregation of platelets, which is the first step in thrombosis. Since low-dose **aspirin** inhibits platelet COX and reduces the $TXA_2$ content, it helps protect against thrombosis. Low-dose aspirin does not affect endothelial COX greatly, so the production of the anti-aggregation factor $PGI_2$ continues, tipping the balance against thrombosis. Therefore, low-dose aspirin is prescribed prophylactically for patients with coronary atheroma.

## Leukotrienes

Leukotrienes are vasoactive eicosanoids produced from AA by the action of arachidonate 5-lipoxygenase (cf. COX) in leukocytes. They contribute to the **inflammatory response** by causing leukocyte margination-emigration and venular hyperpermeability, for example, the bronchial inflammation of asthma. Their gap-inducing action on venules is 1000-fold more potent than that of histamine. Leukotrienes can also cause vasoconstriction or dilatation, depending on the tissue.

## Platelet-activating factor

PAF is a vasoactive lipid generated by activated inflammatory cells, such as polymorphonuclear leukocytes and macrophages. It is produced from acyl-PAF by $PLA_2$. Although its name stems from its ability to promote platelet aggregation, PAF exerts many of its major effects on smooth muscle. It causes bronchoconstriction in asthmatics, and may also contribute to the vasospasm of atheromatous coronary arteries. PAF also contributes to the venular hyperpermeability of **inflammation** (Figure 11.28).

## 13.6 AUTOREGULATION OF BLOOD FLOW

The intrinsic mechanisms described earlier – the myogenic response, endothelial secretions, vasodilator metabolites and autacoids – account for several major circulatory responses without any help from extrinsic nerves or hormones. The most important of these intrinsic responses are the **autoregulation of blood flow**, **metabolic hyperaemia** and **post-ischaemic (reactive) hyperaemia**, as follows.

## Autoregulation keeps blood flow almost constant when pressure changes

The relationship between perfusion pressure and blood flow in the myocardium, brain, kidney, skeletal muscle and intestine is a remarkable one because changes in perfusion pressure over

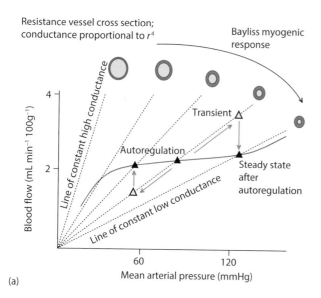

(a)

the physiological range have little effect on the steady-state blood flow. In other words, a plot of flow versus pressure is almost flat over the physiological pressure range, a phenomenon called autoregulation (Figures 13.6a, 13.7 and 8.21). At first acquaintance, this seems to defy the laws of physics, which state that flow is proportional to perfusion pressure (Sections 1.5 and 8.7); however, such laws do not consider the active responses of contractile resistance vessels. A rise in arterial pressure indeed raises flow initially, but within 30–60 s the arterioles respond by contracting. This increases the vascular resistance and reduces the flow to close to its former level. Conversely, a fall in arterial pressure evokes vasodilatation, which reduces the resistance and restores the flow. Thus, active changes in vascular calibre hold flow almost constant in the steady state. Autoregulation nevertheless operates over a limited pressure range, and severe hypotension causes a fall in cerebral, myocardial and renal perfusion. Autoregulation is absent in the pulmonary circulation (as is to be expected!) and in the cutaneous circulation.

The usefulness of autoregulation is that, within its upper and lower limits, it protects organ perfusion against minute-to-minute fluctuations in arterial BP. In the **brain**, autoregulation maintains blood flow during the hypotension caused by spinal anaesthesia. In the **myocardium**, it helps maintain blood flow downstream of a stenosed, atheromatous coronary artery, where pressure is reduced. In the **kidney**, it stabilizes the glomerular filtration rate by maintaining a constant renal perfusion and glomerular capillary pressure. The latter point brings us to the second, less well-recognized function of autoregulation, namely the stabilization of capillary pressure.

## Autoregulation stabilizes capillary pressure

Autoregulation stabilizes not only tissue perfusion but also capillary BP and fluid turnover (Figure 13.6b). When an isolated skeletal muscle is perfused by a pump, elevation of the pump pressure from 30 to 170 mmHg causes only a 2 mmHg rise in capillary pressure. This is because the autoregulatory contraction of the arterioles raises the pre- to postcapillary resistance ratio $R_A/R_V$, and capillary pressure is inversely related to $R_A/R_V$ (Figure 11.4). The bigger pressure drop across the increased resistance $R_A$ prevents capillary BP from increasing substantially when arterial pressure is raised. This protects tissues against oedema when arterial pressure is high. Capillary pressure autoregulation is crucial in the renal glomeruli, where it ensures a virtually **constant glomerular filtration rate** for waste product elimination.

## Autoregulation is due mainly to the myogenic response

The mechanisms underlying autoregulation are the myogenic response (Figure 13.3), vasodilator washout and, in the kidney, tubuloglomerular feedback. Vasodilator washout is the removal of vasodilator metabolites from the tissue by a transiently increased blood flow when arterial pressure rises. Indirect evidence indicates that the **myogenic mechanism**

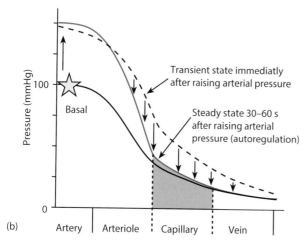

(b)

**Figure 13.6** Autoregulation of (**a**) blood flow and (**b**) capillary pressure in isolated, perfused skeletal muscle. (**a**) Raising or lowering blood pressure transiently raises or lowers blood flow as dictated by Poiseuille's law (lines of constant conductance; grey arrows). The myogenic response then actively changes the resistance vessel radius, producing a new isoconductance line and restoring flow to close to its former level in the steady state (vertical grey arrows). (**b**) The dashed lines show the transient state immediately after changing perfusion pressure from a control level of 100 mmHg (star), before autoregulation has had time to kick in. Over the next 30–60 s, arteriolar contraction readjusts the flow and capillary pressure to a steady-state value like before (solid red curve). ((**a**) Drawn partly from data of Jones RD, Berne RM. *Circulation Research* 1964; 14: 126–38.)

predominates in the brain, intestine, liver and spleen, and contributes to renal autoregulation. For example, autoregulation in the brain and kidney is severely impaired by blocking the formation of 20-HETE, the vasoconstrictor involved in sustaining the myogenic response.

In the kidney, the myogenic response accounts for roughly half of the autoregulation. A specialized, local mechanism called **tubuloglomerular feedback** accounts for the other half. If glomerular BP increases, increased capillary filtration delivers more fluid and salt into the renal tubule. The $Na^+Cl^-$ is sensed by macula densa cells in the ascending loop of Henle, which lie adjacent to the glomerulus in a complex called the **juxtaglomerular apparatus**. Macula densa activation leads, via adenosine and mesangial $A_1$ receptors, to contraction of the adjacent afferent arteriole, reducing glomerular capillary BP to its former level.

## Autoregulated flow can be changed by metabolic factors and sympathetic activity

Autoregulation does not mean that the blood flow is unchangeable; it means that the flow is insensitive to physiological changes in arterial pressure. Changes in metabolic or sympathetic activity can still alter the blood flow, by resetting the autoregulation to operate at a different level of flow. Figure 13.7 illustrates how **autoregulation and changes in blood flow can co-exist**. An increase in cardiac work increases the coronary blood flow (metabolic hyperaemia), but the pressure-flow relation remains relatively flat at each work intensity. In other words, the metabolic vasodilators reset autoregulation to operate at a higher, but still autoregulated, flow.

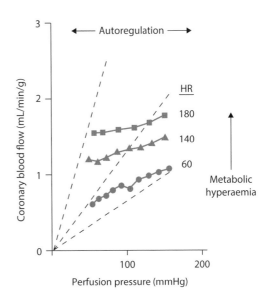

**Figure 13.7** Distinct effects of perfusion pressure and metabolic activity on coronary blood flow in the dog. The dashed lines are theoretical pressure-flow lines at constant conductance; the steepest line has the highest conductance. At any given metabolic rate, that is, heart rate (HR), blood flow increases relatively little with perfusion pressure, due to a shift to a lower conductance line as pressure is raised. This is autoregulation. At any given perfusion pressure, flow increases with metabolic rate (HR). This is metabolic hyperaemia. (Data from Laird. In: Drake-Holland AJ, Noble MIM, eds. *Cardiac Metabolism*. Chichester: Wiley; 1983. pp. 257–78.)

## 13.7 METABOLIC (FUNCTIONAL) HYPERAEMIA

In skeletal muscle, myocardium and brain, blood flow increases almost linearly with the metabolic rate of the tissue, so that blood flow in the steady state is almost directly proportional to $O_2$ consumption (Figures 13.7 and 15.4). This beautiful and striking coupling of supply to demand is called metabolic hyperaemia (also functional hyperaemia, active hyperaemia, metabolic vasodilatation). In the initial few seconds of muscle hyperaemia, vasodilatation may be due to myogenic relaxation in response to intermittent compression by the contracting muscle. In the later, sustained phase, the coupling is probably brought about by the metabolic vasodilators described in Section 13.4, namely **interstitial $K^+$ ions, acidosis, adenosine, ATP, phosphate, hyperosmolarity** and **$H_2O_2$**. Most of these agents not only act directly on resistance vessels but also inhibit noradrenaline release from sympathetic fibres (neuromodulation; Figure 14.2). Studies using inhibitors of eNOS and COX indicate that **NO and prostaglandins** also contribute to skeletal muscle hyperaemia, by ~20%–33%. In limbs with ischaemic arterial disease, bradykinin also contributes. These multiple factors can increase muscle blood flow >20-fold during heavy exercise (Figure 13.1).

It is worth emphasizing that **metabolic hyperaemia is mediated entirely by intrinsic factors, not vasodilator nerves**. Also, much confusion can be avoided by noting that metabolic hyperaemia, which is an increase in flow and a form

---

**CONCEPT BOX 13.1**

### THE HIERARCHY OF VASCULAR CONTROL

- Vascular tone is regulated by a three-tier hierarchy:
  - Bottom tier. The most basic form of regulation is autoregulation. Resistance vessels react to changes in BP so that blood flow varies little with arterial pressure, especially in the brain, myocardium and kidney. Autoregulation is mediated by the Bayliss myogenic response in many tissues.
  - Middle tier. The autoregulated flow can be increased or decreased by intrinsic vasoactive agents produced within the tissue. These include the metabolic vasodilators (adenosine, $K^+$, $CO_2$, lactate, phosphate, hyperosmolarity, $H_2O_2$), endothelial secretions (NO, EDH, $PGI_2$, ET) and the autacoids that mediate inflammation (histamine, bradykinin, PAF, leukotrienes) and vasospasm (serotonin, $TXA_2$).
  - Top tier. The highest level of control is extrinsic regulation by sympathetic and parasympathetic vasomotor nerves, and by circulating hormones (adrenaline, angiotensin II, vasopressin). This enables the brain to regulate BP and blood flow to specific organs.

of automatic regulation, should not be called autoregulation, which is a constancy of flow in the face of pressure changes. The coexistence of these two very different phenomena is illustrated in Figure 13.7.

## Muscle blood flow oscillates during rhythmic exercise

During rhythmic exercise, the mean blood flow through the exercising muscle increases, but the flow falls during each contraction phase because the vessels inside the contracting muscle are compressed (Figure 13.8). The pressure exerted on the outside of the vessels in contracting human skeletal muscle can reach 270–570 mmHg. Similarly, myocardial blood flow falls sharply at the onset of systole (Figure 15.5). Most of the hyperaemia in skeletal and myocardial muscle occurs during the relaxation phases. Muscle myoglobin holds a small reserve of $O_2$ for use during the poorly perfused contraction phase.

## The onset-related $O_2$ debt is repaid by post-exercise hyperaemia

As indicated earlier, the hyperaemia of exercise develops in two phases. There is a moderate increase in blood flow within seconds (Figure 13.8), but the full, sustained response takes a minute or so to develop. Because the muscle's demand for more $O_2$ increases instantly on contraction, the blood flow and $O_2$ supply fail to match demand during the first minute or so, and the muscle must draw on its reserve of high-energy creatine phosphate instead. This metabolic deficit, or '$O_2$ debt', must be repaid at some point by extra $O_2$ consumption. The $O_2$ debt may cease to grow once blood flow has reached a steady state, where blood flow is directly proportional to $O_2$ consumption. When the exercise stops, hyperaemia does

not cease instantly but decays gradually over many minutes (Figure 13.11). This is called **post-exercise hyperaemia**. Post-exercise hyperaemia quickly repays the metabolic debt, and persists for several minutes longer, helping restore muscle pH and temperature to baseline.

## Hyperaemia is impaired by static, isometric exercise

During static, isometric exercise, such as holding a heavy weight, the increase in blood flow through the muscle is much less pronounced than during dynamic exercise. This is because the sustained increase in intra-muscle pressure limits the dilatation of the resistance vessels. Consequently, blood flow fails to match $O_2$ consumption and a large $O_2$ debt accumulates rapidly. This leads to the anaerobic production of lactic acid and rapid muscle fatigue.

## The whole arterial tree undergoes co-ordinated dilatation

The arterial tree supplying a skeletal muscle is shown in Figure 13.9. The resistance of the main conduit artery and its chief branches, the feed arteries, is relatively small under resting conditions, namely <30% of that of the narrow resistance vessels. During metabolic hyperaemia, the resistance of the resistance vessels can fall to 1/20th of normal. Under these conditions, the resistance of the conduit and feed arteries would seriously limit the increase in blood flow, unless these arteries likewise dilated. Happily, the metabolic vasodilatation of the resistance vessel triggers mechanisms that dilate the local conduit and feed the arteries. Thus, a co-ordinated dilatation of arterioles, terminal arteries, feed arteries and conduit arteries contributes to the exercise hyperaemia.

Because the conduit and feed arteries are generally located outside the active muscle, they are beyond the reach of the metabolic factors that mediate resistance vessel dilatation. So, how are they induced to dilate? The mechanisms are:

- **metabolic vasodilatation** of the terminal arteries and arterioles, that is, resistance vessels;
- **ascending (conducted) vasodilatation** of small feed arteries; and
- **flow-induced vasodilatation** of the large conduit artery.

The graded sensitivity of each type of vessel to these mechanisms is illustrated in Figure 13.9.

## Feed arteries exhibit ascending (conducted) vasodilatation, mediated by the endothelium

A feed artery is a vessel with a diameter of up to 0.5 mm located between the terminal resistance arteries and the main arterial supply vessel, the conduit artery (e.g. a branch of the brachial artery). Feed arteries exhibit the strange property of ascending or conducted vasodilatation. When the

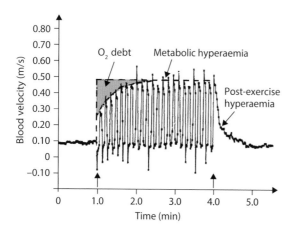

**Figure 13.8** Oscillating increase in blood flow (metabolic hyperaemia) in the human femoral artery during rhythmic quadriceps exercise. Flow was measured with the Doppler ultrasound method. Note the relatively slow initial phase of the hyperaemia, creating an $O_2$ debt. The post-exercise period of hyperaemia repays the nutritional debt. (From Walløe L, Wesche J. *The Journal of Physiology* 1988; 405: 257–73, with permission from Wiley-Blackwell.)

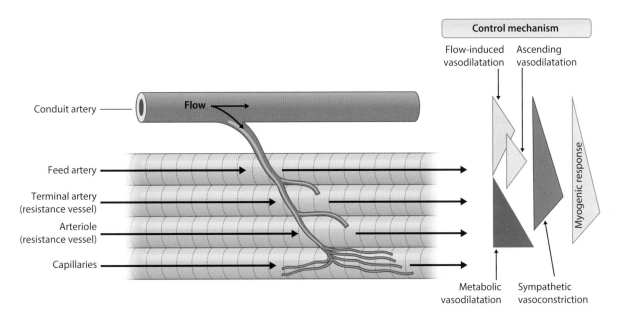

**Figure 13.9** Differential control of the arterial tree. Metabolic vasodilators dominate the terminal arterioles. Sympathetic vasoconstrictor nerves dominate the more proximal resistance vessels. Ascending (conducted) vasodilatation involves endothelial electrical transmission up the arterial tree to the feed arteries. Flow-induced vasodilatation, mediated by nitric oxide, is important in the conduit and proximal feed arteries. (Adapted from Brown MD. In: Jordan D, Marshall J, eds. *Cardiovascular Regulation*. London: Portland Press; 1995. pp. 113–26.)

intra-muscle arteriolar network is dilated by vasoactive metabolites, or in a laboratory setting by a vasodilator such as bradykinin or acetylcholine, the dilatation spreads rapidly up the arterial system in a proximal direction. As a result, feed arteries several millimetres upstream dilate within 30 s or so, even though they may be outside the muscle. Ascending vasodilatation can be blocked by creating a ring of damaged endothelium, indicating that it depends on **endothelial conduction** (Figure 13.10). Fast- and slow-conducted mechanisms are responsible, as follows.

## Fast-conducted, electromechanical response

Metabolic vasodilators in the active tissue cause hyperpolarization of the local ECs, partly by raising intracellular $Ca^{2+}$, which activates small- (SK) and intermediate-conductance (IK) $K_{Ca}$ channels (Section 9.3), and partly by adenosine-mediated activation of the $K_{ATP}$ channels of EC. EC hyperpolarization is rapidly conducted proximally through EC homocellular gap junctions (Figure 9.7), at several mm/s, and is transmitted to the vascular myocytes of feed arteries through **myoendothelial gap junctions** (Figures 1.11, 9.1, 9.7). The endothelium-dependent vascular hyperpolarization causes closure of the vascular myocyte L-type $Ca^{2+}$ channels and hence vasodilatation of the proximal feed artery.

## Slow-conducted, pharmacomechanical response

The endothelial $Ca^{2+}$ release evoked by the agonists triggers an ascending wave of $Ca^{2+}$ release that passes slowly from EC to EC. The ascending EC $Ca^{2+}$ wave causes an ascending wave

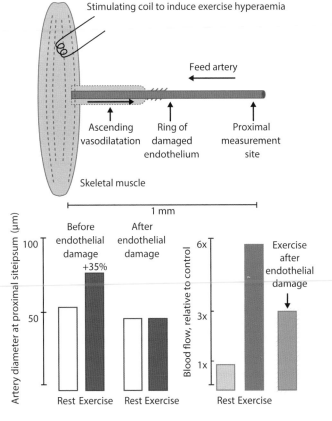

**Figure 13.10** Ascending or conducted vasodilatation in a feed artery following contractions of a hamster muscle. Metabolic hyperaemia caused a sixfold increase in blood flow. After destruction of the ring of endothelium, the ascending dilatation halted at the ring and metabolic hyperaemia fell by 47%. (Adapted from Segal SS, Jacobs TL. *The Journal of Physiology* 2001; 536(Pt 3): 937–46, with permission from Wiley-Blackwell.)

of endothelial NO and PGI$_2$ production, which helps maintain the proximal vasodilatation.

## Conduit arteries undergo flow-induced dilatation mediated by nitric oxide

The human brachial artery can dilate by >10% during forearm exercise. As the resistance vessels undergo metabolic vasodilatation, blood flow through the conduit artery increases. This increases the shear stress on the arterial endothelium, stimulating the production of NO, which dilates the conduit artery. Thus, the widening of the conduit artery is automatically triggered by the downstream metabolic hyperaemia.

## Summary of increased blood flow to exercising muscle

An increase in tissue metabolic activity elicits a co-ordinated dilatation of the arterial system supplying that tissue. The primary event is dilatation of local arterioles within the tissue by locally released vasoactive agents such as adenosine, K$^+$, H$^+$, phosphate, hyperosmolarity and H$_2$O$_2$. The peripheral, metabolic vasodilatation triggers conducted vasodilatation of the feed arteries (mediated by endothelial hyperpolarization) and flow-induced vasodilatation of conduit arteries (mediated by endothelial NO). Both latter changes are necessary for the full expression of hyperaemia. Indeed, one study showed that blocking the ascending vasodilatation reduced exercise hyperaemia by 50%.

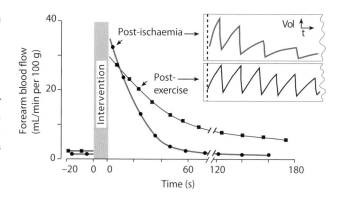

**Figure 13.11** Forearm blood flow measured in a medical student using venous occlusion plethysmography. Release of a brachial artery occlusion cuff that had cut off blood flow for 120 s resulted in post-ischaemic hyperaemia (red line). The black line shows post-exercise hyperaemia following 30 s of strenuous forearm exercise; blood flow remains elevated for longer after exercise. The insets show typical forearm volume traces during these plethysmographic measurements. See Figure 8.5 for venous occlusion plethysmography.

decays exponentially over ~60 s. Even longer occlusions cause a prolonged, post-ischaemic plateau at maximal hyperaemia, before the exponential decay phase sets in. Local anaesthetics substantially reduce cutaneous reactive hyperaemia, implicating the release of sensory nerve **vasodilator neuropeptides** in the response (Section 14.4). Hyperaemia is also reduced in some tissues by the COX inhibitor indomethacin, implicating **prostaglandins** in the response. NO appears to play a minor, sometimes negligible role.

## 13.8 POST-ISCHAEMIC (REACTIVE) HYPERAEMIA

The arterial blood supply to a tissue may sometimes be impeded by external compression, either naturally (e.g. brachial artery compression when the arm is rested over the back of a chair) or by sphygmomanometry or surgery. Blood flow may fall to a level, which no longer supplies the tissue's O$_2$ requirement, a condition called **ischaemia**. When the compression is removed, the tissue blood flow is initially many times faster than normal, followed by a period of exponential decay (Figure 13.11). This is called post-ischaemic or reactive hyperaemia. It is obvious in the skin, which flushes bright pink after a period of compression, and it also occurs in most other tissues. Its value lies in rapidly restoring the supply of O$_2$ and nutrients to ischaemic tissue, and washing out accumulated waste products.

The mechanism of reactive hyperaemia remains incompletely understood. After short arterial occlusions, 30 s, reactive hyperaemia is probably due chiefly to the **myogenic response**; the upstream arterial occlusion reduces pressure in the resistance vessels, causing them to dilate myogenically. After longer occlusions, **vasodilator metabolites** may accumulate. A 3-min occlusion produces maximal vasodilatation in human limbs, and release is followed by a maximal hyperaemia that

## 13.9 ISCHAEMIA-REPERFUSION INJURY

Surgeons sometimes arrest the blood supply to peripheral tissues for an hour or more, for example, during limb orthopaedic surgery, aortic aneurysm repair and organ transplantation (kidney, heart and lung, liver). When the clamped artery is released, instead of the brisk reactive hyperaemia that follows a few minutes of occlusion, the hyperaemia is weak and blood flow falls to abnormally low levels within minutes – the **no-reflow phenomenon**. Moreover, the tissues show biochemical and structural signs of cellular damage soon after the flow is restarted. This is called **ischaemia-reperfusion injury**, and is most marked in the intestine, liver and heart. It can also affect the survival of the rim of tissue around a myocardial or cerebral infarct.

Ischaemia-reperfusion injury is to a large extent caused by the restored blood supply, surprisingly. For example, 3 h of ischaemia followed by 1 h of reperfusion produces more tissue damage than does 4 h of ischaemia. What component of the blood causes the damage? Reperfusion with leukocyte-free blood attenuates reperfusion injury, and reperfusion with hypoxic blood likewise attenuates the injury. Thus, both white cells and O$_2$ contribute to reperfusion injury. A third factor, particularly in the heart, is post-ischaemic Ca$^{2+}$ overload (Section 6.12).

## Leukocyte adhesion contributes to reperfusion injury

In laboratory experiments, antibodies against the leukocyte-endothelial adhesion molecules attenuate reperfusion injury. During a period of prolonged ischaemia, microvascular ECs begin to express selectins and other surface adhesion molecules. When leukocytes arrive in the restored bloodstream, they adhere to the sticky endothelium (Figure 9.12). Since leukocytes are ~100 times stiffer than red cells, the adherent cells physically obstruct microvascular perfusion. The situation is further exacerbated by ischaemic swelling of the ECs. The result is the no-reflow phenomenon. Adherent leukocytes also contribute actively to tissue injury. They release leukotrienes and PAF, which cause inflammation; they release elastase, a potent tissue protease, and they generate $O_2^-$ anions, which damage the tissues.

## Free $O_2^-$ radicals too contribute to reperfusion injury

$O_2$ in the restored bloodstream contributes greatly to tissue injury. On reaching the ischaemic tissue, some $O_2$ molecules are converted into free radicals, which are highly reactive particles with an unpaired electron in the outer shell. The $O_2$ free radicals are $O_2^-$, the hydroxyl radical and, via a reaction with NO, peroxynitrite. The free radicals react with lipids and amino acids to damage cell membranes and enzymes.

The free $O_2$ radicals come from several sources during reperfusion. One is the adherent, activated leukocyte. Leukocytes contains the enzyme **nicotinamide adenine dinucleotide phosphate oxidase**, which generates $O_2^-$ radicals. The normal role of the radicals is to kill pathogens, but in reperfusion injury the tissue itself is damaged.

The other source of radicals is tissue **xanthine dehydrogenase** (XDH), an enzyme that is abundant in the myocardium and intestinal mucosa. Intestinal villi have a high concentration of XDH and are very sensitive to reperfusion injury. During the ischaemic period, a $Ca^{2+}$-triggered protease converts the XDH into **xanthine oxidase** (XO). At the same time, the substrate for this enzyme, hypoxanthine, is generated by the breakdown of adenosine, itself the breakdown product of ATP. When reperfused $O_2$ reaches the metabolically altered tissue, hypoxanthine is oxidized to xanthine by XO, and during this reaction harmless molecular $O_2$ is converted into $O_2^-$ and $H_2O_2$. Thus, reperfusion generates a burst of toxic radicals.

The NO synthase enzyme is also capable of generating $O_2^-$ radicals when its oxidative and reductive domains become 'uncoupled'. This can happen during ischaemia when cofactors (such as tetrahydrobiopterin, $BH_4$) become depleted.

Reperfusion injury can be attenuated by $O_2^-$ **dismutase**, a scavenger of free $O_2$ radicals, confirming their role in reperfusion injury. Reperfusion injury can also be attenuated in many tissues by **allopurinol**, an inhibitor of XO. During coronary bypass surgery, allopurinol can be given before reperfusion and may improve ventricular function after reperfusion.

## Cytosolic $Ca^{2+}$ overload contributes to myocardial reperfusion injury

Reperfusion injury in the heart is further exacerbated by the overloading of the cardiac myocytes with $Ca^{2+}$ during the ischaemic period. This is described under 'The paradox of myocardial ischaemia-reperfusion injury' in Section 6.12.

### SUMMARY

- Though complex in detail, the control of blood vessels can be conceptualized as a hierarchy of three control systems, each of which can override and modify the lower one.
- The **lowest level of control** is the **Bayliss myogenic response,** namely vascular contraction in response to an increase in BP. The myogenic response contributes to basal tone in resistance vessels and to **autoregulation**. Autoregulation is the maintenance of a near-constant blood flow and capillary pressure when arterial pressure changes. Autoregulation is well developed in the brain, myocardium and kidneys.
- A **second level of control** is superimposed by **local vasoactive agents**. Agents released when tissue metabolic rate increases, such as adenosine, $CO_2$, lactate, $K^+$, phosphate, osmolarity and $H_2O_2$, dilate the local arterioles. The resulting **metabolic hyperaemia** couples tissue perfusion to local $O_2$ consumption, particularly in the brain, myocardium and skeletal muscle. **Ascending (conducted) vasodilatation** of the feed arteries ensures upstream vessels do not limit the hyperaemia. **Flow-induced vasodilatation** of the conduit artery, mediated by NO, ensures that the main artery in turn does not limit flow to the feed arteries.

- A short period of reduced perfusion (seconds to minutes) evokes **post-ischaemic (reactive) hyperaemia**, due to the myogenic response and metabolite accumulation. Longer periods of ischaemia (an hour) may be followed by **poor reflow** and **reperfusion injury**, caused by leukocyte adhesion, toxic $O_2$ radical generation and (in the myocardium) cytosolic $Ca^{2+}$ overload.
- **Endothelial NO** exerts a tonic vasodilator influence on basal tone, especially in pregnancy. NO mediates flow-induced vasodilatation in conduit arteries, and the vasodilator action of bradykinin, substance P and acetylcholine. Inducible NOS contributes to endotoxin hypotension. Nitridergic parasympathetic fibres induce the dilatation that drives genital erection.
- **Autacoids** are paracrine, vasoactive agents such as histamine, bradykinin, serotonin, prostaglandins, thromboxane $A_2$, leukotrienes and PAF. Autacoids modify local vascular tone, chiefly in pathological situations such as inflammation (vasodilatation by histamine, bradykinin, prostaglandins) and bleeding (vasoconstriction by serotonin, thromboxane $A_2$).
- The **third level of control** is the neuroendocrine system, which brings the vasculature under central and reflex control for the benefit of the whole organism (Chapter 14).

## FURTHER READING

Shabeeh H, Khan S, Jiang B, et al. Blood pressure in healthy humans is regulated by neuronal NO synthase. *Hypertension* 2017; **69**(5): 970–6.

Ellinsworth DC, Sandow SL, Shukla N, et al. Endothelium-derived hyperpolarization and coronary vasodilation: diverse and integrated roles of epoxyeicosatrienoic acids, hydrogen peroxide, and gap junctions. *Microcirculation* 2016; **23**(1): 15–32.

Mederos Y, Schnitzler M, Storch U, Gudermann T. Mechanosensitive Gq/11 protein-coupled receptors mediate myogenic vasoconstriction. *Microcirculation* 2016; **23**(8): 621–5.

Bendall JK, Douglas G, McNeill E, et al. Tetrahydrobiopterin in cardiovascular health and disease. *Antioxidants & Redox Signaling* 2014; **20**(18): 3040–77.

Schubert R, Lidington D, Bolz SS. The emerging role of $Ca^{2+}$ sensitivity regulation in promoting myogenic vasoconstriction. *Cardiovascular Research* 2008; **77**(1): 8–18.

Canty JM Jr, Iyer VS. Hydrogen peroxide and metabolic coronary flow regulation. *Journal of the American College of Cardiology* 2007; **50**(13): 1279–81.

Hill MA, Davis MJ. Coupling a change in intraluminal pressure to vascular smooth muscle depolarization: still stretching for an explanation. *American Journal of Physiology. Heart and Circulatory Physiology* 2007; **292**(6): H2570–2.

Moncada S, Higgs EA. The discovery of nitric oxide and its role in vascular biology. *British Journal of Pharmacology* 2006; **147**(Suppl. 1): S193–201.

Berry CE, Hare JM. Xanthine oxidoreductase and cardiovascular disease: molecular mechanisms and pathophysiological implications. *The Journal of Physiology* 2004; **555**(Pt 3): 589–606.

Clifford PS, Hellsten Y. Vasodilatory mechanisms in contracting skeletal muscle. *Journal of Applied Physiology* 2004; **97**(1): 393–403.

Roman RJ. P-450 metabolites of arachidonic acid in the control of cardiovascular function. *Physiological Reviews* 2002; **82**(1): 131–85.

Gustafsson F, Holstein-Rathlou N. Conducted vasomotor responses in arterioles: characteristics, mechanisms and physiological significance. *Acta Physiologica Scandinavica* 1999; **167**(1): 11–21.

Marshall JM. The Joan Mott Prize Lecture. The integrated response to hypoxia: from circulation to cells. *Experimental Physiology* 1999; **84**(3): 449–70.

Granger DN, Korthuis RJ. Physiological mechanisms of post-ischemic tissue injury. *Annual Review of Physiology* 1995; **57**: 311–32.

Melkumyants AM, Balashov SA, Khayutin VM. Control of arterial lumen by shear stress on endothelium. *News in Physiological Sciences* 1995; **10**(5): 204–10.

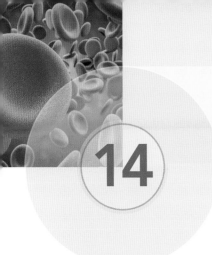

# Control of blood vessels: extrinsic control by nerves and hormones

14

## LEARNING OBJECTIVES

*After reading this chapter, you should be able to:*

- sketch the sympathetic pathway from brainstem to blood vessel and adrenal medulla (14.1);
- name the neurotransmitters and receptors mediating sympathetic vasomotor neurotransmission (14.1);
- list the chief functions of sympathetic vasoconstrictor nerves (14.1);
- state the distribution, roles and neurotransmitters of parasympathetic vasodilator nerves (14.2) and sympathetic vasodilator nerves (14.3);

- explain the meaning of 'sensory axon reflex' (14.4);
- contrast the cardiovascular effects of intravenous adrenaline and noradrenaline (14.6);
- outline the formation, action and regulation of angiotensin II, vasopressin and atrial natriuretic peptide (14.7–14.9);
- state the importance and main mechanisms of venous control (14.10).

The previous chapter focused on the **intrinsic regulation** of vascular tone by mechanisms originating from within the tissue itself, such as metabolic hyperaemia in exercising muscle and myocardium. However, local mechanisms serve local needs. To serve the needs of the whole organism, such as blood pressure (BP) homeostasis or the sentient control of a specific organ (e.g. erectile tissue), the central nervous system (CNS) superimposes a sentient control system, acting through vasomotor nerves and hormones. Since neural and hormonal control is imposed from outside the tissue itself, this is called **extrinsic regulation**. In general, extrinsic regulation is the motor, efferent limb of a vascular reflex. The sensory, afferent limbs of the reflexes are described in Chapter 16.

Extrinsic regulation involves three kinds of autonomic vasomotor nerve:

- sympathetic vasoconstrictor nerves;
- parasympathetic vasodilator nerves;
- sympathetic vasodilator nerves.

Note that the labels 'vasoconstrictor' and 'vasodilator' refer to the effect of an increase in nerve activity. It is important

to remember that **a reduction in vasoconstrictor fibre activity causes vasodilatation**; vasodilatation does not necessarily require vasodilator fibres. The flushed skin of warm hands is an example of vasodilatation brought about by reduced sympathetic vasoconstrictor activity. Of the various autonomic vasomotor nerves, the sympathetic vasoconstrictor fibres are the most widespread and most important physiologically. Students accustomed to associating sympathetic activity with alarm and dilatation should note that **the vast majority of sympathetic vasomotor fibres are vasoconstrictor fibres**.

## 14.1 SYMPATHETIC VASOCONSTRICTOR NERVES

### The sympathetic system comprises bulbospinal, preganglionic and postganglionic fibres

The sympathetic vasoconstrictor system consists of a three-neuron pathway that starts in the brainstem medulla.

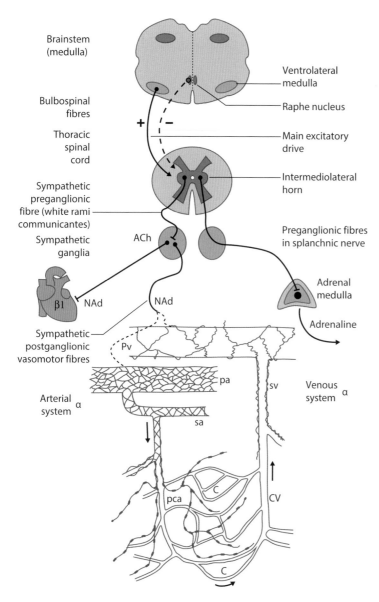

Brainstem
(medulla)

Ventrolateral
medulla

Bulbospinal
fibres

Raphe nucleus

Thoracic
spinal
cord

Main excitatory
drive

Sympathetic
preganglionic
fibre (white rami
communicantes)

Intermediolateral
horn

Sympathetic
ganglia

ACh

Preganglionic fibres
in splanchnic nerve

β1   NAd

NAd

Adrenal
medulla

Adrenaline

Sympathetic
postganglionic
vasomotor fibres

Pv

pa

sv

Venous
system   α

Arterial
system   α

sa

pca

C

CV

C

**Figure 14.1** Sympathetic innervation of the cardiovascular system. α and β refer to the predominant adrenoceptor. One descending tract (bulbospinal tract) excites the sympathetic intermediolateral cells; other bulbospinal fibres inhibit the cell. pa and pv, primary conduit artery and vein to an organ, respectively; sa and sv, small artery and vein, respectively; pca, precapillary arteriole; c, capillary; cv, collecting venule. ACh, acetylcholine; NAd, noradrenaline. (Adapted from Furness JB, Marshall JM. *The Journal of Physiology* 1974; 239(1): 75–88, with permission from Wiley-Blackwell.)

Medullary presympathetic neurons send **bulbospinal fibres** (axons) down the spinal cord (Figure 14.1). The bulbospinal fibres synapse with sympathetic preganglionic neurons in the intermediolateral columns of grey matter, located in thoraco-lumbar segments T1-L3.

## Preganglionic cholinergic fibres activate nicotinic receptors in sympathetic ganglia

The tonically active excitatory and inhibitory bulbospinal fibres, plus local spinal inputs, regulate the output of the preganglionic spinal neurons. Their axons, the sympathetic preganglionic fibres, travel through the ventral roots of the spinal nerves and **white rami communicantes** to enter the prevertebral right and left **sympathetic chains** (Chapter 4.4). The axons may travel up or down the sympathetic chain for several segments before synapsing with postganglionic neurons; some do not synapse until they reach the adrenal medulla or a more distant ganglion (coeliac, hypogastric).

The preganglionic fibres are mostly cholinergic and the **post-ganglionic receptors are nicotinic**. They are blocked by hexamethonium and stimulated by **smoking**, which causes vasoconstriction and BP elevation. Smoking-induced vaso-constriction is compounded by reduced nitric oxide (NO) availability (Concept box 14.1).

## Postganglionic noradrenergic fibres innervate blood vessels

Sympathetic postganglionic neurons send non-myelinated axons through the **grey rami communicantes** into the ventral roots of the spinal nerves, for distribution in mixed peripheral nerves. Some fibres also course directly over the major vessels. Postganglionic fibres terminate in branches that run along the outer border of the tunica media, penetrating it only in veins. Most small arteries and terminal resistance arteries are richly innervated, whereas arterioles are poorly innervated (Figure 14.1), being controlled chiefly by intrinsic

## SMOKING AND THE VASCULAR SYSTEM

- The stimulation of nicotinic receptors on postganglionic neurons increases sympathetic vasoconstrictor activity.
- Smoking-activated leukocytes generate free radicals in oxidative bursts. NO reacts with the free $O_2$ radicals. This forms harmful peroxynitrite and reduces beneficial NO levels.
- Raised sympathetic activity coupled with reduced NO availability cause smoking-induced vasoconstriction.
- Smoking-induced vasoconstriction raises BP and reduces coronary and cutaneous blood flow.
- Low levels of NO and prostacyclin ($PGI_2$) facilitate platelet aggregation, atheroma progression and thrombosis.
- The walls of arterioles are thickened, probably due to the hypertension and to the loss of the inhibitory effect of NO on myocyte proliferation.

mechanisms (Figure 13.9). The venous innervation is similar but less dense, and skeletal muscle veins have almost no sympathetic innervation.

## Terminal varicosities release packets (quanta) of noradrenaline

The terminal axon resembles a string of beads (Figure 1.11). Each bead, or **varicosity**, contains numerous **dense-cored vesicles** (Figure 14.2). Each vesicle is filled with concentrated noradrenaline (NAd) (norepinephrine) at up to 1 molar, and adenosine triphosphate (ATP). NAd is synthesized from the amino acid tyrosine via two intermediate products, dihydroxyphenylalanine (DOPA) and dopamine. Out of the thousands or so varicosities per axon, only a small proportion release a vesicle as an action potential sweeps along the axon; so, only a small fraction of the stored NAd is released per action potential.

Vesicle release, or **exocytosis**, is triggered by a rise in cytosolic $[Ca^{2+}]$ as the action potential activates axonal N-type $Ca^{2+}$ channels. The $Ca^{2+}$ activates a protein on the vesicle membrane, synaptobrevin. If the vesicle is close to the surface membrane, the synaptobrevin binds to the membrane protein syntaxin. This 'docking' process allows the two membranes to fuse and release the vesicle contents. **Guanethidine** blocks exocytosis by acting as a local anaesthetic on sympathetic terminals, and was formerly used to treat hypertension. Conversely, **amphetamines** have a sympathomimetic effect because they displace NAd from the vesicle into the cytosol, from where it escapes into the extracellular fluid.

## Noradrenaline activates vascular α-adrenergic receptors and contraction

The released NAd diffuses rapidly across the junctional gap and binds to α adrenergic receptors on the vascular myocyte membrane, leading to vascular contraction (Figure 12.9). Adrenergic receptor classification is summarized in Table 14.1. $\alpha_1$ receptors are found on most blood vessels. They activate $G_q$ protein, leading to vasoconstriction through depolarization-dependent or depolarization-independent pathways (Figure 12.6). $\alpha_2$ receptors are $G_i$-coupled and more limited in distribution. They occur as prejunctional receptors on sympathetic varicosities, and as postjunctional receptors on resistance vessels in human skin and limbs, additional to the ubiquitous $\alpha_1$ receptors. $\alpha_1$ and $\alpha_2$ contribute roughly equally to sympathetic-mediated vascular resistance in resting human limbs. The $\alpha_2$ receptor is important in the response of skin blood vessels to temperature (Section 15.3).

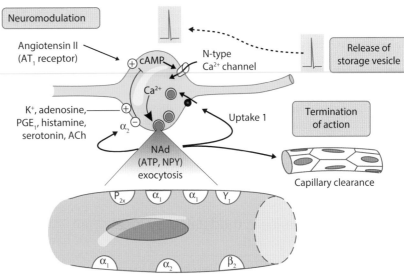

**Figure 14.2** Sympathetic neuromuscular transmission. Only one out of thousands of varicosities per axon is shown here. Noradrenaline (NAd) binds to postjunctional $\alpha_1$ receptors; $\alpha_2$ receptors are generally more remote from the junction. Prejunctional $\alpha_2$ receptors, and receptors for many intrinsic vasodilators, inhibit cyclic AMP (cAMP) production to attenuate $Ca^{2+}$ channel opening and vesicle release (negative sign). Angiotensin receptors promote more transmitter release per action potential (positive sign). Adenosine triphosphate (ATP) and neuropeptide Y (NPY) are co-transmitters in some sympathetic fibres. Not to scale (varicosity 2 μm long × 1 μm wide; axon 0.1–0.5 μm wide; myocyte 4 μm wide centrally). ACh, acetylcholine; NPY, neuropeptide Y; $PGE_1$, prostaglandin $E_1$.

**Table 14.1** Pharmacology of cardiovascular adrenergic transmission

| Receptor | Subtype | Principal location and effect | Agonists: relative potency | Antagonists | Therapeutic use of antagonists |
|---|---|---|---|---|---|
| α | | Vascular myocytes: vasoconstriction | Noradrenaline (NAd) and adrenaline (Ad) | Phentolamine, phenoxybenzamine | Raynaud's vasospasm Acute hypertension (phaeochromocytoma) |
| | | | | Ergotamine | Migraine |
| | α1 | Postjunctional receptor on most vessels. Vasoconstriction via $G_q$, PLC, ↑ $IP_3$ and DAG | NAd = Ad, phenylephrine | Prazosin, doxazosin, tamsulosin | Essential hypertension Benign prostatic hypertrophy |
| | α2 | Autoreceptor of sympathetic varicosity: inhibits NAd release. Abundant postjunctional receptor in human skin vessels and muscle distal arterioles. Vasoconstriction via $G_i$, ↓ cAMP | NAd = Ad, clonidine | Yohimbine | – |
| β | | SA node and myocardium: ↑ heart rate and contractility Arterioles of heart, skeletal muscle and liver; vasodilatation | NAd, Ad, isoprenaline | Propranolol, nadolol, carvedilol (also $α_1$ antagonist) | Angina (↓ cardiac work), hypertension |
| | β1 | SA node and myocardium: ↑ heart rate and contractility via $G_s$, adenylyl cyclase, ↑ cAMP | NAd = Ad Dobutamine (use: acute cardiac failure) | Atenolol, metoprolol, bisoprolol | Angina (↓ cardiac work) Hypertension (↓ cardiac work) Arrhythmias |
| | β2 | Arterioles of heart, skeletal muscle, liver Also, bronchiole smooth muscle. Dilatation via $G_s$, ↑ cAMP | Ad >NAd Salbutamol, terbutaline | – | – |

cAMP, cyclic adenosine monophosphate; DAG, diacylglycerol; $IP_3$, inositol 1,4,5 trisphosphate; PLC, phospholipase C; SA, sinoatrial.

## Noradrenaline is removed quickly after release

The action of NAd is terminated by three processes:

1. Around 80% of the NAd is transported back into the varicosity by a $Na^+$-$Cl^-$-amine co-transporter called **uptake 1**, driven by the $Na^+$ gradient. Uptake 1 can be blocked by **reserpine**, a former antihypertensive drug that causes NAd depletion. Mood enhancers such as **cocaine** and **tricyclic antidepressants** (e.g. desipramine) likewise inhibit uptake 1, and the attendant rise in extracellular NAd in the heart can cause tachycardia or arrhythmia.
2. Significant amounts of NAd also diffuse into the capillary bloodstream. This sympathetic '**spillover**' accounts for much of the circulating plasma NAd in humans.
3. Smaller amounts of transmitter are degraded by a postjunctional, intracellular enzyme, catechol-$O$-methyltransferase.

## Noradrenaline release is modulated by local metabolites and agonists

The amount of NAd that is released depends not only on impulse frequency but also on the chemical environment of the varicosity, a process known as **neuromodulation** (Figure 14.2). Metabolic vasodilators such as adenosine, $H^+$ and $K^+$ ions depress NAd release, thereby enhancing their vasodilator effect. Most vasodilator autacoids have a similar action. NAd itself binds to prejunctional $α_2$ receptors (autoreceptors) to inhibit further exocytosis and thus prevent excessive discharge of vesicles. The $α_2$ receptors, being coupled to inhibitory $G_i$ protein, lower the varicosity cyclic AMP (cAMP) level, which leads to a fall in axonal N-type $Ca^{2+}$ channel opening. By contrast, the hormone **angiotensin II facilitates NAd exocytosis** and thereby amplifies its own direct vasoconstrictor effect.

## ATP and neuropeptide Y contribute to sympathetic neuromuscular transmission

The α adrenergic receptor blockers phentolamine and phenoxybenzamine completely abolish the sympathetic vasoconstrictor response in most veins and the pulmonary artery. However, in many systemic arteries the inhibition is only partial. This led to the discovery of co-transmitters in the sympathetic varicosity, namely the purine ATP and the peptide neuropeptide Y (NPY) (Table 14.2). The contribution of co-transmitters varies from tissue to tissue.

**Table 14.2** Main co-transmitters in perivascular nerve fibres[a]

| Main co-transmitters | |
| --- | --- |
| Sympathetic vasoconstrictor fibre | Noradrenaline |
| | Adenosine triphosphate (ATP) |
| | Neuropeptide Y |
| Parasympathetic dilator fibre | Acetylcholine |
| | Vasoactive intestinal polypeptide |
| | Nitric oxide |
| Sensory dilator fibre (C-fibre) | Substance P |
| | Calcitonin gene-related peptide |
| | ATP |

[a] The ratio of transmitter substances within the fibre varies from tissue to tissue. (From Burnstock G. *Acta Physiologica Scandinavica. Supplementum* 1988; 571: 53–9.)

**ATP** is co-released with NAd in some large and small arteries. ATP stimulates postjunctional $P_{2X}$ purinergic receptors. These '**ionotropic**' receptors are physically part of an ion channel protein (unlike '**metabotropic**' α receptors, which activate enzyme cascades). Ligand-binding to the P2X receptor activates a cation conductance, partially selective for $Ca^{2+}$ over $Na^+$. The cation current causes a fast, brief depolarization of the myocyte (the fast excitatory junction potentials in Figures 14.3 and 12.9).

**NPY** is synthesized in the postganglionic cell body and transported slowly along the axon to the sympathetic terminals in skeletal muscle, kidney, salivary gland, spleen and nasal mucosa. It may be stored in large dense-cored vesicles along with NAd. It is co-released chiefly by the high-frequency sympathetic activity associated with stress; the high frequency raises the neural $[Ca^{2+}]$ sufficiently to dock

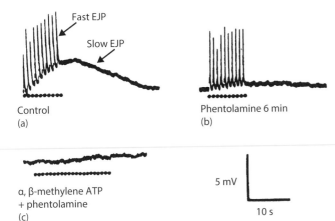

**Figure 14.3** Evidence for co-transmission by noradrenaline and adenosine triphosphate (ATP) in sympathetic fibres innervating rat tail artery. (**a**) Myocyte intracellular potential during repeated sympathetic stimulation (dots), showing fast excitatory junction potentials (EJPs, spike) on top of a slower depolarization (slow EJPs, baseline under spikes). NB: The spikes are not action potentials, as is evident from the voltage scale. (**b**) Phentolamine, an α adrenergic receptor blocker, abolishes the slow EJPs. (**c**) Desensitization of purinergic receptors by α, β-methylene ATP abolishes the fast EJPs. (After Sneddon P, Burnstock G. *European Journal of Pharmacology* 1984; 106(1): 149–52, with permission from Elsevier.)

the NPY-containing vesicles with the varicosity membrane. NPY produces a slower, more prolonged depolarization than ATP and sensitizes the postjunctional membrane to NAd (neuromodulatory effect) via the $Y_1$ receptor.

## Sympathetic fibres are tonically active

Sympathetic vasoconstrictor fibres are continuously active, though the average frequency is low in resting humans (0.5–1 impulses/s) and even maximal activity averages only 8–10 impulses/s. Activity is uneven; it occurs in bursts in muscle and is irregular in skin. Nevertheless, the tonic activity contributes substantially to resting vascular tone, so **a fall in sympathetic vasomotor activity or pharmacological blockade causes vasodilatation**. Sympathetic blockade increases the blood flow to resting skeletal muscle two- to threefold, though this is far from maximal flow, owing to the persistence of basal tone.

## Sympathetic drive to one tissue is independent of that to another tissue

Sympathetic drive to each tissue (skin, muscle, kidney, etc.) appears to be controlled by distinct groups of neurons in the ventrolateral medulla (organotopic organization). Their responsiveness falls into three main classes: barosensitive; thermosensitive; and glucosensitive. The barosensitive sympathetic pathway innervates muscle, kidneys and viscera, and is controlled predominantly by BP sensors (baroreceptors, Chapter 16). Thermosensitive sympathetic vasoconstrictor fibres innervate mainly the skin, and are regulated predominantly by hypothalamic core temperature sensors and emotion. Glucosensitive sympathetic fibres innervate the adrenal medulla, and are activated by hypoglycaemia and exercise, stimulating adrenaline release.

Although a generalized activation of all sympathetic vasomotor fibres occurs in certain circumstances, for example, during a haemorrhage, this is often not the case. For example, during the human **alerting response** to stress, sympathetic vasoconstrictor drive to the skin is increased (causing blanching), while at the same time the vasoconstrictor drive to skeletal muscle is reduced (causing vasodilatation). Activation of the sympathetic system is thus not an 'all-or-none' affair; it is finely graded and is adjusted regionally according to need.

## Reduced sympathetic activity elicits vasodilatation

Although it is natural to think of vasoconstriction as the primary role of vasoconstrictor nerves, vasodilatation by reduced sympathetic activity is also important. Indeed, it was flushing of the rabbit ear on cutting the nervous innervation that led the celebrated French physiologist, Claude Bernard, to discover the sympathetic vasomotor system in 1851. Two examples of vasodilatation in humans through reduced sympathetic activity are as follows:

- If BP rises acutely, the baroreceptor reflex evokes a widespread fall in sympathetic activity (Section 16.2). The resulting vasodilatation helps to bring BP back towards normal.
- When body temperature rises during exercise, the hypothalamic temperature-regulating centre evokes a fall in vasoconstrictor nerve activity to the skin, and the ensuing cutaneous vasodilatation helps to bring the temperature back down (Section 15.3).

## Increased sympathetic activity raises peripheral resistance, reduces local blood flow and boosts central blood volume

The principal effects of an increase in sympathetic vasomotor activity in a tissue are as follows:

- **Tissue blood flow** is reduced by contraction of the local resistance vessels (Figure 14.4, label c).
- **Tissue blood volume** is reduced by contraction of the local veins (Figure 14.5). This can squeeze 28 mL blood/kg out of the intestinal tract and liver, and 15 mL/kg from the skin, into central veins. Skeletal muscle veins lack an effective innervation, but 7.5 mL/kg can nevertheless be expelled as local venous pressure is lowered by the contraction of upstream resistance vessels (Figure 14.4, arrow a).
- **Capillary pressure** is reduced by resistance vessel contraction, as explained in Figure 11.11b. This allows interstitial fluid to be absorbed into the plasma compartment by osmosis in accordance with the Starling principle (Figure 14.4, arrow b).
- **Total peripheral resistance** (TPR) is raised in proportion to the amount of tissue involved and the severity of the vasoconstriction. A global increase in sympathetic outflow to multiple tissues, for example, on standing up, raises TPR substantially. This helps to restore a fallen arterial BP, since arterial pressure = cardiac output × TPR. Indeed, the **regulation of BP through the adjustment of TPR** is a major function of the sympathetic vasomotor system, both normally and in pathophysiological situations. To this end, sympathetic activity is regulated by reflexes initiated by arterial pressure receptors (Chapter 16).

A global increase in sympathetic outflow is a major part of the body's defence against hypovolaemia (low blood volume, e.g. haemorrhage). Reduced peripheral blood flow, displacement of blood from peripheral to central veins, interstitial fluid absorption and increase in TPR are a life-preserving package of responses because they help preserve cardiac output and arterial pressure (Section 18.2).

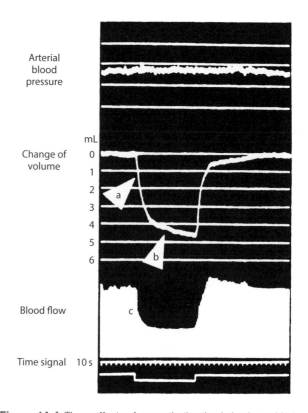

**Figure 14.4** Three effects of sympathetic stimulation in cat hindquarters (two impulses/s, square signal). Arrow 'a' shows a fall in volume of blood, caused by the reduced diameter of capacitance vessels (secondary to a fall in venous pressure following resistance vessel contraction; veins in skeletal muscle have little direct innervation). Arrow 'b' shows a slower fall in tissue volume due to the osmotic absorption of interstitial fluid by the capillaries, as capillary pressure is reduced by resistance vessel contraction. Label 'c' shows a fall in blood flow caused by resistance vessel contraction. (From Mellander S. *Acta Physiologica Scandinavica* 1960; 50(176): 1–86, with permission from Wiley-Blackwell.)

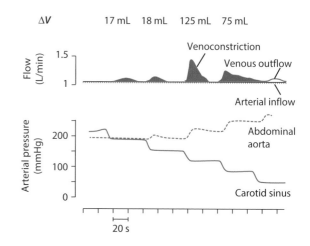

**Figure 14.5** Active splanchnic venoconstriction mediated by increases in sympathetic activity in the dog. Sympathetic activity was raised reflexly by step reductions in pressure in an isolated carotid sinus, while measuring splanchnic arterial inflow and venous outflow. Each transient excess of outflow over inflow marks an episode of venoconstriction. ΔV, displaced blood volume. Aortic pressure rises due to the reflex, sympathetically mediated rise in peripheral resistance. (After Hainsworth R, Karim F. *The Journal of Physiology* 1976; 262(3): 659–77, with permission from Wiley-Blackwell.)

## Sympathetic activity contributes to regular oscillations in blood pressure

The sympathetic drive to skeletal muscle waxes and wanes over the respiratory cycle. Left ventricle output likewise oscillates with respiration, falling during inspiration (Section 2.5, 'split second sound'). These oscillations cause the mean arterial pressure to fall by a few mmHg during inspiration and rise during expiration (**Traube–Hering waves**, Section 8.5, 12–14 cycles/min). Human BP may also oscillate at a slower frequency than the breathing cycle, ~6 cycles/min. These are called **Mayer waves**. Mayer waves are attributed to cyclic changes in sympathetic vasomotor tone, driven by a resonance in the baroreceptor reflex.

## 14.2 PARASYMPATHETIC VASODILATOR NERVES

In a **few, specialized tissues**, the arteries and resistance vessels are innervated by vasodilator fibres **as well as** the ubiquitous sympathetic vasoconstrictor fibres. Vasodilator fibres are found in the parasympathetic, sympathetic and sensory systems. This section deals with the first of these.

## The parasympathetic system comprises long preganglionic fibres and short postganglionic fibres

Parasympathetic vasodilator fibres have a more restricted distribution than sympathetic vasoconstrictor fibres, and are not tonically active; they are only activated when organ function demands a rise in blood flow.

Parasympathetic **preganglionic fibres** are much longer than their sympathetic counterparts; they extend all the way from the CNS to the innervated tissue. They emerge from the CNS in two 'outflows', one carried by the **cranial nerves** (e.g. vagus) and the other by the **sacral spinal nerves**. The cranial outflow innervates the cerebral and coronary arteries, salivary glands, exocrine pancreas and gastrointestinal mucosa. The sacral outflow innervates the genitalia, bladder and colon. Skin and muscle do not have a parasympathetic innervation.

In the target organ, the long, preganglionic fibres synapse with short, **postganglionic neurons**. The short postganglionic axons innervate the resistance vessels. Like sympathetic terminals, the axons have multiple varicosities containing vesicles of neuroeffector. Parasympathetic vesicles are small and clear, and contain acetylcholine (ACh).

## Parasympathetic vasodilatation is mediated by acetylcholine and NANC transmitters

Parasympathetic postganglionic terminals release the classic neurotransmitter **ACh**, which elicits vasodilatation (Figures 9.8, top left and 14.6a). ACh activates the

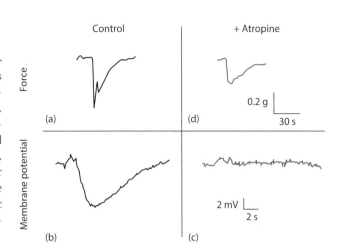

**Figure 14.6** Parasympathetic-mediated vasodilatation of rabbit lingual artery; noradrenergic fibres blocked by guanethidine. (**a**) Mechanical response to perivascular fibre stimulation, showing arterial dilatation. (**b**) Corresponding membrane potential, showing slow hyperpolarization of a myocyte (baseline –51 mV). (**c**) Total abolition of electrical response by atropine, proving that the electrical response is purely cholinergic. (**d**) However, the dilatation was only partly blocked by atropine, indicating the release of a non-cholinergic vasodilator, probably vasoactive intestinal polypeptide. (From Brayden JE, Large WA. *British Journal of Pharmacology* 1986; 89(1): 163–71, with permission from Wiley-Blackwell.)

muscarinic $M_3$ receptor on the vessel endothelium, triggering the endothelial $G_q$–phospholipase C (PLC)–$Ca^{2+}$ pathway to stimulate endothelial NO production (Figure 9.10). The NO diffuses into the myocytes to cause relaxation. By contrast, ACh causes contraction in de-endothelialized vessels (Figure 9.8, top right). This is because myocytes express muscarinic $M_3$ receptors, which raise $[Ca^{2+}]$ via the $G_q$–PLC pathway. The endothelial effect predominates in intact vessels.

The muscarinic receptor blocker, **atropine**, inhibits parasympathetic vasodilatation; however; the inhibition is often incomplete (Figure 14.6d). This is because the parasympathetic fibres in some tissues also release **non-adrenergic, non-cholinergic (NANC) transmitters**. NANC transmitters are **vasoactive intestinal polypeptide** (VIP), **substance P** (another neuropeptide) and **NO**. NO is generated by 'nitridergic' parasympathetic terminal fibres in erectile tissue and possibly cerebral, temporal, mesenteric and coronary arteries.

## Salivary and pancreatic vasodilatation underpins fluid secretion

Blood flow to the submandibular **salivary gland** increases tenfold when the parasympathetic fibres of the chorda tympani nerve are activated. The increase in perfusion supplies the water needed for salivation; a salivary gland can secrete its own weight in fluid in just 1 min. The vasodilatation is mediated partly by ACh and partly by VIP and substance P. In the **pancreas**, VIP seems to be the main parasympathetic transmitter, rather than ACh. Such fibres are said to be 'peptidergic'. In the **intestinal submucosa**, the postganglionic transmitter is mainly ACh, acting via endothelial NO production (since vasodilatation is largely blocked by l-NG-monomethylarginine, an inhibitor of endothelial nitric oxide synthase (NOS).

## Parasympathetic vasodilatation brings about genital erection

Sacral parasympathetic fibres form the nervi erigentes, which innervate the blood vessels of the genital erectile tissue, that is, the penis and clitoris. Therefore, these vasomotor nerves are truly essential to the continuation of the species! In the penis, an artery in the centre of each corpus cavernosum gives rise to helicine resistance arteries, which feed blood into the cavernous venous sinuses. Parasympathetic activity profoundly dilates the resistance arteries, causing the corpora to swell. Since the swelling compresses the outflow veins against the outer coat of the corpora, the tunica albuginea, the usual balance of resistances is reversed; the resistance to inflow becomes smaller than the resistance to outflow. The venous sinuses of the corpora cavernosa therefore fill with blood at a high pressure, creating distension and erection. A fall in sympathetic vasoconstrictor drive reinforces the dilatation. In the absence of sexual excitement, detumescence is maintained by sympathetic α adrenergic tone in the penile arteries and corpus smooth muscle.

Parasympathetic-induced erection is not blocked by atropine, but is blocked by inhibitors of NOS. This shows that the parasympathetic fibres are chiefly **nitridergic** rather than cholinergic. The axons contain NOS and secrete NO on electrical stimulation. **Sildenafil (Viagra)**, a successful treatment for human erectile dysfunction, amplifies the biochemical effect of the NO–cyclic guanosine monophosphate (cGMP) pathway by inhibiting **phosphodiesterase type 5**, the enzyme that normally degrades cGMP (Figure 9.10). A common side effect is vascular headache due to cerebral artery dilatation.

Parasympathetic **VIP** may also contribute to erectile vasodilatation, since VIP is present in penile parasympathetic fibres and appears in penile venous blood following pelvic fibre stimulation.

## 14.3 SYMPATHETIC VASODILATOR NERVES

As emphasized repeatedly, most sympathetic vasomotor fibres are noradrenergic and cause vasoconstriction. However, in certain species and tissues there is a limited distribution of sympathetic **cholinergic** (ACh-releasing) fibres that cause vasodilatation.

## Sympathetic cholinergic fibres mediate sweating and cutaneous vasodilatation

Human sweat glands are innervated by sympathetic cholinergic fibres (sudomotor fibres), which elicit cutaneous vasodilatation as well as sweating. The fibres release ACh, which stimulates the vascular endothelium to produce $PGI_2$ (via cyclooxygenase 1) and endothelium-derived hyperpolarizing factor, along with a little NO (Section 9.5). Since sudomotor-mediated vasodilatation is only partially inhibited by atropine, additional NANC transmitters must also contribute to the dilatation. VIP seems to be one such factor, being demonstrable in vasomotor fibres close to the sweat glands.

## In non-primate muscle, sympathetic cholinergic fibres mediate the vasodilatation of the alerting response

In the cat, dog, goat and sheep, but not primates, the small arteries of skeletal muscle are innervated by sympathetic cholinergic vasodilator nerves, stimulation of which increases muscle blood flow. The sympathetic cholinergic fibres are controlled by the forebrain and are not tonically active, unlike the sympathetic vasoconstrictor fibres (Table 14.3). They play no part in the baroreflex control of BP and are activated solely as part of the **alerting response**, which is a co-ordinated set of cardiac and vascular changes evoked by mental stress, fear and danger (Section 16.8). The cholinergic vasodilatation increases the muscle blood flow in anticipation of exercise, but fails to increase the microvascular permeability-surface area product, probably because cholinergic fibres innervate chiefly the arteries with a diameter of 0.1–0.2 mm rather than arterioles. Metabolic hyperaemia, by contrast, has its greatest effect

**Table 14.3** Contrasting organization of sympathetic vasoconstrictor and vasodilator nervous systems

| Feature | Sympathetic vasoconstrictor fibre | Sympathetic vasodilator fibre |
| --- | --- | --- |
| Main neuroeffector | Noradrenaline (and ATP) | Acetylcholine (and VIP) |
| Distribution | Most organs and tissue | Only sweat glands in humans. Skeletal muscle in non-primates |
| Tonically active? | Yes | No |
| Central control | Brainstem | Forebrain |
| Involvement in baroreceptor reflex | Major role | Negligible |
| Role in blood pressure homeostasis | Very important | Unimportant |
| Duration of effect | Mostly well sustained | Transient |

ATP, adenosine triphosphate; VIP, vasoactive intestinal polypeptide.

on arterioles (Figure 13.9). It recruits capillaries and thus raises the permeability-surface area product as well as blood flow. It cannot be emphasized too strongly that **local metabolic factors cause the functional hyperaemia associated with normal, non-emotional exercise**, not sympathetic vasodilator nerves.

## In human muscle, adrenaline and other mechanisms mediate the vasodilatation of the alerting response

Acute mental stress, such as mental arithmetic, evokes vasodilatation in human forearm muscles (Figure 14.7), though not in the calf. This alerting response was formerly attributed to sympathetic cholinergic innervation; more recent observation indicate otherwise, as follows:

- Primates, as a group, lack a sympathetic cholinergic innervation to the muscle vasculature (cf. skin vasculature).
- Electrode recordings show that the sympathetic activity in human muscle is reduced, not increased, by stress.

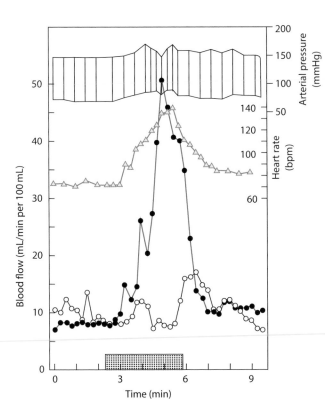

**Figure 14.7** A classic demonstration of the human alerting response. Closed circles, forearm blood flow, mainly to the muscle; open circles, hand blood flow, mainly to the skin; triangles, heart rate. During the time represented by the rectangle, the experimenters made the participant believe that he was bleeding badly through a leak in the apparatus (!). The increase in forearm flow is comparable with that in severe exercise, and greatly exceeds the maximum flow produced by the withdrawal of sympathetic vasoconstrictor tone. (From Blair DA, Glover WE, Greenfield AD, et al. *The Journal of Physiology* 1959; 148: 633–47, with permission from Wiley-Blackwell.)

- Axillary nerve block does not prevent the human forearm vasodilator response to stress. However, β adrenergic receptor blockers significantly attenuate the human response, indicating that it is due in part to circulating **adrenaline**. Plasma adrenaline concentration doubles during the alerting response, due to the sympathetic stimulation of the adrenal medulla.
- An additional factor is a **reduction in sympathetic vasoconstrictor activity** to the muscle, though this alone is insufficient to explain the large increase in flow. (The finding in some, but not all, studies that atropine, a blocker of ACh muscarinic receptors, attenuates human stress-induced vasodilatation remains a puzzle.)

## 14.4 NOCICEPTIVE C-FIBRE MEDIATED VASODILATATION

### Antidromic stimulation of sensory C-fibres causes cutaneous vasodilatation

The curious ability of sensory nerves to cause cutaneous vasodilatation was discovered by William Bayliss early in the 20th century. He stimulated the dorsal root of a spinal nerve antidromically, sending action potentials in the 'wrong' direction down the sensory nerves, and found that this caused cutaneous vasodilatation. Antidromic activity probably contributes to the characteristic segmental cutaneous hyperaemia of **shingles**, a dorsal root infection by herpes zoster (a reactivated form of latent varicella zoster, the chickenpox virus).

### C-fibre-mediated vasodilatation is part of the Lewis triple response

The motor function of nociceptive (harm-sensing) sensory fibres, that is, the C-fibres, was revealed further in the Lewis triple response, described in 1927. Sir Thomas Lewis noted that the reaction of human skin to a mild trauma such as a scratch has three components:

- **Local redness** along the line of the scratch is caused by local vasodilatation, resulting probably from the release of K+ ions and inflammatory autacoids by activated cells.
- **Local swelling** along the line of the scratch (a wheal) is caused by inflammatory oedema resulting from microvascular damage (Section 11.11).
- **The spreading flare** is an area of redness that gradually extends laterally from the line of trauma for 2–3 cm. Humans and rats exhibit this response, but many other species do not. Remarkably, the flare must be mediated by sensory fibres because it abolished by sensory denervation or by local anaesthetics such as lidocaine (Figure 14.8). Since the flare spreads too quickly to be explained by autacoid diffusion, Lewis suggested that it is mediated by a C-fibre **sensory axon reflex**, as follows.

263

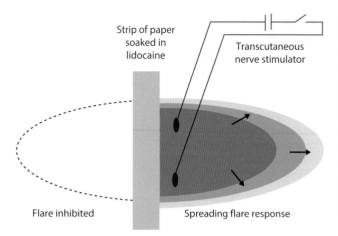

Strip of paper soaked in lidocaine

Transcutaneous nerve stimulator

Flare inhibited

Spreading flare response

**Figure 14.8** Vasodilatation mediated by sensory C-fibres in human skin, seen en face. Nociceptive C-fibres were stimulated by transcutaneous electrical stimulation. The spreading flare was recorded by a laser Doppler imager. The leftward spread of the flare is abolished by the sensory anaesthetic lidocaine. (Based on Schmelz M, Petersen LJ. *News in Physiological Sciences* 2001; 16: 33–7, with permission from the American Physiological Society.)

## The C-fibre sensory axon reflex causes the spreading flare

The flare is mediated by nociceptive (harm-sensing) C-fibres. Trauma triggers a C-fibre action potential, which not only propagates centrally but also passes down an axon side branch, travelling antidromically to blood vessels up to a centimetre away (Figure 14.9). Arrival of the action potential in the axon branch terminal causes it to release vasodilator neuropeptides. These include **substance P**, which activates endothelial $NK_1$ receptors to stimulate NO production; and **calcitonin gene-related peptide** (CGRP), which activates the vascular myocyte cAMP pathway (Figure 12.10). CGRP is extremely potent and its effect lasts many hours. **Mast cell histamine** is also implicated, at least in rat skin and some human dermatological conditions. Many substance P-containing fibres terminate on mast cells, which express $NK_1$ receptors. Receptor activation causes the mast cell to release its histamine granules, exacerbating the vasodilatation.

## C-fibre antidromic activity can lead to neurogenic inflammation

Antidromic stimulation of C-fibres not only causes vasodilatation but also venular hyperpermeability, due to the action of substance P and histamine on the venular endothelium (Section 11.11). The resulting plasma exudation and high-protein oedema is called neurogenic inflammation. Neurogenic inflammation is readily elicited in rat skin and synovial joints. Healthy human skin is not very susceptible to neurogenic inflammation, but becomes susceptible when sensitized by dermatological disorders.

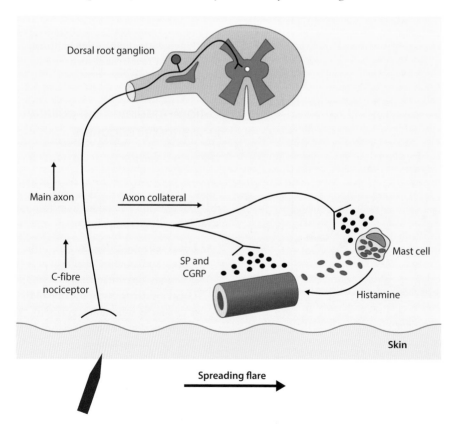

Dorsal root ganglion

Main axon

Axon collateral

Mast cell

SP and CGRP

C-fibre nociceptor

Histamine

Skin

Spreading flare

**Figure 14.9** The sensory axon reflex and spreading flare response to a scratch. Vasodilatation is due to the release of substance P (SP) and calcitonin gene-related peptide (CGRP) from nociceptive C-fibre axon branches. In rat skin and possibly some human dermatological conditions, collateral endings near mast cells also trigger histamine granule release, which augments the flare. (After Foreman JC. *Allergy* 1987; 42(1): 1–11, with permission from Wiley-Blackwell.)

## 14.5 HORMONAL CONTROL OF THE CIRCULATION

Many hormones influence the heart and circulation. Hormones such as adrenaline, vasopressin and angiotensin are in general less important than autonomic nerves for physiological, acute cardiovascular regulation, but become major regulators in pathological situations such as haemorrhagic hypovolaemia or transplanted hearts. The main cardiovascular hormones, **adrenaline**, **vasopressin**, **angiotensin** and **atrial natriuretic peptide (ANP)**, are described in Sections 14.6–14.9. Except for adrenaline, they also regulate renal tubular function to control extracellular fluid volume. Other hormones with significant cardiovascular effects, such as **insulin, thyroxine, oestrogen** and **relaxin**, are described briefly in this section.

### Insulin

Insulin stimulates the endothelium to produce NO, so insulin has vasodilator and antithrombotic actions. It also inhibits vascular smooth muscle growth and migration. These important anti-atheroma effects are reduced in people with diabetes, who either lack insulin or are resistant to it. This may contribute to the high incidence of atheroma, ischaemic heart disease and limb ischaemia in such individuals. Diabetes is a major risk factor for these conditions.

### Thyroxine

Thyroxine induces cardiac myocytes to express a high density of $\beta_1$ adrenergic receptors, and thereby enhances contractility. Hyperthyroidism increases basal metabolic rate, which leads to a generalized vasodilatation, fall in TPR, tachycardia and rise in stroke volume.

### Oestrogen

The ovarian follicle hormone 17β-oestradiol causes vasodilatation in many tissues, including the female genitourinary system (uterus, vagina, kidneys), mammary glands, heart and skin. Its acute vasodilator action is mediated partly by the activation of endothelial NOS via the protein kinase B pathway (Figure 9.10) and partly through activation of vascular myocyte $BK_{Ca}$ channels. During pregnancy, high levels of oestrogen cause a characteristic fall in BP by midterm. Oestrogen reduces the incidence of coronary artery disease in premenopausal women, probably by a genomic upregulation of NOS and $PGI_2$ production.

### Relaxin

Relaxin is a peptide hormone secreted by the ovarian corpus luteum during pregnancy and parturition. It causes vasodilatation in the uterus, mammary gland and heart, and acts by attenuating endothelin-mediated vasoconstriction.

## 14.6 ADRENALINE AND NORADRENALINE

The adrenal gland is situated at the upper pole of the kidney. Its outer part, the cortex, secretes the steroid hormones cortisol and aldosterone. Its inner part, the medulla (10% of the gland) comprises chromaffin cells that secrete the catecholamines adrenaline (epinephrine) and NAd (norepinephrine). NAd is methylated by phenylethanolamine N-methyltransferase (PNMT) to form adrenaline, which accounts for ~80% of catecholamine secretion in humans. In diving mammals, by contrast, NAd is the chief product, contributing to muscle vasoconstriction during dives.

The adrenal vasculature is organized as a **cortico-medullary portal system**; see Section 1.8 for portal systems. This carries cortisol-rich blood from the cortex to many chromaffin cells in the medulla, where the high cortisol concentration induces PNMT expression and hence adrenaline production. Other chromaffin cells are supplied directly via medullary arteries, express less PNMT and secrete NAd.

Although the human medulla secretes mainly adrenaline, the basal plasma adrenaline concentration (0.1–0.5 nM) is lower than the NAd concentration (0.5–3.0 nM). The relatively high-circulating NAd is due mainly to **spillage** from the tonically active, sympathetic vasomotor terminals (Figure 14.2), so it is often used as a measure of sympathetic activity. For example, plasma NAd approximately doubles on standing up because of increased sympathetic activity, while plasma adrenaline changes little. The circulating **half-life** of the catecholamines is only a few minutes, so the circulating concentration can be adjusted rapidly. The catecholamines are taken up by non-neural tissue for **degradation** by catechol-O-methyltransferase, and by nerve endings for degradation by monoamine oxidase.

### Adrenaline secretion is stimulated by sympathetic preganglionic fibres in stress situations

During embryogenesis, the medullary chromaffin cells develop from postganglionic sympathetic neurons. This accounts for their innervation by preganglionic sympathetic fibres in the splanchnic nerve (Figure 14.1). Sympathetic activity thus regulates adrenaline secretion. Secretion is stimulated in response to four main stresses, namely:

- **exercise**;
- **alerting** (the alerting response to 'fight or flight' situations);
- **hypotension**; and
- **hypoglycaemia**.

During exercise, the plasma adrenaline concentration can reach 5 nM, and NAd 10 nM. The latter is due partly to spillover from the increased sympathetic activity.

## Adrenaline has both metabolic and cardiovascular effects

The cardiovascular effects of adrenaline at physiological concentrations are relatively minor compared with those of the autonomic nerves and intrinsic regulators. Consequently, the **metabolic effects of adrenaline are as important as its cardiovascular effects**, albeit not our main concern here. Adrenaline stimulates **glycogenolysis** in skeletal muscle and **lipolysis** in adipose tissue, thereby releasing glucose into the bloodstream. Adrenaline also has the following cardiovascular effects:

- **Cardiac contractility and heart rate are raised** via the activation of the cardiac $\beta_1$ adrenergic receptors (Section 4.5).
- **Arterial and venous constrictions** are induced in tissues with a predominance of vascular **$\alpha$ adrenergic receptors**, such as the **skin and intestines**. The ingrained belief of many students that adrenaline always causes vasodilatation is untrue.
- **Vasodilatation in myocardium, skeletal muscle and liver** is due to their abundance of $\beta_2$ **adrenergic receptors**, along with the high affinity of adrenaline for this class of receptor (Table 14.1). The $\beta_2$ adrenergic receptor is coupled to the vasodilator $G_s$–adenylyl cyclase–cAMP pathway (Figure 12.10). If the $\beta$ receptors are blocked by propranolol, adrenaline causes vasoconstriction, even in skeletal muscle, because it also activates $\alpha$ receptors. NAd vasoconstricts muscle because it has a higher affinity for $\alpha_1$ than $\beta_2$ receptors.

Because myocardial vasodilatation improves coronary perfusion, adrenaline is often injected as an emergency measure during a **cardiac arrest**, though it appears to have relatively little effect on the outcome.

## Adrenaline and noradrenaline have different net effects on the circulation

As explained above, adrenaline and NAd at physiological concentrations have opposite effects on skeletal muscle, which is the most abundant tissue in the body (~40% by weight). Consequently, their effects on the systemic circulation differ substantially (Figure 14.10).

**Intravenous NAd** causes a widespread systemic vasoconstriction, which **greatly increases the TPR** and arterial BP. The raised pressure triggers a baroreceptor reflex, which reduces the sympathetic drive to the heart and increases the parasympathetic drive. This more than offsets the direct stimulatory effect of NAd on the pacemaker and myocardium, resulting in a fall in heart rate and cardiac output.

**Intravenous adrenaline**, by contrast, **reduces the TPR**, because the $\beta_2$ receptor driven vasodilatation in skeletal muscle outweighs the $\alpha_1$ receptor activated vasoconstriction in other tissues. Mean BP changes little (Figure 14.10). Consequently, the stimulation of the heart by adrenaline is not opposed by the baroreflex, and cardiac output increases markedly.

**Phaeochromocytoma**, a rare tumour of the medullary chromaffin cells, secretes a mixture of catecholamines and causes hypertension. The latter can be treated with $\alpha$ antagonists such as phentolamine (reversible antagonist) or phenoxybenzamine (irreversible antagonist with a longer half-life).

## 14.7 VASOPRESSIN (ANTIDIURETIC HORMONE)

Vasopressin is a vasoconstrictor nonapeptide that is synthesized by the magnocellular (big) neurons of the supraoptic and paraventricular nuclei of the hypothalamus (Figure 14.11). Vasopressin is transported along the neuron's axon, which passes down the pituitary stalk into the posterior pituitary gland. The arrival of action potentials stimulates $Ca^{2+}$-dependent secretion of vasopressin from the axon terminals into the bloodstream. The half-life of vasopressin in the bloodstream is only ~5 min, so the circulating level can be rapidly adjusted. Vasopressin secretion is regulated by two kinds of sensory input, one from central osmoreceptors and the other from cardiovascular pressure receptors.

### Osmoreceptors regulate diuresis via vasopressin

Osmoreceptors are neurons in the anterolateral hypothalamus that are sensitive to plasma osmolarity. They are located in the organum vasculosum lamina terminalis and subfornicular organ

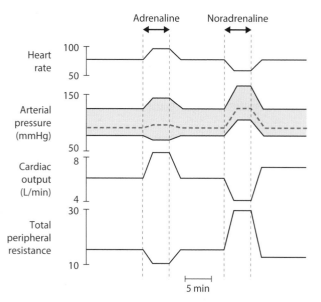

**Figure 14.10** Contrasting effects of intravenous adrenaline and noradrenaline in man. The dashed red line is the mean blood pressure. For explanation, see text. An initial transient drop in blood pressure during adrenaline infusion is not shown on this time scale. (From the classic monograph, Barcroft H, Swan HJC. *Sympathetic Control of Human Blood Vessels*. London: Edward Arnold; 1953. By permission.)

**Figure 14.11** Regulation of vasopressin secretion; relative contribution of arterial baro-receptors and low-pressure atrial receptors varies between species. ABP, arterial blood pressure, regulated by resistance vessel tone; AP, atrial pressure, regulated by renal control of extracellular fluid volume; CVLM, caudal ventrolateral medulla; OVLT, organum vasculosum lamina terminalis; PVN, paraventricular nucleus; SFO, subfornicular organ; SON, supraoptic nucleus. The inset shows sensitivity to plasma osmolarity and increase caused by blood loss.

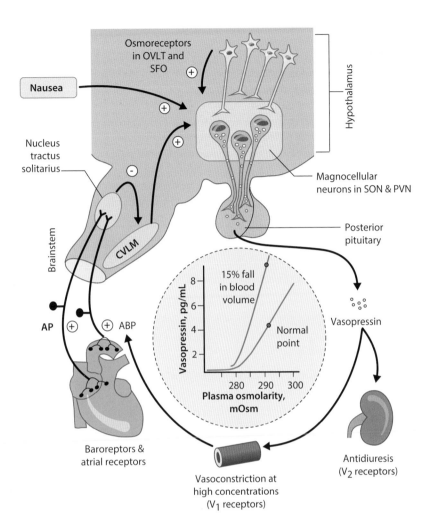

which, appropriately, lack a blood–brain barrier; the capillary endothelium is fenestrated at these sites. The osmoreceptors are excited by a rise in plasma osmolarity above 280–285 mOsm, for example during dehydration. Cholinergic axons extend from the osmoreceptors to synapse with the nearby magnocellular neurons, stimulating them to secrete vasopressin. Since a 2% rise in plasma osmolarity has the same stimulatory effect as a 10% fall in blood volume, vasopressin secretion is more sensitive to plasma osmolarity than blood volume. The osmoreceptors also project to **parvocellular (small) neurons** in the paraventricular nucleus, which influence sympathetic activity; consequently, water deprivation increases peripheral vasoconstrictor sympathetic activity, as well as vasopressin levels.

The main role of vasopressin at its normal, low plasma concentrations is to regulate the amount of water excreted by the kidneys, in order to stabilize plasma volume and osmolarity. This is reflected in its alternative name, 'antidiuretic hormone' (diuresis is urine production). Vasopressin stimulates high-affinity $V_2$ receptors on the renal collecting ducts, leading to increased water reabsorption and the prevention of dehydration. At physiological osmolarity, ~290 milliosmoles/L, the circulating vasopressin concentration is near the middle of the renal dose–response range, so water excretion can be adjusted up or down by changes in circulating vasopressin.

## Cardiovascular pressure receptors stimulate vasopressin secretion during hypovolaemia

Vasopressin secretion is also stimulated by **a fall in blood volume and BP**, for example, during a haemorrhage or severe dehydration. Pressure receptors in the heart and arteries, described in Chapter 16, send information about the central blood volume and arterial pressure to the brainstem. From here, the information is relayed to the magnocellular neurons via an inhibitory synapse. As a result of the inhibitory step, a fall in cardiovascular receptor traffic leads to a rise in vasopressin secretion (Figure 14.11). Once the blood volume falls by >10%, vasopressin secretion increases steeply. Vasopressin causes peripheral vasoconstriction, though this requires a higher circulating concentration than the antidiuretic action because the vascular $V_1$ receptors have a lower affinity than the renal duct $V_2$ receptors. The low-affinity vascular $V_1$ receptors are coupled to the $G_q$–PLC pathway that leads to vasoconstriction (Figure 12.7).

Vasopressin-induced vasoconstriction helps to support the arterial BP in hypovolaemic patients, and contributes to the characteristic pallor of their skin. However, in cerebral and coronary vessels vasopressin stimulates the endothelium, leading to NO-mediated vasodilatation. Vasopressin thus redistributes the limited cardiac output of hypovolaemia in favour of the brain and heart. At the same time, urine production is reduced to a minimum to conserve body fluids. If vasopressin is absent, as in **diabetes insipidus** and Brattleboro rats, BP is abnormally depressed during dehydration or haemorrhage.

**Nausea** is a further potent stimulus for vasopressin secretion. During nausea and vomiting, vasopressin levels can reach 50 times that required for antidiuresis. The resulting vasoconstriction contributes to the characteristic grey pallor of nausea. The vasoconstrictor action of injected vasopressin can also be used in an emergency to reduce the bleeding from oesophageal varices, a common feature of portal hypertension.

## 14.8 RENIN–ANGIOTENSIN– ALDOSTERONE SYSTEM

Angiotensin II is a vasoconstrictor peptide, production of which increases when BP falls. Its role is to help maintain the extracellular fluid volume and arterial BP. It achieves this through three principal actions:

1. Angiotensin II stimulates **aldosterone** secretion by the adrenal cortex. Aldosterone promotes renal salt and water retention to maintain the extracellular fluid and plasma volume, and is essential to life.
2. Angiotensin II causes a generalized **vasoconstriction**, partly by direct action and partly by boosting sympathetic activity. This raises peripheral resistance and BP.
3. Angiotensin II stimulates the sensation of **thirst**, and hence fluid intake.

The half-life of angiotensin II in the circulation is ~20 min, and it is inactivated by the liver. Circulating angiotensin II levels are normally low, and angiotensin II inhibitors cause only a small fall in BP in healthy humans. However, in patients with clinical hypertension angiotensin II inhibitors reduce BP markedly. In general, angiotensin II becomes important in pathological situations, namely hypovolaemia, cardiac failure and clinical hypertension.

## Angiotensin II production is mediated by renin and endothelial angiotensin-converting enzyme

Angiotensin II production is initiated by the secretion of **renin** into the renal bloodstream (Figure 14.12). Renin is a proteolytic enzyme that is synthesized, stored and secreted by specialized cells in the wall of renal afferent arterioles, called **juxtaglomerular (JG) cells** ('juxta'-glomerular, close to glomeruli). Renin attacks a plasma $\alpha_2$-globulin, angiotensinogen, to cleave off a decapeptide called angiotensin I. Angiotensin I has little activity, but it is cleaved further by an ecto (outside)-enzyme on the surface of endothelial cells, **angiotensin-converting enzyme (ACE)**, to generate an active octapeptide, angiotensin II. This process takes place mainly in the lungs because

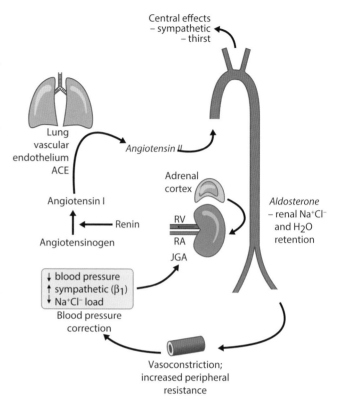

**Figure 14.12** Renin–angiotensin–aldosterone system. ACE, angiotensin-converting enzyme; JGA, juxtaglomerular apparatus; RA, renal artery; RV, renal vein. Central effects are the stimulation of sympathetic outflow, reduction in sensitivity of baroreceptor reflex and stimulation of thirst.

this is the first major expanse of endothelium encountered by venous angiotensin I. **ACE inhibitors** such as captopril, enalapril and ramipril block the formation of angiotensin II; however, as ACE normally also degrades circulating bradykinin, ACE inhibitors also raise circulating bradykinin levels, with unwanted side effects. These can be avoided by using the **angiotensin II receptor blocker**, losartan. Cleavage of one more amino acid from some angiotensin II molecules by aminopeptidase forms a heptapeptide, angiotensin III.

## Angiotensin II supports blood pressure via aldosterone secretion

At normal physiological concentrations, angiotensin II and III help stimulate the secretion of the steroidal hormone **aldosterone** by the outermost adrenal cortex (zona glomerulosa). Over the course of an hour or so, aldosterone stimulates the renal distal convoluted tubules to increase the rate of $Na^+$ reabsorption, in exchange for $K^+$ and $H^+$. The response is slow because it requires the synthesis and insertion of $Na^+/K^+$ pumps into the basal membrane and epithelial $Na^+$ channels into the apical membrane of the tubule cells. The $Na^+$ reabsorbed from the tubular fluid draws water with it by osmosis. In this way, the renin–angiotensin–aldosterone system (RAAS) maintains the plasma volume and therefore arterial BP. Failure of the adrenal cortex to secrete aldosterone leads to severe hypotension and hyperkalaemia, a potentially fatal condition called **Addison's disease**. Conversely, an adrenal tumour may secrete excessive amounts of aldosterone, leading to salt and water retention and hypertension (**Conn's syndrome**).

## Angiotensin II also supports blood pressure through direct vasoconstriction

Angiotensin II binds to $AT_1$ receptors on vascular myocytes. Since $AT_1$ receptors are coupled to the $G_q$–PLC–diacyl glycerol pathway, they trigger depolarization-independent and depolarization-dependent contraction (Figures 12.6 and 12.7). This tonic, vasoconstrictor action of angiotensin II contributes to the peripheral resistance, and thus to BP maintenance, though the contribution is quite modest at basal concentrations. However, angiotensin II makes a much greater contribution at the raised concentrations found in **hypovolaemia, clinical shock, cardiac failure** and **hypertension**. In hypovolaemia, shock and cardiac failure, angiotensin II causes pronounced vasoconstriction of skin, splanchnic and renal vessels. In clinical shock and renal artery stenosis, angiotensin II contracts the renal **glomerular efferent arterioles** (Figure 1.5), which helps maintain the glomerular capillary pressure and filtration rate. Many, but not all, patients with essential hypertension have raised renin and angiotensin II levels, so **ACE inhibitors** (captopril, enalapril, ramipril) and **$AT_1$ blockers** (losartan) are valuable antihypertensive drugs.

Angiotensin II also increases cardiac contractility during hypovolaemia and shock, partly by enhancing the plateau $Ca^{2+}$ current, and partly by stimulating sympathetic activity, as described next.

## Angiotensin II supports blood pressure by peripheral and central sympathetic amplification and by eliciting thirst

Angiotensin II raises the peripheral resistance not only by direct vasoconstrictor action but also by interacting with the brainstem, sympathetic ganglia and sympathetic terminals to boost sympathetic-induced vasoconstriction. Angiotensin II diffuses into the area postrema of the brainstem, where the blood–brain barrier is deficient. The area postrema is rich in angiotensin II receptors and their activation **increases the sympathetic preganglionic outflow**. $AT_1$ receptors on the postganglionic neurons of the **sympathetic ganglia** further facilitate the generation of sympathetic action potentials. **Sympathetic terminal varicosities** likewise have $AT_1$ receptors, activation of which facilitates the release of NAd by sympathetic action potentials (neuromodulation; Figure 14.2). In cardiac failure, raised angiotensin II levels contribute to the increased sympathetic activity, fluid retention (via aldosterone) and high cardiac filling pressures (Section 18.5).

In addition to its pro-sympathetic actions, angiotensin III acts on the hypothalamus to stimulate the sensation of **thirst**,

a common symptom in patients with hypovolaemia. Fluid intake helps to restore plasma volume in such patients.

## Negative feedback loops regulate the renin–angiotensin–aldosterone system

The concentration of circulating angiotensin II depends on the rate at which renal JG cells secrete renin. Renin exocytosis is controlled by multiple factors, which create negative feedback loops to support arterial BP during hypovolaemia, as follows:

- **Hypotension** activates the RAAS directly because the JG cells of afferent arterioles are inhibited by stretch. In patients with **renal artery stenosis**, the low pressure beyond the stenosis activates the RAAS inappropriately, causing hypertension.
- The increased **renal sympathetic activity** and circulating adrenaline during hypotension stimulates $\beta_1$ adrenergic receptors on JG cells. The resulting rise in intracellular cAMP stimulates renin secretion and thus helps to correct the hypotension.
- **A fall in $Na^+Cl^-$ concentration at the macula densa** stimulates renin production. The macula densa is a $Na^+Cl^-$-sensitive group of cells in the renal tubule (ascending loop of Henle) directly adjacent to the JG cells, forming the **juxtaglomerular apparatus**. Hypotension and increased sympathetic activity reduce the glomerular filtration rate, which reduces the amount of $Na^+Cl^-$ reaching the macula densa. This stimulates the macula densa, leading to RAAS activation. The resulting rise in aldosterone stimulates the distal tubules to reabsorb more $Na^+$ and water, to maintain extracellular fluid volume.
- **ANP** and angiotensin II both inhibit the secretion of renin. The natriuretic effect of ANP is partly due to RAAS inhibition.

## 14.9 NATRIURETIC PEPTIDES

Natriuretic peptides (NPs), as the name implies, stimulate renal salt excretion. They act as a counterweight to the salt-retaining RAAS, and have an antihypertensive action. Thus, the inactivation of NP receptors by gene-targeting in mice results in hypertension (see Chapter 18, Section 18.4). NPs come in three main forms: ANP, brain NP (BNP), which is also produced by some atrial and ventricular cells and C-type NP. ANP is the chief circulating form normally, but ventricular BNP secretion increases greatly in heart failure. ANP and BNP are secreted by specialized cardiac myocytes in response to high cardiac filling pressures, and their multiple actions help reduce plasma volume, return the filling pressure to normal and reduce arterial pressure. The actions are as follows:

- NPs cause a **moderate dilatation** of resistance vessels.
- NPs improve sympathovagal balance by increasing acetylcholine release and inhibiting NAd release from postganglionic autonomic nerve endings.

- NPs **increase renal salt and water excretion (natriuresis and diuresis)** through three mechanisms: (1) afferent arteriole dilatation raises the glomerular filtration rate; (2) Na$^+$ reabsorption in the proximal and distal tubules is inhibited; (3) renin and aldosterone secretion is inhibited.

- The lowering of plasma volume by NPs is greater than can be accounted for by the rather moderate diuresis. This is because NPs also cause **fluid transfer from the plasma to the interstitial compartment**. This is due partly to precapillary vasodilatation, which raises the capillary filtration pressure, and partly to an increase in venular permeability, up to twofold.

NPs bring about the above effects by binding to NP receptors on vascular myocytes, endothelium and tubular epithelium. The NP receptor is a transmembrane protein with guanylyl cyclase activity in its cytoplasmic section. Consequently, the activated receptor raises the intracellular cGMP level, which induces vasodilatation (Section 12.7) and venular hyperpermeability (Figure 11.30). ANP and BNP bind to the type A NP receptor, and CNP binds to the type B receptor. The type C receptor was thought to be a clearance receptor that binds all three NPs, but it has recently been shown to have biological activity linked to inhibitory G proteins (G$_i$) and a reduction in adenylyl cyclase activity.

Plasma ANP concentration is normally extremely low. Even when increased two- to fourfold, for example, by central venous pressure elevation during whole-body immersion in water, there is little consistent change in renal excretion. However, in heart failure circulating NP levels can increase 10- to 30-fold, and ventricle-derived BNP 200-fold. This probably helps to mitigate the accumulation of extracellular fluid in heart failure (Chapter 18). BNP can be used as a biochemical index of heart failure, and high levels correlate with a poor prognosis.

## 14.10 SPECIAL FEATURES OF VENOUS CONTROL

The venous system has been called 'the Cinderella of the circulation, because it is often neglected. However, the control of peripheral veins (capacitance vessels) is important, because peripheral venous tone regulates the distribution of blood between peripheral vessels and the thorax, and thereby **regulates cardiac filling pressure** and stroke volume.

### Differentiation of the venous system

The venous system has four distinctive compartments functionally (Figure 14.13). The **central, thoracic compartment**, consisting of the great veins, right heart and pulmonary vessels, is essentially passive. The central blood volume determines the cardiac filling pressure, which influences the stroke volume (Frank–Starling mechanism). The three **peripheral compartments** have differing characteristics as follows.

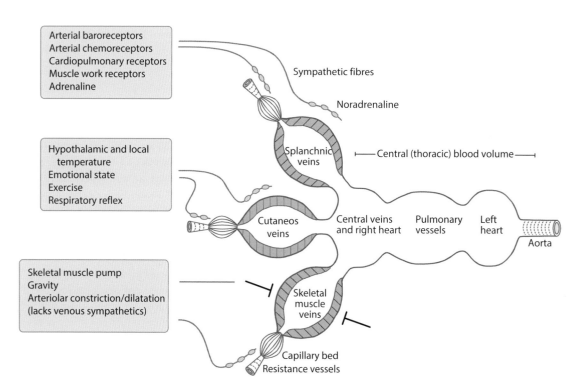

**Figure 14.13** Differentiation within the venous system. Changes in central blood volume and cardiac filling pressure are brought about by contraction of peripheral veins, especially splanchnic veins. The factors regulating the different venous beds are listed on the left.

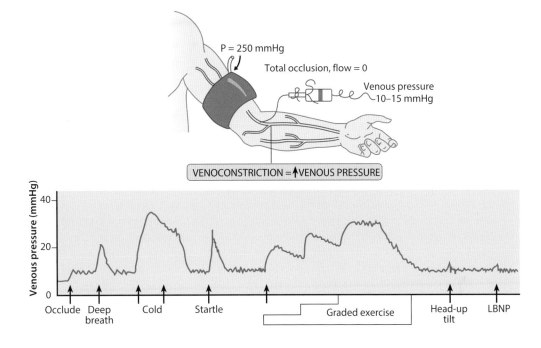

**Figure 14.14**
Sympathetic control of human cutaneous veins. Blood flow was arrested by a sphygmomanometer cuff. A rise in the pressure of station-ary blood trapped in the veins signals venoconstriction. LBNP, lower-body negative pressure. (After Rowell LB. *Human Circulation: Regulation during Physical Stress*. New York: Oxford University Press; 1986. With permis-sion from Oxford University Press.)

## Splanchnic veins

The veins of the gastrointestinal tract, liver and spleen contain ~20% of the total blood volume at rest. They are innervated by sympathetic constrictor nerves and express α adrenergic receptors. During exercise or hypotension, increases in sym-pathetic activity and adrenaline stimulate splanchnic vein contraction (Figure 14.5). This displaces blood into the cen-tral veins and helps to maintain the cardiac filling pressure at times of circulatory stress.

## Skeletal muscle veins

The veins inside skeletal muscles are poorly innervated. Their volume is influenced chiefly by the muscle pump and posture (gravity). Although direct sympathetic control of these veins is almost non-existent, their volume is nevertheless affected indirectly by sympathetic vasomotor activity, because arte-riolar constriction reduces venular pressure. This causes the venous system to recoil elastically and displace blood centrally (Figure 14.4, arrow a).

## Cutaneous veins

The veins of the skin are richly innervated by sympathetic nor-adrenergic fibres. High core temperatures reduce cutaneous sympathetic activity, leading to venodilatation and a flushed appearance. Conversely, during cold weather or clinical hypotension, cutaneous sympathetic activity increases, lead-ing to venoconstriction and blanching of the skin. Cutaneous sympathetic activity is also increased by emotional stress, deep inspiration and exercise (Figure 14.14).

## Comparison of venous and arteriolar control

Veins and resistance vessels respond in similar ways to many stimuli; in the skin, for example, both constrict during hypo-tension. However, there are also differences in behaviour, as follows:

- Most venules and veins have **little basal tone** in the absence of sympathetic activity (though the portal vein is actively contractile in many species).
- Veins generally show **little myogenic response** to stretch (though there are exceptions).
- Veins and arterioles may respond differently to agonists, due to differences in receptor expression. **Angiotensin II** for example, has little direct effect on veins but a powerful effect on arterioles. (However, angiotensin II contributes to the intense venoconstriction of patients in cardiac failure, acting indirectly by sympathetic potentiation.) **Glyceryl trinitrate** has a greater dilator effect on veins than on arterioles, and its efficacy in relieving angina is due partly to the reduction of cardiac filling pressure, and therefore cardiac work, following venodilatation.

## SUMMARY

- Vascular tone is regulated by a three-tier hierarchy of interacting controls. The lowest level of control is the Bayliss myogenic response, which provides autoregulation. The next level of control involves intrinsic (locally produced) vasoactive agents, for example, endothelial secretions, metabolic vasodilators, autacoids. The highest level of control is the **neuroendocrine system**, which brings the vasculature under central control for the benefit of the organism as a whole.

- **Sympathetic vasoconstrictor fibres** to the skin, muscle, kidney and gut are tonically active. Their terminal varicosities release NAd to activate $\alpha$ adrenergic receptors, which raise vascular tone. Sympathetic drive to resistance vessels is varied to stabilize arterial BP, regulate tissue perfusion and adjust fluid partitioning between plasma and the interstitium. Sympathetic drive to splanchnic and cutaneous veins is varied to maintain central blood volume and cardiac filling pressure. Sympathetic drive is regulated by bulbospinal fibres descending from the brainstem to the thoracic preganglionic neurons.

- **Parasympathetic vasodilator fibres** travel in the cranial and sacral outflows. The cranial outflow innervates the salivary glands, pancreas and gut, and evokes secretory hyperaemia. The sacral outflow innervates the genitalia (erectile tissue), bladder and colon. The main parasympathetic effectors are ACh, VIP and NO.

- **Nociceptive C-fibres** in the skin cause the spreading flare component of the Lewis triple response to trauma. This is an axon reflex, mediated by substance P, CGRP and mast cell histamine. C-fibres also mediate neurogenic inflammation.

- **Hormonal control** by adrenaline, angiotensin II and vasopressin supports BP, especially under stressful conditions such as hypovolaemic shock.

- **Adrenaline** is secreted by the adrenal medulla in response to exercise, the alerting response, hypotension and hypoglycaemia. Secretion is triggered by preganglionic sympathetic activity. Adrenaline promotes glucose release into the bloodstream, helps to raise cardiac output, causes $\beta$ adrenergic receptor-mediated vasodilatation in skeletal muscle and myocardium and $\alpha$ adrenergic receptor-mediated vasoconstriction in the skin, intestinal tract and other tissues.

- **Angiotensin II** is formed in the lungs by the action of endothelial ACE on angiotensin I. The latter is generated in renal plasma by the enzyme renin. Renin is secreted by renal JG cells in response to low BP, renal sympathetic activity and a low $Na^+Cl^-$ load. Angiotensin II stimulates aldosterone secretion and it causes vasoconstriction both directly and by enhancing sympathetic activity. Angiotensin II thus supports plasma volume and BP.

- **Vasopressin** (antidiuretic hormone) is produced by hypothalamic magnocellular neurons and is released from the posterior pituitary. Secretion is stimulated by hypertonicity (central osmoreceptors) and hypotension (cardiovascular receptors). The vasoconstrictor action supports BP during hypovolaemic shock.

- **Atrial natriuretic peptide** is secreted by the atria in response to distension. It reduces plasma volume by a mild diuretic action and by enhancing microvascular filtration through vasodilatation and increased permeability. Levels are high in heart failure.

## FURTHER READING

Burnstock G. Purinergic signalling in the cardiovascular system. *Circulation Research* 2017; **120**(1): 207–28.

Kuhn M. Molecular physiology of membrane guanylyl cyclase receptors. *Physiological Reviews* 2016; **96**(2): 751–804.

Shanks J, Herring N. Peripheral cardiac sympathetic hyperactivity in cardiovascular disease: role of neuropeptides. *American Journal of Physiology. Regulatory, Integrative and Comparative Physiology* 2013; **305**(12): R1411–20.

Potter LR. Natriuretic peptide metabolism, clearance and degradation. *FEBS Journal* 2011; **278**(11): 1808–17.

McDermott BJ, Bell D. NPY and cardiac diseases. *Current Topics in Medicinal Chemistry* 2007; **7**(17): 1692–703.

Holmes CL, Landry DW, Granton JT. Science Review: Vasopressin and the cardiovascular system part 2 – clinical physiology. *Critical Care* 2004; **8**(1): 15–23.

Huang A, Kaley G. Gender-specific regulation of cardiovascular function: estrogen as key player. *Microcirculation* 2004; **11**(1): 9–38.

Persson PB, Skalweit A, Thiele BJ. Controlling the release and production of renin. *Acta Physiologica Scandinavica* 2004; **181**(4): 375–81.

Wiers WG, Morgan KG. Alpha1-adrenergic signaling mechanisms in contraction of resistance arteries. *Reviews of Physiology, Biochemistry and Pharmacology* 2003; **150**: 91–139.

Simonsen U, García-Sacristán A, Prieto D. Penile arteries and erection. *Journal of Vascular Research* 2002; **39**(4): 283–303.

Mather K, Anderson TJ, Verma S. Insulin action in the vasculature: physiology and pathophysiology. *Journal of Vascular Research* 2001; **38**(5): 415–22.

Schmelz M, Petersen LJ. Neurogenic inflammation in human and rodent skin. *News in Physiological Sciences* 2001; **16**: 33–7.

Lehr HA. Microcirculatory dysfunction induced by cigarette smoking. *Microcirculation* 2000; **7**(6 Pt 1): 367–84.

Grassi G, Esler M. How to assess sympathetic activity in humans. *Journal of Hypertension* 1999; **17**(6): 719–34.

Fitzsimons JT. Angiotensin, thirst, and sodium appetite. *Physiological Reviews* 1998; **78**(3): 583–686.

Folkow B, Nilsson H. Transmitter release at adrenergic nerve endings: total exocytosis or fractional release? *News in Physiological Sciences* 1997; **12**(1): 32–6.

Monos E, Bérczi V, Nádasy G. Local control of veins: biomechanical, metabolic, and humoral aspects. *Physiological Reviews* 1995; **75**(3): 611–66.

Brock JA, Cunnane TC. Neurotransmitter release mechanisms at the sympathetic neuroeffector junction. *Experimental Physiology* 1993; **78**(5): 591–614.

Marshall JM. The venous vessels within skeletal muscle. *News in Physiological Sciences* 1991; **6**: 11–15.

Hainsworth R. The importance of vascular capacitance in cardiovascular control. *News in Physiological Sciences* 1990; **5**(6): 250–4.

Jänig W. Pre- and postganglionic vasoconstrictor neurons: differentiation, types, and discharge properties. *Annual Review of Physiology* 1988; **50**: 525–39.

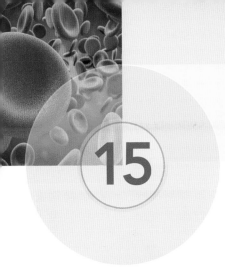

# Specialization in individual circulations

## LEARNING OBJECTIVES

*In this chapter, the learning objectives and summary are combined into a 'Key features' box after each section.*

Very many factors regulate vascular tone (Chapters 12–14). However, their relative importance varies from organ to organ, as explained in this chapter. $CO_2$, for example, is a major regulator of cerebral but not cutaneous blood flow. This chapter also explains how the different circulations exhibit specializations that underpin the function of a tissue. A major function of skin, for example, is to regulate body temperature, so its circulation exhibits specializations for heat exchange. The five special circulations described here – myocardium, skeletal muscle, skin, brain and lung – were chosen partly for their clinical importance and partly for their contrasting characteristics. The splanchnic circulation is described briefly under 'Feeding and digestion' in Section 17.5. The same unifying approach is adopted for each system as follows:

1. **Special tasks** imposed on the circulation by the tissue's functions are outlined first.
2. **Adaptations** that help the circulation accomplish its special tasks are considered under the headings 'Structural adaptation' and 'Functional adaptation'.
3. **Vascular problems** specific to the organ/tissue are described.
4. Finally, **techniques** for assessing each circulation are outlined.

## 15.1 CORONARY CIRCULATION

Coronary blood flow, resting human 70–80 mL/min/100 g

Coronary blood flow during heavy exercise (maximal cardiac work), 300–400 mL/min/100 g

The right and left coronary arteries arise from the aorta immediately above the aortic valve cusps, in dilatations called the sinuses of Valsalva (Figures 1.4, 1.6). Branches of the **left coronary artery** supply mainly the left ventricle and interventricular septum; the **right coronary artery** supplies mainly the right ventricle, although the distribution is variable (Figure 15.1).

The right coronary artery passes from the anterior aortic sinus in the atrioventricular (AV) groove to the inferior border of the heart. Seventy per cent of people have a **right dominant circulation**, where the posterior descending artery arises from the right coronary artery, whereas in 10%, this branch arises from the left circumflex artery (**left dominant circulation**). It is possible for both the right and left circumflex arteries to supply the posterior descending artery in a **co-dominant system** (20% of people). A branch of the right coronary artery supplies the AV node in 90% of people. The left main stem passes from the posterior aortic sinus and divides to give the left anterior descending artery and left circumflex artery. The left anterior descending artery supplies the septum (via septal branches), apex and anterior wall (via diagonal branches) of the left ventricle. The left circumflex artery supplies the lateral wall (via oblique marginal branches) and the inferior wall is supplied by either the left circumflex or right coronary artery depending on which artery is dominant.

About 95% of the coronary venous blood returns through the **coronary sinus**, which runs in the posterior AV groove and receives blood from the great cardiac vein (anteriorly), posterior lateral cardiac veins and middle cardiac vein (from the inferior interventricular groove) and then drains into the right atrium (Figure 1.4). Posterior lateral cardiac veins and branches of the middle cardiac vein are common sites for

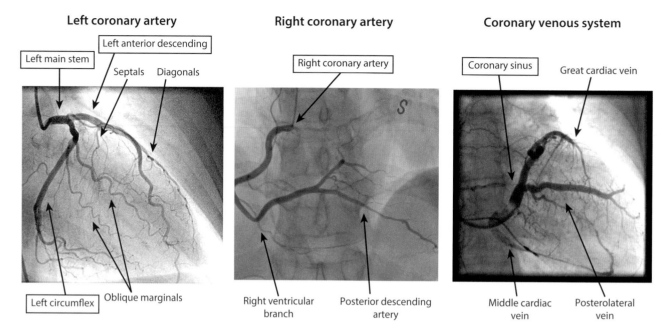

**Left coronary artery**

- Left main stem
- Left anterior descending
- Septals
- Diagonals
- Left circumflex
- Oblique marginals

**Right coronary artery**

- Right coronary artery
- Right ventricular branch
- Posterior descending artery

**Coronary venous system**

- Coronary sinus
- Great cardiac vein
- Middle cardiac vein
- Posterolateral vein

**Figure 15.1** Radiographic images taken during percutaneous coronary angiography. Catheter-based contrast injection demonstrates the left and right coronary arteries, the coronary venous system and their major branches. Note that the left circumflex artery runs in the atrio-ventricular groove around the back of the heart as viewed in this projection.

placement of left ventricular pacing leads of cardiac resynchronization pacemakers and defibrillators (see Chapter 18.5). The rest drains into the cardiac chambers through the anterior coronary and Thebesian veins. Some **Thebesian veins** drain into the left side of the heart, contributing to the slight deoxygenation of arterial blood (saturation ~97%). The coronary circulation is the shortest in the body, with a mean transit time of only 6–8 s in a resting human.

## Special tasks

- The coronary circulation must deliver $O_2$ at a high rate to match the basal myocardial demand (~8 mL $O_2$ $min^{-1}$ 100 $g^{-1}$ in a resting human), which is 20× that of resting skeletal muscle.
- During exercise, the coronary circulation must increase $O_2$ delivery to match the increase in cardiac work (≥5×); that is, coronary blood flow must be coupled to cardiac work.

## Structural adaptation

**Myocardial capillary density** is very high, roughly one capillary per myocyte (3000–5000 $mm^{-2}$ section; Figure 15.2). This creates a large endothelial surface area and reduces the maximum diffusion distance to ~9 μm (myocytes being 18 μm wide), thereby facilitating $O_2$ and nutrient transfer to the myocytes. **Myoglobin** (3.4 g/L) facilitates $O_2$ transport within the cardiac myocytes (Section 10.11). **Exercise training** increases coronary artery width and the number of arterioles and capillaries, to keep pace with the increase in ventricular mass.

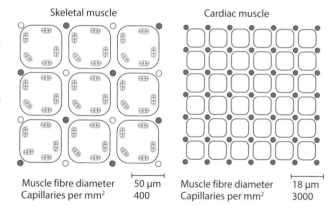

Skeletal muscle — Muscle fibre diameter 50 μm; Capillaries per $mm^2$ 400

Cardiac muscle — Muscle fibre diameter 18 μm; Capillaries per $mm^2$ 3000

**Figure 15.2** Capillary density (number/area) in skeletal and cardiac muscle, on the same scale. Each tissue has approximately one capillary (red circle) per muscle fibre; but myocardial fibres are smaller, so myocardial capillary density is greater and diffusion distance correspondingly shorter. Open circles in skeletal muscle are capillaries not (or poorly) perfused with blood at any given moment in resting muscle. (From Renkin EM. In: Marchetti G, Taccardi B, eds. *Coronary Circulation and Energetics of the Myocardium*. Basel: Karger; 1967. pp. 18–30.)

## Functional adaptations

### High basal flow and $O_2$ extraction

To satisfy the high metabolic demand, coronary blood flow per gram of tissue is about 10 times the whole-body average. Endothelium-dependent **nitric oxide** production helps maintain this high flow, since flow is reduced by 60% by nitric oxide synthase inhibitors. Despite the high flow, the myocardium must extract 65%–75% of the $O_2$ to meet its

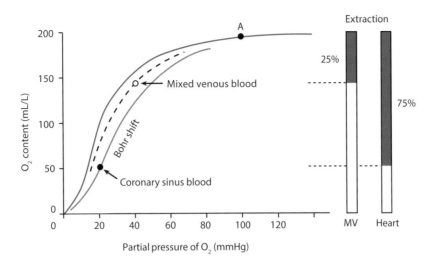

**Figure 15.3** $O_2$ dissociation curves of arterial blood ($P_{CO_2}$ 40 mmHg), mixed venous blood ($P_{CO_2}$ 46 mmHg) and coronary sinus blood ($P_{CO_2}$ 58 mmHg). $CO_2$ shifts the dissociation curve to the right (Bohr shift), which enhances myocardial $O_2$ unloading. A, arterial values. Mixed venous (MV) blood refers to resting human.

needs (cf. whole-body average 25% at rest). This reduces the blood $O_2$ content from 195 mL/L (arterial) to 50–70 mL/L (coronary sinus) (Figure 15.3). During heavy exercise, the extraction can rise to 90%. **Fatty acid** extraction is likewise high (40%–70%), but **glucose** extraction is usually low (2%–3%), showing that fatty acids are the preferred substrate of the myocardium.

## Metabolic hyperaemia is the dominant form of vascular regulation

The extra $O_2$ required at high cardiac work rates is supplied mainly by increases in coronary blood flow rather than extraction, because extraction is already high at basal work rates. The coupling between coronary blood flow and myocardial work is remarkable; flow increases almost linearly with cardiac $O_2$ consumption at light-to-moderate work rates (Figure 15.4), while at high work rates $O_2$ extraction also rises. This is a classic example of metabolic hyperaemia (Section 13.7).

The elegant coupling between supply and demand is achieved by the myocardium releasing vasodilator substances in proportion to its work rate. However, the nature of the vasodilators remains a well-sought but carefully guarded secret of nature. One contender is **adenosine**, generated by the breakdown of adenosine triphosphate (ATP) (Section 13.4). Adenosine binds to vascular $A_{2A}$ receptors, activating the $G_s$–adenylyl cyclase–cAMP vasodilator pathway (Figure 12.10). However, the effects of adenosine inhibitors on myocardial hyperaemia have proved variable, ranging from little to a ~50% reduction. Other factors, such as increases in $H_2O_2$ **production, interstitial** $K^+$ **and** $H^+$ also contribute to resistance vessel dilatation. Upstream dilatation of the coronary arteries is mediated by **NO**, produced by the shear-stimulated endothelium (Figure 13.9).

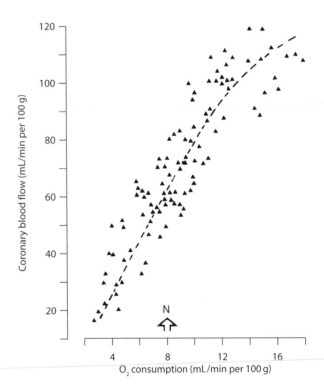

**Figure 15.4** Effect of cardiac work, as measured by myocardial $O_2$ consumption, on coronary blood flow in the dog. N, normal resting level. Cardiac work was altered by adrenaline or blood withdrawal. (From Berne RM, Rubio R. In: Berne RM, Sperekalis N, eds. *The Cardiovascular System. Vol. 1. The Heart*. Bethesda, MD: American Physiological Society; 1979. pp. 873–952. By permission.)

**Autoregulation** is also well developed in the coronary circulation (Figure 13.7). This stabilizes myocardial perfusion when blood pressure (BP) fluctuates, and can prevent underperfusion, down to ~50 mmHg. When myocardial work increases, the metabolic vasodilators **reset** autoregulation to operate at a higher flow.

## Sympathetic vasomotor activity maintains high vascular tone at rest

Sympathetic vasoconstrictor fibres innervate myocardial arteries and arterioles, and the tonic α adrenergic receptor activation contributes to coronary vascular tone and resistance. During exercise, cardiac sympathetic activity increases, and β₁ adrenergic receptor-mediated tachycardia and increased contractility raise the cardiac work rate. The latter elicits a metabolic vasodilatation, which overcomes the concomitant α adrenergic receptor-mediated vasoconstriction. Thus, sympathetic activity normally raises rather than reduces myocardial blood flow.

## Adrenaline causes coronary vasodilatation

Adrenaline (epinephrine) levels increase during the alerting response, exercise and hypovolaemia. This activates β₁ adrenergic receptors on cardiac myocytes, raising cardiac work, and activates β₂ adrenergic receptors on coronary vascular myocytes, causing vasodilatation (Figure 12.10). Adrenaline thus increases coronary blood flow. The increase can precede exercise (feed forward), before the more powerful metabolic hyperaemia is triggered.

## Ischaemic vasodilatation limits damage by coronary artery disease

Myocardial ischaemia elicits marked vasodilatation, due partly to the breakdown of ATP to adenosine, a powerful coronary vasodilator. Also, the fall in ATP/adenosine diphosphate (ADP) ratio activates $K_{ATP}$ channels in the vascular smooth muscle, leading to hyperpolarization and further vasodilatation (Table 12.2). Ischaemic vasodilatation, downstream from a coronary artery stenosis, helps to maintain the restig coronary flow in angina patients (Concept box 15.2). Also, ischaemic vasodilatation at the margins of an infarct helps to limit its extent.

## Special problems

### Systole obstructs coronary blood flow

About two-thirds of the coronary arterial system is intramural, that is, inside the myocardium. Intramural vessels are compressed during systole, especially during the isovolumetric contraction phase, when coronary BP is at its minimum (~80 mmHg) and stress within the left ventricle wall is maximal (~240 mmHg). At this point, coronary artery flow stops briefly or even reverses (Figure 15.5). Full flow is only restored in diastole. About **80% of coronary blood flow occurs during diastole** at basal heart rates, so coronary perfusion is driven chiefly by **diastolic BP**, not systolic pressure. The timing of the reflected pulse wave, by augmenting either diastolic or systolic pressure, affects the ratio of coronary perfusion to cardiac work (Figure 8.10). The beneficial effect of β blockers

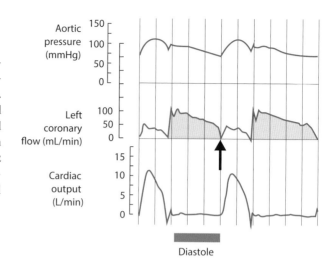

**Figure 15.5** Blood flow in the left coronary artery of conscious dog, recorded by electromagnetic flow meter. Note the sharp curtailment of flow at the onset of systole (arrow). Most coronary flow occurs during diastole (shaded area). Time lines 0.1 s. (After Khouris EM, Gregg DE, Rayford CR. *Circulation Research* 1965; 17(5): 427–37.)

in heart failure is partly due to the bradycardic lengthening of diastole, and hence the interval of good perfusion.

In **aortic valve stenosis**, the high resistance to ejection further increases the systolic stress within the left ventricle wall, especially during exercise. This exacerbates the systolic impairment of myocardial perfusion, leading to angina-like chest pain and collapse during exercise; see Clinical Case 1, 'Elderly man with a murmur'.

## Human coronary arteries are functional end arteries prone to atheroma

Coronary arteries are a common site for atheroma (atherosclerosis). Section 9.10 outlined the pathology of atheroma, Concept box 15.1 shows the risk factors, and Table 17.4 highlights the distinction from arteriosclerosis. Briefly, atheroma is a cholesterol-rich, subintimal plaque that narrows the coronary artery lumen, limiting blood flow and causing ischaemic pain (angina) during exercise. Atheroma may also trigger arterial thrombosis (the formation of an organized blood clot), which blocks a coronary artery and causes myocardial infarction.

The narrowing of even one branch of a coronary artery is serious because human coronary arteries are **functional end arteries**, that is, they have ineffective anastomoses. This is not so in all species; dogs have relatively good arterio-arterial anastomoses, and are less prone to myocardial infarction (Figure 15.6, upper panel). Although humans have some arterio-arterial anastomoses between distal branches of the coronary tree, they are only 20–350 μm wide and transmit relatively little flow. Consequently, an upstream obstruction reduces distal tissue perfusion to a few per cent of normal, causing myocardial ischaemia (Figure 15.6, lower panel).

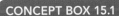

## CONCEPT BOX 15.1

### EPIDEMIOLOGY OF ISCHAEMIC HEART DISEASE

- The main modifiable risk factors for coronary atheroma are:
  - hypercholesterolaemia (high low-density lipoprotein);
  - hypertension;
  - smoking;
  - diabetes mellitus;
  - obesity and physical inactivity.
- Acute ischaemic incidents (infarction, arrhythmia) are around nine times more common during strenuous exercise than at rest. This is attributed to catecholamine-triggered arrhythmias, rupture of atheromatous plaques by mechanical stress and increased blood coagulability in exercise.
- Nevertheless, the risk of developing symptomatic ischaemic heart disease is about halved in fit compared with unfit humans. The benefits of regular, moderate dynamic exercise outweigh the risks.

**Arterio-arterial anastomoses**

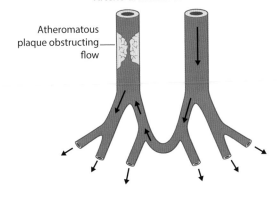

Atheromatous plaque obstructing flow

**End arteries, e.g. coronary arteries**

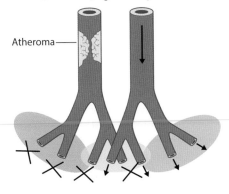

Atheroma

| Zone of necrosis (infarction) | Peripheral rim of partial ischaemia | Healthy normoxic tissue |

**Figure 15.6** Arterio-arterial anastomoses affect susceptibility to infarction following arterial obstruction. (**Lower panel**) Human, baboon, rabbit and pig coronary arteries are functional end-arteries. Acute ligation of a major vessel in the pig heart reduces perfusion to 0.6% in the downstream territory. (**Upper panel**) Dog coronary circulation has better arterio-arterial anastomoses. Acute ligation of a major canine coronary artery reduces myocardial perfusion less severely, to ~16%.

## Acute coronary obstruction by a thrombus causes myocardial infarction (a heart attack)

The sudden obstruction of an atheromatous coronary artery by plaque rupture and thrombosis is the most common cause of death in the West (see Section 9.10). The downstream zone of ischaemic myocardium is called a **myocardial infarct** (Figure 1.2). Here, the accumulation of interstitial $K^+$, $H^+$, adenosine and other factors stimulates nociceptors (Section 16.3). This causes a band of **crushing chest pain**, often radiating into the arms and neck. Contractility is impaired (Section 6.12), causing **acute cardiac failure**. **Sympathetic activity** increases due to the pain and clinical shock. **Arrhythmias** are common (Sections 3.11, 4.8 and 5.11). The pathophysiological changes are brought together in Figure 6.22. Residual coronary blood flow is often so low that myocytes begin to die after a few hours (**necrosis**). The region affected (e.g. anterior, lateral, inferior) depends on which branch of the coronary artery is obstructed. The subendocardium (inner tissue) is often affected more than the subepicardium, because systolic wall stress is greater in the subendocardium, curtailing subendocardial perfusion at low BPs.

**Diagnosis** is based on the characteristic history, electrocardiogram (ECG) changes (Figure 5.9), leakage of myocardial intracellular enzymes (particularly troponin) into the bloodstream (Section 6.14), as well as coronary angiography, echocardiography, cardiac magnetic resonance imaging and nuclear imaging. **Treatment** includes:

- supplementary $O_2$;
- morphine, to reduce the pain and the pro-arrhythmogenic sympathetic activity;
- low-dose aspirin, together with a second antiplatelet agent (such as clopidogrel, prasugrel or ticagrelor; see Section 9.11);
- percutaneous coronary intervention to reopen the occluded coronary artery with angioplasty and stenting. This is performed on an emergency basis with ST-elevation myocardial infarctions (see Section 5.9) and urgently for non-ST-elevation myocardial infarctions, unstable or crescendo angina;
- β adrenergic receptor blockers, to reduce cardiac work and the risk of subsequent arrhythmias;
- angiotensin-converting enzyme (ACE) inhibitors to reduce cardiac work;
- statins to lower blood lipids and stabilize plaques.

## Chronic coronary stenosis causes stable angina

Arteries normally offer negligible resistance to flow compared with arterioles. Even severe atheromatous stenosis of the artery, if it develops slowly, may have little effect on flow during rest, because the rise in proximal resistance is offset by a fall in distal resistance. This is brought about partly by **distal arteriogenesis** (proliferation and widening of small, distal arterial vessels under the influence of growth factors), and partly by **distal vasodilatation**, due to vasodilator metabolite accumulation (Section 13.4) and the myogenic response to the reduced distal pressure (Sections 13.2 and 13.6).

The above compensations often maintain an adequate perfusion at rest. However, during **exercise** the fixed resistance of the stenosed artery prevents flow from increasing sufficiently to meet the increase in myocardial $O_2$ demand. Even if the distal resistance vessels undergo maximal metabolic and ischaemic vasodilatation, the **proximal stenosis** now dominates the total resistance to flow; for a worked example, see Concept box 15.2. Therefore, exercise precipitates local myocardial ischaemia, leading to nociceptor activation and a crushing chest pain, reversible on rest, called angina pectoris. Correspondingly, the **exercise ECG test** shows acute ST-segment depression during exercise, resolved by rest (Figure 5.11a).

---

**CONCEPT BOX 15.2**

## EXERCISE-INDUCED ANGINA

- Resistances in series summate. If a healthy coronary artery has a resistance of 1 unit and coronary resistance vessels have a resistance of 19 units, the total resistance is 20 units.

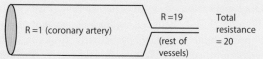

- During exercise, metabolic vasodilatation of the myocardial resistance vessels reduces their resistance, for example, to four units. Total resistance of the healthy coronary circulation is now five units. Myocardial blood flow increases fourfold (20/5), meeting the increased $O_2$ demand.

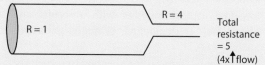

- Consider a severely stenosed coronary artery, of resistance 10 units, in a resting individual. Distal arteriogenesis and dilatation reduces the distal coronary resistance from 19 to, say, 10 units. Total resting vascular resistance is still 20 units, so **resting** flow is normal.

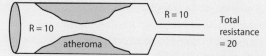

- When the patient **exercises**, the reserve dilatation of coronary resistance vessels reduces the distal resistance further, for example, to three units. But total resistance, 13 units, is now dominated by the stenosis. Myocardial blood flow increases only about one-and-a-half-fold (20/13). This fails to meet the increased $O_2$ demand, leading to ischaemia and angina during exercise.

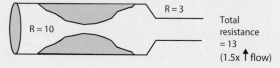

---

Other triggers for angina include mental stress and cold. **Mental stress** increases coronary sympathetic vasomotor activity, leading to the contraction of atheromatous coronary arteries. The resulting regional ischaemia causes angina. The **stress ECG test** shows a corresponding, reversible ST-segment depression. As the eminent anatomist John Hunter once remarked in relation to his own stress-induced angina, "My life is at the mercy of any rascal who chooses to annoy me"; Hunter indeed died during a stressful medical committee meeting. Severe **cold** can likewise trigger a reflex sympathetic constriction of ischaemic coronary vessels, triggering angina or exacerbating exercise-induced angina.

Different forms of angina are recognized. **Stable angina** is exercise-induced angina that is predictable for a given level of exercise. **Crescendo angina** is exercise-induced angina occurring at progressively lower levels of exertion. This usually leads to **unstable angina** occurring at rest with minimal increase in cardiac metabolic demand and is likely to progress to a myocardial infarction. **Variant angina** (Prinzmetal's angina) is relatively rare. It is caused by an episode of coronary artery **vasospasm**, that is, intense, prolonged contraction of the artery. Vasospasm usually occurs downstream of an atheromatous plaque that is not flow-limiting, due to the release of serotonin (5-hydroxytryptamine, 5HT) and thromboxane from atheroma-activated platelets. Thus, variant angina is precipitated by reduced myocardial $O_2$ supply, whereas exercise-induced angina is precipitated by increased myocardial $O_2$ demand. Variant angina is usually treated with vasodilators such as dihydropyridine $Ca^{2+}$ channel blockers.

Another rare cause of extreme coronary artery vasoconstriction arises from conditions associated with sudden and excessive adrenergic drive, such as severe emotional trauma (stress-related cardiomyopathy/broken heart syndrome), phaeochromocytoma, subarachnoid haemorrhage or overdose with drugs such as amphetamines or cocaine. The dramatic surge in plasma catecholamines is thought to result in direct myocyte stunning and toxicity combined with small vessel vasoconstriction, which leads to a deterioration in cardiac contractile ability and potentially cardiogenic shock. An unusual pattern of contractile dysfunction in the heart often occurs where the left ventricular base contracts while the apex balloons. This phenomenon is called **Takotsubo cardiomyopathy**, named after a Japanese ceramic 'octopus trap' whose shape resembles that of the left ventricle (see Figure 15.7). The pattern of wall motion abnormalities seen may be related to the distribution of adrenergic receptors in the myocardium and vasculature.

**Treatment of stable angina** is based on physiological principles. The following pharmacological and surgical therapies are available:

- **Glyceryl trinitrate** (GTN) dilates systemic veins and conduit arteries, but not the stenosed artery. It has relatively little effect on arterioles and peripheral resistance. The venodilatation reduces cardiac filling pressure (preload). Conduit artery relaxation reduces the pulse wave velocity, which delays the wave reflection and thereby reduces systolic pressure (afterload) (Figure 8.10). The fall in preload and afterload reduces cardiac work and therefore $O_2$ demand. Nitrodilators may also dilate coronary collateral vessels that bypass the stenosis. GTN can be used as a sublingual spray or tablet for the acute relief of angina pain.

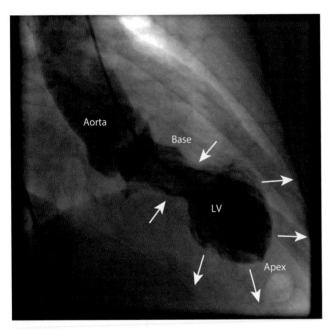

**Figure 15.7** Takotsubo cardiomyopathy. Still image of a left ventriculogram in the right anterior oblique view taken at peak contraction demonstrating apical ballooning. This was accompanied by posterolateral segment akinesis in the left anterior oblique view. The white arrows demonstrate the movement of the walls of the left ventricle (LV) moving inwards at the base but outwards (ballooning) at the apex.

- **Low-dose aspirin** reduces platelet aggregation and is taken as a prophylaxis against progression to thrombosis.
- **Predisposing factors** (Concept box 15.1) should be treated, for example, **statins** to reduce hypercholesterolaemia, stopping smoking and controlling BP and diabetes mellitus.
- **Antianginal medications** are listed in Table 15.1. These include medications that vasodilate (such as long-acting nitrates, $K^+$ channel openers and dihydropyridine $Ca^{2+}$ channel blockers) and medications aimed at lowering heart rate or reducing cardiac metabolic demand (such as β blockers, hyperpolarization-activated cyclic nucleotide-gated (HCN) channel blockers, non-dihydropyridine $Ca^{2+}$ channel blockers and $Na^+$ channel blockers). These are often used in combination.
- **Percutaneous coronary intervention** (PCI) involves dilatation of a localized coronary stenosis by coronary catheterization followed by angioplasty with a balloon. A small expandable tube, or **coronary stent**, is then inserted to maintain patency. Stents can be made of 'bare-metal' or they can be 'drug-eluting', that is, impregnated with an anti-proliferative drug (such as sirolimus (rapamycin) or paclitaxel) to prevent subsequent smooth muscle proliferation and restenosis from occurring. Treatment with aspirin and another antiplatelet drug is required until the stent becomes endothelialized to prevent thrombosis occurring on the stent. This is usually for 1 month for a bare-metal stent, and 1 year for a drug-eluting stent because the endothelialization process is slowed due to anti-proliferative medication. Clinical trials have shown that PCI is more effective than antianginal drugs at treating

**Table 15.1** Medications used as antianginals

| Drug class | Example (trial name) | Mechanism of action | Side effects |
|---|---|---|---|
| Nitrates | Short-acting: GTN Long-acting: isosorbide mononitrate | Coronary and systemic vasodilatation and venodilatation via release of nitric oxide | Hypotension, headaches |
| $K^+$ channel opener | Nicorandil (IONA) | Nitrodilator and vascular smooth muscle $K^+$ channel opener causing coronary and systemic vasodilatation | Hypotension, headaches, mouth and perianal ulcers |
| Dihydropyridine $Ca^{2+}$ channel blockers | Amlodipine | Coronary and systemic vasodilatation | Hypotension, ankle swelling, constipation |
| Non-dihydropyridine $Ca^{2+}$ channel blockers | Diltiazem Verapamil | Reduction in heart rate and cardiac metabolic demand | Bradycardia, hypotension |
| β blockers | Atenolol Bisoprolol | Reduction in heart rate and cardiac metabolic demand | Bronchospasm, bradycardia, hypotension, depression, type II diabetes, Raynaud's syndrome, erectile dysfunction |
| HCN channel blocker | Ivabradine (BEAUTIFUL) | Inhibition of the pacemaking current $I_f$ to reduce heart rate | Bradycardia, AV block, visual disturbances |
| $Na^+$ channel blocker | Ranolazine (MERLIN-TIMI 36) | $Na^+$ channel blocker reduces myocardial $O_2$ demand | Bradycardia, hypotension, constipation |

*Note:* AV, atrioventricular; BEAUTIFUL, Ivabradine for patients with stable coronary artery disease and left-ventricular systolic dysfunction; GTN, glyceryl trinitrate; HCN, hyperpolarization-activated cyclic nucleotide-gated; IONA, Impact Of Nicorandil in Angina; MERLIN-TIMI 36, Metabolic Efficiency with Ranolazine for Less Ischemia in Non-ST Elevation Acute Coronary Syndromes.

**THE CORONARY CIRCULATION**

**Special tasks**

- Maintain a high basal rate of $O_2$ supply
- Increase the $O_2$ supply in proportion to the cardiac work rate

**Functional adaptations**

- High $O_2$ extraction (>60% at rest)
- Metabolic vasodilatation dominates regulation
- Good autoregulation
- Vascular $\beta_2$ adrenergic receptors, so adrenaline causes vasodilatation

**Special problems**

- Flow during systole is obstructed by systolic wall stress; it is aggravated by aortic stenosis
- Functional end arteries in man, so thrombosis → infarction (heart attack)
- Chronic stenosis by atheroma → exercise-induced angina
- Sympathetic vasoconstrictor activity plus atheroma → stress-induced angina
- Coronary artery vasospasm downstream of atheroma → variant (resting) angina

**Assessment in man**

- Coronary angiography locates the stenosed segment(s)
- Coronary sinus thermal dilution method measures absolute flow
- Isotope imaging shows distribution of perfusion
- Exercise/stress ECG assesses latent ischaemia (ST depression during test)

the symptoms of chronic stable angina, but does not improve mortality rates.

- **Coronary artery bypass grafting** is the treatment of choice when stenoses occur proximally in multiple coronary arteries or the left main stem. During open heart surgery, a stenosed length of artery is bypassed from the ascending aorta with a segment of saphenous vein or radial artery, or an internal mammary artery (typically on the left) is dissected and rerouted beyond the coronary artery stenosis.

## Assessment of human coronary circulation

**Coronary sinus thermodilution** measures coronary blood flow quantitatively, as described in Chapter 7 (Section 7.2). **Coronary angiography** is used to locate atheromatous obstructions, often as a guide to vascular surgery. The artery is perfused with a radio-opaque contrast medium, which is imaged by X-ray (see Figure 15.1). **Cardiac computed tomography** (CT) images the dense calcification associated with atheroma, and is highly predictive of future ischaemic heart disease (Figure 2.12). **Gamma scans** (nuclear imaging) assess the distribution of myocardial perfusion (Figure 2.11). A gamma-emitting isotope such as thallium or technetium is infused into the circulation and its appearance in myocardium is imaged by a gamma-camera at rest and following exercise. Due to the similarity to $K^+$, thallium and technetium are

pumped into the myocytes by the $Na^+/K^+$ pump. Regions with inadequate perfusion are revealed by patches of defective uptake. Coronary perfusion can also be assessed using cardiac magnetic resonance imaging (Figure 2.10), as described in Chapter 2 (Section 2.6).

## 15.2 SKELETAL MUSCLE CIRCULATION

Flow, rest, postural (tonic) muscle, 15 mL/min/100 g

Flow, rest, phasic muscle, 3–5 mL/min/100 g

Maximum flow, phasic exercise, sedentary person, 250 mL/min/100 g

Maximum flow, phasic exercise, endurance athlete, 400 mL/min/100 g

The skeletal muscle and coronary circulations have much in common, notably the important role of metabolic hyperaemia in each; however, there are also important differences, such as the major contribution of the skeletal muscle circulation to the reflex regulation of BP.

## Special tasks

- During exercise, the muscle circulation must increase the $O_2$ and glucose delivery to match the increase in work, that is, blood flow must be coupled to exercise intensity.
- Since skeletal muscle constitutes ~40% of the body mass, its vascular resistance has a major effect on total peripheral resistance, and must help regulate arterial BP.

## Structural adaptations

Muscle capillary density is adapted to the muscle's function. **Postural muscles** (e.g. soleus) tend to be continuously active, with tonically active, slow oxidative (red) fibres, so they have a higher capillary density than phasic muscles. **Phasic muscles** (e.g. forearm, gastrocnemius) consist chiefly of fast, glycolytic white fibres. **Endurance training** stimulates capillary angiogenesis via growth factors. The number of capillaries per muscle fibre increases in proportion to the mitochondria per fibre. The arterial vessels likewise adapt to conduct a staggering maximal blood flow of 400 mL/min/100 g in endurance-trained muscles.

## Functional adaptations

### Vascular tone is high at rest

Vascular tone is a prerequisite for dilatation, since dilatation is simply a loss of tone. The high tone of the resistance vessels in resting muscle is evident from the 50- to 100-fold increase in vascular conductance in active muscle. The basal tone is mainly non-neural in origin, since sympathetic denervation merely doubles vascular conductance.

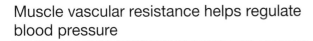

## Muscle vascular resistance helps regulate blood pressure

The arterial vessels of human muscle are richly innervated by tonically active, sympathetic vasoconstrictor fibres. Proximal vessels (feed arteries to first-order arterioles) express predominantly $\alpha_1$ adrenergic receptors, while the more distal second- and third-order arterioles express $\alpha_2$ adrenergic receptors. **Muscle sympathetic activity** is regulated by a reflex from **baroreceptors** that sense BP (Chapter 16); the baroreflex raises sympathetic activity when BP falls (e.g. orthostasis, hypovolaemia). Sympathetic activity reaches its maximum after a severe haemorrhage (mean: 6–10 impulses/s). The attendant rise in vascular resistance reduces muscle blood flow to about one fifth of normal and helps maintain the arterial blood pressure.

During **exercise** the resistance vessels dilate, but tonic sympathetic vasoconstrictor activity continues to modulate the tone of the $\alpha_1$ adrenergic receptor-rich feed arteries and proximal resistance vessels, guided by the baroreflex. This prevents an excessive fall in total peripheral resistance; unrestrained vasodilatation in a large mass of intensively used muscle (e.g. cross-country skiing) would otherwise cause arterial hypotension. The dilated terminal arterioles, with $\alpha_2$ receptors, become unresponsive to sympathetic activity during exercise hyperaemia (**functional sympatholysis**).

## Metabolic vasodilatation increases blood flow in active muscle

Muscle blood flow begins to increase within ~1 s of starting exercise and reaches a sustained level in ~40 s (Figure 13.8). In phasic muscle, the increase can reach 50-fold and account for 80%–90% of the cardiac output (cf. 18% at rest). Indeed, if all the muscles of the body dilated maximally at the same time, demand would exceed the heart's output capacity. The hyperaemia is due almost entirely to the fall in muscle vascular resistance, not the small rise in arterial pressure associated with exercise. The sustained phase is brought about by **metabolic vasodilatation** of the resistance vessels, accompanied by a permissive **ascending dilatation** of feed arteries and **flow-induced dilatation** of conduit arteries (Figure 13.9). The rapid initial phase is due partly to the venous muscle pump and partly to the myogenic response to compression, while by 4 s the $K^+$ ions released by the contracting muscle begin to contribute.

As in the myocardium, $O_2$ supply is tightly coupled to demand; blood flow increases in almost direct proportion to muscle metabolic rate. The identity of the metabolic vasodilators remains controversial. Over the first few minutes, muscle $K^+$ efflux during action potential repolarization raises the local **interstitial $[K^+]$** in proportion to exercise intensity. Interstitial $[K^+]$ can reach 11 mM in exhausting exercise, sufficient to produce near maximal vasodilatation in some muscles. This, along with increases in interstitial **osmolarity** (by 20–30 mOsm), **inorganic phosphate**, **adenosine** and **acid** (released by contracting muscle), probably accounts for much of the early hyperaemia. NO and prostaglandins also make a moderate contribution.

As exercise continues, the elevated interstitial $K^+$ and osmolarity decay, though not to basal levels, so other factors must sustain the vasodilatation. Interstitial **adenosine** concentration increases in proportion to exercise intensity, and some studies using blockers indicate that adenosine accounts for up to 40% of the sustained vasodilatation. Mitochondrial production of the vasodilator $H_2O_2$ likewise increases as $O_2$ consumption increases.

The skeletal muscle circulation has two further special adaptations, namely $\beta_2$ adrenergic receptor-mediated vasodilatation to **adrenaline** (Section 14.6) and, in non-primates only, sympathetic cholinergic activation during the alerting response (Section 14.3).

## Capillary recruitment improves solute exchange in active muscle

In resting muscle, the terminal arterioles contract intermittently and asynchronously (vasomotion). As a result, only a half to a third of muscle capillaries is well perfused at any one instant (Figure 15.2, left). During metabolic hyperaemia, arteriolar dilatation increases the fraction of capillaries that is well perfused with blood (capillary recruitment, Figure 10.14). This raises the effective **surface area** for gas exchange and shortens the extravascular **diffusion distance**.

## $O_2$ extraction rises. $O_2$ debt and lactate accumulate

The diffusion gradient in resting muscle (arterial $P_{O_2}$ 100 mmHg; intracellular $P_{O_2}$ ~20 mmHg) drives the extraction of 25%–30% of the $O_2$ from the perfusing blood. During exercise, muscle intracellular $P_{O_2}$ falls, so $O_2$ extraction increases, and can reach 80%–90% (Figure 10.16). In severe exercise, the intracellular $P_{O_2}$ falls so low that the muscle fibre switches to anaerobic glycolysis, generating **lactic acid**. Interstitial lactic acid helps stimulate muscle metaboreceptors, which drive the exercise pressor reflex (Section 16.6). Plasma lactate rises from 0.5 mM at rest (plasma pH 7.4) to ≤20 mM in extreme exercise (pH 6.9). The amount of lactate formed is a biochemical index of the deficit in muscle $O_2$ supply – the '$O_2$ debt' – which can reach several litres. When the exercise terminates, blood flow remains raised for several minutes (Figures 13.8 and 13.11). This **post-exercise hyperaemia** resupplies the muscle with $O_2$ and washes out the accumulated lactic acid. The circulating lactate is taken up by the heart as a primary substrate, and by the liver for resynthesis into glycogen.

## The venous muscle pump enhances perfusion during rhythmic exercise

Exercise hyperaemia is due primarily to a rise in vascular conductance, but perfusion is also enhanced modestly

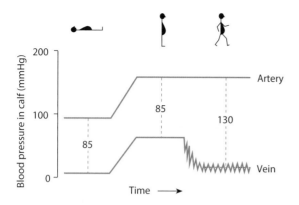

**Figure 15.8** Effect of posture and muscle pump on absolute pressures and on the difference in pressure driving blood through the calf.

in rhythmic exercise by the intermittent compression of deep veins, particularly in the calf. In a stationary, standing adult, gravity raises the arterial and venous pressures in the calf equally, by ~70 mmHg, to 165 mmHg and 80 mmHg, respectively (Figure 15.8). The pressure difference driving blood through the resting calf muscle is therefore (165 − 80) = 85 mmHg. During walking, running or cycling, the calf muscle pump reduces the venous pressure to ~35 mmHg (Figure 8.27), which increases the pressure difference to 130 mmHg, a 50% rise. This contributes to the immediate onset of exercise hyperaemia over a time interval that is too brief to invoke metabolic vasodilators (Figure 13.8).

## Special problems

### Muscle contraction compresses intramuscle blood vessels

When a muscle contracts at >30%–70% maximum force, the internal stress compresses the intramuscle vessels. Consequently, perfusion oscillates during rhythmic exercise (Figure 13.8). During a sustained contraction, perfusion is markedly impaired. The $O_2$ stored as oxymyoglobin is only sufficient for 5–10 s of muscle contraction, so the muscle quickly becomes hypoxic and switches to anaerobic glycolysis, producing lactate. This leads to rapid fatigue, a scenario familiar to anyone who has carried a heavy suitcase any distance.

### Active muscle swells, due to increased capillary filtration

Increased fluid translocation across the capillary bed of an exercising muscle causes the muscle to swell, creating the 'pumped' muscle of intense exercise. The forces responsible are described in Section 11.9. During whole-body exercise, the fluid translocation into active muscle can reduce the plasma volume by 10%–15%.

---

**KEY FEATURES BOX 15.2**

### THE SKELETAL MUSCLE CIRCULATION

**Special tasks**

- Deliver $O_2$ and nutrients in proportion to the muscle work rate
- Help regulate arterial BP, muscle being 40% of body mass

**Structural adaptations**

- High capillary density, especially in postural muscles

**Functional adaptations**

- Metabolic vasodilatation couples flow to exercise intensity
- Vasodilatation to adrenaline during stress
- Capillary recruitment boosts solute transfer during exercise
- Skeletal muscle pump boosts the local pressure gradient driving flow
- Fractional $O_2$ extraction increases with exercise intensity
- Sympathetically mediated participation in the baroreflex

**Special problems**

- Flow is mechanically impaired, especially during isometric contraction
- Increased capillary filtration causes swollen, 'pumped' muscle in severe exercise
- Ischaemia due to leg artery atheroma causes intermittent claudication, ulcers, gangrene

**Assessment in man**

- Venous occlusion plethysmography measures limb blood flow
- Doppler velocity meter and ankle–brachial pressure index (ABPI) assess vessel patency clinically
- Kety's isotope clearance method measures local capillary perfusion

### Intermittent claudication is due to ischaemic leg artery disease

The major arteries of the leg are common sites for atheroma, particularly in diabetic patients and smokers, leading to chronic stenosis. Similar arguments apply as in Concept box 15.2 (heart). At first, ischaemic leg pain occurs only on walking, and is relieved by rest (intermittent claudication). Severe cases progress to chronic pain at rest, **arterial ulcers** and **gangrene**, at which point amputation becomes necessary.

### Measurement of human muscle perfusion

The soft tissue of a human limb consists mainly of skeletal muscle. Limb blood flow can be measured by **venous occlusion plethysmography** (Figures 8.5 and 13.11) or **Doppler velocimetry** of the principal artery (Figure 13.8). The **ABPI** assesses artery patency (Section 8.5). The local capillary perfusion rate can be estimated with the **Kety's radioisotope clearance method** (Figure 8.6).

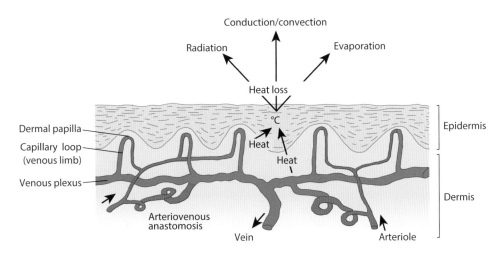

**Figure 15.9** Dermal vascular arrangement and heat flux in a human extremity (e.g. fingers, earlobe [acral skin]). Non-acral skin of limbs and trunk lacks arteriovenous anastomoses. Red cell volume and oxygenation in the subpapillary venous plexus influence skin colour.

## 15.3 CUTANEOUS CIRCULATION

> Blood flow, thermoneutral (27 °C), 10–20 mL/min/100 g
>
> Minimal blood flow, 1 mL/min/100 g
>
> Maximum blood flow, 150–200 mL/min/100 g

The skin is the organ of temperature regulation in humans, with a blood flow that can change >100-fold. The adult skin surface area is ~1.8 m², weight 2–3 kg and thickness 1–2 mm (epidermis plus dermis). The epidermis is avascular, but the dermis is well vascularized (Figure 15.9). Unlike the muscle and myocardium, the skin has a relatively constant, low metabolic rate, so its $O_2$ needs are satisfied by a low blood flow, aided by the direct diffusion of $O_2$ into the superficial ~100 μm epidermis. Temperature, not metabolic rate, is the principal factor regulating skin blood flow.

## Special tasks

### Cutaneous blood flow must regulate core temperature

The temperature of the human core (brain, thorax, abdominal organs) is held constant at 37.0 °C–37.5 °C by adjusting cutaneous heat loss to match core heat production. The main heat-dissipating surface is the skin in humans, and the tongue in many furry mammals. In a thermoneutral environment, namely 27 °C–28 °C for a naked human, the skin temperature is ~33 °C. Heat is dissipated by three processes: radiation, conduction/convection and evaporation (Figure 15.9):

- The rate of heat loss by **radiation** is proportional to the difference between ambient temperature and skin temperature. The latter depends on the rate at which cutaneous blood flow delivers heat.

- During **conduction/convection**, warm skin heats up the adjacent air by conduction, and the warmed air is removed by convection (air currents). Conductive heat loss increases with skin temperature, so this form of heat loss is again dependent on cutaneous blood flow.
- The **evaporation of sweat** consumes 2.4 kJ heat energy per gram (latent heat of evaporation), and both water and heat are delivered to the skin by the bloodstream.

Cutaneous blood flow is thus the key factor regulating heat loss by all three physical processes. The skin itself is **poikilothermic**, not homeothermic; its temperature varies widely, with extremes of 0 °C and 45 °C possible for short periods without causing tissue damage.

### Cutaneous vessels must participate in the defence against the environment

The other major role of skin is to provide a defence against the environment. The vasculature contributes to this through the Lewis triple response to trauma.

In addition, emotion-related changes in human skin colour contribute to **non-verbal communication**.

## Structural adaptations

### Arteriovenous anastomoses abound in the extremities

**Acral** or glabrous skin is specialized skin with numerous direct connections between dermal arterioles and venules, called arteriovenous anastomoses (AVAs) (Figure 15.9). AVAs are coiled, muscular-walled vessels, ~35 μm wide, discovered originally in the rabbit ear by RT Grant in 1930. In humans, they occur in exposed regions with a high surface area/volume ratio (fingers, toes, palm and sole, lips, nose, ear pinna). AVAs have little basal tone and are controlled almost exclusively by sympathetic vasoconstrictor fibres, whose activity is influenced by the **hypothalamic temperature-regulating centre**. AVAs also respond directly to ambient temperature, being dilated by heat and constricted by cold.

In a thermoneutral environment, the sympathetic drive to acral skin is high, so the AVAs are contracted and conduct little blood. By contrast, basal sympathetic drive to the skin of the limbs and trunk is low. Thus, sympathectomy or a local nerve block causes greater cutaneous hyperaemia in the extremities than proximally. When the core temperature exceeds 37.5 °C, the hypothalamus reduces the vasoconstrictor drive to the AVAs, allowing them to dilate. This creates a low-resistance shunt into the dermal venous plexus, raising the cutaneous blood flow and heat delivery (Figure 15.9). Since heat readily crosses the vein wall, skin temperature rises, and heat loss increases. Conversely, under cold conditions the AVAs are constricted to conserve heat. It is worth reiterating that the **dilatation** of AVAs **increases heat loss**, since the contrary is still taught in some school biology textbooks. The following aide-memoire might well have been sung by the mud-loving hippopotamus in Flanders and Swan's famous comic song:

> *A – V – A's, let 'em flood,*
> *There's nothing quite like them*
> *For cooling the blood.*
> *So dilate them widely,*
> *Let's lose heat right blithely –*
> *But close them up tightly*
> *When chill is the mud.*

### Venous-arterial countercurrent exchanger in the limbs conserves heat

The flippers of whales and the feet of wading birds possess an elaborate countercurrent heat-conserving mechanism. The cooled blood returning from the cold extremity drains into deep veins that ramify around the main artery. Heat passes from the warm arterial blood into the cool venous blood, so the extremity receives pre-cooled arterial blood, which reduces heat loss to the environment. This also occurs in human limbs to a minor degree.

## Functional adaptations

Cutaneous blood flow is affected by both **ambient** and **core** temperature.

### Cutaneous vascular tone is inversely related to ambient temperature

Cutaneous arterioles, venules and small veins dilate in response to local warming and contract in response to cooling, down to 10 °C–15 °C (Figure 15.10a). **Skin colour** is affected by the volume and $O_2$ content of blood in the dermal venous plexus, so warmth causes flushing (increased flow of well-oxygenated blood into the dilated venular plexus) and cold causes pallor. Warmth-induced vasodilatation promotes heat loss, while cold-induced vasoconstriction promotes heat conservation, thereby

contributing to core temperature homeostasis. The mechanisms mediating the local heat and cold responses differ, as follows.

**Heat-induced vasodilatation** is due in part to increased eNOS activity. Also, at >30 °C, sensory C-fibres release substance P and calcitonin gene-related peptide (CGRP) (Figure 14.9). Consequently, heat-induced flushing is blocked by local anaesthesia.

**Cold-induced vasoconstriction** is greatly attenuated by $\alpha_2$ adrenergic receptor blockers (yohimbine, rauwolscine) and by sympathetic inhibition, showing that it depends on tonic sympathetic activity and $\alpha_2$ **adrenergic receptors**, which are expressed by cutaneous vascular myocytes. Cold induces the insertion of more $\alpha_2$ adrenergic receptors from the myocyte Golgi apparatus into the plasma membrane, raising the apparent affinity for the sympathetic transmitter noradrenaline (NAd). Also, eNOS activity declines. These changes lead to cold-induced vasoconstriction.

The immersion of one hand in cold water elicits a small contralateral **reflex vasoconstriction** in the opposite hand. This is due partly to a spinal sympathetic reflex and partly to cooled blood affecting the hypothalamic temperature sensors. **Facial cold** causes a peripheral vasoconstriction and a rise in systolic pressure, due partly to increased wave reflection. This can aggravate angina and may contribute to the well-documented rise in heart attacks and deaths in cold weather.

### Severe ambient cold causes paradoxical cold vasodilatation

When a hand is placed in water at 10 °C or lower, the initial cold-induced vasoconstriction gives way to dilatation after 5–10 min (paradoxical cold vasodilatation), with flushing and pain relief (Figure 15.10c). This occurs in regions rich in AVAs, and contributes to the cold, red noses and hands seen in frosty weather. The phenomenon is attributed to the paralysis of noradrenergic neurotransmission by the cold and the release of vasodilators such as prostacyclin. Cold-induced vasodilatation is well developed in Arctic people (Inuit) and Norwegian fishermen, and helps prevent skin damage during prolonged cold exposure. If the exposure persists, vasoconstriction recurs after a while. During prolonged exposure, the skin oscillates between periods of vasoconstriction and vasodilatation at 15–20 min intervals. This is called the **hunting reaction** and is an adaptive response to cold that was discovered by Thomas Lewis in the 1930s. However, activating the hunting response with ice can be detrimental when treating sports injuries that involve muscle tears. Prolonged ice compressions (>10 min) will cause dilatation, exacerbate internal bleeding and promote haematoma.

### Core temperature strongly influences cutaneous sympathetic vasomotor activity

A rise in core temperature (e.g. during exercise) is sensed by **warmth receptors** in the anterior hypothalamus, which project to pre-sympathetic neurons in the brainstem. These evoke changes in the sympathetic vasomotor and sudomotor

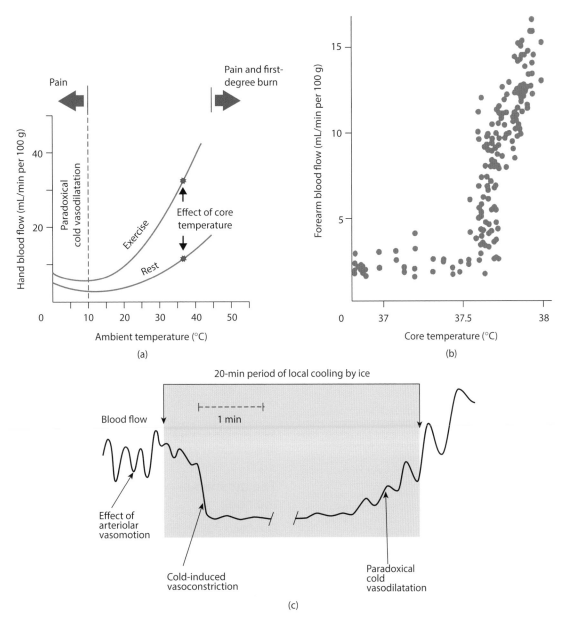

**Figure 15.10** Effect of external (ambient) temperature and internal (core) temperature on skin blood flow. **(a)** Response of immersed hand to water temperature, when internal heat load is low (rest) or high (exercise). Note the paradoxical cold vasodilatation at <10 °C. **(b)** Response of forearm blood flow, measured by plethysmography, to rise in core temperature induced by leg exercise. The hyperaemia is due to cutaneous vasodilatation; flow in the forearm muscles actually fell (xenon clearance method). **(c)** Cold-induced vasoconstriction in human calf skin recorded by laser Doppler fluxmeter, changing to paradoxical cold vasodilatation after 10–20 min. The oscillation in arteriolar tone at normal temperature is an example of vasomotion. (a: After Greenfield ADM. In: Hamilton WF, Dow P, eds. *Handbook of Physiology. Section 2. Circulation. Vol. III*. Bethesda, MD: American Physiological Society; 1963. pp. 1325–52; b: From Johnson JM, Rowell LB. *Journal of Applied Physiology* 1975; 39(6): 920–4, with permission of the American Physiological Society; c: Based on Van den Brande P, De Coninck A, Lievens P. *International Journal of Microcirculation* 1997; 17(2): 55–60.)

drive to the skin, resulting in cutaneous vasodilatation and sweating (Figures 15.10b and 15.11). The 'thermosensitive' sympathetic pathway (responsive also to emotion) is mediated by different neurons to the 'barosensitive' sympathetic pathway regulating BP (Chapter 16); cutaneous arterioles have a relatively sparse innervation by the latter. In **acral skin**, the thermoregulatory vasodilatation is brought about mainly by **reduced sympathetic vasoconstrictor** drive to the AVAs. In **non-acral skin** (limbs, trunk, scalp), the dilatation is closely associated with sweating and is due mainly

to **increased sympathetic cholinergic vasodilator activity**, being inhibited by local nerve block (Figure 15.11) or botulinum toxin, an inhibitor of cholinergic vesicle release. Pharmacological inhibitor studies indicate that the neuroeffector is partly acetylcholine (ACh), partly vasoactive intestinal polypeptide (VIP) and partly NO. Both VIP and the neuronal isoform of NOS are present in cutaneous cholinergic nerves and in sweat glands.

The above response is finely **graded** and spans a massive flow range (Figure 15.10b). During **cold stress**, the entire skin

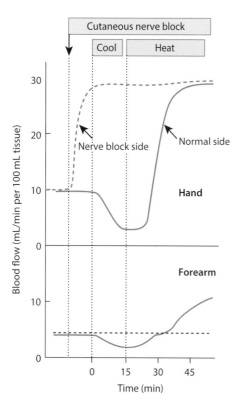

**Figure 15.11** Contrast between cutaneous vascular control in the hand and arm. The dashed line shows the marked effect in the hand, but not forearm, of sympathetic fibre block by local anaesthetic. Core temperature was then cooled, followed by heating, by placing legs in cold/hot water (upper limbs at room temperature). The results show that, in the hand, sympathetic restraint of arteriovenous flow is great at thermoneutrality, and heat-mediated dilatation is due chiefly to abolition of this restraint. In more proximal skin (arm), sympathetic-induced tone is slight and vasodilatation depends on increased sympathetic cholinergic fibre activity. (After Roddie IC. In: Geiger SR, Shepherd JT, Abboud FM, eds. *The Cardiovascular System. Vol. 3. Peripheral Circulation and Organ Blood Flow.* Bethesda, MD: American Physiological Society; 1983. pp. 285–317.)

perfusion can fall to just 20 mL/min, which allows the full insulating action of the subcutaneous fat to protect the core temperature. During **heat stress**, adult human skin perfusion can reach 7–8 L/min. This necessitates a major increase in the cardiac output, to ~13 L/min, of which more than half goes to the skin. A compensatory vasoconstriction in the splanchnic, renal and skeletal muscle circulations helps maintain arterial BP.

## The cutaneous circulation helps regulate arterial and central venous pressure

If BP falls (e.g. during hypovolaemia), acute cardiac failure and other cases of clinical shock, there is an intense cutaneous venoconstriction and arteriolar constriction, causing the characteristic **pale, cold skin of patients in clinical shock**. The constriction is driven by angiotensin, vasopressin, adrenaline and increased sympathetic vasoconstrictor activity. The increase in cutaneous vascular resistance helps to support arterial pressure, while venoconstriction helps to support central venous pressure. The importance of cutaneous vaso-constriction was noted during World War I; wounded men

who were rescued quickly and warmed in blankets (producing cutaneous dilatation) survived haemorrhage less well than the men who could not be reached for some time and retained their reflex cutaneous vasoconstriction.

**Exercise** evokes an initial, sympathetic-mediated cutaneous vasoconstriction, but this changes to dilatation when core temperature rises. Stimuli that elicit the **alerting (defence) response**, such as mental arithmetic, cause a transient cutaneous venous and arteriolar constriction (Figure 14.14). **Deep inspiration** has the same effect.

## Orthostasis elicits the cutaneous veni-arteriolar response

Lowering a limb below heart level (dependency) causes a marked vasoconstriction of cutaneous resistance vessels (Figures 8.6 and 11.5). Indeed, cutaneous perfusion in the dependent foot falls by two-thirds. This response to dependency helps to maintain central arterial pressure during standing, and to minimize dependent oedema formation. The arteriolar contraction is somehow triggered by the dependency-induced venous congestion, the **veni-arteriolar response**; however, the link is poorly understood. The Bayliss myogenic response may contribute, but in addition local nerve fibres seem to be involved since the response is abolished by local anaesthetics. The former view that the veni-arteriolar response is a 'sympathetic axon rflex' is now questioned, because the response is not prevented by a blocking dose of the α antagonist phentolamine.

## The cutaneous circulation as the mirror of the soul

Poets and playwrights have long emphasized the way skin colour responds to emotional state. Skin colour is strongly affected by vascular tone because pinkness/pallor depends on the mass and oxygenation of red cells in the subpapillary venous plexus. We blush with embarrassment (vasodilatation) and blanch with fear or stress (vasoconstriction elicited by the alerting response).

Juliet was evidently a blusher. Her nurse, announcing Romeo's desire to marry her, remarked:

> *There stays a husband to make you a wife:*
> *Now comes the wanton blood up in your cheeks,*
> *They'll be in scarlet straight at any news.*

**(*Romeo and Juliet*, Act 2, Scene 5)**

The defence or alerting response has the opposite effect. When Salisbury tells King Richard of his army's desertion, the King pales, crying:

> *But now the blood of twenty thousand men*
> *Did triumph in my face, and they are fled;*
> *And till so much blood thither comes again,*
> *Have I not reason to look pale and dead?*

**(*Richard II*, Act 3, Scene 2)**

Blushing is poorly understood because it is difficult to produce on demand. Folkow and Neil, in their classic textbook *Circulation*, recall how they could not make a habitual blusher blush in a laboratory setting, either by insults or rude jokes, but when they disconnected their equipment and thanked the participant, she blushed violently. Blushing is often associated with emotional sweating and is probably mediated by sympathetic cholinergic fibres innervating the face, neck and upper chest. Emotional stimuli can also evoke hyperaemia in the gastric and colonic mucosa.

## Trauma increases skin blood flow

The cutaneous vascular response to trauma is summarized by the **Lewis triple response** (Figures 14.8 and 14.9). Both blood flow and capillary permeability increase, thereby boosting the delivery of white cells and immunoglobulins to the injured site.

## Special problems

### Compression leads to pressure ulcers

Skin gets sat on and leaned on for long periods, causing vascular compression. **Pressure-induced vasodilatation** (dilatation evoked by innocuous external pressure) delays the onset of ischaemia, and skin tolerates ischaemia better than most tissues. Pressure-induced vasodilatation may be mediated by vasoactive peptides (e.g. CGRP) released by skin sensory fibres, since it is blocked by local anaesthetics. If the compression is maintained, increasing discomfort normally triggers a shift in position. This relieves the compression and allows **reactive (postischaemic) hyperaemia** to increase cutaneous perfusion for a while. The associated flush is obvious in white-skinned people. For mechanisms, see Section 13.8.

In patients who are old, frail, paraplegic or comatose, there is little or no voluntary shifting of position to relieve skin compression. If major pressure areas such as the heels and buttocks are not relieved by regularly turning the patient, the skin undergoes ischaemic necrosis over days and weeks, resulting in deep **pressure ulcers** (**bed sores**). The elderly are particularly prone to bed sores because the skin becomes thin and frail with ageing. A low incidence of bed sores in a geriatric ward is a sign of good nursing care.

### Cutaneous vasodilatation contributes to fainting and heat exhaustion in hot weather

The dilatation of cutaneous veins in hot weather reduces central venous pressure, which predisposes the individual to **postural fainting**. The classic example is the guardsman who faints while standing to attention on a hot day. Resistance vessel vasodilatation increases capillary filtration pressure, leading to **tissue swelling**, hence the common experience that a ring often feels tight on the finger during hot weather. Heavy exercise in a hot environment can lead

---

**KEY FEATURES BOX 15.3**

**THE CUTANEOUS CIRCULATION**

**Special tasks**
- Regulate body temperature
- Respond to traumatic breaches of the integument

**Structural adaptations**
- AVAs in acral skin (fingers, palms, toes, lips, nose, ears) dilate to dissipate heat

**Functional adaptations**
- Sympathetic nerves, not metabolic hyperaemia, are the dominant control system
- Core temperature receptors in the hypothalamus control sympathetic vasoconstrictor fibres to acral skin (AVAs) and sympathetic vasodilator fibres to non-acral skin
- Ambient cold causes veno- and vasoconstriction ($\alpha_2$-mediated), followed by paradoxical cold vasodilatation. Heat causes dilatation
- Cutaneous veno- and vasoconstriction driven by the baroreflex support the circulation during hypotension or acute cardiac failure
- The veni-arteriolar response reduces the perfusion of dependent skin
- Stress causes vasoconstriction, embarrassment vasodilatation
- The Lewis triple response enhances perfusion and immunoglobulin escape in damaged skin
- Reactive hyperaemia restores nutrition rapidly after compression

**Special problems**
- Prolonged compression → pressure ulcers (bed sores)
- Heat → tissue swelling and venodilatation, aggravating postural hypotension, which may cause fainting. Heat-induced cutaneous dilatation plus strenuous exercise → heat exhaustion
- Ambient cold → sustained, damaging vasoconstriction in fingers of Raynaud's patients

**Assessment in man**
- Laser Doppler probe assesses red cell flux
- Kety's isotope clearance method measures local dermal perfusion

---

to **heat exhaustion**. The combination of cutaneous vasodilatation (for heat loss) and muscle vasodilatation reduces the peripheral resistance profoundly, while plasma volume and cardiac filling pressure are lowered by sweating, fluid filtration into the exercising muscle and cutaneous venodilatation. The resulting fall in cardiac output, combined with the excessive fall in peripheral resistance, leads to arterial hypotension and collapse (heat exhaustion).

### Cold triggers Raynaud's disease

During cold weather, paradoxical cold vasodilatation normally prevents any tissue damage. However, in **Raynaud's disease** the vessels of the fingers show an exaggerated, sustained vasoconstriction to cold, usually in women. This leads to severe blanching, numbness, tingling or pain in the finger tips, and local tissue ischaemia.

In severe **eczema and psoriasis**, the skin's normal vaso-constrictor response to cold is prevented by inflammatory vasodilatation. Temperature regulation becomes unstable and occasionally necessitates hospitalization.

## Measurement of human cutaneous blood flow

The **laser Doppler 'flowmeter'** (really a cell flux meter) provides a rapid, semi-quantitative measure of red cell flux in a patch of superficial dermis.

**Thermography**, the imaging of surface temperature by an infrared camera, has been used as an indirect index of flow; however, epidermal temperature depends on ambient temperature and skin thickness as well as blood flow.

**Venous occlusion plethysmography** (Figure 8.5) can be adapted to a single digit, where most of the blood flow is cutaneous.

**Kety's isotope clearance technique** measures nutritive flow (Figure 8.6).

### 15.4  CEREBRAL CIRCULATION

Mean blood flow, whole brain, 55 mL/min/100 g

Basal blood flow, grey matter, 100 mL/min/100 g

The human brain (~1.5 kg) forms only 2% of the total body mass. Nevertheless, it receives 14% of the resting cardiac output and accounts for nearly 20% of resting $O_2$ consumption. Most of the blood goes to the neuron-rich grey matter (40% of brain mass) and a smaller proportion to the white matter (chiefly myelinated axon tracts). The cerebral arterioles are unusually short and thin-walled, so large cerebral arteries account for an unusually high fraction of the vascular resistance (40%–50%) and have a rich autonomic innervation.

## Special tasks

### Maximum security of $O_2$ supply

Grey matter has a very high rate of oxidative metabolism, ~7 mL $O_2$/min/100 g, which raises jugular venous blood temperature by ~0.3 °C. Because of its high $O_2$ demand, grey matter is exquisitely sensitive to hypoxia; consciousness is lost after a few seconds of cerebral ischaemia, and irreversible neuronal damage follows within ~4 min. Therefore, the primary task of the cerebral circulation is to maintain $O_2$ delivery at all costs.

### Local cerebral perfusion must adapt to changes in neuronal activity

Many mental functions are well localized, such as visual interpretation in the occipital cortex. Increased local neuronal activity raises the local metabolic rate, as shown by increased uptake of radiolabelled glucose and $O_2$. For example, illumination of the retina raises the metabolic rate of the occipital visual cortex. The cerebral vessels must therefore adjust blood flow locally, to match the varying local demand for $O_2$.

## Structural adaptations

### The circle of Willis helps safeguard the arterial supply

The **basilar** and **internal carotid arteries** enter the cranial cavity and anastomose to form a circle around the optic chiasma, the circle of Willis (Figure 15.12). (The young assistant

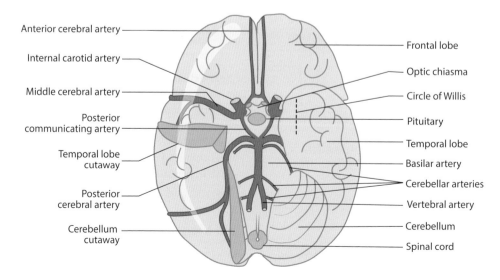

**Figure 15.12** Circle of Willis and main cerebral arteries in man, viewed from the underside of the brain. The blood reaches the circle of Willis via the basilar artery and two internal carotid arteries.

employed by Thomas Willis to draw the circle later designed St Paul's Cathedral in London, being one Christopher Wren.) **Anterior, middle** and **posterior cerebral arteries** arise from the circle of Willis. This arrangement helps preserve cerebral perfusion if a carotid artery is obstructed, at least in the young; in older individuals, the anastomoses are less effective. The main cerebral arteries divide into **pial arteries** that run over the surface of the brain. Pial artery pressure is unusually low, ~50% of systemic pressure, because the distal/proximal resistance ratio is low. Pial arteries give off fine arteries that penetrate the parenchyma and divide into short arterioles.

## A high capillary density optimizes $O_2$ transport

Grey matter contains ~3000–4000 capillaries per $mm^2$ cross section, similar to the myocardium. This creates a large surface area for $O_2$ diffusion and reduces the extravascular diffusion distance to <10 μm. Cerebral capillaries have exceptionally tight endothelial junctions, which create a blood–brain barrier for lipid-insoluble solutes (see later).

## Functional adaptations

Cerebral blood flow is regulated chiefly by intrinsic mechanisms, namely autoregulation and functional hyperaemia, rather than vasomotor nerves and hormones.

## Grey matter has a very high basal blood flow

Blood flow to the grey matter is very high, ~100 mL/min/100 g, which is over 10 times the whole-body average. Fractional $O_2$ extraction, ~35%, is likewise above average.

## Cerebral perfusion pressure is safeguarded by brainstem regulation of other circulations

As in any tissue, blood flow depends on vascular conductance and arterial pressure. However, unlike other tissues the brain can safeguard its blood supply by strangling the blood supply to other, less vital tissues, while sparing itself – a selfish organ, but wisely so! When necessary (e.g. acute hypovolaemia, clinical shock), the perfusion of the peripheral tissues, except the myocardium, is restricted via sympathetic-mediated vasoconstriction, to maintain arterial BP and hence cerebral perfusion. The brain also has control over the cardiac output via the autonomic nerves.

## Cerebral autoregulation maintains perfusion during hypotension

A further safeguard against underperfusion is provided by autoregulation, which is very well developed in the brain (Figure 15.13). If arterial BP falls, cerebral resistance vessels dilate to maintain perfusion. However, below the

limit of ~60 mmHg, cerebral blood flow declines steeply. Hypotension of this severity therefore leads to mental confusion and syncope. The upper limit of autoregulation is ~150–160 mmHg.

## Cerebral vessels are dilated by arterial $CO_2$ and hypoxia

Cerebral resistance vessels are unusually sensitive to arterial $CO_2$ (Figure 15.13). **Hypercapnia** causes cerebral vasodilatation, which helps to maintain $O_2$ supply during asphyxia. The vasodilatation is partly mediated by endothelial NO and partly by a fall in vascular myocyte pH due to carbonic acid. Conversely, **hypocapnia** causes cerebral vasoconstriction. If the arterial $P_{CO_2}$ is reduced to 15 mmHg by hyperventilation (normal $P_{CO_2}$ 40 mmHg), vasoconstriction halves the cerebral blood flow, and can be observed in the retina, which is embryologically an extension of the brain. Thus, **panic hyperventilation** in adults, or hyperventilation for fun by children, can reduce cerebral perfusion sufficiently to cause disturbed vision, dizziness and even fainting. The traditional remedy is to breathe in and out of a paper bag (not plastic), so that expired $CO_2$ is rebreathed.

**Local hypoxia** causes cerebral vasodilatation, due partly to adenosine formation. However, **systemic hypoxia** stimulates ventilation, and the resulting hypocapnia causes a counteracting cerebral vasoconstriction. Because of these two opposite effects, systemic hypoxia has only a minor effect on human cerebral blood flow.

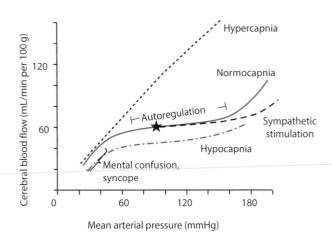

**Figure 15.13** Autoregulation of cerebral perfusion at normal arterial $P_{CO_2}$ (solid line); the star marks the normal operating point. Over the autoregulated range, flow changes by only 6% per 10 mmHg pressure change. A raised arterial $CO_2$ causes cerebral vasodilatation (upper dashed line); a low $CO_2$, usually due to hyperventilation, causes vasoconstriction (lower dashed line). Local sympathetic stimulation affects flow significantly only when arterial pressure is high (lower dashed line). (After Heistad DD, Kontos HA. In: Geiger SR, Shepherd JT, Abboud FM, eds. *The Cardiovascular System. Vol. 3. Peripheral Circulation and Organ Blood Flow*. Bethesda, MD: American Physiological Society; 1983. pp. 137–81, by permission.)

## Regional neuronal activity evokes regional metabolic hyperaemia

Shining a light into one eye increases the local blood flow and temperature in the corresponding occipital cortex and lateral geniculate body. Cerebral vessels thus display excellent functional/active/metabolic hyperaemia. Increased mental activity evokes hyperaemia in many other regions too (Figure 15.14). Functional hyperaemia is mediated partly by **interstitial [K⁺]**, which is raised initially by the outward, repolarizing K⁺ currents of active neurons (Figure 15.15). However, the rise in K⁺ is not well maintained. Sustaining factors include interstitial adenosine and astrocyte activation. Interstitial **adenosine**, a powerful cerebral vasodilator, increases rapidly in response

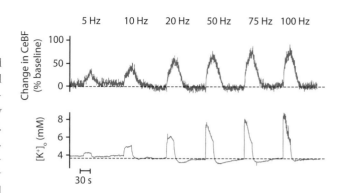

**Figure 15.15** Effect of neuronal activity on rat cerebellar blood flow (CeBF), monitored by laser Doppler; an example of metabolic hyperaemia. Concomitant interstitial K⁺ concentration $[K^+]_o$ was monitored by an ion-sensitive electrode. Neurons were activated by remote electrical stimulation of a parallel fibre system at the frequency indicated in Hertz. (From Caesar K, Akgören N, Mathiesen C, et al. *The Journal of Physiology* 1999; 520(Pt 1): 281–92, by permission.)

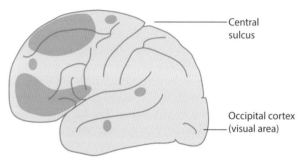

(a) Control, resting

Central sulcus

Occipital cortex (visual area)

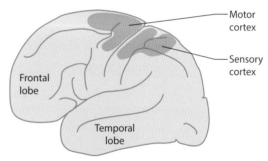

(b) Movement of contralateral hand

Motor cortex

Sensory cortex

Frontal lobe

Temporal lobe

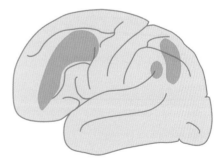

(c) Reasoning test

**Figure 15.14** Functional/metabolic hyperaemia in the human cortex shown by xenon-133 imaging. The red areas show raised flow, 20% above mean. (**a**) Frontal lobe hyperaemia in resting, pensive participant. (**b**) Hyperaemia of the hand area of the upper motor, premotor and sensory cortex during voluntary movement of the contralateral hand. (**c**) Hyperaemia in precentral and postcentral areas during a reasoning test. (Data from Ingvar DH. *Brain Research* 1976; 107(1): 181–97; and Lassen NA, Ingvar DH, Skinhøj E. *Scientific American* 1978; 239(4): 62–71.)

to electrical stimulation and hypoxaemia, and is well sustained. **Astrocytes** are located between the neurons and blood vessels, and are thought to be stimulated by active neurons. As Ca²⁺ rises in the stimulated astrocytes, they release vasodilators such as eicosatrienoic acids (Section 9.5) close to the vessel. This results in the vasodilatation of both local resistance vessels and upstream, pial vessels (**neurovascular coupling**).

## Extracerebral arteries are innervated by both sensory and motor fibres

Intracerebral arterioles are poorly innervated, but the cerebral arteries on the brain surface are innervated by nociceptive C-fibres, parasympathetic vasodilator fibres and sympathetic vasoconstrictor fibres.

**Perivascular nociceptive C-fibres** are abundant and probably mediate the pain of **vascular headaches**, including the severe pains of meningitis, migraine and strokes. These sensory fibres also have a motor function, for they contain the vasodilator neurotransmitters **CGRP** and **substance P**, which in the skin are involved in several vasodilator responses (Section 14.4). C-fibre-mediated vasodilatation probably contributes to the hyperaemia of meningitis, seizures and the headache phase of migraine.

**Parasympathetic vasodilator fibres** contain ACh and VIP, and may likewise contribute to the vasodilatation of vascular headaches.

**Sympathetic vasoconstrictor fibres** release NAd and neuropeptide Y (NPY), but the NAd has only a weak effect because cerebral vessels express few α adrenergic receptors. **NPY** is abundant in cerebral sympathetic varicosities and probably accounts for much of the evoked vasoconstriction. Even so, the maximal effect of sympathetic stimulation in humans is only a 37% rise in cerebral vascular resistance (cf. 500% in skeletal muscle). Its chief role may be to protect the blood–brain barrier against disruption by sudden rises in arterial pressure.

## Cerebral capillaries form a tight blood–brain barrier

Lipid-soluble molecules, such as $O_2$, $CO_2$ and general anaesthetics, diffuse freely across cerebral capillaries, whereas lipid-insoluble solutes, such as plasma salts, L-glucose, mannitol, catecholamines and angiotensin, fail to permeate the cerebral capillary wall in most regions of the brain (cf. free permeation in most tissues). This 'blood–brain barrier' to lipophobic solutes was discovered through the simple observation that an intravenous injection of an ionic dye stains almost every tissue in the body except the nervous system and testis.

The **functions** of the blood–brain barrier are to:

- protect the delicate neuronal circuits from interference by circulating solutes such as catecholamines, which are also neurotransmitters;
- maintain a tight control of pH and $K^+$ concentration in the cerebrospinal and interstitial fluid; and
- prevent the washout of synaptic neurotransmitters from the brain parenchyma.

As J Barcroft eloquently remarked in his book, *Features in the Architecture of Physiological Function*, 'To look for high intellectual development in a milieu whose properties have not become stabilized is to seek music among the crashings of a rudimentary wireless, or ripple patterns on the surface of the stormy Atlantic.'

The blood–brain barrier is created by specialized endothelial cell junctions (Section 10.8). Multiple junctional strands, composed of cadherin-10, claudin-1, occludin and tight junction protein ZO-1/2, form an unbroken seal between the cells (Figure 9.3). Also, the caveola-vesicle system is very scanty. These structural specializations are probably induced by the astrocytes, the 'feet' of which envelop over 80% of the abluminal surface of a brain capillary.

In certain specific locations, the blood–brain barrier is **physiologically defective**. Here plasma solutes can gain access to intracerebral receptors. In the **circumventricular region**, fenestrated capillaries allow $Na^+Cl^-$ access to the osmoreceptors of the laminae terminalis and subfornicular organ, and angiotensin access to the subfornicular thirst centre. In the **area postrema** of the lateral medulla, angiotensin accesses presympathetic neurons, and circulating emetics access the vomiting centre. **Pathological breakdown** of the normal barrier is described in Key features box 15.4 under 'Special problems'.

## The cerebral endothelium expresses special carriers that transport metabolites and potassium

The main neuronal energy source is D-**glucose** (dextrose, $C_6H_{12}O_6$), as demonstrated by the neuronal $O_2$/glucose consumption ratio of almost 6:1. Unlike the impermeant stereoisomer L-glucose, D-glucose crosses the blood–brain barrier rapidly by **facilitated diffusion**. The D-glucose binds reversibly to a specific carrier protein in the endothelial cell membrane, glucose transporter type 1. Consequently, uptake exhibits typical carrier-based phenomena, such as saturation and stereospecificity. Transport is nevertheless passive, being driven by the glucose concentration gradient created by neuronal consumption. The cerebral endothelium also expresses carriers for **adenosine**, **metabolic acids** (lactate, pyruvate), **neutral amino acids** (e.g. phenylalanine), **anionic amino acids** (e.g. glutamate) and **cationic amino acids** (e.g. arginine).

There is also **active $K^+$ transport** across the cerebral endothelium. When interstitial $[K^+]$ is raised by neuronal electrical activity, a $Na^+/K^+$ ATPase in the abluminal endothelial membrane expels $K^+$ ions from the interstitium. Interstitial $K^+$ homeostasis is of course vital for the neuron resting potential. This active role of the cerebral endothelium is supported by five to six times as many mitochondria as in muscle endothelium.

## Special non-lymphatic pathways drain fluid from the brain

The brain lacks a lymphatic system. Instead, the cerebral interstitial fluid communicates with the cerebrospinal fluid (CSF), which drains through two specialized pathways: (1) the **arachnoid granulations** in the walls of the cranial venous sinuses transmit CSF directly into the venous system; (2) some CSF flows along the sheath of the olfactory nerve, exiting the skull through the perforated cribriform plate. This fluid is then absorbed by the **lymphatics of the olfactory mucosa**.

## Special problems

### Blood–brain barrier breakdown

Disorganization of the endothelial junctional protein causes barrier breakdown in numerous pathological conditions, including severe, acute hypertension, cerebral haemorrhage, ischaemia (strokes), hypoxia (high-altitude exposure) and inflammation (meningitis, multiple sclerosis). The attendant rise in paracellular permeability leads to cerebral oedema, which impairs brain function and can induce fits (e.g. pre-eclamptic toxaemia of pregnancy). These changes can be ameliorated with glucocorticoids and blockers of inflammatory mediator receptors.

### Standing up can cause transient cerebral hypoperfusion and dizziness

The pull of gravity during orthostasis (upright position) has no direct effect on cerebral blood flow, because the cerebral circulation becomes an inverted U-tube siphon; the effect of gravity on the carotid and vertebral arteries is offset by its effect on the jugular and vertebral veins and CSF (Figures 8.2 and 8.25, bottom panel). However, standing up reduces cerebral perfusion transiently through a fall in cardiac output. Venous pooling in the legs lowers the CVP and hence cardiac output (Frank–Starling mechanism), which causes transient postural hypotension. Although this is quickly corrected by the baroreflex (Chapter 16), it can reduce cerebral perfusion sufficiently to cause a passing dizziness or even fainting (postural syncope, Section 17.1). The internal jugular vein collapses above heart level during orthostasis, because gravity reduces its internal pressure to below atmospheric pressure (Figure 8.20). Consequently, much of the venous drainage is shunted into the vertebral venous plexus.

## Space-occupying lesions elicit Cushing's reflex

Unlike other organs, the brain is confined within a rigid case, the cranium. Consequently, a large space-occupying lesion, such as a cerebral tumour or haemorrhage, raises the intracranial pressure and displaces the brainstem down into the foramen magnum, the opening in the base of the skull that admits the spinal cord. The brainstem contains the vasomotor control centres, and compression triggers an increase in their activity. This raises peripheral sympathetic vasomotor activity and hence arterial BP (**Cushing's reflex**). The raised BP helps to maintain cerebral perfusion despite the raised intracranial pressure and it also evokes a bradycardia through the baroreflex. The combination of **bradycardia** and **acute hypertension** is recognized by neurologists as the hallmark of a large, space-occupying lesion.

## Carotid/cerebral artery atheroma causes thromboembolic strokes

Around 80% of strokes (cerebral infarcts) are caused by a **thrombus** forming on an atheromatous plaque in the internal carotid artery or a major cerebral vessel, or by **embolism**, the lodging of a detached thrombus at a downstream vascular narrowing. An internal carotid thrombus often embolizes into the middle cerebral artery, due to their close anatomical relation (Figure 15.12). Thromboembolism causes characteristic patterns of neurological deficit due to the infarction of the grey matter in the artery's territory. For example, obstruction of the left middle cerebral artery (generally the dominant side, containing the language centres) causes a right-sided hemiplegia and sensory loss plus aphasia, that is, loss of language-related skills (speech, comprehension, reading, writing).

## Arterial vasospasm causes haemorrhagic strokes

Around 20% of strokes are caused by a haemorrhage. **Subarachnoid haemorrhage** is bleeding on the surface of the brain, under the arachnoid membrane. This accounts for ~10% of cerebrovascular cases, and is often caused by the rupture of a saccular ('berry') aneurysm in the circle of Willis. **Intracerebral haemorrhage** is bleeding within the brain parenchyma. It is often caused by the rupture of microaneurysms (Charcot–Bouchard aneurysms) in patients with hypertension. The haemorrhage may trigger **cerebral artery vasospasm**, which reduces perfusion sufficiently to cause a stroke. Factors contributing to the vasospasm include **serotonin** from shed platelets and perivascular nerves,

**NPY** from sympathetic varicosities, **endothelin-1** and **$Ca^{2+}$ sensitization**. The vasospasm is usually treated with the $Ca^{2+}$-channel blocker nimodipine, which has some selectivity for cerebral vessels. $ET_A$ receptor antagonists also ameliorate the vasospasm.

## Cerebral vasodilatation contributes to migraine headaches

Migraine headache is preceded, in ~20% of cases, by a **visual prodrome** – flickering wavy lines in the visual field. This used to be attributed to vascular contraction in the visual pathway; however, it now seems that it may be due to a neuronal phenomenon, cortical spreading depression. The ensuing

---

### KEY FEATURES BOX 15.4

#### THE CEREBRAL CIRCULATION

**Special tasks**

- Maintain a high $O_2$ delivery to $O_2$-hungry, hypoxia-intolerant grey matter
- Increase regional $O_2$ supply in response to regional activity
- Maintain a tightly regulated neuronal environment

**Structural adaptations**

- Anastomosis of major arteries forms the circle of Willis
- High capillary density facilitates gas exchange
- Tight endothelial junctions form the blood–brain barrier

**Functional adaptations**

- High basal blood flow due to low arteriolar resistance
- Brain controls the rest of the circulation through the baroreflex to safeguard its own perfusion pressure. Cerebral vessels are 'excused' from the baroreflex and have only a weak sympathetic innervation
- Good autoregulation of flow if BP falls
- Strong vasodilatation to $CO_2$ and asphyxia
- Well-developed regional metabolic hyperaemia in response to neuronal activity, mediated by interstitial $K^+$, adenosine and astrocyte neurovascular coupling
- Blood–brain barrier creates a well-regulated neuronal environment, with specific carriers for facilitated diffusion of D-glucose and amino acids

**Special problems**

- Blood–brain barrier breakdown (paracellular junction leakage) → cerebral oedema in severe hypertension, cerebral haemorrhage, strokes, high-altitude hypoxia, inflammatory disorders
- Postural syncope if baroreflex is impaired
- Space-occupying lesions (tumours, haemorrhage) → bulbar ischaemia and Cushing's reflex
- Atheroma of carotid/cerebral arteries → thromboembolic strokes
- Subarachnoid/intracerebral aneurysm bleeding → vascular spasm → haemorrhagic strokes
- Vascular dilatation → headaches, migraine

**Assessment in man**

- Carotid angiography
- Transcranial Doppler velocimetry
- Xenon-133 and SPECT imaging

severe **headache** is associated with dilatation of the large extracerebral vessels, such as the middle cerebral artery, and perivascular inflammation. The vascular headache is mediated by perivascular nociceptive C-fibres and the dilatation is attributed to the **release of substance P and CGRP** from the perivascular fibres (jugular venous CGRP rises), coupled with local **depletion of the vasoconstrictor serotonin** (urinary serotonin metabolite excretion rises). Cerebral vessels express serotonin $5HT_{1D}$ receptors, and the agonist **sumatriptan** is an effective treatment for migraine headaches.

The other major nociceptor-rich intracranial structure, besides the major arteries, is the dura mater, which contributes to the severe headache of meningitis.

## Measurement of human cerebral blood flow

**Carotid angiography** (arteriography) is the X-ray imaging of the major cerebral arteries during the infusion of radio-opaque contrast medium into the internal carotid artery. This assesses cerebral vessel patency, aneurysms and the anatomical course deviations caused by tumours.

**Transcranial Doppler velocimetry** assesses flow in the major cerebral arteries.

**Single-photon emission computerized tomography (SPECT) imaging** (single-photon emission compound tomography) assesses regional perfusion by imaging the brain with a gamma-camera after the intra-arterial injection of a lipophilic, high-energy, gamma-emitting isotope.

## 15.5 PULMONARY CIRCULATION

Blood flow (cardiac output), resting human, 4–6 L/min

Maximum flow, exercising non-athlete, 20–25 L/min

The pulmonary circulation differs markedly from the other systemic circulations:

- Pressures are low and flows high because of the low pulmonary vascular resistance.
- Autoregulation of flow is absent and basal tone is low.
- Sympathetic vasomotor nerves have no major role.
- Metabolic vasodilatation has no role; alveolar perfusion vastly exceeds metabolic demand.
- Pulmonary hypertension readily causes failure of the thin-walled right ventricle (~3 mm).

The metabolic needs of the alveoli are grossly oversupplied by the pulmonary blood flow, and the bronchi are supplied with systemic, arterial blood through a separate **bronchial circulation**. Some bronchial venous blood drains into the pulmonary veins (Figure 1.5). This, coupled with Thebesian vein drainage into the left heart, reduces the arterial $O_2$ saturation to ~97%.

## Special tasks

Since the role of the lungs is gas exchange, the pulmonary circulation must (1) allow blood to equilibrate with the gas phase, and (2) perfuse each alveolus in proportion to its ventilation; that is, local blood flow must match local gas supply. A secondary task of the pulmonary endothelium is the enzymatic modification of circulating peptides, such as angiotensin and bradykinin.

## Structural adaptations

### Dense capillary packing and ultrashort diffusion distance produce efficient gas exchange

The density of capillaries in the alveolar wall is extraordinary; blood flows over the alveolar surface almost as a continuous sheet, because there is so little tissue separating adjacent capillaries (Figure 15.16). Moreover, the endothelium-epithelium layer separating the plasma and alveolar gas is extremely thin, ~0.3 μm. The short diffusion distance and massive capillary surface area (90–126 $m^2$ for the two human lungs) allow very high $O_2$ transfer rates. Consequently, $O_2$ transfer is limited chiefly by blood flow, that is, by cardiac output (**flow-limited exchange**, Section 10.10).

### Numerous short arterioles create a low resistance to flow

Pulmonary arteries and arterioles are shorter and thinner-walled than their systemic counterparts, so they offer less hydraulic resistance. Consequently, a small pressure gradient and thin right ventricle wall (~3 mm) suffice to drive pulmonary perfusion (Table 15.2). Due to the low arteriolar resistance, pulmonary capillary pressure is pulsatile and the pre/postcapillary resistance ratio, which determines capillary pressure (Figure 11.4), is ~1, in contrast ~4 in systemic circulations. A ratio of 1 means that pulmonary capillary pressure is midway between the arterial and venous pressures. The low pulmonary capillary pressures (9–18 mmHg) prevent stress damage to the extremely thin alveolar membrane.

## Functional adaptations

### Blood gases equilibrate despite short transit times

The volume of blood in the pulmonary capillaries of a resting human is ~100 mL, and blood flow is ~5000 mL/min (cardiac output). Therefore, blood traverses the pulmonary capillaries in 100/5000 min, or ~1 s, the mean **transit time**. Although the transit time is very short, 1 s is more than long enough for the blood gases to equilibrate with the alveolar gas (see curves 1–3 of Figure 10.13).

During **exercise**, the increased right ventricular output shortens the transit time. It also raises pulmonary pressure

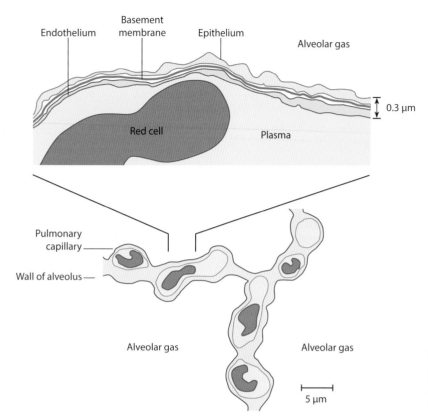

**Figure 15.16** Ultrastructure of alveolar wall and pulmonary capillaries, based on electron micrographs. Note the high ratio of blood to tissue and extreme thinness of membrane separating the plasma from alveolar gas, ~0.3 μm.

**Table 15.2** Typical pressures in human pulmonary circulation

| | Pulmonary artery (mmHg) | | | Pulmonary capillary (mmHg)[a] | Pulmonary vein (mmHg) |
|---|---|---|---|---|---|
| | Systolic | Diastolic | Mean | | |
| **Rest** | | | | | |
| Supine | 25 | 12 | 17[b] | 13 | 9 |
| Upright | 22 | 9 | 14 | 9 | 5 |
| **Heavy exercise** | | | | | |
| Upright[c] | 40 | 24 | 30 | 18 | 6 |

*Sources:* Nichols WW, O'Rourke MF, eds. *McDonald's Blood Flow in Arteries: theoretical, experimental and clinical principles*, 5th edn. London: Hodder Arnold; 2005. pp. 307–20; Stickland MK, Welsh RC, Haykowsky MJ, et al. *The Journal of Physiology* 2004; 561(Pt 1): 321–9; Caro CG, Pedley TJ, Schroter RC, et al. *The Mechanics of the Circulation*. Oxford: Oxford University Press; 1978.

[a] Pulmonary capillary pressure is midway between arterial and venous pressures because the pulmonary pre- to post-capillary resistance ratio *RA/RV* is ~1 (cf. 4 in systemic circulation); see Pappenheimer–Soto-Rivera equation, Figure 11.4.

[b] Pulmonary hypertension is a resting mean pulmonary arterial pressure of ≥25 mmHg.

[c] Submaximal treadmill exercise, cardiac output 17.5 L/min, $O_2$ consumption 2.35 L/min.

(Figure 15.17), which distends the vessels and increases pulmonary capillary volume by about one-and-a-half-fold. Since transit time is volume/flow, the increase in volume helps limit the shortening of the transit time to ~0.3 s. The blood still equilibrates with the alveolar gas, or very nearly so, during the shortened time in the pulmonary capillary. Since equilibration is achieved by the end of the capillary bed, gas exchange is **flow-limited** (Section 10.10) and the **uptake of $O_2$ is directly proportional to the pulmonary blood flow** (Fick's principle, Section 7.1).

**Endurance athletes** generate exceptionally high cardiac outputs during extreme performance, and this causes a marked fall in arterial $P_{O_2}$ and $O_2$ saturation. The same is true of racehorses, though not all mammals. Non-athletes also display a small fall in saturation during heavy exercise (Figure 15.17). A likely explanation is that the pulmonary transit time becomes so short that full gaseous equilibration is no longer achieved (**diffusion-limited exchange**, curve 4 of Figure 10.13). An additional, possibly minor factor may be the opening of pulmonary arteriovenous shunts that bypass the capillaries.

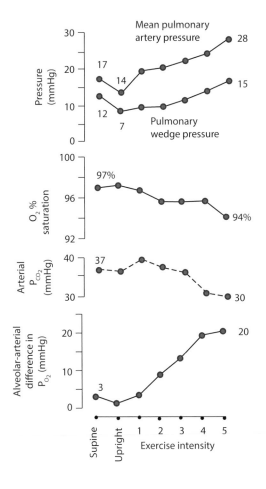

**Figure 15.17** Effect of orthostasis (standing) and exercise on pulmonary blood pressures and arterial $O_2$ saturation in healthy non-athletes; wedge pressure is a clinical measure of venular pressure (see text). Orthostasis reduces pulmonary blood pressure, exercise increases it. High-intensity exercise reduced arterial saturation, despite the hyperventilation revealed by the fall in arterial $P_{CO_2}$. The desaturation is attributed to reduced transit time (diffusion limitation), ventilation/perfusion mismatch and arteriovenous shunt vessels, which have been demonstrated in human lungs postmortem. (Data from Stickland MK, Welsh RC, Haykowsky MJ, et al. *The Journal of Physiology* 2004; 561(Pt. 1): 321–9.)

pulmonary vessels and whole lung. There is growing agreement that hypoxia is 'sensed' by the vessel mitochondria, which generate reactive $O_2$ species, but how this leads to vasoconstriction is not fully understood. One mechanism involves myocyte depolarization as $K^+$ channels are inhibited (a $K_V$ isoform and a potassium channel subfamily K member 3, or TASK channel isoform). A second mechanism is sarcoplasmic reticulum $Ca^{2+}$ store release via ryanodine receptors (for example, via cyclic adenosine diphosphate ribose or reactive $O_2$ species) and $Ca^{2+}$ entry through voltage-gated and store-operated channels, a process shown to be critical for early HPV. Over the next 20–40 min, HPV increases further, but cytosolic $[Ca^{2+}]$ does not, indicating a third, slower mechanism, $Ca^{2+}$ sensitization. The slow phase is partly endothelium-dependent and is mediated by the $Ca^{2+}$-sensitizing kinase, Rho-associated protein kinase (Section 12.5). Sustained HPV is largely blocked by inhibitors of Rho-associated protein kinase.

## Hypoxic pulmonary vasoconstriction optimizes local ventilation/perfusion ratios

In the systemic circulation, local hypoxia causes vasodilatation (Section 13.4), but in the pulmonary circulation it causes vasoconstriction (hypoxic pulmonary vasoconstriction [HPV]). The role of HPV is to preserve an optimum, uniform alveolar ventilation/perfusion ratio, $\dot{V}/\dot{Q}$, throughout the lungs, in normal and pathological states. For efficient oxygenation, each alveolus requires the same $\dot{V}/\dot{Q}$ ratio, namely 0.8 at rest (alveolar ventilation 4 L/min, cardiac output 5 L/min). HPV helps to maintain this ratio throughout the lung in supine humans. (Changes during orthostasis are considered in Key features box 15.5, under 'Special problems'.) If a group of alveoli is underventilated and therefore hypoxic, perhaps due to slight airway narrowing or mucus, the resistance vessels supplying that region undergo HPV (Figure 15.18). This reduces the local alveolar blood flow to match the reduced local alveolar ventilation, and diverts blood away from hypoxic alveoli, so that relatively little under-oxygenated blood is added to arterial blood. Thus, although pulmonary HPV is the opposite response to the hypoxic vasodilatation of systemic vessels, both responses are well adapted to the local needs.

Multiple controversial mechanisms have been suggested to underlie HPV. HPV has been studied in isolated

## Pulmonary vascular pressure-volume and pressure-flow relations are passive, lacking autoregulation

Because of its great vascularity and distensibility, the pulmonary circulation contains **12%–16% of the total blood volume** in a supine human, that is, ~600 mL. On standing, venous pooling in the legs reduces pulmonary blood volume by ~20% and pulmonary pressures by 3–4 mmHg (Table 15.2 and Figure 15.17). The pulmonary blood volume can be increased transiently to ~1 L by a forced inspiration, because inspiration reduces intrathoracic pressure. Pulmonary blood volume can be reduced to ~300 mL by a forced expiration because expiration raises intrathoracic pressure (Valsalva manoeuvre, Section 17.2).

Pulmonary vascular resistance is about one-sixth of the systemic resistance, so resting pulmonary arterial pressure is only 22–25 mmHg systolic, 9–12 mmHg diastolic (Table 15.2). The pressure-flow relation in an isolated, perfused lung is typical of passive, slightly distensible tubes; the curve steepens slightly with pressure because vascular distension increases vascular conductance (Figure 15.19a). This contrasts with the highly autoregulated relations in brain, myocardium and kidney; autoregulation would be counterproductive in the lungs because it would prevent pulmonary flow from increasing with pressure.

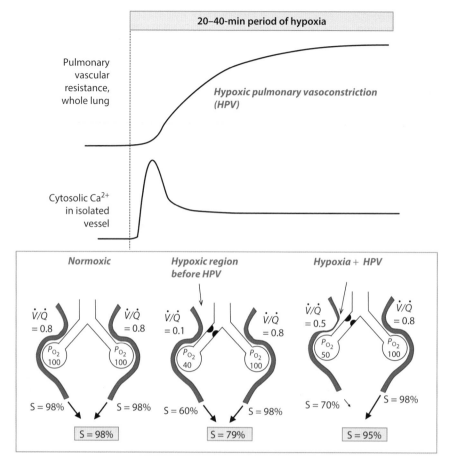

**Figure 15.18** (**Top**) Hypoxic pulmonary vasoconstriction (HPV) in a perfused whole lung exposed to hypoxia. (**Middle**) Corresponding change in vascular myocyte cytosolic $Ca^{2+}$ in an isolated rat pulmonary artery exposed to hypoxia. (**Bottom**) Effect of local alveolar hypoxia and HPV on gas exchange. HPV prevents extremely low ventilation/perfusion ratios $\dot{V}/\dot{Q}$, and thus preserves the $O_2$ saturation (S) of mixed arterial blood. $P_{O_2}$ in mmHg; arrow size indicates flow magnitude. (Based on Robertson TP, Aaronson PI, Ward JP. *American Journal of Physiology* 1995; 268(1 Pt. 2): H301–7, with permission from the American Physiological Society.)

## Exercise increases pulmonary artery pressure and flow

During exercise, the increased right ventricular output raises the pulmonary artery pressure (Figure 15.17 and Table 15.2). In **young adults** performing supine exercise, pulmonary blood flow increases almost linearly with the pressure gradient (pulmonary artery pressure minus left atrial pressure) (Figure 15.19b, middle line). In **endurance-trained athletes**, the pressure-flow relation is steeper because the 'trained' pulmonary vessels have a higher conductance; that is, they transmit more flow per unit pressure (Figure 15.19b, left). Conversely, at **high altitude** the pressure-flow relation becomes flatter because chronic HPV reduces vascular conductance (Figure 15.19b, right).

## Increased pulmonary pressure during exercise improves apical perfusion and O₂ transfer capacity

In standing/sitting humans, the lung apices are not well perfused at rest due to the effect of gravity (Figure 15.20).

During exercise, the rise in pulmonary artery pressure greatly improves apical perfusion, boosting the $O_2$ transfer capacity of the lungs. Mean pulmonary artery pressure reaches ~30 mmHg during strenuous upright exercise, cf. ~14 mmHg at rest.

## Low capillary pressure reduces alveolar membrane stress and fluid filtration

As noted earlier, **pulmonary capillary pressure** is only ~9 mmHg at heart level in the upright position. This reduces the tension in the alveolar-endothelial membrane to a low level, obviating rupture of this ultra-thin membrane. Although capillary pressure is much lower than plasma colloid osmotic pressure, pulmonary capillaries are nevertheless in a state of filtration (Figure 11.12, lowest point) because lung interstitial fluid has a high plasma protein concentration and colloid osmotic pressure (Table 11.2).

Capillary filtrate is prevented from accumulating within the alveoli and airways by epithelial ion channels and pumps,

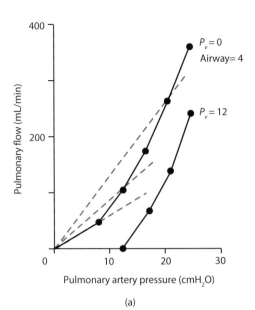

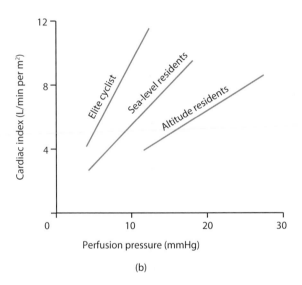

Figure 15.19 Pressure-flow relations in pulmonary circulation. (a) Isolated cat lung perfused with plasma, with venous pressure ($P_v$) set to zero or 12 cmH$_2$O and airway pressure to 4 cmH$_2$O. The dashed lines are lines of constant conductance; actual pulmonary conductance increases as arterial pressure rises. Consequently, a 4× increase in right cardiac output requires less than a 4× increase in pressure. (b) Human curves during supine exercise. 'Perfusion pressure' is pulmonary artery pressure minus left atrial pressure; airway pressure is atmospheric. ((a) From Banister RJ, Torrance RW. *Quarterly Journal of Experimental Physiology and Cognate Medical Sciences* 1960; 45: 352–67, with permission from Wiley-Blackwell; (b) from Grover RF, et al. Pulmonary circulation. In: Geiger SR, Shepherd JT, Abboud FM, eds. *The Cardiovascular System. Vol. 3. Peripheral Circulation and Organ Blood Flow.* Bethesda, MD: American Physiological Society; 1983. pp. 103–36, by permission.)

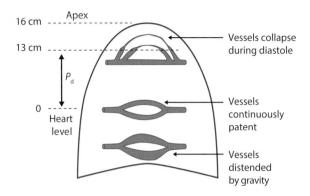

Figure 15.20 Gradient of perfusion in the human lung in an upright position at rest. The scale shows vertical distance above the heart. Diastolic artery pressure $P_d$ is 13 cmH$_2$O (~9 mmHg) at heart level, falling to zero (atmospheric) 13 cmH$_2$O above the heart. Vessels higher than this are perfused only during systole. Perfusion was measured by external gamma counting following an injection of radioisotope into the right heart.

contrast, a Cl$^-$ pump causes water to flow into the airways; the switch to Na$^+$-driven water absorption occurs at birth.)

**Pulmonary oedema** is a life-threatening excess of interstitial fluid, arising from left ventricular failure, mitral stenosis, high-altitude exposure or sepsis. Its clinical manifestations are cough, dyspnoea, crepitation (airways crackles), and in the worst cases pink, frothy sputum, with arterial desaturation. Causes include alveolar-endothelial barrier breakdown, impaired epithelial Na$^+$ clearance (e.g. high-altitude hypoxia) and haemodynamic abnormalities (raised pulmonary capillary pressure, cardiogenic oedema). Left atrial pressure elevation to >20 mmHg raises capillary pressure sufficiently to generate pulmonary oedema; smaller increases are within the safety margin against oedema (Section 11.10), but nevertheless cause **dyspnoea** (difficulty in breathing). Dyspnoea results from distension of the lung vasculature by a raised pulmonary venous pressure (**pulmonary congestion**), which makes the lungs stiff and difficult to inflate.

## The pulmonary endothelium modifies circulating vasoactive agents

As blood passes through the lungs, it is exposed to 90–126 m$^2$ of endothelium. This huge surface area facilitates the chemical modification of circulating vasoactive substances by endothelial ectoenzymes. ACE converts angiotensin I to angiotensin II and degrades circulating bradykinin. Many other vasoactive substances (serotonin, prostaglandin E, leukotrienes) are also removed by the lung endothelium.

## Special problems

### Orthostasis causes a vertical perfusion gradient

When humans adopt an upright position, the distribution of pulmonary blood flow is distorted by gravity. Mean pulmonary

and is cleared as **lung lymph**. Airway epithelial cells express amiloride-sensitive, epithelial Na$^+$ channels (**ENaCs**) on the luminal surface and **Na$^+$/K$^+$ pumps** on the basolateral surface. As Na$^+$ is absorbed from the airways through these channels, water follows it by osmosis. Mice lacking functional ENaCs die from pulmonary oedema soon after birth. (In the fetus, by

arterial pressure is ~14–15 mmHg at heart level (Table 15.2), but gravity raises this to ~21 mmHg in the lung bases, and reduces it to ~3 mmHg in the apices. The high pressure at the base distends the vessels there, raising their vascular conductance and hence the basal perfusion (Figure 15.20). Conversely, vessels at the apex collapse during diastole, because these vessels are ~16 cm above heart level, whereas diastolic pressure is only 13 cmH$_2$O (9 mmHg, Table 15.2). The apex is therefore perfused only during systole at rest (Figure 15.20), and the **mean flow through the apex is about one tenth of the flow through the base**. As noted earlier, efficient gas exchange requires a uniform ventilation perfusion ($\dot{V}/\dot{Q}$) ratio of 0.8 throughout the lung. Although alveolar ventilation $\dot{V}$ is likewise greater at the base than apex, the ventilation gradient does not fully compensate for the even bigger gradient of flow $\dot{Q}$. A standing human, therefore, has a higher $\dot{V}/\dot{Q}$ at the apex than the base. This $\dot{V}/\dot{Q}$ mismatch slightly impairs the efficiency of blood oxygenation during orthostasis.

## Pulmonary arterial hypertension leads to right ventricular failure

Although HPV is valuable in minimizing local $\dot{V}/\dot{Q}$ mismatch, it can be deleterious when the whole lung becomes hypoxic, as happens when low-altitude dwellers move to high altitude. The chronic hypoxia raises the pulmonary vascular resistance, which causes chronic pulmonary arterial hypertension, defined as a resting mean of >25 mmHg. Because the wall of the right ventricle is only ~3 mm thick, its ability to withstand a chronic increase in afterload is poor. Consequently, hypoxic chronic pulmonary hypertension can lead to right ventricular failure in mountaineers. Pulmonary arterial hypertension also occurs at low altitudes, where its aetiology is poorly understood. There is evidence that some cases are due to the proliferation of pulmonary arterial myocytes under the influence of serotonin.

## Pulmonary embolism impairs right ventricular output

A venous thrombus in a deep leg vein (often arising during a period of immobility) or pelvic veins (e.g. after surgery) may become detached (embolize). The embolus is washed through the right heart into the pulmonary artery, until it jams in a branch. This raises pulmonary vascular resistance, hence pulmonary arterial pressure and right ventricular afterload. A rise in arterial pressure reduces stroke volume (Figure 6.11b, loop 3). Thus, embolism causes a sharp fall in right ventricular output, which in turn reduces left ventricular output, leading to collapse.

## High stresses in the thin alveolar-endothelial membrane may rupture it

The blood–gas barrier is extremely thin, ~0.3 µm, so the tensile force per unit thickness of membrane (stress) is substantial,

even though capillary pressure is low. The stress is probably carried mainly by type IV collagen in the basement membrane, which is only ~50 nm thick in places (Figure 15.16). If the stress is raised by pulmonary capillary hypertension, as in patients with **mitral valve stenosis**, the membrane may break down in places, causing **pulmonary oedema** and, in severe cases, **alveolar haemorrhage**. This occurs most dramatically in thoroughbred racehorses. Racehorses are capable of extremely high cardiac outputs, ~300 L/min, which raises the pulmonary arterial pressure to 120 mmHg and left atrial pressure to 70 mmHg! This can lead to race-induced pulmonary haemorrhage. In strenuous human exercise, fortunately, the rise in pulmonary pressure is considerably more modest (Table 15.2).

---

**KEY FEATURES BOX 15.5**

### THE PULMONARY CIRCULATION

**Special tasks**

- Respiratory gas exchange
- Enzymatic modification of circulating peptides, notably angiotensin I and II

**Structural adaptations**

- Extremely high capillary density and extremely short diffusion distance
- Short arterioles of low resistance allow large flow (right ventricular output) under a low-pressure head

**Functional adaptations**

- Transit time of 0.3–1.0 s is long enough to allow blood-alveolar gas equilibration
- HPV matches local alveolar blood perfusion to local ventilation
- Flow increases in proportion to pressure; no autoregulation
- Low capillary pressure reduces membrane stress and fluid filtration
- Endothelial enzymes modify/degrade circulating vasoactive peptides

**Special problems**

- Apices not well perfused in orthostasis, but this improves during exercise
- At extreme flows (athletes), a capillary transit time of <0.3 s causes arterial under-oxygenation
- Chronic hypoxia causes chronic vasoconstriction. The resulting pulmonary arterial hypertension can lead to right heart failure, as can other forms of pulmonary arterial hypertension
- Pulmonary embolism can cause a sudden fall in cardiac output and collapse
- Ultra-thin alveolar/endothelial membrane (0.3 µm). In mitral stenosis, pulmonary capillary hypertension raises membrane stress and leads to leakage

**Assessment in man**

- Fick's principle based on O$_2$ uptake measures pulmonary blood flow (cardiac output)
- Indicator and thermal dilution methods likewise measure pulmonary blood flow
- Pulmonary wedge pressure indicates pulmonary venular pressure

## Assessment in man

The measurement of pulmonary blood flow is, of course, the measurement of right ventricle cardiac output. This can be measured by the **Fick's principle**, **indicator dilution method** and **thermal dilution method** (Chapter 7). Pulmonary microvascular pressure is estimated clinically by advancing a catheter through the pulmonary artery until the tip wedges in a narrow arterial vessel, blocking the downstream flow. The pressure of the stationary distal column of blood, the **pulmonary wedge pressure**, equals that in the nearest distal perfused vessel, usually a venule.

## FURTHER READING

### Coronary circulation

Duncker DJ, Koller A, Merkus D, et al. Regulation of coronary blood flow in health and ischemic heart disease. *Progress in Cardiovascular Disease* 2015; **57**(5): 409–22.

Beyer AM, Gutterman DD. Regulation of the human coronary microcirculation. *Journal of Molecular and Cellular Cardiology* 2012; **52**(4): 814–21.

Deussen A, Ohanyan V, Jannasch A, et al. Mechanisms of metabolic coronary flow regulation. *Journal of Molecular and Cellular Cardiology* 2012; **52**(4): 794–801.

Duncker DJ, Bache RJ, Merkus D. Regulation of coronary resistance vessel tone in response to exercise. *Journal of Molecular and Cellular Cardiology* 2012; **52**(4): 802–13.

Schaper W. Collateral circulation: past and present. *Basic Research in Cardiology* 2009; **104**(1): 5–21.

### Skeletal muscle circulation

Joyner MJ, Casey DP. Regulation of increased blood flow (hyperemia) to muscles during exercise: a hierarchy of competing physiological needs. *Physiological Reviews* 2015; **95**(2): 549–601.

Zoladz JA, Majerczak J, Duda K, et al. Coronary and muscle blood flow during physical exercise in humans; heterogenic alliance. *Pharmacology Reports* 2015; **67**(4): 719–27.

Joyner MJ. Exercise hyperaemia: are there any answers yet? *The Journal of Physiology* 2007; **583**(Pt 3): 817.

Marshall JM. The roles of adenosine and related substances in exercise hyperaemia. *The Journal of Physiology* 2007; **583**(Pt 3): 835–45.

Joyner MJ. Feeding the sleeping giant: muscle blood flow during whole body exercise. *The Journal of Physiology* 2004; **558**(Pt 1): 1.

### Cutaneous circulation

Smith CJ, Johnson JM. Responses to hyperthermia. Optimizing heat dissipation by convection and evaporation: neural control of skin blood flow and sweating in humans. *Autonomic Neuroscience: Basic & Clinical* 2016; **196**: 25–36.

Johnson JM, Minson CT, Kellogg DL Jr. Cutaneous vasodilator and vasoconstrictor mechanisms in temperature regulation. *Comprehensive Physiology* 2014; **4**(1): 33–89.

Braverman IM. The cutaneous microcirculation: ultrastructure and microanatomical organization. *Microcirculation* 1997; **4**(3): 329–40.

Folkow B, Neil E. *Circulation*. New York: OUP; 1971.

### Cerebral circulation

Willie CK, Tzeng YC, Fisher JA, et al. Integrative regulation of human brain blood flow. *The Journal of Physiology* 2014; **592**(5): 841–59.

Filosa JA, Iddings JA. Astrocyte regulation of cerebral vascular tone. *American Journal of Physiology. Heart and Circulatory Physiology* 2013; **305**(5): H609–19.

Duelli R, Kuschinsky W. Brain glucose transporters: relationship to local energy demand. *News in Physiological Sciences* 2001; **16**: 71–6.

Heistad DD. What's new in the cerebral microcirculation? Landis Award lecture. *Microcirculation* 2001; **8**(6): 365–75.

Faraci FM, Heistad DD. Regulation of the cerebral circulation: role of endothelium and potassium channels. *Physiological Reviews* 1998; **78**(1): 53–74.

Bradbury MW. The blood–brain barrier. *Experimental Physiology* 1993; **78**(4): 453–72.

Barcroft J, Sir. *Features in the Architecture of Physiological Function*. Cambridge: CUP; 1934.

### Pulmonary circulation

Frise MC, Robbins PA. Iron, oxygen, and the pulmonary circulation. *Journal of Applied Physiology* 2015; **119**(12): 1421–31.

Sylvester JT, Shimoda LA, Aaronson PI, et al. Hypoxic pulmonary vasoconstriction. *Physiological Reviews* 2012; **92**(1): 367–520.

West JB. Comparative physiology of the pulmonary circulation. *Comprehensive Physiology* 2011; **1**(3): 1525–39.

Maina JN, West JB. Thin and strong! The bioengineering dilemma in the structural and functional design of the blood-gas barrier. *Physiological Reviews* 2005; **85**(3): 811–44.

Dorrington KL, Talbot NP. Human pulmonary vascular responses to hypoxia and hypercapnia. *Pflügers Archiv: European Journal of Physiology* 2004; **449**(1):1–15.

Olver RE, Walters DV, Wilson S. Developmental regulation of lung liquid transport. *Annual Review of Physiology* 2004; **66**: 77–101.

Butler J. The bronchial circulation. *News in Physiological Sciences* 1991; **6**(1): 21–5.

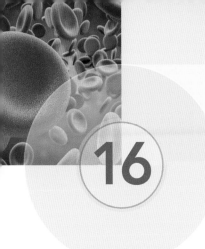

# Cardiovascular receptors, reflexes and central control

## 16

## LEARNING OBJECTIVES

*After reading this chapter, you should be able to:*

- outline the locations and properties of arterial baroreceptors (16.1);
- state the reflex effects of baroreceptors and their role in hypovolaemia (16.2);
- outline the properties and roles of veno-atrial stretch receptors (16.3, 16.4);
- state the neural origin of ischaemic cardiac pain (16.3);
- outline the reflex responses to a rise in central venous pressure (CVP) and fluid volume in humans (16.4);
- explain the role of the kidneys in long-term blood pressure (BP) regulation (16.5);

- outline the location and role of peripheral arterial chemoreceptors (16.6);
- state the cardiovascular reflex evoked by lung stretch receptors (16.6);
- outline the role of muscle work receptors during exercise (16.6);
- list the roles of medulla oblongata in cardiovascular control (16.7);
- define the alerting response and central command (16.8);
- explain how inspiration affects vagal outflow to the pacemaker (16.9).

The activity of the cardiovascular sympathetic and parasympathetic nerves is controlled by the brain; and the brain is guided by sensory information coming from neural receptors both inside and outside the circulation. (The term 'receptor' in this context means a sensory nerve ending, not a drug-binding molecule.) The afferent sensory fibres, central relays and efferent motor fibres together form cardiovascular reflex arcs (Figure 16.1). Key **sensors** include pressure receptors in the walls of specific systemic arteries (arterial baroreceptors) and pressure receptors in the heart (cardiopulmonary receptors). Their afferent fibres transmit information about arterial BP and cardiac filling to the **brainstem**, where the information is integrated with information from muscle receptors, arterial chemoreceptors and other sensors. The integration of information and computation of an appropriate response involves much up-and-down traffic between the brainstem,

hypothalamus, cerebellum and cortex. **Pre-sympathetic and parasympathetic outflows** from the brainstem are then adjusted to initiate an appropriate cardiovascular response.

The reflexes are often, but not invariably, directed at stabilizing BP. For example, the reflex response to a rise in BP is a bradycardia and peripheral vasodilatation, which restore BP to its original level (a **depressor reflex**). This is an example of **negative feedback**; a change in the sensed variable (BP) triggers an inhibitory response that returns the variable towards its control value, or **set point**. Other reflexes, such as those from arterial and muscle chemoreceptors, are excitatory; that is, they raise rather than stabilize pressure (**pressor reflexes**). The brain can also initiate non-reflex changes. For example, at the start of exercise a signal from the cerebral cortex, called the **central command**, increases heart rate (HR) almost instantly. This process is termed **feedforward** (cf. feedback).

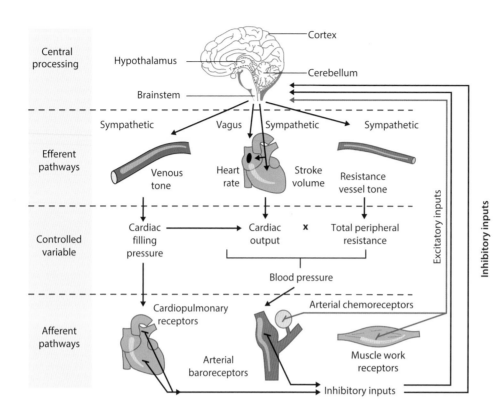

**Figure 16.1** Overview of neural reflex control of the circulation; 'inhibitory' and 'excitatory' refer to the net effect on cardiac output and blood pressure. Inhibitory reflexes are depressor and excitatory reflexes are pressor.

## 16.1 ARTERIAL BARORECEPTORS

The prefix 'baro' means pressure. A baroreceptor is a spray-type sensory fibre ending, packed with mitochondria and connected to a myelinated or non-myelinated afferent axon. Baroreceptors occur in the adventitia of arteries at two main locations: the carotid sinus and aortic arch (Figure 16.2).

The **carotid sinus** is a thin-walled dilatation at the origin of the internal carotid artery. Afferent fibres from the carotid

sinus baroreceptors form the carotid sinus nerve. This joins the **glossopharyngeal nerve** (ninth cranial nerve) to reach the petrous ganglion, where the parent neurons are located. Like all afferent neurons, the petrous neurons are bipolar. Their central axons continue up the glossopharyngeal nerve to the brainstem and terminate in the **nucleus tractus solitarius**.

**Aortic baroreceptors** are found mainly on the transverse arch of the aorta. Their fibres form the aortic or 'depressor'

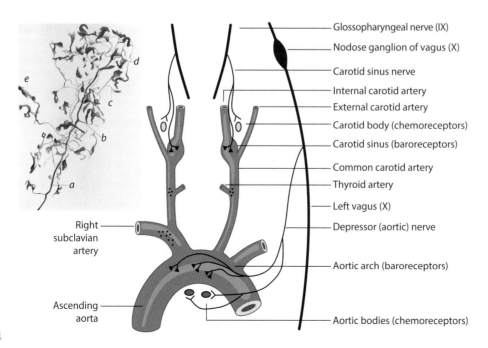

**Figure 16.2** Main reflexogenic zones of the arterial system; minor baroreceptor regions are shown as dots. The right vagus nerve is not shown. (Inset) Single baroreceptor ending in the human carotid sinus. (From Abraham A. *Microscopic Innervation of the Heart and Blood Vessels in Vertebrates Including Man.* Oxford: Pergamon Press; 1969. With permission from Elsevier.)

nerve in some species, then ascend in the **vagus** (tenth cranial nerv) to the sensory neurons of the nodose ganglion. The central axons again terminate in the nucleus tractus solitarius of the brainstem. **Coronary arteries** also possess baroreceptors, at least in dogs, and the coronary baroreflex is of similar potency to the carotid sinus baroreflex.

## Baroreceptors are stretch receptors

Baroreceptors are mechanoreceptors that respond to stretch (not blood flow). A rise in arterial pressure stretches the artery wall, which deforms and excites the receptor terminals. The wall of the carotid sinus is relatively thin, and the sinus diameter changes by ~15% with each pulse. If distension is prevented by a plaster cast, the baroreceptors no longer respond to changes in BP.

## Baroreceptors exhibit static and dynamic sensitivity

Arterial baroreceptors respond not only to the magnitude of the pressure (static sensitivity) but also to its rate of change (dynamic sensitivity). If the carotid sinus is distended rapidly in an experiment, an individual baroreceptor fibre first fires off a volley of action potentials at a high frequency (**dynamic response** to the pressure change), then the firing frequency declines (**adaptation**) until it stabilizes at a lower, but still raised, frequency that signals the new pressure level (**static response**) (Figure 16.3, fibre 1). The adaptation may be due to mechanical creep of the receptor within its stretched environment, or ion channel adaptation.

Conversely, when pressure is reduced, the baroreceptor fibre transiently falls silent (dynamic 'off' response), then resumes activity at a new, lower rate (static 'off' response) (Figure 16.3, fibre 2). Because of its dynamic sensitivity, a baroreceptor fibre *in vivo* characteristically fires a burst of action potentials in systole and falls silent in diastole (Figure 16.3, fibre 3).

## A-fibres have lower thresholds and are more sensitive than C-fibres

There are two kinds of arterial baroreceptor, A-fibres and C-fibres. The distinction is based on myelination, conduction velocity and threshold. The **threshold** of a baroreceptor is the lowest pressure that triggers an action potential in its axon.

**A-fibres** are large-diameter, fast-conducting, myelinated fibres with low thresholds, in the range 30–90 mmHg (Figure 16.4a). A-fibres are active at normal BP and fire a burst of impulses with each arterial pulse. A-fibres are less numerous than C-fibres.

**C-fibres** are the more abundant. They are small-diameter, slow-conducting, unmyelinated fibres with high thresholds, in the range 70–140 mmHg. Only a quarter or so of C-fibres are active at normal BPs. The active fibres fire in phase with the pulse, but at a low frequency.

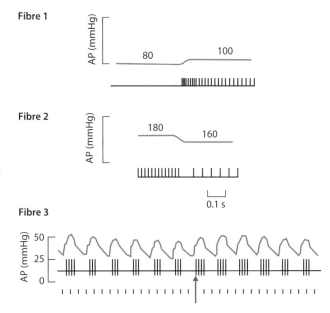

**Figure 16.3** Firing characteristics of baroreceptor afferents. (Fibres 1 and 2) Action potentials in myelinated afferents of cat carotid sinus when non-pulsatile arterial pressure (AP) is raised (Fibre 1) or reduced (Fibre 2). (Fibre 3) Single baroreceptor fibre from rabbit aorta responding to a normal, pulsatile pressure. There are four impulses per pulse when pulse pressure is high (arrow) and three when it is lower. Time intervals 0.1 s. (Fibres 1 and 2 after Landgren S. *Acta Physiologica Scandinavica* 1952; 26(1): 1–34, with permission from Wiley-Blackwell; fibre 3 from Downing SE. *The Journal of Physiology* 1960; 150: 210–13, with permission from Wiley-Blackwell.)

The mean discharge frequency in a baroreceptor fibre increases with mean BP, above threshold. The steepness of the relation is called the **sensitivity** of the fibre. A-fibres are two to three times more sensitive than C-fibres in the middle of their respective operating ranges (Figure 16.4a). A-fibres can also achieve higher discharge frequencies than C-fibres.

## C-fibres are important at high blood pressures, when A-fibre activity saturates

When BP reaches a high level, A-fibre activity reaches a maximum frequency (**saturation**), whereas C-fibres remain responsive to pressure at these levels (Figure 16.4a). Therefore, C-fibres of high threshold are important for signalling graded information about high BPs. A-fibres are important for signalling changes around normal BP, aided by ~25% of C-fibres with low enough thresholds.

## Recruitment extends the signalling range of multifibre nerves

The carotid sinus nerve and aortic nerve contain large numbers of A- and C-fibres. When BP rises, not only does the discharge frequency increase in previously active fibre, but also previously silent fibres of high threshold begin to fire (**recruitment**). Due to recruitment, the multifibre nerve has a wider operating range than a single fibre, and can keep the brainstem informed about a wider range of pressures (Figure 16.4b).

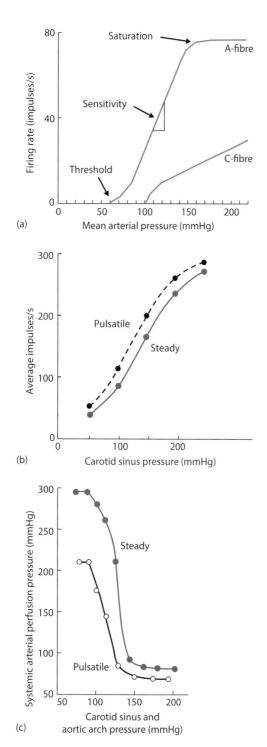

(a)

(b)

(c)

**Figure 16.4** Effect of arterial blood pressure on baroreceptor traffic and reflex change in systemic blood pressure in anaesthetized dogs. (**a**) Response of a single A-fibre and C-fibre to increasing pressure. (**b**) Average discharge rate in multifibre carotid sinus nerve: pulsatile pressures evoke higher activity. (**c**) Raising pressure in a vascularly isolated, perfused baroreceptor region triggers a reflex fall in systemic arterial blood pressure, mediated by bradycardia and peripheral vasodilatation. Pulsatility strengthens this depressor reflex. ((**a**) Coleridge HM, Coleridge JC, Schultz HD. *The Journal of Physiology* 1987; 394: 291–313; (**b**) Korner PI. *Physiological Reviews* 1971; 51(2): 312–67, with permission from the American Physiological Society; and (**c**) James JE, Daly Mde B. *The Journal of Physiology* 1970; 209(2): 257–93, with permission from Wiley-Blackwell.)

## Baroreceptors signal pulse pressure and mean pressure

Carotid baroreceptors signal not only the mean pressure but also the size of the oscillation about the mean, that is, the pulse pressure. The greater the oscillation in pressure about a given mean, the greater the average baroreceptor activity (Figure 16.4b). Consequently, a pulsating pressure has a greater reflex effect than a steady pressure (Figure 16.4c). The difference is due partly to the dynamic sensitivity of the receptors, partly to recruitment of extra fibres during each systole and partly to the gradual adaptation of brainstem neurons to a steady signal. The signalling of pulse pressure is particularly important during **orthostasis** and **moderate haemorrhage**, when there is a fall in pulse pressure (due to the fall in cardiac stroke volume), but often little fall in mean arterial pressure (Figure 18.2).

## Carotid sinus and aortic baroreceptors have similar properties

Carotid sinus A-fibres have slightly lower thresholds than aortic arch A-fibres; otherwise, the receptors and reflexes elicited by the two reflexogenic zones are broadly similar. Both regions have strong reflex effects on human HR, but the aortic baroreceptors have a stronger effect on vasomotor nerve activity. What, then, are the reflexes elicited by baroreceptors?

## 16.2 THE BAROREFLEX

The baroreflex adjusts the cardiac output and peripheral vascular tone to stabilize the arterial BP. The reflex response to an acute rise in arterial BP is described first, then the medically important response to a fall in pressure, such as occurs during hypovolaemia.

## Acute pressure elevation triggers a depressor reflex

In 1866, Ludwig and Cyon noted that electrical stimulation of the aortic nerve causes a reflex fall in HR and BP – the depressor reflex. Hering later discovered that stimulation of the carotid sinus nerve elicits the same reflex (Figure 16.5). In normal life, an acute rise in arterial pressure increases the baroreceptor traffic, which is conveyed by the vagi and glossopharyngeal nerves to the brainstem, where it activates polysynaptic central pathways. These **enhance the vagal parasympathetic output** to the heart and **inhibit the sympathetic output** to the heart and systemic vasculature (Figure 16.6), with the following effects:

- A fall in sympathetic vasomotor activity causes **peripheral vasodilatation**, which **reduces total peripheral resistance**. Human sympathetic vasomotor activity ceases entirely if BP is raised rapidly to >150/90 mmHg.

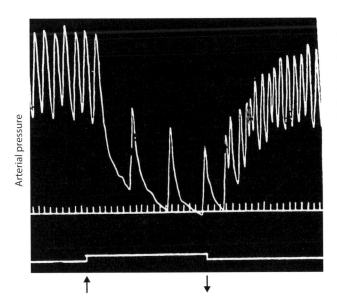

**Figure 16.5** Electrical stimulation of the carotid sinus nerve of the dog elicits reflex hypotension and bradycardia. This is the classic smoked-drum record of Hering, who discovered the carotid baroreflex in 1923. Time intervals 0.2 s. (From Hering HE. *Die Karotissinusreflexe auf Herz und Gefässe: vom normal-physiologischen, pathologischen und klinischen Standpunkt (Gleichzeitig über die Beutung der Blutdruckzügler für den normalen und abnormen Kreislauf).* [Monograph in German]. Dresden: T. Steinkopf, 1927.)

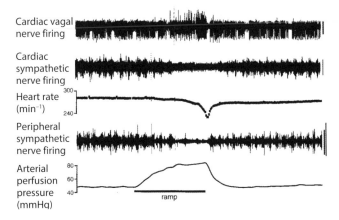

**Figure 16.6** Effect of raising arterial pressure (bottom trace) in the artificially perfused carotid arteries and aorta of a rat. Cardiac vagal activity increased, cardiac sympathetic fibre activity decreased and heart rate slowed. Peripheral sympathetic vasoconstrictor activity decreased (sympathetic chain, level T12). (Adapted from Simms AE, Paton JF, Pickering AE. *Journal of Physiology* 2007; 579(Pt 2): 473–86, with permission from Wiley-Blackwell.)

- A fall in cardiac sympathetic activity and rise in vagal parasympathetic activity cause **bradycardia** and **reduced myocardial contractility**, which together reduce cardiac output.

Since mean BP equals cardiac output × peripheral resistance, these changes return the raised arterial pressure towards normal (Figure 16.1). The baroreflex is thus a buffer against acute changes in BP. The buffering process is rapid; the latency between baroreceptor stimulation and the onset of bradycardia is only 0.5 s, and the latency for vascular dilatation is ~1.5 s.

Knowledge of the carotid sinus reflex can occasionally be put to practical use in patients experiencing a suspected supraventricular tachycardia. **Massage of the carotid sinus** region, which is located just below the angle of the jaw, stimulates the baroreceptors. The resulting reflex increase in parasympathetic drive to the atrioventricular node can sometimes terminate an atrioventricular nodal re-entrant tachycardia (see Chapter 5).

## Hypovolaemia triggers multiple compensatory reflexes

Acute hypovolaemia is a fall in blood volume, a common cause of which is a serious haemorrhage (Section 18.2). Because this is a common emergency in nature, the reflex responses are important for survival, both clinically and in evolutionary terms. Hypovolaemia reduces the cardiac stroke volume and arterial pulse pressure, and in severe cases it also reduces mean arterial BP. The fall in baroreceptor traffic triggers the following reflex responses:

- Increased cardiac sympathetic activity and reduced vagal parasympathetic activity cause a **tachycardia** and **increased myocardial contractility**. These changes help restore the depressed cardiac output.
- Increased sympathetic vasomotor activity causes **vasoconstriction of peripheral resistance vessels**. The resulting rise in total peripheral resistance helps to maintain the mean arterial pressure. In humans, the splanchnic circulation, kidneys and forearm muscles participate strongly in the carotid sinus reflex, the skin to a lesser degree.
- Increased sympathetic vasomotor activity also causes **splanchnic venoconstriction**, which displaces blood from the gut and liver into the central veins (Figures 14.5 and 14.13). Blood is also displaced from the poorly innervated skeletal muscle veins, because arteriolar contraction reduces local venous pressure (Figure 14.4) and because circulating adrenaline, vasopressin (antidiuretic hormone [ADH]) and angiotensin cause widespread venoconstriction. The displaced venous blood helps to restore the **CVP** and hence stroke volume (Frank–Starling mechanism).
- Increased sympathetic splanchnic nerve activity stimulates **adrenaline secretion** by the adrenal medulla. Adrenaline stimulates the heart and enhances glycogenolysis.
- The sympathetic-induced contraction of precapillary resistance vessels reduces the capillary pressure. This initiates a gradual **osmotic absorption of interstitial fluid**, which partially restores the depleted plasma volume (Figures 11.4 and 11.11b).
- Increased renal sympathetic activity activates the **renin–angiotensin–aldosterone system (RAAS)** (Figure 14.12). The circulating Ang II contributes to the generalized vasoconstriction. The aldosterone promotes

renal salt and water retention, which helps correct the hypovolaemia in the long term.

- Baroreceptor unloading (fall in activity) in primates evokes a reflex rise in **vasopressin (ADH) secretion** from the posterior pituitary gland (Figure 14.11). Vasopressin causes an antidiuresis and boosts the peripheral vasoconstriction.

The baroreflex evoked by acute hypovolaemia thus stimulates the heart, raises peripheral resistance, attenuates the fall in CVP, partially restores plasma volume and promotes renal fluid retention (Section 18.2). Together, these responses support arterial BP and cerebral perfusion. It is estimated that the rise in peripheral resistance accounts for about three-quarters of the initial BP recovery.

## The baroreflex 'gain' and 'setting' can be changed

In animal studies, the operating characteristics of the baroreflex can be assessed by measuring the changes in HR and systemic BP when a vascularly isolated baroreceptor region is distended (Figure 16.4c). In humans, the baroreflex is assessed by measuring the change in HR when arterial BP is raised by intravenous phenylephrine, a vasoconstrictor drug, or by measuring both arterial pressure and HR when the carotid sinus is distended by external suction. Using these techniques, a stimulus–response curve can be plotted to determine the gain and setting of the human baroreflex (Figure 16.7). 'Gain' (**sensitivity**) is the maximum slope of the response curve. Gain is reduced by ageing and chronic hypertension because the distensibility of the artery

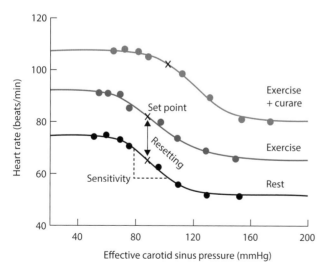

**Figure 16.7** Resetting of the human baroreflex during cycling (red line). The carotid sinus was distended with a suction collar around the neck to evaluate the reflex. 'X' shows the increase in set point during exercise; sensitivity (slope) was unchanged. After partial neuromuscular blockade by curare, a greater central command was needed to achieve the same level of exercise, and this reset the curve further. This shows that central command contributes to exercise resetting. (Based on Gallagher KM, Fadel, PJ, Strømstad M, et al. *The Journal of Physiology* 2001; 533(Pt 3): 861–70, with permission from Wiley-Blackwell.)

wall declines. **Set point** is the pressure that the reflex strives to maintain. This can be altered by neural interactions in the central nervous system (CNS) (central resetting) or by physical changes around the receptor (peripheral resetting), as follows.

## Central resetting

During **exercise**, impulses from the higher regions of the brain (central command), and from afferents in the active muscle, reset the baroreflex to operate around a higher pressure so HR is allowed to increase (Figure 16.7, middle curve). Part of this response is driven by the activity of C-fibres (group III and IV afferents) in muscle that are free nerve endings stimulated by movement itself and the metabolic by-products of contraction. If the muscle afferent input is blocked by epidural anaesthesia, quadriceps exercise induced by electrical stimulation (no central command) no longer resets the baroreflex. The degree of resetting is proportional to work intensity. This allows arterial pressure to rise without evoking a reflex inhibition of HR. The baroreflex is nevertheless active throughout the exercise period, striving to maintain the BP at its new set point. The brain is essential in resetting the exercise baroreflex, because even before the muscle contracts, both HR and arterial BP increase in anticipation of exercise. Moreover, if individuals are totally paralysed (and ventilated) and attempt to contract their muscles, both HR and arterial BP increase proportionally to the mental effort involved (with no feedback from muscle). Neuroimaging studies indicate the insular cortex is a key part of the neurocircuitry in resetting the reflex, because projections from it inhibit cardiac vagal structures via γ-aminobutyric acid (GABA)ergic pathways.

A different form of central modulation occurs with every breath and accounts for **sinus arrhythmia**, the tachycardia associated with each inspiration in humans. The brainstem neurons that drive inspiration also inhibit the cardiac vagal motor neurons, rendering them briefly unresponsive to the baroreceptor input (Figure 16.17). The resulting fall in vagal activity causes a tachycardia during each inspiration.

## Peripheral resetting

If BP is raised for a substantial period, the baroreceptor threshold shifts to a new, higher pressure over hours and days. This causes a rightward shift of the stimulus–response curve and reinstates the receptors on a steep part of the stimulus–response curve, where they operate most effectively, though the resetting is not perfect. Peripheral resetting has the advantage of **extending the range** over which the reflex can operate effectively. Its **disadvantage** is that the baroreceptors cannot inform the brain reliably about absolute BP over extended periods; after peripheral resetting, a high pressure may produce little more baroreceptor traffic than an earlier lower pressure.

The ambiguity of baroreceptor information over extended periods is exacerbated by sympathetic fibres that innervate the carotid sinus and enhance its baroreceptor activity. Because the baroreceptors fail to provide unambiguous information about absolute BP, it is thought that they are not sufficient, unaided, to control BP in the long term. The major role of arterial baro-receptors appears to be the short-term stabilization of BP over seconds to minutes.

## The baroreflex provides short-term homeostasis of blood pressure

When an experimental animal is deprived of its baroreceptor input, its arterial pressure becomes very unstable from minute to minute. For example, in a normal dog walking up a 21-degree incline, BP rises by only ~10 mmHg; however, when the dog is deprived of the baroreflex, the same exercise raises the BP by 50 mmHg (Figure 16.8). The major role of the baroreflex is thus to buffer short-term fluctuations in arterial pressure.

When the baroreceptor nerves of a dog are first cut, the animal becomes very hypertensive for the first few days, but the time-averaged BP then settles down to a level only ~11 mmHg above normal, albeit with fluctuations around the mean over a wider range than normal (Figure 16.9a). The fact that the average BP settles down to a near-normal level indicates that additional factors help regulate BP in the long term. Nevertheless, the small rise in time-averaged pressure indicates that arterial baroreceptors make some long-term contribution to BP regulation, despite partial resetting.

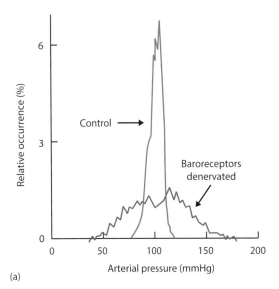

(a)

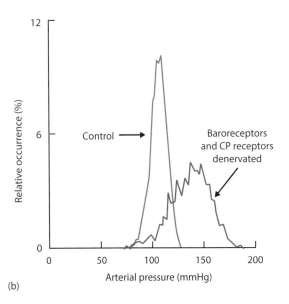

(b)

**Figure 16.9** Contribution of baroreceptors to arterial pressure level and stability. (**a**) In a normal dog, range of arterial pressure over time was narrow (control). A few days after chronic arterial baroreceptor denervation, mean pressure was only moderately raised, but the fluctuations about the mean increased markedly; that is, pressure was less stable. (**b**) After denervation of the cardiopulmonary receptors (CP) as well as arterial baroreceptors, there was a marked rise in mean pressure, as well as pressure instability. (a: From Cowley AW Jr, Liard JF, Guyton AC. *Circulation Research* 1973; 32(5): 564–76; b: Persson PB, Ehmke H, Kirchheim HR. *News in Physiological Sciences* 1989; 4: 56–9, by permission.)

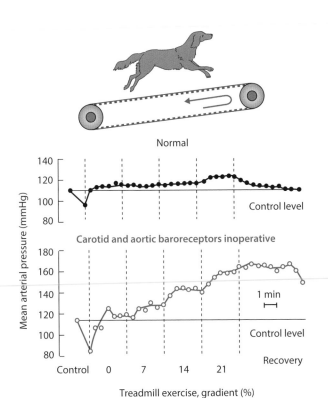

**Figure 16.8** A dog walking up an increasingly steep slope normally experiences only a small rise in arterial pressure (mean increase 12 mmHg). After elimination of the carotid sinus and aortic arch reflexes, exercise caused much bigger increases in pressure (mean 51 mmHg). (Data from Walgenbach SC, Donald DE. *Circulation Research* 1983; 52(3): 253–62.)

## 16.3 RECEPTORS IN THE HEART AND PULMONARY ARTERIES

The heart and pulmonary artery are richly innervated by afferent fibres (Figure 16.10), 80% of which are small-diameter, unmyelinated fibres. These afferent fibres mediate a variety of reflexes via feedback loops which influence the behaviour of the

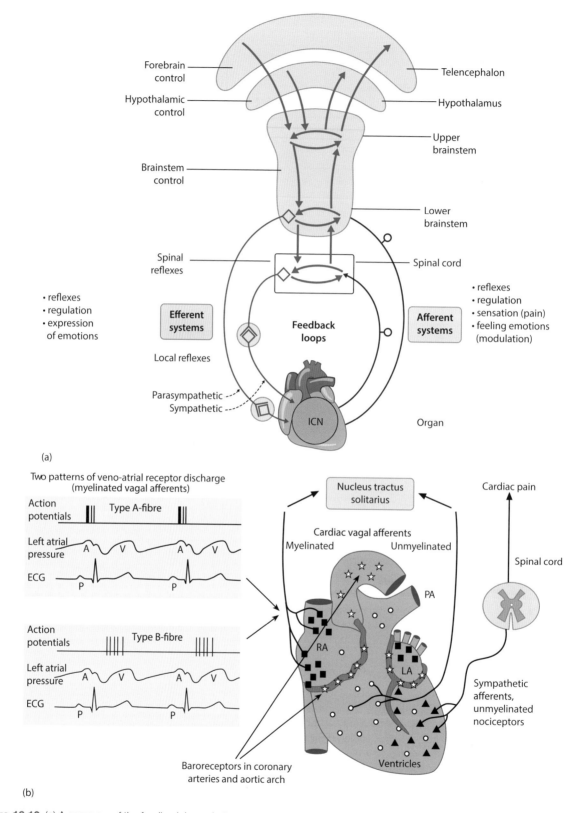

(a)

(b)

**Figure 16.10** (**a**) A summary of the feedback loops between sensory afferent fibres (in blue) and the autonomic efferent fibres (in red) which modulate the intrinsic cardiac nervous system (ICN) as described in Chapter 4.4. Note that the feedback loops can be local and intrinsic to the heart, at the level of the spinal cord, or brainstem. These are modulated by ascending and descending neural signalling from the fore-brain, hypothalamus and brainstem. (Modified from Fukuda K, Kanazawa H, Aizawa Y, et al. *Circulation Research* 2015; 116(12): 2005–19.) (**b**) Distribution of cardiopulmonary afferent endings. Squares, myelinated veno-atrial stretch receptors; circles, unmyelinated mechano-receptors; stars, arterial baroreceptors; triangles, nociceptive chemosensors; RA and LA, right and left atria, respectively; PA, pulmonary artery. Recordings of veno-atrial receptor activity in dogs are shown on the left. (Based on Kappagoda CT, Linden RJ, Sivananthan N. *The Journal of Physiology* 1979; 291: 393–412, with permission from Wiley-Blackwell.)

intrinsic cardiac nervous system (see Chapter 4, Section 4.4). The cardiopulmonary afferents fall into four main categories:

1. **Ventricular chemosensors** mediate cardiac pain and make up most of the non-myelinated afferents. They travel in the cardiac sympathetic nerves and vagi, which are 'mixed nerves', that is, they carry both motor and sensory fibres.
2. **Myelinated veno-atrial mechanoreceptors** are mechanoreceptors distributed around the right and left veno-atrial junctions, served by myelinated vagal afferent fibres. They signal central blood volume.
3. **Non-myelinated cardiac mechanoreceptors** are mechanoreceptors in the ventricles, atria and pulmonary artery served by non-myelinated fibres. They travel in both the vagus and cardiac sympathetic nerves.
4. **Coronary artery baroreceptors** function much like other arterial baroreceptors and travel in the vagi. Their reflex potency is several times greater than that of left ventricular mechanoreceptors.

Cardiac deafferentation studies show that the cardiopulmonary afferents have a net tonic inhibitory effect on HR and peripheral vascular tone, similar to arterial baroreceptors. Thus, the non-selective stimulation of the cardiac receptors by intracoronary injections of veratridine causes a reflex bradycardia, vasodilatation and hypotension (Bezold–Jarisch reflex). However, this kind of mass unphysiological stimulation obscures the fact that the different receptors can elicit different reflexes.

## Ventricular chemosensitive fibres mediate ischaemic heart pain

Most unmyelinated, left ventricular fibre endings are chemosensitive. They can be activated by adenosine, bradykinin, prostaglandins, histamine, 5-hydroxytryptamine (serotonin), platelet-released thromboxane, lactic acid, $K^+$ ions and reactive $O_2$ species. These are substances released by ischaemic myocytes. The axons, mainly C-fibres and some A delta (A$\delta$) fibres, travel in the cardiac sympathetic nerves and vagi. The chemosensitive sympathetic fibres are known to mediate the pain of angina and heart attacks, since surgical interruption of the pathway relieves chronic ischaemic cardiac pain in >80% of cases. The sympathetic afferents ascend the spinal cord in the cervical spinothalamic tract, where there is **convergence** with somatic afferents, that is to say, a neuron receives inputs from both the cardiac nociceptors and somatic afferents. This is probably why cardiac pain seems to emanate from the chest wall, shoulders and arms (**referred pain**). The excitatory reflex effect is an **increase in sympathetic activity** (which is pro-arrhythmogenic), causing tachycardia and a rise in BP.

## Myelinated veno-atrial stretch receptors monitor atrial filling

Veno-atrial fibres are normally the most active of the non-coronary afferents in animals; human data are lacking.

The receptors are branched, endocardial sprays, resembling arterial baroreceptors, served by large, myelinated vagal afferent fibres. Activity is pulsatile, coinciding with atrial systole (A wave, type A pattern) or atrial filling (V wave, type B pattern), as shown in Figure 16.10b. An increase in **cardiac blood volume** stretches the veno-atrial receptors and increases the discharge frequency. Thus, veno-atrial receptors transmit information about CVP and cardiac filling. When stimulated experimentally, by inflating a small balloon at the veno-atrial junction, two reflexes are elicited, namely tachycardia and diuresis (increased urine production).

The **tachycardia** is mediated, unusually, by a selective increase in sympathetic drive to the pacemaker with no fall in vagal parasympathetic activity. The tachycardia shifts blood from the congested venous system into the arterial system. The '**Bainbridge reflex**', discovered in 1915 by Francis Arthur Bainbridge, is a tachycardia induced by the rapid infusion of a large volume of saline into the venous system. The response is mediated partly by the veno-atrial stretch receptors and partly by pacemaker distension.

The **diuresis** and natriuresis (increased salt excretion) establish a negative feedback loop that helps to regulate plasma volume and hence atrial distension. The diuresis is brought about partly by a fall in sympathetic nerve activity specifically to the kidneys (not to other tissues), causing renal vasodilatation, and partly by changes in the circulating levels of vasopressin (ADH), angiotensin II, aldosterone and atrial natriuretic peptide (ANP).

## Unmyelinated cardiac mechanoreceptors signal overdistension

A minority of small-diameter, unmyelinated cardiac fibres are mechanoreceptors, located in the left ventricle and atria. The activity of the unmyelinated left ventricular mechanoreceptors is weak unless the heart is distended. Similarly, unmyelinated atrial mechanoreceptors fire only when atrial filling is at its highest, for example, during the V wave of inspiration. Like the baroreceptors, the unmyelinated cardiac mechanoreceptors elicit a depressor reflex, that is, bradycardia and peripheral vasodilatation. In laboratory animals, the reflex is weak and probably of little importance, but the situation may be different in humans, as described next.

## 16.4 REFLEXES FROM CARDIAC RECEPTORS IN HUMANS

Most of our knowledge of cardiac mechanoreceptors and reflexes comes of necessity from laboratory animals. In humans, cardiac transplantation involves some afferent denervation, and reflex studies in these patients indicate that humans also possess **central volume receptors** (atrial stretch receptors and left ventricular mechanoreceptors).

## Cardiac volume receptors reflexly regulate peripheral vascular tone in humans

Raising the legs above heart level increases intrathoracic venous pressure and central blood volume, with little rise in arterial pressure. This elicits a graded reflex vasodilatation in the skin and skeletal muscle (Figure 16.11). Conversely, if central blood volume is reduced by applying suction to the lower body in a sealed container, there is reflex vasoconstriction in the muscle and splanchnic circulations, a rise in circulating noradrenaline and stimulation of the RAAS. This occurs even when the lower body negative pressure is so mild that arterial pressure does not change detectably, thus excluding the baroreflex. Moreover, the reflex is greatly attenuated in **cardiac transplant patients with denervated ventricles**, indicating that human left ventricular mechanoreceptors may be important in the reflex regulation of peripheral vascular tone (cf. minor role in laboratory animals).

## Cardiac and arterial receptors reflexly influence the renal regulation of extracellular fluid volume

Plasma is the only component of extracellular fluid whose volume and pressure are sensed, and the cardiovascular sensors initiate reflexes to maintain a normal extracellular fluid volume. The cardiopulmonary stretch receptors and arterial

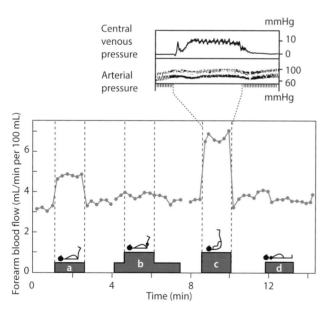

**Figure 16.11** Reflex vasodilatation in human forearm muscle evoked by a rise in intrathoracic blood volume. (**a**) Intrathoracic blood volume increased by raising the legs. (**b**) Legs raised but pneumatic cuff around thigh at 180 mmHg prevented translocation of blood into the thorax; no change in forearm perfusion. (**c**) Legs and lower trunk elevated, to raise central venous pressure further (inset). This increased the reflex vasodilatation. (**d**) Pneumatic cuff around neck inflated to 30 mmHg to reduce carotid sinus distension; very little reflex change in forearm blood flow. (From Roddie IC, Shepherd JT, Whelan RF. *The Journal of Physiology* 1957; 139(3): 369–76, with permission from Wiley-Blackwell.)

baroreceptors can be stimulated experimentally by immersing a human feet-down in water; the water pressure displaces ~700 mL blood into the thorax (Figure 8.24), which distends the heart by ~180 mL in diastole and raises arterial BP by ~10 mmHg. These stimuli elicit a substantial diuresis, which helps reduce the raised filling pressures and arterial pressure. The diuresis is mediated by **renal vasodilatation** (selective inhibition of renal sympathetic activity), reduced **vasopressin**, reduced **RAAS** activation and increased **ANP**. Similarly, astronauts subjected to zero gravity experience a redistribution of venous blood from legs to thorax, provoking a reflex diuresis. When the astronaut returns to earth, the reduced plasma volume, coupled with a weakened baroreflex, causes orthostatic intolerance (postural hypotension). It is clear from these examples that cardiovascular receptors influence renal fluid excretion to maintain a normal cardiac filling pressure and arterial pressure. This link is important for the long-term regulation of BP, as described next.

## 16.5 LONG-TERM REGULATION OF ARTERIAL BLOOD PRESSURE: THE KIDNEY LINK

As indicated earlier, the arterial baroreflex is primarily a short-term buffer of arterial BP, effective over seconds to minutes. The preservation of a normal, time-averaged BP over longer periods – days and weeks – also requires the maintenance of a normal blood volume, because blood volume influences cardiac filling pressure and output (Frank–Starling mechanism), and hence arterial BP (equation 8.5). Blood comprises mainly red cells and plasma, both of which are influenced by the kidneys. Consequently, **the kidneys are crucial to long-term BP regulation**, as illustrated in Figure 16.12. For example, when renal function is manipulated in a dog to raise the extracellular salt mass, the plasma volume and time-averaged arterial BP likewise increase, in direct proportion to the increase in body salt and water masses.

To regulate **red cell mass**, the kidneys secrete a haemopoietic hormone, **erythropoietin**. To regulate **plasma volume**, the kidneys adjust the rate of **excretion of salt** via RAAS (Figure 14.12). The extracellular water mass closely matches the extracellular $Na^+$ mass because the osmoreceptor–vasopressin system preserves isotonicity (Figure 14.11). Plasma is, of course, part of the extracellular fluid compartment. In **Addison's disease**, where adrenal failure reduces the concentration of circulating aldosterone, $Na^+$ loss results in a reduced extracellular fluid volume, leading to life-threatening hypotension.

Through what mechanisms is the kidney informed of the state of the circulation? The mechanisms fall into two classes: (1) cardiac stretch receptors and arterial baroreceptors monitor central blood volume and arterial BP, and reflexly regulate the secretion of **hormones** controlling renal function; (2) arterial pressure also affects renal excretion directly, by a process termed **pressure natriuresis**.

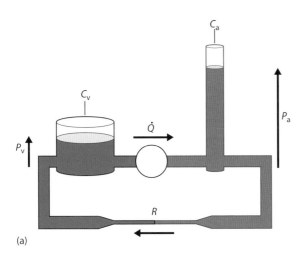

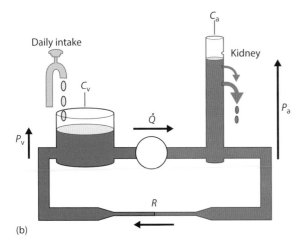

**Figure 16.12 (a)** Representation of the circulation in which the heart and lungs are represented by a circular pump generating a cardiac output ($\dot{Q}$), the veins and arteries are represented by open reservoirs of fluid and the peripheral resistance by a single tube (*R*). The heights of the reservoirs respectively represent venous pressure ($P_v$) and arterial pressure ($P_a$), while the compliance of the veins ($C_v$) and arteries ($C_a$) are represented by the cross-sectional area of the reservoirs. **(b)** The open circulation in which, over long periods of time, mean arterial pressure ($P_a$) is independent of cardiac output ($\dot{Q}$) and peripheral resistance (*R*). $P_a$ depends instead on the kidney and daily intake. The daily intake is represented by a tap pouring liquid into the venous reservoir. The kidney is presented as a series of holes in the arterial reservoir, by which fluid leaves the circulation under the influence of gravity. The distribution of holes can be modified to represent the pressure-natriuresis relationship. (Modified from Dorrington KL, Pandit JJ. *Anaesthesia* 2009; 64(11); 1218–28.)

## Cardiovascular pressure receptors reflexly regulate hormones that act on the nephron

The circulating levels of all the hormones controlling renal salt and water excretion are influenced by cardiovascular receptors, as follows.

The **RAAS**, which promotes salt and water retention, is inhibited by a rise in arterial pressure, partly through renal afferent arteriole sensors and partly through a baroreflex-mediated fall in renal sympathetic activity (Figure 14.12).

RAAS inhibition results in natriuresis and diuresis, which reduces extracellular fluid volume and returns the raised BP to normal. Conversely, if BP falls, RAAS activation promotes salt and water retention, leading to the restoration of the depressed BP.

**ADH** (vasopressin), which promotes water retention, is secreted when plasma osmolarity rises (Figure 14.11). This ensures that water excretion matches $Na^+$ excretion, keeping the plasma isotonic. ADH secretion is also stimulated by a fall in central blood volume and arterial pressure, via reduced arterial baroreceptor traffic in primates, or reduced veno-atrial receptor traffic in other species. The resulting fluid retention helps restore the reduced extracellular fluid volume and BP to normal.

**ANP**, which promotes salt excretion and diuresis, is released in response to atrial distension. This links renal function directly to central blood volume. However, the effect of ANP at physiological concentrations is weak (Section 14.9).

## Pressure natriuresis: a rise in renal arterial pressure directly increases salt and water excretion

Pressure natriuresis is an increase in renal salt and water excretion in response to a rise in renal arterial pressure. A rise in renal arterial pressure has little effect on glomerular capillary pressure or filtration rate, because these parameters are subject to excellent autoregulation. Therefore, the proposed mechanism is that the pressure rises in the renal medullary capillaries, which are thought to be less well autoregulated. A rise in medullary capillary pressure increases the renal interstitial fluid pressure, which impairs the reabsorption of tubular fluid. Thus, a diuresis and natriuresis follow. There is controversy over the importance of pressure natriuresis relative to the powerful RAAS.

The important role of the kidney in setting the arterial BP over periods of time from days to weeks and months can be demonstrated by a model system that compares the behaviour of the cardiovascular system when it contains a fixed volume of fluid with its behaviour when the volume can vary. (Figure 16.12a,b). A circle represents the heart and pulmonary circulation combined, pumping an output of $\dot{Q}$ against a systemic vascular resistance *R*. When circulating volume is fixed, $P_a$ becomes a function of *R*, the ratio of the vascular compliances ($C_v/C_a$, commonly around 10–20), and the Frank–Starling mechanism; the latter is the relationship between $\dot{Q}$ and the filling pressure $P_v$.

Over longer periods, the behaviour of the circulation, when it becomes an open system with intake and output of fluid, is very different indeed (Figure 16.12b). Here, a daily intake of salt and water has eventually to be balanced by an equal output, most of which is via the kidney. The pressure the kidney requires to achieve this output is set by many factors, including the hormones mentioned, the sympathetic nerve supply to the kidney and drugs acting on the kidney, either directly or indirectly. This working pressure is depicted in Figure 16.12b by the position and distribution of the holes in the arterial reservoir, which are set to model the pressure natriuresis behaviour of the kidney. We see now that, in the steady state, $P_a$ becomes entirely independent of $R$, the compliances and even the Frank–Starling mechanism. However, $P_a$ can depend on the daily salt and water intake in some cases, as you can imagine from the behaviour of the holes representing the kidney function. The conclusion that, over a long period, $P_a$ is independent of $R$ and the Frank–Starling mechanism can come as a bit of a surprise to many readers, but is entirely in keeping with all realistic models of the circulation from Guyton's model in the 1970s, to complex computer models of the present day. All are based on the requirement of mass balance: 'what goes in must come out', and the kidney, the main route out, requires a pressure to do its work that becomes $P_a$ when the system is in equilibrium. Of course, this is a physical model based on linearity that does not model the non-linear dynamics of the physiology. In particular, neurohumoral balance must also be considered. Cardiac stretch receptors and baroreceptors monitor central blood volume and arterial BP, and reflexly regulate the secretion of hormones controlling renal function. In addition, the CNS integrates these afferent inputs and may determine the baseline secretion of these hormones. Some cases of hypertension may therefore be neurally mediated; as hypertension progresses to diastolic and then systolic heart failure, the neurohumoral balance is dramatically changed. For example, RAAS and brain natriuretic peptide levels are raised affecting the kidney, heart and autonomic nervous system (see Chapter 18).

## Renal pressure natriuresis with neural control of circulating hormones together underpin long-term pressure homeostasis

To summarize, cardiac mechanoreceptors and arterial baroreceptors regulate the levels of circulating angiotensin, aldosterone, vasopressin and ANP, which in turn regulate renal salt and water excretion, and hence plasma volume. Thus, **cardiovascular receptors and their neural pathways, aided by renal pressure natriuresis, are important for the long-term regulation of mean BP**. If the input from one group of receptors alone is interrupted, BP rises only a little in the long term (Figure 16.9a). This is fortunate for patients with transplanted hearts, who lose their ventricular mechanoreceptor input but have little problem regulating their BP. Evidently, one group of receptors can largely compensate for lack of the other group. This illustrates the Comroe's principle: if a job is worth doing, the body has more than one way of doing it! If both the cardiac and arterial receptors are denervated, there is a sustained elevation of renin–angiotensin–aldosterone levels and sustained hypertension (Figure 16.9b).

---

**CONCEPT BOX 16.1**

### REGULATION OF ARTERIAL BLOOD PRESSURE

- In the short term, mean arterial pressure is determined by total peripheral resistance and cardiac output. The arterial baroreflex adjusts both determinants to stabilize the arterial pressure over seconds to minutes.
- A rise in arterial pressure stimulates the arterial baroreceptors. This evokes a reflex fall in sympathetic outflow and rise in cardiac vagal parasympathetic outflow. The ensuing peripheral vasodilatation and bradycardia lower the raised arterial pressure, returning it to its set point (depressor reflex).
- Conversely, hypovolaemia unloads the baroreceptors, leading to a reflex rise in sympathetic outflow, which helps maintain BP.
- The set point of the baroreflex can be raised by central command and muscle afferents (metaboreceptors). This raises BP during exercise.
- In the longer term, BP homeostasis depends on the renal regulation of extracellular fluid volume. Renal excretion is enslaved to BP through two kinds of mechanism: (1) the circulating level of excretion-regulating hormones (vasopressin, angiotensin II, aldosterone, ANP) is controlled by cardiovascular receptors; (2) pressure natriuresis causes an increase in salt and water excretion when renal artery pressure rises.

---

## 16.6 EXCITATORY INPUTS: MUSCLE WORK RECEPTORS, ARTERIAL CHEMORECEPTORS, LUNG STRETCH RECEPTORS

As well as depressor reflexes to stabilize arterial BP, there are excitatory reflexes that help stimulate the cardiovascular system during challenges such as exercise and hypoxia. Excitatory reflexes raise BP (pressor reflexes) and are initiated by several classes of sensory receptor:

- muscle work receptors (metaboreceptors and mechanoreceptors);
- arterial chemoreceptors;
- lung stretch receptors;
- the external senses.

## Work receptors in skeletal muscle help drive the exercise pressor response and tachycardia

During exercise, arterial BP rises and HR increases. These changes are driven predominantly by 'central command' from the cortical-subcortical networks (premotor areas linked to the subthalamic nucleus and periaqueductal grey [PAG] matter), and partly by a reflex from work-activated receptors in skeletal muscle, that is, C-fibre nerve endings activated by muscle contraction (excluding muscle spindles, which do not contribute to cardiovascular control). There are two types of work receptor, the mechnoreceptor (group III) and the chemosensitive (metaboreceptor, group IV). The role of the peripheral reflex (i.e. exercise pressor reflex) becomes increasingly important during isometric or static muscle contractions compared to dynamic exercise.

**Muscle mechanoreceptors** are stimulated by local pressure and muscle contraction, and are served mainly by small, myelinated axons (group III). They modestly influence HR. The reflex effect is to **inhibit cardiac vagal tone**, which helps increase HR quickly in the first few seconds of exercise, complementing the central command (Figure 16.13).

**Muscle metaboreceptors** are chemosensitive endings of unmyelinated group IV axons (mainly). They reflexly **increase sympathetic vasomotor activity** and thus contribute to the exercise pressor response. They also boost cardiac contractility at high levels of activation. The human muscle metaboreflex was demonstrated in a simple, ingenious experiment by Alam and Smirk, in 1937 (Figure 16.14). The participant performed a forearm exercise and, just before the end of the exercise, a pneumatic cuff was inflated around the upper arm to trap local chemical stimulants in the forearm. The exercise pressor response (though not the tachycardia) was then partly maintained after the active exercise finished, and only subsided fully when the cuff was released.

Metaboreceptors are activated by numerous chemicals released by contracting muscle fibres (adenosine triphosphate (ATP), $K^+$, $H_2PO_4^-$, prostaglandin E2, bradykinin, 20-hydroxyeicosatetraenoic acid and, to a lesser degree, adenosine and lactic acid acting on acid-sensing ion channels). These agents accumulate to higher levels during **isometric (static) exercise** than dynamic exercise, because an isometric contraction restricts local blood flow (Section 15.2). Consequently, metaboreceptors act as **sensors of underperfusion**; that is, they sense a mismatch between $O_2$ supply and demand, and they cause BP to rise much higher during isometric than dynamic exercise (Figure 17.6). Underperfusion is higher in patients with heart failure, presumably due to impaired muscle perfusion. The reflex, sympathetic-mediated peripheral vasoconstriction raises arterial BP without impeding flow in the active muscle itself, because metabolic vasodilatation predominates locally (Section 15.2). The rise in arterial pressure is particularly advantageous in isometric exercise because it helps counteract the maintained compression of the intramuscular blood vessel by contracted muscle. In this way, the pressor reflex can maintain muscle perfusion at isometric contractions up to 50% of maximum voluntary contraction. However, more forceful contractions impede the local perfusion. This type of exercise increases muscle discomfort and is painful if sustained; therefore, it should come as no surprise that C-fibres also transduce nociception. These afferents synapse into the nucleus tractus solitarius. They also connect to the lateral PAG matter, which is a major centre for the integration of both pain and sympathetic outflow. Neurosurgical techniques in awake humans during activation of the muscle pressor reflex, has shown that the PAG matter is a major integrator of the exercise pressor reflex.

In human studies, both metaboreceptors and mechanoreceptors can be blocked by a local anaesthetic (epidural anaesthesia), while essentially preserving motor axon function. This markedly reduces the exercise pressor response, but does

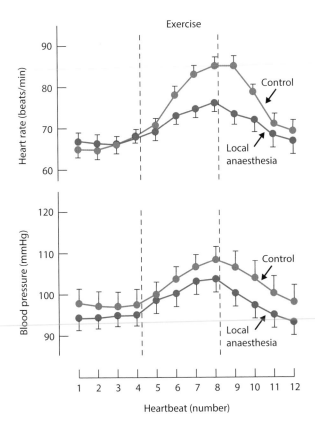

**Figure 16.13** Evidence that a reflex from muscle work receptors (mechanoreceptors and metaboreceptors) contributes to exercise tachycardia and the exercise pressor response in humans. The response to 4 s of maximal voluntary handgrip was attenuated when muscle afferent traffic was blocked by local anaesthesia of the axillary and radial nerves, leaving motor function unimpaired. Note the rapidity with which the heart responds at the onset of exercise. (From Lassen A, Mitchell JH, Reeves DR Jr, et al. *The Journal of Physiology* 1989; 409: 333–41, with permission from Wiley-Blackwell.)

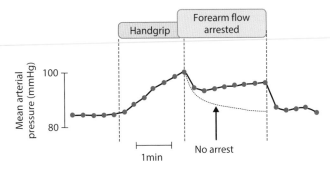

**Figure 16.14** Evidence that human muscle metaboreceptors contribute to the exercise pressor response. Isometric handgrip raises blood pressure. If blood is then trapped in the exercised arm by inflating a brachial cuff to suprasystolic pressure, the exercise pressor response is partly maintained, until the cuff is released. (Data from Rusch NJ, Shepherd JT, Webb RC, et al. *Circulation Research* 1981; 48(6 Pt 2): 118–30, by permission.)

not abolish the overall blood pressure response completely (Figure 16.13) illustrating the importance of both central command and peripheral reflex control. However, this experiment is difficult to interpret because epidural anaesthesia also decreases sympathetic efferent drive to muscle, causing vasodilatation as sympathetic vasoconstrictor tone is lost (the legs feel warm).

## The arterial chemoreflex supports blood pressure during asphyxia and clinical shock

Arterial chemoreceptors monitor respiratory gas levels, being stimulated by arterial hypoxaemia (low), hypercapnia (high), acidosis and hyperkalaemia. They are located mainly in the **carotid bodies** (not the carotid sinus) and the **aortic bodies**, small, highly vascularized nodules adjacent to the carotid sinus and aorta (Figure 16.2). The carotid bodies have such an extremely high blood flow, 20 mL/g/min, that the venous blood has near-arterial gas levels. The aortic bodies have a somewhat lower blood flow and their chemoreceptors can be stimulated by hypotension and anaemia, as well as changes in blood chemistry. The chemoreceptor afferent fibres travel in the ninth and tenth cranial nerves (glossopharyngeal and vagus), along with the baroreceptor afferents.

The arterial chemoreceptors normally regulate alveolar ventilation, but they also drive important circulatory reflexes during **asphyxia** (hypoxia plus hypercapnia) and **clinical shock**. The arterial chemoreflex elicits the following cardiovascular changes:

1. **Peripheral resistance increases** because of a reflex increase in peripheral sympathetic vasomotor drive to skeletal muscle, renal and splanchnic vascular beds.
2. **Splanchnic veins constrict** because of a reflex increase in sympathetic activity. This helps support CVP and hence stroke volume.
3. **BP rises**, due to the previous two effects.
4. **Tachycardia** is an indirect consequence of the increased breathing. If chemoreceptors are stimulated during artificial ventilation at a fixed rate, the chemoreflex actually elicits a moderate **bradycardia**. However, when an individual breathes spontaneously the chemoreflex stimulates deeper, more rapid breathing, and this stimulates stretch receptors within the lungs. These evoke a **lung inflation reflex**, which causes a marked tachycardia, overriding the moderate chemoreflex bradycardia.

The cardiovascular effects of the arterial chemoreflex are particularly important in the following situations:

- **Asphyxia** (concomitant hypoxaemia and hypercapnia) stimulates arterial chemoreceptors very strongly, causing a reflex rise in sympathetic activity and BP. The latter, along with the hypercapnic vasodilatation of the cerebral circulation, raises cerebral perfusion and hence $O_2$ delivery (Figure 15.13). In **obstructive sleep apnoea**, repeated episodes of airway blockage trigger chemoreflex-mediated episodes of nocturnal hypertension.
- **Clinical shock** is a syndrome (group of signs and symptoms, see Section 18.2) resulting from hypovolaemia (e.g. severe haemorrhage), hypotension and circulatory failure. Carotid and aortic body perfusion falls during clinical shock, with particularly marked effects on the less vascular aortic bodies. The chemoreceptors are excited by the resulting 'stagnant hypoxia', and by the arterial metabolic acidosis of clinical shock (Figure 18.3). The chemoreflex drives the **rapid breathing** of patients in hypotensive shock, and raises sympathetic vasomotor activity to increase **peripheral resistance** and support arterial BP. This is particularly **important when BP falls below the operating range of the baroreflex**. Most baroreceptor fibres fall silent below ~70 mmHg, whereas arterial chemoreceptor activity continues to increase at pressures <70 mmHg. The importance of the chemoreflex during severe haemorrhage has been confirmed experimentally in dogs; cutting the chemoreceptor nerves caused a sharp fall in BP and large increase in mortality rate.
- **Hypertension**. Emerging evidence indicates that arterial chemoreceptor denervation can reduce BP. It is possible that a dysfunctional arterial chemoreflex may contribute to some cases of essential hypertension (see Chapter 18, Section 18.4), since hypoxia activates the sympathetic nervous system.
- **The diving reflex**. The important contribution of arterial chemoreceptors to the bradycardia and peripheral vasoconstriction of diving is described in Section 17.6.

## Lung stretch receptors cause reflex tachycardia

The lung mechanoreceptors are excited by inspiration. Their afferent fibres inhibit the cardiac vagal parasympathetic neurons in the brainstem and thus cause a reflex tachycardia, for example, during **asphyxia**. The lung mechanoreceptor reflex is powerfully reinforced by inspiratory neurons in the brainstem, which likewise inhibit the cardiac vagal neurons. Consequently, each inspiration is associated with both reflex and central inhibition of the cardiac vagal neurons. This causes **sinus arrhythmia**, a regular increase in human HR during the inspiration phase of breathing. A sudden, deep inspiration also elicits a reflex vaso- and venoconstriction in human skin, called the **inspiratory gasp reflex** (Figure 14.14), a convenient reflex for testing human sympathetic function.

## External sensory receptors can affect heart rate and blood pressure

Cardiovascular responses are often evoked by receptors not concerned primarily with cardiovascular control. **Somatic pain** causes tachycardia and hypertension. Severe **visceral** pain causes bradycardia, hypotension and even fainting. **Ambient cold** causes a rise in BP, which increases left ventricular work and can trigger angina in susceptible patients. The **special senses** can also influence the cardiovascular system. The alerting response, for example, to a sudden loud noise or the sight of a charging bull, produces a brisk tachycardia. Sexual stimulation evokes tachycardia and hypertension (Figure 8.13). Stimulation of facial receptors by cold water elicits a strong bradycardia (diving reflex, Section 17.6).

## 16.7 CENTRAL PATHWAYS: ROLE OF THE MEDULLA OBLONGATA

In 1852, the celebrated French physiologist, Claude Bernard, reported that transection of the cervical spinal cord causes a peripheral vasodilatation and an abrupt fall in BP to ~40 mmHg. This shows that the normal, tonic activity of the sympathetic vasomotor fibres and their spinal neurons depends on a tonic, net excitatory drive from the brain (Figure 14.1). This presympathetic excitatory drive comes from the medulla oblongata, the most caudal (tail end) part of the brainstem (Figure 16.15). However, the medulla is by no means the only region involved in cardiovascular regulation. The hypothalamus, limbic system, PAG matter, cerebellum and cerebral cortex all play a role, though the pathways are as yet incompletely understood.

The traditional notion that the medulla has a dorsal 'vasomotor centre' is no longer tenable. The modern view emphasizes transverse traffic between a number of different regions of the medulla, and up-and-down traffic between the medulla and higher regions, as follows.

## The nucleus tractus solitarius receives and integrates all cardiovascular receptor traffic

The dorsomedial region of the medulla contains an elongated grouping of neurons called the **nucleus tractus solitarius (NTS)** (Figures 16.15 and 16.16). Virtually all the cardiovascular afferents – baroreceptors, cardiopulmonary afferents, muscle mechano- and metaboreceptors, arterial chemoreceptors and pulmonary stretch receptors – terminate in the NTS. Consequently, destruction of this nucleus causes a sustained hypertension. Muscle work receptors also project to the lateral reticular nucleus and to the PAG matter of the pons (midbrain), which are regions that help organize the exercise pressor response.

The processing of sensory information begins in the NTS. An individual neuron receives many different inputs, so its output is influenced by many different signals. This is called **sensory integration**. The integrated information is then **relayed** by NTS neurons to other regions, as follows.

## Nucleus tractus solitarius relays integrated, afferent information to other regions

The NTS relays information to the hypothalamus, cerebellum and other parts of the medulla (Figure 16.15). Within the medulla, a polysynaptic path projects to the **nucleus ambiguus**, which contains the vagal cardiac motor neurons. Another path projects to the **caudal vasodepressor area of the medulla**, located in the caudal ventrolateral medulla (CVLM), which influences sympathetic output (Figure 16.16). The **hypothalamus** receives projections to the vasopressin-producing **magnocellular neurons** of the supraoptic and paraventricular

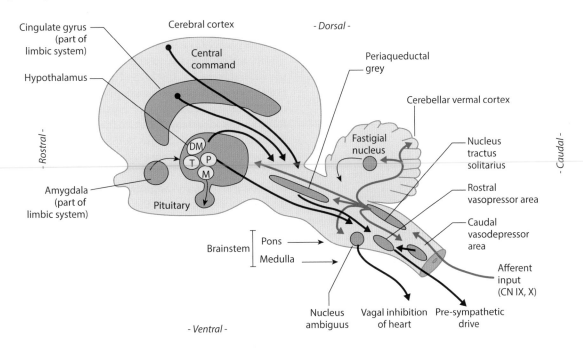

**Figure 16.15** Longitudinal pathways mediating cardiovascular regulation in cat brain. DM, dorsomedial nucleus and perifornical hypothalamus (alerting response); M, magnocellular neurons of supraoptic and paraventricular hypothalamic nuclei (synthesize vasopressin); P, parvocellular neurons of paraventricular nucleus (modulate sympathetic activity); T, temperature-regulating centre, anterior hypothalamus.

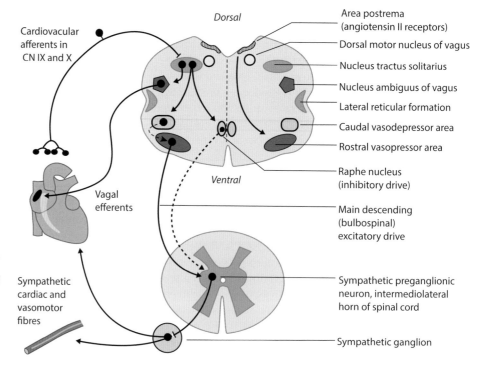

**Figure 16.16** Schematic transverse section through the medulla, showing reflex pathways and relative positions of cardio-vascular nuclei in the dorsoventral plane. Dashed lines indicate inhibitory pathways. The various neuron groups occur at different rostrocaudal levels, so in reality they would not all be seen in a single anatomical section.

nuclei, and to the sympathetic-regulating **parvocellular neurons of the paraventricular nucleus** (Figure 16.15). The **cerebellum** receives projections to the **fastigial nuclei** and **vermal cortex**, which are important during exercise.

## The nucleus ambiguus generates tonic vagal parasympathetic outflow to the heart

The cell bodies of the vagal parasympathetic fibres controlling the HR are located chiefly in the **nucleus ambiguus** of the brainstem, and to a lesser extent in the dorsal motor nucleus (Figures 16.15 and 16.16). These vagal nuclei used to be known collectively as the 'cardioinhibitory centre'. Their activity is regulated by inputs from the NTS, the inspiratory neurons and the hypothalamus.

## The rostral vasopressor area generates a tonic pre-sympathetic outflow to the spinal cord

If the anaesthetic pentobarbitone is applied to the surface of the **rostral ventrolateral medulla (RVLM)**, there is a sharp fall in BP, similar to that produced by cervical cord transection. Conversely, stimulation of this area raises BP. These observations revealed a zone of tonically active vasomotor neurons, the **rostral vasopressor area**. The neurons are glutaminergic (excitatory), and ~70% are also adrenergic (C1 neurons). The vasopressor neurons may be organized organotopically, with some neurons controlling renal sympathetic activity, others controlling the output to the heart, muscle and so on. This allows independent control of

the sympathetic activity to different organs. The vasopressor neurons send **bulbospinal fibres** down the dorsolateral funiculus of the spinal cord to synapse with the barosensitive sympathetic preganglionic neurons of the **thoracic spinal cord**, providing a tonic, excitatory drive (Figure 16.16). (Thermosensitive-type spinal sympathetic neurons, by contrast, are regulated from the hypothalamus via the rostroventral medial medulla (RVMM).) The spinal sympathetic neurons also receive a descending inhibitory input from **raphe nuclei** near the brainstem midline. The raphe nuclei receive an excitatory input from the NTS.

The tonically active, rostral vasopressor neurons are regulated, indirectly, by the NTS. The NTS sends an excitatory projection to the **caudal vasodepressor area** in the **CVLM**, and the caudal vasodepressor area sends a tonically inhibitory input, mediated by GABA, to the rostral vasopressor area, restraining its output (Figure 16.16).

The blood–brain barrier is absent in the **area postrema** on the floor of the fourth ventricle (dorsal surface of medulla). Here, circulating emetics and **angiotensin II** gain access to area postrema neurons, increasing their activity. Projections from the area postrema to the RVLM boost vasomotor presympathetic outflow. Thus, a rise in circulating angiotensin II increases sympathetic vasomotor activity (Figure 14.12). Central angiotensin II also plays a prominent role in the enhanced central sympathetic outflow seen in heart failure. This occurs as a consequence of increased reactive $O_2$ stress, upregulation in glutamate signalling and N-methyl-D-aspartate subtype 1 receptors driving sympathetic outflow from areas such as the paraventricular nucleus. Exercise training attenuates this response, by decreasing angiotensin II signalling and facilitating nitric oxide (NO) activity. This also results in enhanced vagal responsiveness, which protects against the potentially deleterious effect of high sympathetic drive. NO is thought to play a dominant role here as training increases neuronal NO synthase expression. NO bioavailability increases acetylcholine release to facilitate a fast heart recovery on cessation of exercise.

## 16.8 CENTRAL PATHWAYS: ROLE OF HIGHER REGIONS

Many central areas of the brain contribute to a specific, organized cardiovascular response (Figure 16.15). The central long axis of the brain, the limbic system, the hypothalamus, the cerebellum and the cerebral cortex contribute as follows.

### The central long axis organizes the alerting response

'Alerting' is a stereotyped pattern of responses to a sudden, unusual environmental stimulus, such as a sudden noise or danger; this is a vital response for survival in the wild. The alerting response has a behavioural component (head raised, ears pricked in dog and cats) and a cardiovascular component that prepares the animal for action. The alerting response was first described by Cannon in 1929, and is often called the defence or **fight-or-flight response**; however, alerting response seems a better description in humans, because the cardiovascular manifestations can be elicited by quite mild stimuli, such as performing mental arithmetic to the beat of a metronome. The human cardiovascular alerting response is illustrated in Figures 14.7 and 14.14 and comprises:

- **tachycardia** and increased cardiac output;
- **skeletal muscle vasodilatation**;
- sympathetic-mediated **vasoconstriction** of the cutaneous, splanchnic and renal circulations, along with cutaneous venoconstriction;
- **a rise in BP**, accompanied by central inhibition of the baroreflex.

The vasodilatation in skeletal muscle is mediated partly by circulating adrenaline, partly by reduced sympathetic vasoconstrictor activity to the muscle, and in many non-primates by sympathetic cholinergic nerves (Section 14.3).

Brain stimulation experiments show that the alerting response is generated by an extensive system of neurons distributed along the **central long axis** of the brain. The neurons are located in three zones: the amygdala, which is part of the **limbic system** (the generator of emotional behaviour patterns); the dorsomedial/perifornical region of the **hypothalamus**; and the **PAG matter** of the pons (Figure 16.15). Electrical stimulation of the PAG matter evokes characteristic cardiac and vasomotor alerting responses and also, in conscious animals, the behavioural manifestations of fear and rage, such as spitting, snarling and piloerection. The central long axis is itself influenced by inputs from the cortex. The output of the

central long axis modulates the NTS, cardiac vagal motor neurons and rostral vasopressor neurons to produce the characteristic tachycardia and increased BP of the alerting responses.

Hypertensive humans show greater renal vasoconstriction to mental stress test than normal individuals, and less habituation to repeated stress. This led to the suggestion that an overdeveloped alerting response may contribute to the development of some forms of clinical hypertension (neurogenic hypertension).

### The limbic system also co-ordinates the 'playing dead' response

The opossum, famously, and many other young creatures play dead when faced with danger. This entails a profound **bradycardia** and **hypotension**, and as such is the opposite of the alerting response. The response originates in the **cingulate gyrus of the limbic system** (Figure 16.15). It is thought that **human emotional fainting** in response to an intolerable psychological stimulus ('swooning') is a manifestation of the same response, namely the avoidance of a threatening situation by collapse (see Chapter 18).

### The hypothalamus influences temperature control, vasopressin secretion, the baroreflex and sympathetic outflow

In addition to the dorsomedial nucleus and adjacent perifornical region of the hypothalamus (see 'alerting response' described earlier), several other parts of the hypothalamus contribute to cardiovascular regulation, including:

- the temperature-regulating area;
- vasopressin-secreting magnocellular neurons; and
- sympathetic-regulating parvocellular neurons in the paraventricular nuclei (Figure 16.15).

The **temperature-regulating area** in the anterior hypothalamus receives information from peripheral and core temperature receptors. Its output controls the sympathetic vasodilator and sudomotor outflow to skin (Section 15.3), partly via the RVMM neurons.

The **magnocellular neurons** in the supraoptic and paraventricular nuclei synthesize vasopressin. They have two main inputs: baroreceptor information, transmitted by the NTS–CVLM pathway; and osmolarity information transmitted by local osmoreceptors (Figure 14.11). The magnocellular neurons respond with appropriate changes in vasopressin output via the pituitary gland.

The **paraventricular nucleus** contains not only magnocellular neurons but also small, glutaminergic **parvocellular neurons**, which regulate sympathetic activity. Baroreceptor and veno-atrial receptor information is relayed to the parvocellular neurons by the NTS. The parvocellular neurons project to the RVLM and spinal cord to modulate sympathetic outflow. For example, increased parvocellular neuron activity in heart failure contributes to the excessive renal and cardiac sympathetic activity, which in turn contributes substantially to the pathophysiology. Parvocellular neurons also mediate the selective activation of renal sympathetic fibres by veno-atrial volume receptors.

## The cerebellum co-ordinates cardiovascular changes during exercise

The main function of the cerebellum is to co-ordinate movement; it also co-ordinates the cardiovascular changes of exercise. Muscle afferents relay in the lateral reticular nucleus, which projects to the cerebellar fastigial nucleus and the associated vermal cortex, as does the NTS (Figures 16.15 and 16.18). Destruction of the fastigial nucleus reduces the tachycardia and pressor response to exercise in dogs. Stimulation of the vermal cortex in laboratory animals elicits renal vasoconstriction and muscle vasodilatation, the characteristic pattern observed during exercise. Such observations indicate that projections from the cerebellum to the medullary cardiovascular areas help co-ordinate the cardiovascular response to exercise.

## The cerebral cortex provides 'central command' during exercise

To explain the rapid onset of the cardiovascular response to exercise, Krogh and Lindhard (1913) postulated that the cerebral cortex not only initiates muscular exercise, but also initiates cardiovascular responses through 'cortical irradiation' to the brainstem (Figure 16.15). This is now called the central command hypothesis. The hypothesis is supported by the finding that electrical stimulation of several areas of cerebral cortex, including the prefrontal, insular and cingulate cortices, elicits multiple cardiovascular changes. Moreover, if the arm muscles are paralysed by anaesthetizing the motor nerve, voluntary attempts to carry out handgrip exercise cause an immediate rise in HR and BP independent of afferent feedback. Several midbrain nuclei are also involved, namely the mesencephalic locomotor region and PAG matter. Recordings in the PAG matter of conscious humans asked to anticipate (but not perform) exercise show potential changes coincident with changes in HR and BP. As well as playing a role in anticipatory 'central command' at the onset of exercise, it is interesting to note that the PAG matter also receives input from the exercise pressor reflex (see Chapter 16, Section 16.6). Therefore, it may serve as a 'comparator' or 'calibration centre' for future central command instructions, depending on how well its previous feed forward message matched the actual work done, as indicated by the exercise pressor reflex.

## 16.9 OVERVIEW OF CENTRAL CONTROL

Figures 16.17 and 16.18 offer a highly simplified overview of the central, cardiovascular-regulating pathways; those that regulate the vagal outflow to the heart, and those that regulate the sympathetic outflow to the heart and peripheral blood vessels.

## Control of the vagal outflow to the heart

Two main pathways link the baroreceptor input to the vagal motor neurons, whose activity restrains the HR. One pathway, of short latency, remains within the medulla and passes from the NTS to the vagal motor nuclei, possibly via interneurons (Figure 16.17). The other, of longer latency, passes from the NTS to a hypothalamic depressor area (dorsal anterior hypothalamus) and from there to the vagal motor neurons.

The vagal nuclei also receive an important projection from the inspiratory centre of the brainstem. During **inspiration**, the inspiratory neurons elicit hyperpolarization of the vagal cardiac motor neurons. This reduces the vagal neuron responsiveness to the baroreflex during inspiration, a process termed baroreflex '**gating**'. The resulting fall in vagal activity causes a tachycardia synchronous with inspiration, that is, **sinus arrhythmia**. The inspiratory tachycardia helps to compensate for the fall in left ventricular stroke volume during inspiration, which is itself caused by the expansion of the pulmonary vascular capacity during inspiration.

## Control of the sympathetic outflow

The baroreceptor-stimulated output of the NTS has a net inhibitory effect on the spinal sympathetic neurons, but the intermediate pathways are more complex and less well understood than the vagal pathway (Figure 16.18). One pathway passes

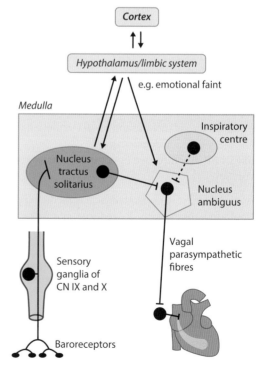

**Figure 16.17** Central pathways by which the baroreflex regulates vagal parasympathetic drive to the heart. Inspiratory inhibition (dashed line) generates sinus arrhythmia. Inputs from muscle work receptors (exercise pressor reflex) and face (diving reflex) are not shown. (Based on Spyer KM. *The Journal of Physiology* 1994; 474(1): 1–19, with permission from Wiley-Blackwell.)

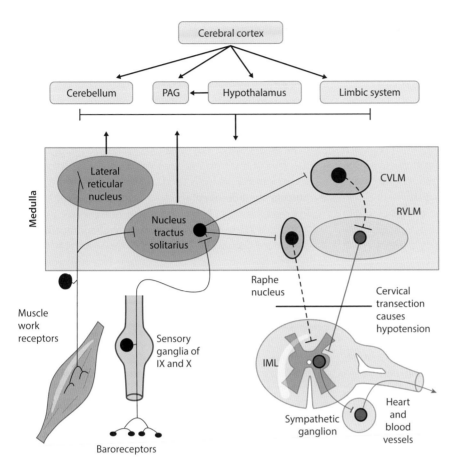

**Figure 16.18** Sympathetic drive to the heart and blood vessels (red neurons) and regulatory pathways. Dashed lines denote inhibitory pathways; excitatory arterial chemoreceptors are not shown. CVLM, caudal ventrolateral medulla containing caudal vaso-depressor area; IML, intermediolateral horns of thoracic spinal cord with sympathetic preganglionic neurons. PAG, periaqueductal grey (matter of pons); RVLM, rostral ventrolateral medulla containing rostral vasopressor areas.

via the hypothalamic paraventricular nuclei. Another pathway projects from the NTS to the caudal vasodepressor area, which in turn inhibits the tonically active rostral vasopressor area (Figure 16.19). The net effect is that many rostral vasopressor neurons fall silent during the pulse. The baroreflex thus inhibits the descending excitatory drive from the rostral vasopressor area to the spinal preganglionic sympathetic neurons. The spinal neurons are also inhibited by bulbospinal fibres from the brainstem raphe nuclei, which are activated by the baroreflex.

## Blood pressure is labile in spinal patients

The activity of spinal, sympathetic, preganglionic neurons is determined chiefly by the descending excitatory and inhibitory bulbospinal fibres, and to a lesser degree by local inputs within the spinal cord. The net descending influence is normally excitatory, so cervical cord transection causes an abrupt hypotension, as demonstrated by Claude Bernard. However, Sherrington and others pointed out that, over the course of several weeks, **BP gradually recovers following spinal transection,** because local spinal pathways gradually take over the excitation of the sympathetic preganglionic neurons, once brainstem control is removed. Local spinal pathways also mediate a degree of reflex modulation of sympathetic activity in cervical transection patients; for example, a full bladder or somatic pain can cause a reflex rise in BP. Although a spinal patient retains the baroreflex control of the HR via the vagus nerve, the patient **lacks the vasomotor component of the baroreflex.** Consequently,

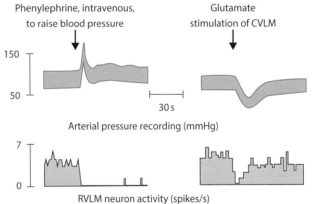

**Figure 16.19** Reflex control of vasopressor pre-sympathetic neurons in rostral ventrolateral medulla (RVLM). (Left) Raising blood pressure by intravenous phenylephrine evokes a baroreflex inhibition of RVLM. (Right) Stimulation of the caudal vasodepressor area of the caudal ventrolateral medulla (CVLM) by a glutamate injection (excitatory neurotransmitter) inhibits the RVLM, leading to a fall in spinal sympathetic activity and blood pressure. This sequence mimics the baroreflex. (After Blessing WW. *News in Physiological Sciences* 1991; 6: 139–41, with permission from the American Physiological Society.)

they have an excessively labile BP and are prone to postural hypotension during orthostasis, although some vascular compensation is provided by the myogenic constrictor response to dependency (Figures 8.6 and 11.5) and by angiotensin formation when renal artery pressure falls.

## SUMMARY

- HR, contractility, vascular tone and BP are regulated by cardiovascular reflexes. The reflex can be **depressor** (pressure-lowering, e.g. baroreflex) or **pressor** (pressure-raising, e.g. arterial chemoreceptors, muscle metaboreceptors). The afferent input from the cardiovascular receptors relays in the brainstem and modifies the autonomic outflow to the heart and vessels.

- **Arterial baroreceptors** in the wall of the carotid sinus and aortic arch are dynamically sensitive stretch receptors that signal pulse pressure and mean pressure. The myelinated, low-threshold A-fibres and non-myelinated, higher-threshold C-fibres travel in the glossopharyngeal and vagal nerves to the medulla. Baroreceptor excitation elicits a depressor reflex comprising bradycardia, reduced contractility and relaxation of resistance vessels and some peripheral veins.

- During **hypovolaemia**, baroreceptor unloading elicits tachycardia, increased contractility, vaso- and venoconstriction, interstitial fluid absorption and renal fluid retention (mediated by renin–angiotensin–aldosterone and vasopressin). These responses help maintain arterial BP.

- The baroreflex is thus a negative feedback loop that **stabilizes BP** over seconds to minutes. 'Resetting' enables the baroreflex to buffer the pressure around a higher level during exercise (central resetting) or clinical hypertension (peripheral resetting).

- **Cardiac receptors** fall into several classes. **Chemosensitive ventricular afferents** mediate ischaemic heart pain. **Myelinated veno-atrial stretch receptors** monitor atrial distension and evoke reflex tachycardia and diuresis, which reduces the cardiac distension and extracellular fluid volume. **Non-myelinated mechanoreceptors** in the left ventricle, atria and pulmonary artery elicit a depressor reflex (vasodilatation), which is weak in dogs but may be important in humans.

- In humans, **increases in extracellular fluid volume and hence CVP** lead to increased cardiopulmonary and arterial baroreceptor activity. This elicits a reflex vasodilatation in skin, muscle and kidneys, reduced vasopressin secretion and reduced renin–angiotensin–aldosterone production. Atrial distension also stimulates ANP secretion.

- **Long-term homeostasis of arterial pressure** depends on the regulation of extracellular salt and water mass by the kidneys. Renal salt and water excretion is controlled by aldosterone, vasopressin and pressure natriuresis. Aldosterone and vasopressin levels are regulated reflexly by baroreceptor and cardiopulmonary receptors and their neural pathways.

- **Muscle metaboreceptors** are group IV chemoreceptors that are excited by chemicals released locally within exercising muscle. Along with group III **muscle mechanoreceptors**, they evoke the exercise pressor reflex (vasoconstriction and tachycardia). These 'work receptors' help to drive the cardiovascular response to exercise, especially isometric exercise.

- **Peripheral arterial chemoreceptors** in the carotid and aortic bodies are excited by hypoxia, acidosis, asphyxia, hyperkalaemia and underperfusion. Besides stimulating ventilation, they elicit hypertension through peripheral vasoconstriction. This supports the BP during severe haemorrhage and asphyxiation. A reflex from **lung stretch receptors** elicits a concomitant tachycardia.

- These afferent inputs relay in the **nucleus tractus solitarius** of the brainstem (medulla). The latter projects to the hypothalamus, cerebellum and other parts of the medulla, which modulate (1) cardiac vagal motor neuron activity in the **nucleus ambiguus**, and (2) the pre-sympathetic excitatory outflow from the **rostral vasopressor area** of the medulla.

- Higher regions mediate co-ordinated responses. The **central defence axis** elicits the alerting response (tachycardia, muscle vasodilatation, splanchnic, renal and cutaneous vasoconstriction) in preparation for fight or flight. The **hypothalamic temperature-regulating area** controls cutaneous sympathetic outflow. The **cerebral cortex** issues a 'central command' to raise HR and BP rapidly at the start of exercise.

## FURTHER READING

Ardell JL, Armour JA. Neurocardiology: Structure-Based Function. *Comprehensive Physiology* 2016; **6**(4): 1635–53.

Hart EC. Human hypertension, sympathetic activity and the selfish brain. *Experimental Physiology* 2016; **101**(12): 1451–62.

McBryde FD, Hart EC, Ramchandra R, et al. Evaluating the carotid bodies and renal nerves as therapeutic targets for hypertension. *Autonomic Neuroscience* 2016; **S1566–0702**(16): 30123–30.

Fukuda K, Kanazawa H, Aizawa Y, et al. Cardiac innervation and sudden cardiac death. *Circulation Research* 2015; **116**(12): 2005–19.

Haack KK, Zucker IH. Central mechanisms for exercise training-induced reduction in sympatho-excitation in chronic heart failure. *Autonomic Neuroscience* 2015; **188**: 44–50.

Mitchell JH. Neural circulatory control during exercise: early insights. *Experimental Physiology* 2013; **98**(4): 867–78.

Basnayake SD, Green AL, Paterson DJ. Mapping the central neurocircuitry that integrates the cardiovascular response to exercise in humans. *Experimental Physiology* 2012; **97**(1): 29–38.

Dorrington KL, Pandit JJ. The obligatory role of the kidney in long-term arterial blood pressure control: extending Guyton's model of the circulation. *Anaesthesia* 2009; **64**(11): 1218–28.

Montani JP, Van Vliet BN. Understanding the contribution of Guyton's large circulatory model to long-term control of arterial pressure. *Experimental Physiology* 2009; **94**(4): 382–8.

Osborn JW, Averina VA, Fink GD. Current computational models do not reveal the importance of the nervous system in long-term control of arterial pressure. *Experimental Physiology* 2009; **94**(4): 389–96.

Green AL, Paterson DJ. Identifying neurocircuitry controlling cardiovascular function in humans using functional neurosurgery: Implications for exercise control. *Experimental Physiology* 2008; **93**: 1022–8.

Guyenet PG. The sympathetic control of blood pressure. *Nature Reviews Neuroscience* 2006; **7**: 335–46.

Joyner MJ. Baroreceptor function during exercise; resetting the record. *Experimental Physiology* 2006; **91**: 27–36.

Brooks VL, Sved AF. Pressure to change? Re-evaluating the role of baroreceptors in the long-term control of arterial pressure. *American Journal of Physiology* 2005; **288**: R815–18.

Danson EJF, Paterson DJ. Enhanced neuronal nitric oxide synthase expression is central to cardiac vagal phenotype in exercise-trained mice. *The Journal of Physiology* 2003; **546**(1): 225–32.

Foreman RD. Mechanisms of cardiac pain. *Annual Review of Physiology* 1999; **61**: 143–67.

Andresen MC. Nucleus tractus solitarius – gateway to neural circulatory control. *Annual Reviews of Physiology* 1994; **56**: 93–116.

Marshall JM. Peripheral chemoreceptors and cardiovascular regulation. *Physiological Reviews* 1994; **74**: 543–94.

Spyer KM. Central nervous system mechanisms contributing to cardiovascular control. *The Journal of Physiology* 1994; **474**: 1–19.

Schwartz PJ, Vanoli E, Stramba-Badiale M, et al. Autonomic mechanisms and sudden death. New insights from analysis of baroreceptor reflexes in conscious dogs with and without a myocardial infarction. *Circulation* 1988; **78**(4): 969–79.

Krogh A, Lindhard J. The regulation of respiration and circulation during the initial stages of muscular work. *The Journal of Physiology* 1913; **47**(1–2): 112–36.

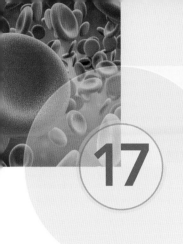

# Co-ordinated cardiovascular responses

**17**

## LEARNING OBJECTIVES

*After reading this chapter, you should be able to:*

**Regarding posture (orthostasis):**

- explain how orthostasis reduces cardiac output;
- describe the compensatory reflexes that prevent postural dizziness.

**Regarding the Valsalva manoeuvre:**

- explain how forced expiration affects cardiac output and blood pressure.

**Regarding exercise, physical training and performance:**

- explain how pulmonary $O_2$ uptake is increased during exercise;
- explain how stroke volume and heart rate are raised during exercise;
- outline how solute exchange is boosted between the active muscle and blood;
- contrast the effects of static and dynamic exercise on blood pressure;
- state the roles of central command and peripheral reflexes during exercise;

- list the cardiovascular changes induced by endurance training.

**Regarding feeding, digestion and splanchnic circulation:**

- state how a meal alters cardiac output, splanchnic and limb blood flow.

**Regarding the diving response:**

- list the three key features of the diving response and state the afferents responsible.

**Regarding ageing:**

- define arteriosclerosis;
- state how mean, systolic and diastolic arterial pressure change with ageing;
- outline the changes in cardiac performance with ageing.

**Regarding sleep and alerting:**

- contrast the cardiovascular responses to sleep and alerting (stress).

All the individual components of the circulation have been covered in the preceding chapters. However, as with a jigsaw puzzle, what really matters is how the components fit together to produce a functional whole. The purpose of this chapter is to show how the numerous components of the cardiovascular system respond in a co-ordinated way to the demands of everyday life. One general principle will emerge, the **principle of adaptation by integration**; that is, each major response is achieved by the integration of several smaller responses. For example, a 13-fold increase in the rate of $O_2$ absorption by the pulmonary circulation during strenuous exercise is achieved, typically, by the combination of a one-and-a-half-fold rise in stroke volume, a threefold rise in heart rate (HR) and a threefold increase in the arteriovenous concentration difference for $O_2$. Many further examples of adaptation by integration will be encountered in these last two chapters.

## 17.1 POSTURE (ORTHOSTASIS)

### Orthostasis causes an initial postural hypotension

Orthostasis, the adoption of an upright position, presents a serious challenge to the human circulation, because gravity causes a redistribution of our venous blood. Gravity increases the transmural pressure about tenfold in the most dependent human veins (Figures 8.2 and 11.5), and the resulting venous distension increases the volume of blood in the lower body by ~500 mL (Figure 8.24). This reduces the intrathoracic blood volume by 20% over ~15 s and lowers central venous pressure (CVP) from 5 to 6 mmHg (supine) to ~0 (upright). The resulting fall in cardiac contractile energy, mediated by the Frank–Starling's mechanism (Figure 6.10b), lowers the stroke volume, initially by 30%–40% (70 to 45 mL). This reduces the pulse pressure and, before compensatory responses, the mean arterial pressure.

Although the mean arterial pressure is normally restored quickly by the baroreflex, the hypotensive episode can be severe enough to impair cerebral perfusion transiently, resulting in dizziness and visual fading for a few seconds. Most healthy individuals will experience this postural giddiness occasionally. It is exacerbated by **warmth**, for example, a hot bath (because the attendant cutaneous venodilatation lowers CVP) and **prolonged bed rest**. Postural hypotension only progresses to **postural syncope** (fainting) if the baroreflex is impaired, usually by drugs (e.g. α adrenergic receptor blockers), autonomic neuropathy, or, in the case of returning astronauts, life under zero gravity.

During prolonged space flight, the cardiovascular system adapts to the environment of microgravity because orthostasis is not a problem in weightlessness. High-pressure receptors decrease their responsiveness over time, which is why astronauts like to undertake regular exercise in space to prevent muscle and autonomic deconditioning. As the astronaut experiences zero gravity, the 1 G effect forcing blood to the periphery is lost, resulting in a headward movement of fluid that increases cardiac filling and CVP, resulting in facial periorbital puffiness. As a result of the high CVP, natriuretic peptides are released into the circulation, which facilitates the loss of Na$^+$ and water in the urine.

### Neuroendocrine reflexes quickly restore mean arterial pressure

On earth, the unloading of arterial baroreceptors and cardiopulmonary mechanoreceptors during orthostasis triggers reflexes that quickly restore mean arterial pressure in healthy individuals (Figure 17.1). **Carotid baroreceptor traffic** is reduced by a fall in both pulse pressure and mean sinus pressure. Being situated near the base of the skull, the carotid sinus is elevated 25 cm or so above heart level during orthostasis, reducing the carotid sinus pressure (Figure 8.2). **Cardiopulmonary receptor traffic** is reduced by the fall in cardiac blood volume. The reduced inputs to the nucleus tractus solitarius inform the brain of the gravity of the situation (!) and elicit a reduction in cardiac vagal outflow and increase in sympathetic outflow, with the following effects:

- **HR increases** by 15–20 beats/min (Figure 17.2);
- **stroke volume** remains depressed, despite a reflex increase in myocardial contractility and splanchnic venoconstriction. Pulse pressure therefore remains low for the duration of the orthostasis (Figure 17.2);

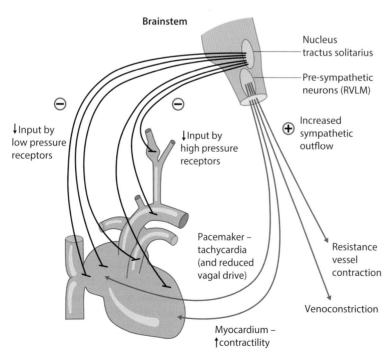

**Figure 17.1** Reflex sympathetic response to orthostasis in humans. RVLM, rostral ventrolateral medulla (site of rostral vasopressor area).

- **cardiac output falls** because of the low stroke volume; however, the reflex tachycardia limits the fall to ~20%;
- **peripheral resistance increases** by 30%–40% due to sympathetic-mediated vasoconstriction in the skeletal muscle, splanchnic and renal vascular beds;
- **mean arterial pressure** is not only restored by the rise in peripheral resistance but is raised by 10–14 mmHg above the supine value (Figure 17.2).

These responses normally take less than a minute to complete. Over the next half hour or so, the orthostasis-induced rise in capillary filtration pressure in the lower body causes a **12%–13%** (375 mL) **fall in plasma volume** (Section 11.9). This reduces the systolic pressure and elicits additional tachycardia. To compensate for the fall in plasma volume, the **excretion of salt and water is reduced** through sympathetic activation of the renin–angiotensin–aldosterone system and reflex vasopressin secretion.

The net result of the combined neuroendocrine responses is that the arterial blood pressure (BP) perfusing the brain is safe-guarded. It seems perverse that, despite all this physiological effort, cerebral blood flow declines by 10%–20% during orthostasis. The decline is caused by an increase in cerebral vascular resistance, brought about by multiple factors: reduced arterial $P_{CO_2}$ due to increased ventilation during orthostasis; the gravitational collapse of the jugular veins in the neck; and a slight sympathetic-mediated cerebral vasoconstriction.

## 17.2 THE VALSALVA MANOEUVRE

Antonio Maria Valsalva was a noted 18th-century Italian physiologist. His name is associated with the Valsalva manoeuvre, which is used as a test of circulatory function. However, the eponymous manoeuvre is not an ancient physiological rite but a natural event performed daily by all of us. It is a forced expiration against a closed or narrowed glottis, and this is a normal accompaniment to defecation, coughing, lifting heavy weights, singing a top A or playing the trumpet. Forced expiration creates a high intrathoracic pressure, which evokes a complex circulatory response with four phases (Figure 17.3):

1. **Phase 1**. Arterial BP increases as the thoracic aorta is compressed by the high intrathoracic pressure.

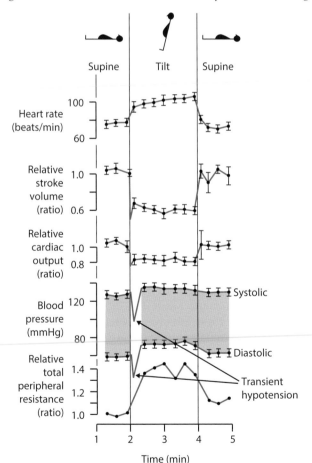

**Figure 17.2** Response of young adults to a 20 min head-up tilt. Stroke volume, cardiac output and peripheral resistance are expressed as a fraction of the supine control values. Bars show the standard error of mean. (From Smith JJ, Bush JE, Wiedmeier VT, et al. *Journal of Applied Physiology* 1970; 29(1): 133, with permission from the American Physiological Society.)

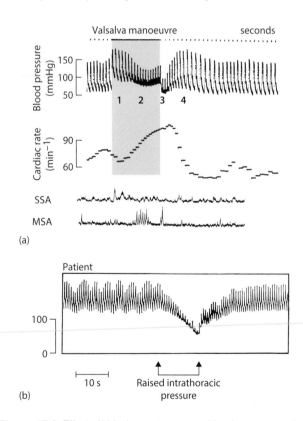

**Figure 17.3** Effect of Valsalva manoeuvre on blood pressure and heart rate. (**a**) Normal individual. (**b**) Patient with idiopathic orthostatic hypotension caused by an autonomic neuropathy. Pressure failed to stabilize in phase 2; no reflex bradycardia in phase 4. MSA, muscle sympathetic activity; SSA, skin sympathetic activity. (a: From Bannister Sir R. In: Sleight P, ed. *Arterial Baroreceptors and Hypertension (Oxford Medical Publications)*. Oxford: Oxford University Press; 1980. pp. 117–21; and Wallin BG, Elam M. *News in Physiological Sciences* 1994; 9: 203–7; b: From Johnson RH, Spalding JMK. *Disorders of the Autonomic Nervous System*. Oxford: Blackwell; 1974. With permission from Wiley-Blackwell.)

2. **Phase 2**. Arterial pulse pressure and mean pressure begin to decline, because the high intrathoracic pressure impedes venous return, reducing stroke volume. However, over the next 5–10 s a reflex increase in sympathetic outflow causes **tachycardia** and **peripheral vasoconstriction**, which halts the fall in mean BP (Figure 17.3a).

3. **Phase 3**. On terminating the Valsalva manoeuvre, intrathoracic pressure falls to normal and the thoracic aorta is decompressed, so arterial BP falls abruptly.

4. **Phase 4**. Pulse pressure and mean pressure quickly increase from their depressed levels, because venous blood surges into the thorax as intrathoracic pressure falls to normal. The increased venous return distends the heart, causing an overshoot in the stroke volume, pulse pressure and MAP. This in turn stimulates the baroreflex, causing a characteristic, transient **reflex bradycardia**.

The sudden bradycardia during phase 4 of the Valsalva response is used as a **clinical test of baroreflex competence** in humans. If the baroreflex is blocked by a neurological disorder such as autonomic neuropathy, the Valsalva manoeuvre shows a continuing pressure fall in phase 2 and neither pressure overshoot nor bradycardia in phase 4 (Figure 17.3b). Individuals with such a response are very prone to postural hypotension.

## 17.3 EXERCISE

Probably the most important circulatory response for an animal's survival in the wild is the response to physical exercise. Exercise imposes three tasks on the circulation:

- **pulmonary blood flow** must increase, to boost $O_2$ uptake and $CO_2$ removal;
- **blood flow in active muscles** must increase to boost $O_2$, glucose delivery and $CO_2$ removal. Vasodilatation is also critical to dissipate the heat generated by muscle contraction;
- **arterial pressure** must be stabilized, despite the huge changes in cardiac output and peripheral vascular resistance occasioned by the above two requirements.

## Raised pulmonary blood flow and reduced venous $O_2$ boost alveolar $O_2$ uptake

During exercise, the $O_2$ uptake by pulmonary blood ($\dot{V}_O$) must increase to satisfy the increased demands of active muscle. This is achieved partly through increased pulmonary blood flow, that is, cardiac output ($\dot{Q}$), and partly through an increase in the amount of $O_2$ that is added to each litre of pulmonary blood, since:

$$\dot{V}_{O_2} = \dot{Q} \times (C_A - C_V)$$

where $C_A$ and $C_V$ are the $O_2$ contents of arterial and mixed venous blood respectively (**Fick's principle**; Section 7.1).

The cardiac output of an untrained human can increase about fourfold, from 5 L/min at rest to 20 L/min during heavy exercise. The $O_2$ uptake per litre of blood, $(C_A - C_V)$, can increase around threefold, not because there is any increase in arterial $O_2$, but because the mixed venous blood entering the lungs has a reduced $O_2$ content, due to the increased extraction by active muscle (Figure 17.4). The mixed venous $O_2$ concentration ($C_V$) falls from ~145 mL $O_2$/L at rest to 40 mL $O_2$/L during heavy exercise. The arterial $O_2$ concentration, ~195 mL $O_2$/L, is unchanged at most exercise intensities.

Substituting the above values into Fick's equation, we see that pulmonary oxygen uptake, $\dot{V}_{O_2}$, increases ~13-fold during maximal exercise in an untrained human; the basal level is 0.25 L $O_2$/min and the maximum, termed $\dot{V}_{O_2max}$, is just over 3 L $O_2$/min (Table 17.1). $O_2$ uptake is widely used as a measure of work intensity; light work, such as level walking at 3 km/h, raises $\dot{V}_{O_2}$ to 0.4–0.8 L/min; moderate work corresponds to 0.8–1.6 L/min; hard work to 1.6–2.4 L/min; and severe work, such as running at 12 km/h, to 2.4–3.3 L/min.

## Pulmonary blood flow is increased through changes in heart rate and stroke volume

Cardiac output, and hence pulmonary blood flow, increases in almost linear proportion to total $O_2$ consumption rate (Figure 17.4). This tight coupling implies that the brainstem regulatory centres receive information about $O_2$ consumption; how this is achieved is not well understood. The increased cardiac output is brought about mainly through an increase in HR, and to a lesser degree stroke volume.

**HR** is a linear function of work rate, in the steady state (Figure 17.4). The tachycardia commences very rapidly, within a second or so of starting the exercise, then climbs to its steady-state level (Figure 16.13). The initial tachycardia is brought about by the withdrawal of the vagal inhibition of the pacemaker (as atropine blocks this response), which is predominantly under the direction of central command. Later, sympathetic drive to the pacemaker adds to the tachycardia. Maximum HR is 180–200 min$^{-1}$ in a young, human adult. If these HRs were experienced at rest, then cardiac failure would occur. The reason this does not happen during exercise is because of the positive inotropic support of the sympathetic drive, including circulating catecholamines.

**Stroke volume** is raised partly through increased **filling pressure**, which increases the ventricular end-diastolic volume (EDV), and partly through increased **ejection fraction**, which reduces the end-systolic volume (ESV) (Figure 6.24 and Table 17.2). However, it is the increase in rate that provides the major component of the increase in cardiac output. The exception to this is following heart transplantation. These patients can still undertake considerable exercise despite being denervated. They increase their cardiac output mainly by increasing stroke volume.

**Table 17.1** Cardiovascular and pulmonary function during maximal exercise in five college students and six Olympic athletes[a]

| | Exercising students | | | |
| --- | --- | --- | --- | --- |
| | Control | After bedrest | After training | Olympic athletes |
| Maximal $O_2$ uptake $\dot{V}_{O_2max}$ (L/min) | 3.30 | 2.43 | 3.91 | 5.38[b] |
| Maximal voluntary ventilation (L/min) | 191.0 | 201.0 | 197.0 | 219.0 |
| Lung transfer coefficient for $O_2$ (mL min$^{-1}$ mmHg$^{-1}$) | 96.0 | 83.0 | 86.0 | 95.0 |
| Arterial $O_2$ capacity (mL $O_2$/100 mL blood) | 21.9 | 20.5 | 20.8 | 22.4 |
| Maximal cardiac output (L/min) | 20.0 | 14.8 | 22.8 | 30.4[b] |
| Maximal stroke volume (mL) | 104.0 | 74.0 | 120.0 | 167.0[b] |
| Maximal heart rate (beats/min) | 192.0 | 197.0 | 190.0 | 182.0 |
| Maximal systemic arteriovenous $O_2$ difference (mL $O_2$/100 mL blood) | 16.2 | 16.5 | 17.1 | 18.0 |

*Source:* After Blomqvist CG, Saltin B. *Annual Review of Physiology* 1983; 45: 169–89.
[a] Similar age, height and weight.
[b] Significantly different from trained college students, $P < 0.05$.

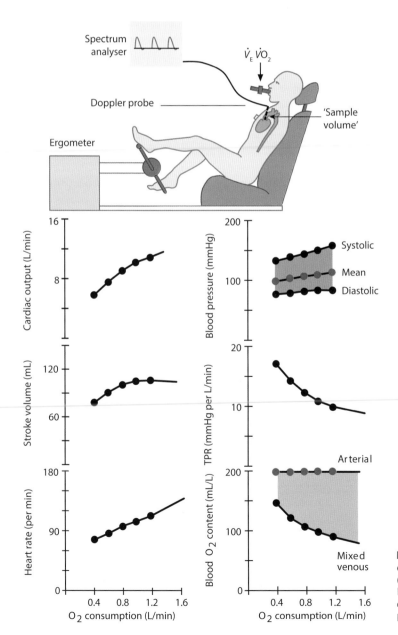

**Figure 17.4** Human cardiovascular response to exercise, measured by the pulsed Doppler method (Section 6.3) and expired gas analysis. (Adapted from Innes JA, Simon TD, Murphy K, et al. *Quarterly Journal of Experimental Physiology* 1988; 73(3): 323–41, by permission.)

**Right ventricle filling pressure**, that is, CVP, rises by ~1 mmHg during moderate, sustained, upright exercise. The rise is brought about by the skeletal muscle pump and sympathetically mediated splanchnic venoconstriction. However, during an explosive burst of cycling the muscle pump can raise right atrial pressure by 12 mmHg transiently. Thus, increases in EDV make a greater contribution in sudden, maximal effort than in sustained, moderate exercise. Increases in EDV are also relatively more important in older individuals; see Section 17.7 on 'Ageing'.

**Ejection fraction** increases because cardiac sympathetic activity increases. This raises ventricular contractility, which reduces the ESV and thus increases stroke volume. Ejection fraction can exceed 80% during heavy exercise. However, ischaemic heart disease prevents such increases in ejection fraction, leading to a poor cardiac output during exercise (Table 17.2).

The contribution of increased stroke volume depends very much on whether the exercise is upright or supine (Table 17.3). In **supine exercise**, CVP and EDV start from a high resting value, and stroke volume increases at most by 10%–20%, brought about mainly by a reduction in ESV. The increased cardiac output is thus due almost entirely to tachycardia. In **upright exercise**, by contrast, the stroke volume starts from a lower value because CVP is low, and can increase by 50%–100% due to a combination of increased EDV and reduced ESV. Most of this increase in stroke volume occurs at low work rates (Figure 17.4).

## Blood flow to active muscle is increased by metabolic vasodilatation

Blood flow increases in the active skeletal muscles (Figure 17.5). In a fit man, the total muscle blood flow can increase from 1 L/min at rest (20% of cardiac output) to ~19 L/min during heavy dynamic exercise (>80% of cardiac output). Many muscle groups are used only lightly, even in heavy exercise (e.g. arm muscles during running), so blood flow to the most active muscles probably increases as much as 40-fold. This is brought about primarily by the dilatation of the local resistance vessels (arterioles and terminal arteries) in the active muscle. The fall in vascular resistance enhances $O_2$ and glucose delivery specifically to the active muscle. It also permits cardiac output to increase optimally, because without a fall in peripheral resistance the rising cardiac output would cause severe hypertension, which would limit the cardiac output (see Section 6.9).

The hyperaemia of active muscles is brought about chiefly by **metabolic vasodilatation**, aided by the calf muscle pump during upright exercise (Figure 15.8). Metabolic dilatation of the resistance vessels increases **flow**, and causes **capillary recruitment**. Capillary recruitment greatly increases the rate of gas and nutrient diffusion between the blood and active muscle fibres, by increasing the surface area available for exchange and by shortening the diffusion distance (Figure 10.14). The increases in $O_2$ and glucose and transport are described more fully in Sections 10.10 and 10.11.

The arteriolar dilatation of metabolic hyperaemia raises not only blood flow but also capillary pressure (Figure 11.4). This, along with the hyperosmolarity of the interstitial fluid in active muscles, increases the capillary filtration rate. As a result, **plasma volume falls** by as much as 600 mL during prolonged, heavy exercise (Section 11.9). The attendant haemoconcentration modestly increases the $O_2$-carrying capacity of the blood. This counteracts a slight fall in arterial $O_2$ saturation (Figure 15.17), which is caused by the Bohr effect (increased acidity and temperature), short pulmonary capillary transit times and shunts. As a result, the arterial $O_2$ content changes little during sustained heavy exercise in non-athletes, though it can fall in athletes.

As emphasized earlier, the vasodilatation inside active muscles is induced by intrinsic metabolic control, not by extrinsic autonomic control. If mental stress is involved (e.g. start of a race), the alerting response is also evoked. **Feedforward** by the alerting response leads to an anticipatory, autonomic-mediated tachycardia and muscle vasodilatation (Figure 14.7).

**Table 17.2** Ventricular volume during upright, submaximal bicycle exercise in normal participants and patients with multiple coronary artery disease

|  | Normal | | Coronary disease | |
| --- | --- | --- | --- | --- |
|  | Rest | Exercise | Rest | Exercise |
| Cardiac output (L/min) | 6.0 | 17.5 | 5.7 | 11.3 |
| Heart rate (beats/min) | 81 | 170 | 75 | 119 |
| Stroke volume (mL)[a] | 76 | 102 | 76 | 96 |
| End-diastolic volume (mL)[a] | 116 | 128 | 138 | 216 |
| End-systolic volume (mL)[a] | 40 | 26 | 62 | 120 |
| Ejection fraction[a] | 0.66 | 0.8 | 0.6 | 0.46 |

*Source:* After Rerych SK, Scholz PM, Newman GE, et al. *Annals of Surgery* 1978; 187(5): 449–64.

[a] Left ventricle dimensions determined by radionuclide angiocardiography.

**Table 17.3** Supine versus upright exercise in eight healthy participants

|  | Stroke volume (mL) | Heart rate (beats/min) | Cardiac output (L/min) |
| --- | --- | --- | --- |
| **Supine** | | | |
| Rest | 111 | 60 | 6.4 |
| Exercise | 112 | 91 | 9.7 |
| **Upright** | | | |
| Rest | 76 | 76 | 5.6 |
| Exercise | 92 | 95 | 8.4 |

*Source:* After Loeppky JA, Greene ER, Hoekenga DE, et al. *Journal of Applied Physiology: Respiratory, Environmental and Exercise Physiology* 1981; 50(6): 1173–82.

*Note:* Response to pedalling at 30% of maximum $O_2$ consumption, $\dot{V}_{O_2max}$. Stroke volume was measured by the aortic Doppler flow technique.

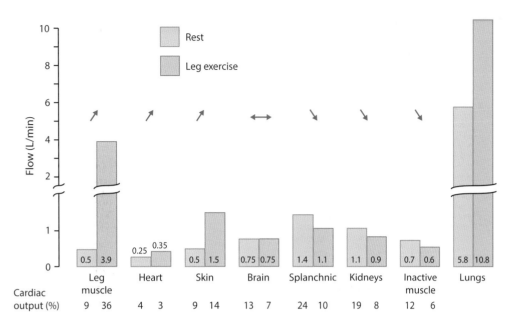

| Cardiac output (%) | Leg muscle | | Heart | | Skin | | Brain | | Splanchnic | | Kidneys | | Inactive muscle | | Lungs | |
|---|---|---|---|---|---|---|---|---|---|---|---|---|---|---|---|---|
| | 9 | 36 | 4 | 3 | 9 | 14 | 13 | 7 | 24 | 10 | 19 | 8 | 12 | 6 | | |

**Figure 17.5** Redistribution of human cardiac output during light leg exercise at room temperature. The number at the base of each column is blood flow in L/min. (Based in part on data from Wade OL, Bishop JM. *Cardiac Output and Regional Blood Flow.* Oxford: Blackwell; 1962. With permission from Wiley-Blackwell.)

## Blood flow to other tissues is altered during exercise: the 'diversion' misconception

Blood flow is also readjusted in most other tissues of the body during exercise; it is raised in some and reduced in others, as follows (Figure 17.5):

- **Coronary blood flow** increases in proportion to cardiac work, due to local metabolic vasodilatation (Figure 15.4).
- **Respiratory muscle perfusion** increases, due to the increased work of breathing. This can account for up to 16% of the cardiac output during heavy exercise.
- **Skin** is a battleground of conflicting demands. Initially, the cutaneous vessels are constricted; as core temperature rises, the thermoregulatory role of skin supervenes, and dilatation ensues (Figure 15.10a,b). This requires a further increase in cardiac output. Moreover, since the cutaneous venodilatation reduces cardiac filling pressure, the stroke volume tends to decline during prolonged hard exercise, so the HR increases further to compensate.
- Sympathetic vasoconstrictor outflow to the **splanchnic, renal** and **non-exercising muscle vascular beds** increases substantially during exercise, due to baroreflex resetting by central command, muscle work receptors and arterial chemoreceptors. During leg exercise, for example, vascular resistance increases in forearm muscles. The vasoconstriction of the inactive vascular beds is needed to maintain BP; without it, the vasodilatation in active muscles, myocardium and skin would lower BP by 12–40 mmHg during intense exercise. Increased sympathetic activity also constrains the metabolic vasodilatation in the contracting muscle to maintain BP.

Textbooks commonly state that the vasoconstriction in the resting tissues 'diverts' blood to working muscle; however, a simple audit of the changes in Figure 17.5 shows that the diverted flow, 0.6 L/min, makes a trivial contribution to the active hyperaemia. The true importance of the sympathetic vasoconstrictor response lies in adjusting the total peripheral resistance to maintain arterial BP.

## Static exercise raises arterial pressure more than dynamic exercise

Mean arterial pressure normally increases during exercise. The size of the increase depends on exercise intensity (Figure 17.4), duration, muscle mass involved and especially the type of exercise, whether dynamic or static (Figure 17.6).

**Dynamic exercise** is exercise in which a muscle alternately shortens and lengthens, under a relatively low load. The rise in mean arterial pressure is quite moderate because the rise in cardiac output is almost offset by the fall in total peripheral resistance. Typically, mean arterial pressure rises by 20 mmHg or less, and rarely exceeds 120 mmHg. Systolic pressure and pulse pressure increase much more than mean arterial pressure because ejection velocity and stroke volume increase; indeed, systolic pressure can reach 200 mmHg. Diastolic arterial pressure increases relatively little (Figure 17.5), and may even fall, because of increased run-off through the increased peripheral conductance (Figure 17.6, right panel). During the **post-exercise period**, arterial pressure is depressed by ~6 mmHg for up to 30 min. Post-exercise hypotension is caused by the persistence of the increased vascular conductance and by a temporary resetting of the baroreflex to a lower level.

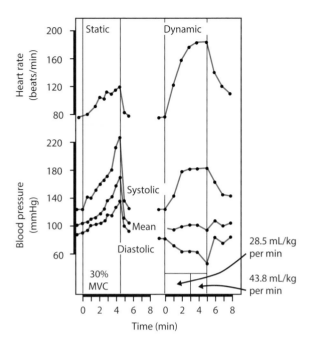

**Figure 17.6** Effect of static exercise compared with dynamic exercise. Static exercise caused a bigger increase in arterial blood pressure. Dynamic exercise caused a bigger rise in pulse pressure and heart rate. MVC, maximal voluntary contraction; the arrowed numbers refer to $O_2$ consumption. (From Lind RA, McNicol GW. *Canadian Medical Association Journal* 1967; 96(12): 706–15.)

**Static exercise**, such as a sustained handgrip, causes a much bigger increase in arterial BP than dynamic exercise (Figure 17.6, left panel). For example, supporting a 20-kg suitcase for 2–3 min can raise diastolic pressure by 30 mmHg, due mainly to a rise in total peripheral resistance. Isometric (static) contraction compresses the intra-muscle blood vessels. This attenuates the fall in muscle vascular resistance and causes a relative underperfusion, which strongly activates the muscle metaboreflex, that is, the exercise pressor reflex (Section 16.6). Because arterial pressure dominates the work of the left ventricle, isometric exercise is best avoided by patients with ischaemic heart disease and atherosclerosis; in these patients, any increase in arterial pressure above the limit of autoregulation will increase blood flow to tissue that may be prone to infarction.

**Resistive exercise** is a combination of static and heavily loaded dynamic exercise, for example, weightlifting. BPs up to 350/250 mmHg (truly!) have been recorded in young adults during maximum effort. Such high pressures are the result of the Valsalva phase 1 (aortic compression by a raised intrathoracic pressure), exercise pressor reflex and intra-muscle vessel compression. Fortunately, a concomitant rise in cerebrospinal fluid pressure protects cerebral vessels during these extreme exertions. Nevertheless, hard resistive exercise is best avoided by patients with ischaemic heart disease.

**Pulmonary arterial pressure** increases substantially during exercise (Figure 15.17 and Table 15.2). Indeed, in percentage terms, the rise is bigger than in the systemic circulation because there is no active vasodilatation in the pulmonary circulation.

## Circulating catecholamines help transplanted hearts respond to exercise

Under normal circumstances, the increased cardiac output during exercise is driven chiefly by the cardiac autonomic nerves. Nevertheless, animals and humans with transplanted, denervated hearts still increase their cardiac output during exercise, owing to a **redundancy of control mechanisms**. The chief backup mechanisms are the circulating catecholamines and the skeletal muscle pump.

The contribution of **circulating catecholamines** was demonstrated in racing greyhounds subjected to chronic cardiac denervation. Exercise still caused a tachycardia in these animals, albeit of smaller magnitude and slower onset (Figure 17.7). The tachycardia is mediated by a rise in plasma adrenaline and noradrenaline (NAd), due to which the greyhound's track speed is only 5% slower than normal. However, if the backup catecholamines are blocked by a β adrenergic receptor antagonist, the exercise tachycardia is abolished, track speed falls markedly and the greyhound becomes exhausted (Figure 17.7b). During strenuous human exercise, **plasma NAd** increases from ~1 nM to 10–20 nM, chiefly because of spillage from peripheral sympathetic vasomotor terminals. **Plasma adrenaline** shows little change during light to moderate exercise (0.2 nM), but rises to 2–5 nM

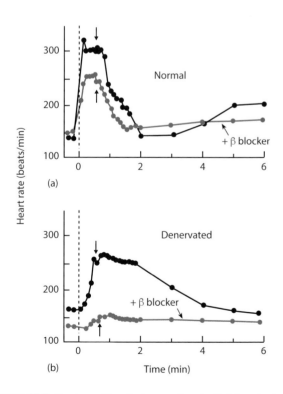

**Figure 17.7** Greyhound heart rate, monitored with telemetry (radio transmitter) during a race: (**a**) normal; (**b**) after cardiac denervation. Red lines show the effect of β adrenergic receptor blockade by propranolol. The response of the denervated heart depends on circulating catecholamines. The arrows show time to the 5/16th mile mark. (From Donald DE, Ferguson DA, Milburn SE. *Circulation Research* 1968; 22(2): 127–34, by permission.)

during maximal dynamic exercise, due to adrenal medulla secretion. The positive inotropic action of the catecholamines more than offsets the negative inotropic effects of exercise-induced hyperkalaemia (up to 8 mM) and lactic acidosis (plasma pH as low as 6.9).

Cardiac transplant patients also benefit from backup by the **skeletal muscle pump**. This raises the cardiac filling pressure during upright exercise, which in turn raises the stroke volume by the Frank–Starling mechanism. These examples of redundant mechanisms illustrate a general principle enunciated by the respiratory physiologist, Julius H Comroe Jr: if a job is worth doing, the body generally has more than one way of doing it.

## What initiates the circulatory adjustments during exercise?

With the major exception of metabolic vasodilatation, the cardiovascular responses to exercise are brought about by the autonomic nervous system. But what induces the brainstem cardiovascular centres to change the autonomic outflow? Two main hypotheses have been put forward: the central command hypothesis; and the peripheral reflex hypothesis. Both processes contribute, but their relative contribution depends on the type of exercise.

### Central command

The central command hypothesis, proposed by Krogh and Lindhard (1913), states that parts of the cerebral cortex (insular cortex, anterior cingulate cortex) or related motor regions of the thalamus, and midbrain nuclei (e.g. periaqueductal grey – PAG), not only initiate voluntary movement but also command the cardiovascular and respiratory centres of the medulla. This is supported by several observations:

- The HR increases at the first beat after the onset of exercise (Figure 16.13), so early that it implies 'feedforward' by the central nervous system; there is insufficient time for feedback to operate.
- After partial neuromuscular blockade by curare, voluntary attempts to contract the partially paralysed muscle require an exaggerated central command signal, and this is accompanied by an enhanced tachycardia, bigger pressor response and greater resetting of the baroreflex (Figure 16.7).

Although central command can account for the early cardiac response, it less readily explains the quintessential feature of the steady-state response, namely the linear relation between cardiac output and total $O_2$ consumption during dynamic exercise (Figure 17.4). This coupling may be underpinned by information from the active muscle itself, telling the brain about the work rate. However, this interpretation could be challenged by the observation that total body paralysis results in a proportional increase in HR and arterial BP depending on the effort involved, even though the muscles are not working. This would suggest that effort *per se* and the motor response are tightly coupled to the cardiovascular response independent of feedback. This does not prove the muscle pressor reflex is unimportant because there is compelling evidence that it contributes significantly to static (isometric)-induced rises in arterial BP.

## Muscle work receptors link cardiac output to work rate

Group III muscle mechanoreceptors and group IV muscle metaboreceptors reflexly increase HR and BP during exercise (Figures 16.13 and 16.14). The mechanoreceptors contribute to the initial vagal inhibition and rapid onset of tachycardia. The local accumulation of interstitial chemicals then activates the metaboreceptors and helps drive further increases in HR and BP that occur in the initial 1–2 min (Figure 17.6).

Thus, **central command feedforward** and **work receptor feedback** together drive the cardiac response to exercise. The central command and muscle mechanoreceptors produce the initial, rapid-onset tachycardia by suppressing the cardiac vagal motor neurons; the muscle metaboreflex contributes to the subsequent slower, sympathetically mediated rise in cardiac output and peripheral vasoconstriction. **Joint mechanoreceptors** also contribute slightly, perhaps 10%, to the increased reflex drive to the heart. Although many still debate the relative contribution of feedforward and feedback control, emerging evidence suggest that both systems are highly dynamic and coupled; indeed, group III/IV muscle afferents can sensitize the neural outflow from midbrain nuclei (e.g. subthalamic and PAG structures).

## 17.4 PHYSICAL TRAINING AND PERFORMANCE

Brief **power events**, such as sprinting or shot-putting, are not critically dependent on cardiovascular performance, because aerobic muscle metabolism is not essential for a brief burst of power. Nevertheless, power training evokes left ventricular wall hypertrophy, probably in response to the strong exercise pressor response.

In an **endurance event**, such as a medium-distance race, the continuous work depends on aerobic muscle metabolism. Consequently, performance is influenced by the maximum rate of $O_2$ transport from the lungs to the muscle mitochondria. This depends on (1) $\dot{V}_{O_2max}$, the maximum rate of $O_2$ uptake by pulmonary blood, (2) muscle perfusion and (3) the diffusive resistance from muscle capillary to mitochondrion. All three aspects are enhanced by endurance training; a rise in maximum cardiac output improves $\dot{V}_{O_2max}$, and changes in the skeletal muscle arteries and capillaries optimize local perfusion and gas exchange.

## Endurance training improves maximum cardiac output and $\dot{V}_{O_2MAX}$

$\dot{V}_{O_2max}$ is determined by maximum cardiac output and haematocrit, and can increase from ~3 L/min in an untrained student to >5 L/min in an endurance-trained Olympic athlete (Table 17.1). This is achieved mainly through a rise in maximal **cardiac output**, from 10–15 L/min (untrained) to 30–36 L/min in athletes. At such high outputs, a red cell's residence time in the alveolus is so short as to curtail gas equilibration, and arterial $O_2$ saturation can fall to ~90%.

It is interesting to compare humans with athletic animals such as dogs and horses. Unlike humans, many athletic animal species have a contractile spleen that pumps red cells into the circulation during exercise, raising the **haematocrit**. In a galloping racehorse, the spleen can inject several litres of red cells into the circulation, raising the haematocrit by 50%, to 0.65%. Selective breeding in racehorses has increased the heart size disproportionately, relative to the lungs, reducing the pulmonary transit time. This leads to a fall in arterial $O_2$ saturation to ~77% during maximum effort. Moreover, the huge pulmonary blood flow in a galloping racehorse generates an alarmingly high pulmonary artery pressure, ~120 mmHg, which can lead to pulmonary haemorrhage during extreme exertion.

## Endurance training boosts stroke volume: eccentric versus concentric hypertrophy

### Endurance training

Big hearts win long races! Dynamic endurance training leads to:

- ventricular enlargement and increased stroke volume;
- bradycardia at rest and a fast recovery of heart rate after termination of exercise;
- a 5%–10% increase in blood volume, raising the CVP;
- increased myocardial vascularity.

Endurance training enlarges the cavities of both the right and left ventricles. New sarcomeres are added in series within each myocyte, increasing the myocyte length but not width. Consequently, the ventricle expands, with little increase in wall thickness. This growth pattern is called **eccentric hypertrophy**. It is driven by local growth factors such as insulin-like growth factor, and can increase the left ventricle mass by 20%. Myocyte contractility also increases, at least in endurance-trained rats. Eccentric hypertrophy is accompanied by increases in the number of capillaries and arterioles, and by an increase in coronary artery calibre.

**Resting ventricular EDV** in endurance-trained athletes increases from ~120 mL to 160–220 mL, due to eccentric hypertrophy, an increase in blood volume and an increase in CVP. **Resting stroke volume** increases from 70–80 mL to 100–125 mL. **Resting cardiac output** is unchanged because

the high stroke volume is offset by a **resting bradycardia** of 40–50 min$^{-1}$, or in extreme cases 35 min$^{-1}$. The resting bradycardia is brought about by three factors: increased tonic vagal activity; increased local acetylcholine release (mediated by a nitric oxide (NO) pathway in the fibre terminals); and a fall in the intrinsic pacemaker rate. Sinus arrhythmia is enhanced by the increased vagal tone. A third and fourth heart sound may be audible, along with a benign systolic ejection murmur. The electrocardiogram shows a resting bradycardia. Mean BP is little changed.

During **maximal exercise**, endurance-trained athletes achieve up to 60% bigger stroke volumes than untrained individuals (Table 17.1). The maximal HR is unaltered, 180–190 min$^{-1}$; however, because athletes have lower resting HRs, they can achieve a proportionately greater increase in rate, for example, 4.5-fold from 40 min$^{-1}$ to 180 min$^{-1}$ (cf. untrained 2.6-fold, from 70 min$^{-1}$ to 180 min$^{-1}$). Because of these adaptations, endurance-trained athletes can increase the right and left ventricular output up to sevenfold, substantially improving $\dot{V}_{O_2max}$ (Table 17.1). Maximal cardiac outputs as high as 35 L/min have been recorded in some individuals.

## Strength training

An increase in cardiac chamber size is specific to endurance training. Strength training (isometric exercise), by contrast, causes short bouts of greatly raised BP (Figure 17.6), which evokes left ventricular wall hypertrophy (thickening), with no increase in internal chamber diameter. This growth pattern is called **concentric hypertrophy**. Some training disciplines (e.g. triathletes) evoke both concentric and eccentric hypertrophy. Concentric hypertrophy also occurs in **hypertensive patients**. It arises from the fact that sarcomeres are replicated in parallel to normalize the stress on them (stress = tension/thickness). Severe myocardial hypertrophy predisposes the ventricle to arrhythmia, and may account for around half of **sudden deaths in young athletes**. The pro-arrhythmogenic changes include prolonged mid-myocardial and subepicardial action potentials, altered repolarization patterns (with ECG T-wave inversion in some cases) and frequent ventricular ectopic beats due to afterdepolarization. If a high sympathetic drive is superimposed on this structural abnormality, then there is a high risk of arrhythmia.

## High-intensity training

Short periods (90 s) of supramaximal exercise to improve cardiovascular fitness have regained popularity. This type of exercise can improve insulin sensitivity and is associated with modest associated cardiovascular benefits. However, high-intensity training (HIT) may also carry significant cardiovascular risk in older patients and those with underlying vascular disease. HIT drives arterial BP to levels in excess of the normal limits of brain and heart autoregulation of blood flow.

## Vascular changes enhance muscle blood flow capacity and gas exchange

Endurance training increases maximal muscle blood flow and local $O_2$ transport through two adaptations: local arterial expansion; and increased number of capillaries. **Muscle conduit arteries** expand with training; the femoral artery of a trained human, for example, has a 7%–9% wider lumen and thinner wall than in a sedentary individual. The **number density of arterioles** increases (it can double in endurance-trained rats), probably through the arterialization of capillaries. Such changes are driven, presumably, by the increases in endothelial shear stress during training. Basic regulatory processes such as the myogenic response and metabolic hyperaemia are not materially changed by training. **Capillary angiogenesis**, induced by vascular endothelial growth factor, increases the surface area for gas exchange and reduces diffusion distance. If the muscle fibre diameter hypertrophies, capillary angiogenesis prevents an increase in diffusion distance. Muscle mitochondria become more abundant, especially at subsarcolemmal sites close to capillaries, and muscle myoglobin concentration increases.

## 17.5 FEEDING, DIGESTION AND THE SPLANCHNIC CIRCULATION

The splanchnic circulation comprises the gastrointestinal (GI) tract, spleen and pancreas, which are fed by the coeliac, superior mesenteric and inferior mesenteric arteries (Figure 1.6). The arrival of food in the GI tract triggers **mucosal hyperaemia**, lasting 1–3 h. The hyperaemia is initiated partly by local hormones (gastrin, cholecystokinin), partly by digestive products (glucose, fatty acids) and partly by vagal parasympathetic activity. Also, parasympathetic-mediated **pancreatic hyperaemia** accompanies pancreatic secretion (Section 14.2). Because of these changes, human splanchnic blood flow increases from a basal 1.5 L/min to 2.5 L/min after a carbohydrate meal. Conversely, sympathetic-mediated vasoconstriction can reduce the splanchnic blood flow to as little as 0.3 L/min during hypovolaemia.

The postprandial splanchnic vasodilatation elicits **tachycardia** and an **increase in cardiac output**, by ~1 L/min for 30–60 min after the meal. Carbohydrate meals cause the greatest hyperaemia and cardiac changes, and may cause **postprandial angina** in patients with severe ischaemic heart disease. **Reflex vasoconstriction** in other vascular beds (e.g. forearm, calf) normally prevents postprandial hypotension. Failure of this response and the reflex tachycardia in patients with autonomic dysfunction (e.g. people with diabetes) or some older patients can result in **postprandial hypotension** after a carbohydrate meal or oral glucose.

**Ethanol** is absorbed rapidly from the GI tract and causes cutaneous vasodilatation (facial flushing) and coronary vasodilatation; 0.2% ethanol (2.5 times the UK driving limit)

doubles the coronary blood flow in guinea pigs. The vasodilatation is mediated by calcitonin gene-related peptide, which is released from sensory terminals on activation of the capsaicin receptor transient receptor potential cation channel subfamily V member 1 (TRPV1). Moderate, daily ethanol consumption reduces deaths from coronary atheroma, but higher consumption contributes to hypertension, alcoholic cardiomyopathy and hepatic cirrhosis. The excessive flushing of many Chinese and Japanese people to alcohol is caused by two liver enzyme isoforms; one converts alcohol unusually rapidly into acetaldehyde, and the other is unusually slow at degrading acetaldehyde.

## 17.6 THE DIVING RESPONSE

Diving animals such as the duck, seal and whale undergo remarkable cardiovascular changes during a dive. Humans also exhibit a diving response, albeit a less well-developed one. The diving response comprises three reflex changes, namely:

- apnoea;
- intense bradycardia;
- peripheral vasoconstriction.

The cardiovascular changes conserve $O_2$ for use by the heart and brain during prolonged dives (pearl divers 40–50 s; competitive free divers a few minutes; Weddell seals <70 min; whales <2 h, although feeding dives are usually shorter). The superior performance of seals and whales is due to their large store of $O_2$ in blood and muscle myoglobin (Figure 17.8, bottom), more extreme cardiovascular responses and greater toleration of asphyxia. The arterial gas values in a harbour (common) seal after a prolonged dive, namely 10 mmHg $O_2$ and 100 mmHg $CO_2$, vastly exceed the human breath-hold breaking point and would probably kill us.

The diving response is initiated by cold water touching **trigeminal nerve facial receptors**, particularly around the eyes, nose and nasal mucosa. Immersion of the body but not the face, or immersion of the face wearing a breathing tube, fails to elicit the reflex. As the dive progresses, asphyxia develops, and **arterial chemoreceptors** reinforce the cardiovascular responses.

## Facial immersion causes bradycardia in humans

A seal's HR falls to ~20 min$^{-1}$ during a dive, due to vagal inhibition of the pacemaker (Figure 17.8). Many humans likewise display a pronounced reflex bradycardia to facial immersion in cold water (Figure 17.9). Indeed, some patients find this simple procedure can terminate a supraventricular tachycardia. The reflex may contribute to sudden deaths associated with water or foreign bodies in the airways.

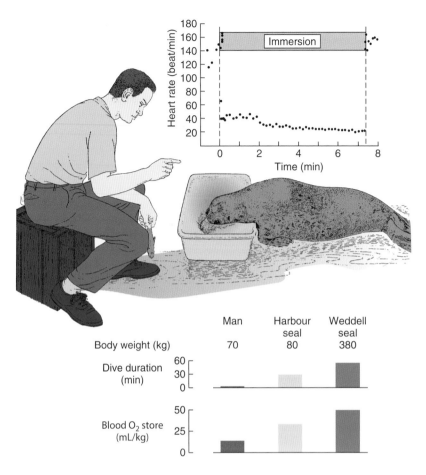

Body weight (kg)

| | Man | Harbour seal | Weddell seal |
|---|---|---|---|
| Body weight (kg) | 70 | 80 | 380 |

Dive duration (min)

Blood O$_2$ store (mL/kg)

**Figure 17.8** Physiological adaptation of the seal to breath-hold diving. The heart rate response of a seal trained to perform voluntary head immersion is shown at the top.

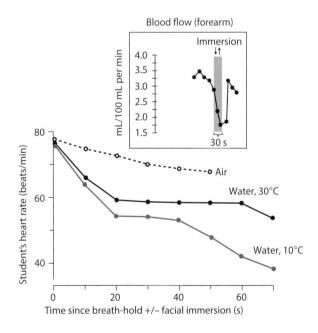

**Figure 17.9** The diving response in humans; bradycardia in a medical student following breath-hold facial immersion in cold water. The experiment was stopped abruptly when the heart rate fell to ~40 beats/min! (**Inset**) Concomitant vasoconstriction in the forearm. (Courtesy of Henderson JR, unpublished). (Inset from Heistad DD, Abboud FM, Eckstein JW. *Journal of Applied Physiology* 1968; 25(5): 542–9, with permission from the American Physiological Society.)

## Peripheral vasoconstriction diverts blood to the heart and brain

Facial immersion triggers vasoconstriction in human skin and skeletal muscles, as in diving mammals (Figure 17.9, inset). Diving mammals show a profound, sympathetically mediated vasoconstriction of the splanchnic, renal and skeletal muscle circulations. Arteries upstream of local metabolic vasodilator agents contract strongly, overriding the usual metabolic hyperaemia. The peripheral vasoconstriction maintains arterial pressure despite the extreme bradycardia, and diverts the remaining cardiac output to the heart and brain. A large quantity of lactic acid accumulates in the swimming muscles, leading to a sharp vasodilatation when the animal resurfaces.

## 17.7 AGEING

Ageing is associated with changes in artery wall structure, a rise in BP (especially systolic pressure), reduced baroreflex sensitivity and impaired cardiac performance during exercise. These changes are due to the ageing process, not atheroma.

## Elastic arteries develop sclerosis of the tunica media (arteriosclerosis)

The elasticity of ageing elastic arteries is reduced by diffuse changes in the media. The elastic lamellae (Figure 1.11) become thin, broken and disordered, due possibly to repetitive strain injury. This diffuse fracturing of elastic lamellae weakens the artery wall, leading to **structural dilatation**; the aorta, for example, dilates by ~50% between the ages of 40 and 70 years. As the elastin fragments and the wall stretches, wall stress is transferred to the **collagen fibres**. More collagen is laid down, and because collagen is much stiffer than elastin, the vessel becomes **stiffer**, as well as dilated (Figure 18.11). $Ca^{2+}$ salts may also be deposited in the media, and there is intimal hyperplasia. These degenerative changes are called arteriosclerosis; 'sclerosis' means fibrous hardening, hence the common expression 'hardening of the arteries'. Arteriosclerosis affects primarily the elastic vessels, and is important because it raises the pulse pressure and cardiac work.

## Arteriosclerosis is not atheroma

Arteriosclerosis is distinct from atheroma (Section 9.10), both biochemically and pathologically. Confusingly, atheroma is often called 'atherosclerosis', a self-contradictory term meaning 'porridge-like hardening'. Even worse, and generating maximum confusion, atheroma is sometimes called arteriosclerosis, in which case one must look at the context to see which pathology the author really means. The differences are summarized in Table 17.4. They include **distribution** (arteriosclerosis is diffuse, atheroma forms plaques), **location** (media versus intima), **biochemistry** (elastin fragmentation versus subintimal cholesterol deposit), effect on **vessel diameter** (arteriosclerotic dilatation versus atheromatous narrowing), **pathological consequence** (raised pulse pressure in arteriosclerosis, distal ischaemia in atheroma) and **epidemiology** (loss of elasticity with ageing in all societies, cf. atheroma associated with a Western diet).

## Arterial blood pressure increases with age

The pattern of pressure change with age is the same in Eastern and Western populations, and has changed little from the early 20th century to the present day; Figure 17.10, based on UK health statistics for 2003, shows the same pattern as the 1936 data in earlier editions of this book.

**Mean arterial pressure** increases moderately with age due to a rise in total peripheral resistance (Figure 17.10). This may be due partly to an increase in sympathetic vasomotor activity, as indicated by neural recordings, and an enhanced dilator response to the α adrenergic receptor blocker phentolamine.

**Systolic pressure** increases much more than the mean pressure because the compliance of the elastic vessels is reduced by arteriosclerosis. In the **brachial artery**, where BP is normally measured, systolic pressure increases steeply from childhood until age 20, levels off until age 30–40 and climbs steadily thereafter. The levelling off of brachial systolic pressure between 20 and 40 years is caused by the gradual loss of distal pressure amplification with age (Figure 8.11). In the **aorta**, systolic pressure probably pursues a steadier climb;

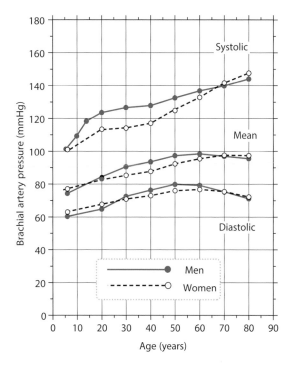

**Figure 17.10** The effect of ageing on brachial artery pressure in the English population. Recent Australian and American surveys show the same pattern, as did the 1936 survey of South Wales. Blood pressure was measured with an automated cuff device (Section 8.5) (Public data from the Department of Health National Statistics. *Health Survey for England 2003. Vol. 2. Risk Factors for Cardiovascular Disease.*)

**Table 17.4** Arteriosclerosis contrasted with atheroma (atherosclerosis)

|  | Arteriosclerosis of ageing | Atheroma |
|---|---|---|
| Epidemiology | All societies, West and East | Western lifestyle and diet |
| Distribution along artery | Diffuse | Focal |
| Layer primarily affected | Media | Intima |
| Key biochemical change | Elastin fragmentation and loss | Cholesterol plaque |
| Effect on lumen | Dilatation | Stenosis |
| Effect on blood flow | None | Impaired |
| Resulting pathophysiology | ↑ Systolic pressure ↑ Ventricular $O_2$ consumption | Distal tissue ischaemia |

consequently, the afterload on the ventricular myocardium increases progressively with age.

**Diastolic pressure**, which drives most of the coronary blood flow (Figure 15.5), begins to decline beyond 60 years.

## Systolic pressure rises due to reduced arterial compliance and rapid wave reflection

Systolic and pulse pressures increase disproportionately with ageing because of two biomechanical consequences of arteriosclerosis, as follows:

1. Pulse pressure depends on stroke volume divided by arterial compliance (Section 7.4). Because arteriosclerosis reduces arterial compliance, pulse pressure increases. Clinical hypertension has a similar effect, and has been likened to accelerated vascular ageing (Figure 18.11).
2. The velocity of propagation of the pulse depends on artery wall stiffness. In the aorta, where the increase in wall stiffness is greatest, the wave velocity more than doubles, from ~4 m/s at 25 years to ~10 m/s at 70 years. The wave now travels so fast that its reflected component returns to the aorta during late systole, adding to the late systolic pressure (Figure 8.10). This systolic augmentation is estimated to add ~25 mmHg to systolic pressure between age 30 and age 60.

## High systolic pressures impair left ventricular performance

The systolic pressure in the aorta governs the afterload on the contracting left ventricle, and this affects cardiac performance (Figures 6.2 and 6.15). Also, by increasing cardiac work, a high systolic pressure raises myocardial $O_2$ demand. Therefore, arteriosclerosis can contribute to heart failure in older patients. The severity of cardiovascular disease is more closely related to systolic than diastolic pressure, and the incidence of cardiovascular disease is reduced by treating systolic hypertension.

## Exercise-related cardiac performance and skeletal muscle hyperaemia are impaired by ageing

Ageing has little effect on resting HR or stroke volume, despite age-associated myocardial fibrosis. The fibrosis increases ventricular wall stiffness, which slows relaxation and early diastolic filling (diastolic dysfunction). Myocardial $O_2$ demand increases for the reasons explained earlier. However, the major effect of ageing on the heart emerges when it is stressed, for example, by physical exercise. The ability to increase the cardiac output and muscle blood flow during exercise declines substantially with ageing, reducing $\dot{V}_{O_2max}$ and exercise tolerance.

## Maximum heart rate in exercise is impaired

The maximum attainable HR falls as we get older. As a very approximate rule of thumb, the maximum is 220 $min^{-1}$ minus age (in years). The decline is caused by a fall in the responsiveness of the pacemaker to $\beta_1$ adrenergic receptor stimulation. Cardiac responsiveness to the baroreflex is also reduced.

## Maximum stroke volume in exercise is impaired

The ability to reduce ESV, by raising the ventricular ejection fraction, declines with age. Although the stroke volume can still be increased, this is brought about chiefly by raising EDV (Frank–Starling mechanism) rather than by raising contractility to reduce ESV. The decline in maximum HR and ejection fraction are both due to an impaired response to $\beta$ adrenergic receptor stimulation. There is ample sympathetic activity and catecholamine release, but the $\beta_1$ adrenergic receptors trigger less of a rise in intracellular cyclic adenosine monophosphate (cAMP) (due to reduced receptor coupling). In addition, counts of myocardial nuclei show that many millions of myocytes are lost each year, although there is some compensatory hypertrophy of the remaining myocytes.

## Skeletal muscle active hyperaemia is impaired

Microvascular density in skeletal muscles appears to be maintained during ageing; however, leg muscles nevertheless show ~20% less increase in blood flow in older humans than in young ones, for the same degree of exercise. This is due partly to a substantial, two- to threefold increase in sympathetic vasoconstrictor activity in older individuals, and partly to a fall in endothelial NO availability (mediating shear-dependent vasodilatation of conduit arteries). Conducted vasodilatation of the feed arteries is also reduced, at least in mice.

## 17.8 SLEEP AND THE ALERTING RESPONSE

### Sleep

During sleep, the metabolic rate and $O_2$ consumption decline. This is accompanied by a characteristic pattern of cardiovascular and respiratory changes, namely:

- bradycardia and a low cardiac output;
- a fall in BP (e.g. 80/50 mmHg; Figure 8.13);
- splanchnic vasodilatation;
- reduced ventilation.

On first falling asleep, during the non-rapid eye movement (REM) phase, bradycardia accounts for the fall in BP. Later, during REM sleep, dilatation of the splanchnic circulation also contributes to hypotension. Cerebral blood flow is increased in many parts of the brain despite the low BP.

## The alerting response

The response to an unusual or threatening environmental stimulus is in many respects the opposite of the sleep response, being characterized by:

- tachycardia;
- a rise in BP;
- splanchnic, renal and cutaneous vasoconstriction;
- muscle vasodilatation;
- increased ventilation.

The alerting response is clearly an appropriate preparation for imminent physical action. It originates from the central long axis of the brain, and is described further in Section 16.8.

## SUMMARY

### POSTURE (ORTHOSTASIS)

- During standing, the distension of dependent veins by gravity redistributes ~500 mL blood from the thorax into the lower limbs. The reduced cardiac filling pressure leads, via the Frank–Starling mechanism, to a 30%–40% fall in stroke volume and arterial pulse pressure. A transient fall in mean pressure can cause postural hypotension and dizziness in warm, venodilated individuals.

- The fall in pulse pressure and carotid sinus mean pressure reduce arterial baroreceptor activity. This evokes a reflex peripheral vasoconstriction, splanchnic venoconstriction and increase in HR by 15–20 beats/min, which together restore mean arterial pressure.

- Over a longer period, an increase in capillary filtration into the dependent limbs reduces the plasma volume by ~12%. Reflex increases in plasma vasopressin and renin–angiotensin–aldosterone reduce the excretion of salt and water.

### VALSALVA MANOEUVRE

- Forced expiration against a closed glottis raises intrathoracic and arterial pressure by mechanical compression (phase 1).

- The impeded venous return results in a fall in stroke volume and arterial pressure. The latter elicits a baroreflex tachycardia and peripheral vasoconstriction, leading to pressure stabilization (phase 2).

- On resumption of normal breathing, intrathoracic and arterial pressure immediately fall (phase 3).

- The inrush of accumulated peripheral venous blood raises the stroke volume (Frank–Starling mechanism). The resulting rise in pulse pressure triggers a baroreflex bradycardia (phase 4). This is used as a clinical test of autonomic function.

### EXERCISE

- **Metabolic hyperaemia** in the active muscle (increased blood flow), along with **capillary recruitment** and **steepened diffusion gradients**, speed up $O_2$ and glucose delivery to active fibres. The increased blood flow is due chiefly to metabolic vasodilatation, aided by the muscle pump during upright exercise and by a relatively small rise in arterial pressure.

- **A rise in cardiac output** supplies the increased flow to active muscle, and increases pulmonary gas exchange (Fick's principle). Output is proportion to muscle $O_2$ consumption and can increase fourfold to ~20 L/min in untrained individuals. Pulmonary $O_2$ uptake can increase much more (12–13-fold) because mixed venous $O_2$ content falls (Fick's principle).

- **Tachycardia** (maximum 180–190 $min^{-1}$) is initiated quickly by withdrawal of vagal tone, followed by increased sympathetic activity. **Stroke volume** increases during upright, dynamic exercise; less so when supine. Increases of 50%–100% result from a rise in EDV (due to muscle pump and peripheral venoconstriction) and a fall in ESV (due to sympathetic-mediated increased contractility).

- The autonomic outflow that drives the cardiac response is elicited by **central command** from the forebrain (feedforward) and by a **pressor reflex from muscle mechano- and metaboreceptors** (feedback).

- **Sympathetic-mediated vasoconstriction** in inactive circulations (splanchnic, renal, inactive muscles) counters the hypotensive effect of vasodilatation in active limb muscles, respiratory muscles, myocardium and, later, skin (heat dissipation). The baroreflex is reset, allowing mean arterial pressure to rise by ~20% during hard, dynamic exercise. Pressure climbs much higher during static (isometric) exercise, due to a stronger muscle metaboreflex; so, isometric/resistive exercise is best avoided by patients with ischaemic heart disease.

### PHYSICAL TRAINING AND PERFORMANCE

- Enhancement of cardiovascular performance by training is advantageous in dynamic endurance events (cf. brief, strength events).

- Endurance training enlarges the ventricular cavities through sarcomere addition. EDV and stroke volume are increased at rest and in exercise.

- Resting cardiac output is unaltered, because a vagus-mediated bradycardia (40–50 $min^{-1}$) offsets the increased resting stroke volume. Since the maximum heart rate remains 180–190 $min^{-1}$, HR can increase fourfold (cf. normal two-and-a-half-fold). Cardiac output can reach 30–35 L/min in athletes.

- Arterial changes and capillary angiogenesis in the endurance-trained muscle and myocardium raise the local maximum perfusion and facilitate solute exchange.

## FEEDING, DIGESTION AND SPLANCHNIC CIRCULATION

- Mucosal hyperaemia is most pronounced after a carbohydrate meal, but more prolonged after a fatty meal. The hyperaemia is mediated by digestion products, local hormones (gastrin, vasoactive intestinal polypeptide) and vagal parasympathetic activity.
- The hyperaemia, up to 1 L/min, necessitates a rise in cardiac output. BP is further supported by vasoconstriction in the limbs. If the latter fails, as in patients with autonomic neuropathy and some older patients, postprandial hypotension can develop.

## DIVING RESPONSE

- Stimulation of trigeminal facial and nasal mucosa afferents by cold water evokes a reflex bradycardia, peripheral vasoconstriction and apnoea.
- As asphyxia develops, the arterial chemoreflex reinforces the bradycardia and vasoconstriction.
- The cardiovascular changes conserve the $O_2$ store for the benefit of the brain and heart. In humans, dives of up to a few minutes are possible; in whales, these last for up to 2 h.

## AGEING

- Arteriosclerosis is diffuse elastin fragmentation and fibrosis (collagen deposition) in the tunica media of ageing elastic arteries. The reduced compliance (increased stiffness) and early return of the reflected wave raise systolic arterial pressure and hence cardiac work.
- Also, mean arterial pressure rises, probably because of a sympathetic-mediated increase in total peripheral resistance.
- The cardiac response to exercise is impaired. Maximum HR and the ability to raise the ejection fraction decline, due to impaired responsiveness to $\beta_1$ adrenergic receptor stimulation (reduced coupling of receptors to cAMP production). Stroke volume is raised instead by increasing the EDV.
- Skeletal muscle maximum flow capacity declines, due to increased sympathetic vasoconstrictor activity and reduced endothelial NO production.

## SLEEP AND THE ALERTING RESPONSE

- Sleep evokes bradycardia, reduced cardiac output, reduced BP, splanchnic vasodilatation and reduced ventilation.
- The alerting response to stress is the opposite to sleep; it involves tachycardia, increased BP, splanchnic, renal and cutaneous vasoconstriction, muscle vasodilatation and increased ventilation.

## FURTHER READING

### Posture (orthostasis)

Chisholm P, Anpalahan M. Orthostatic hypotension: pathophysiology, assessment, treatment, and the paradox of supine hypertension. *Internal Medicine Journal* 2017; **47**(4): 370–9.

Gibbons CH, Schmidt P, Biaggioni I, et al. The recommendations of a consensus panel for the screening, diagnosis, and treatment of neurogenic orthostatic hypotension and associated supine hypertension. *Journal of Neurology* 2017; **264**(8): 1567–82.

### Valsalva manoeuvre

Pstras L, Thomaseth K, Waniewski J, et al. The Valsalva manoeuvre: physiology and clinical examples. *Acta Physiologica* 2016; **217**(2): 103–19.

### Exercise, Physical training and performance

Coote JH, White MJ. CrossTalk proposal: bradycardia in the trained athlete is attributable to high vagal tone. *The Journal of Physiology* 2015; **593**(8): 1745–7.

D'Souza A, Sharma S, Boyett MR. CrossTalk opposing view: bradycardia in the trained athlete is attributable to a downregulation of a pacemaker channel in the sinus node. *The Journal of Physiology* 2015; **593**(8): 1749–51.

D'Souza A, Bucchi A, Johnsen AB, et al. Exercise training reduces resting heart rate via downregulation of the funny channel HCN4. *Nature Communications* 2014; **5**: 3775.

Ellison GM, Waring CD, Vicinanza C, et al. Physiological cardiac remodelling in response to endurance exercise training: cellular and molecular mechanisms. *Heart* 2012; **98**(1): 5–10.

Basnayake SD, Hyam JA, Pereira EA, et al. Identifying cardiovascular neurocircuitry involved in the exercise pressor reflex in humans using functional neurosurgery. *Journal of Applied Physiology* 2011; **110**(4): 881–91.

Krogh A, Lindhard J. The regulation of respiration and circulation during the initial stages of muscular work. *The Journal of Physiology* 1913; **47**(1–2): 112–36.

### Feeding, digestion and the splanchnic circulation

Kearney MT, Cowley AJ, Macdonald IA. The cardiovascular responses to feeding in man. *Experimental Physiology* 1995; **80**(5): 683–700.

### The Diving response

Pendergast DR, Moon RE, Krasney JJ, et al. Human physiology in an aquatic environment. *Comprehensive Physiology* 2015; **5**(4): 1705–50.

Panneton WM. The mammalian diving response: an enigmatic reflex to preserve life? *Physiology* 2013; **28**(5): 284–97.

## Ageing

Alfaras I, Di Germanio C, Bernier M, et al. Pharmacological strategies to retard cardiovascular aging. *Circulation Research* 2016; **118**(10): 1626–42.

Nakayama H, Nishida K, Otsu K. Macromolecular degradation systems and cardiovascular aging. *Circulation Research* 2016; **118**(10): 1577–92.

## Sleep

Penzel T, Kantelhardt JW, Bartsch RP, et al. Modulations of heart rate, ECG, and cardio-respiratory coupling observed in polysomnography. *Frontiers in Physiology* 2016; **7**: 460.

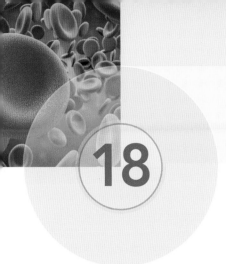

# Cardiovascular responses in pathological situations

## LEARNING OBJECTIVES

*After reading this chapter, you should be able to:*

- state the key cardiovascular responses to hypoxia (18.1);
- list the principal causes of acute circulatory failure (clinical shock) (18.2);
- describe the reflexes that support blood pressure (BP) during hypovolaemia (18.2);
- explain the cardiovascular basis of fainting (18.3);
- define 'clinical hypertension' and list its main ill effects (18.4);
- draw the hypertensive pressure pulse and explain (1) the rise in mean pressure; and (2) the disproportionate increase in systolic pressure (18.4);

- outline the chief aetiological theories for hypertension (18.4);
- define chronic heart failure and sketch the altered ventricular function curve (18.5);
- outline the changes in excitation-contraction coupling and electrophysiology of failing myocytes (18.5);
- list the changes in cardiac performance and peripheral circulation associated with heart failure (18.5);
- explain dyspnoea and how oedema arises in heart failure (18.5).

The previous chapter described co-ordinated cardiovascular responses to the challenges of everyday life; in this final chapter, we consider how the circulation reacts to pathological situations. **Atheroma,** a major pathology of large arteries, was covered in earlier chapters (*pathogenesis*, Section 9.10; *risk factors*, Concept box 15.1; *distinction from arteriosclerosis*, Table 17.4; *myocardial infarction and angina*, Section 15.1; *intermittent claudication/gangrenous necrosis*, Section 15.2; *thromboembolic strokes*, Section 15.4). The present chapter opens with systemic hypoxaemia, a pathological situation encountered not only in chronic lung disease but also by healthy individuals at high altitude.

## 18.1 SYSTEMIC HYPOXAEMIA

Systemic hypoxaemia is a subnormal $O_2$ content in arterial blood. The causes of hypoxaemia can be thought of in terms of the steps content in the cascade of $O_2$ delivery from atmosphere to arterial blood and include:

1. low inspired partial pressure of $O_2$ ($P_{O_2}$) as observed at high altitude;

2. low alveolar $P_{O_2}$, which represents a problem with alveolar ventilation. This could be due to obstructive airways disease (which may be reversible in the case of asthma, or irreversible in the case of chronic obstructive airways disease), restrictive airways disease (due to small lung volumes) or inappropriately suppressed respiratory rate (due to opioid toxicity);

3. a large alveolar–arterial (A–a) gradient. This could be due to impaired diffusion across the alveolar wall (e.g. pulmonary fibrosis) or ventilation-perfusion mismatch (from increased pulmonary dead space or increased right-to-left shunting of blood);

4. reduced $O_2$ carrying capacity of the blood. This may be due to anaemia, carbon monoxide poisoning or a high percentage of methaemoglobin in the blood. While 1, 2 and 3 lead to hypoxia, that is, a low partial pressure of $O_2$ in arterial blood, 4 can lead to hypoxaemia with a normal arterial $P_{O_2}$.

The following account focuses on high-altitude hypoxaemia, which can be simulated in the laboratory by reducing the $O_2$ content of the inspired air (Figure 18.1).

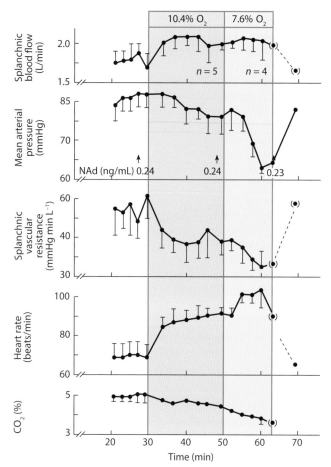

**Figure 18.1** Human cardiovascular responses to hypoxaemia. Inspired $O_2$ of 21% at sea level was reduced to 10.4% (equivalent altitude 5500 m), then 7.6% (equivalent to a major Himalayan summit). Arterial $P_{O_2}$ fell from 100 mmHg to 27 mmHg. Hyperventilation reduced alveolar $CO_2$. NAd, noradrenaline. (After Rowell LB. *Human Circulation Regulation During Physical Stress*. New York: Oxford University Press; 1986. With permission from Oxford University Press and the American Physiological Society.)

## Arterial $P_{O_2}$ falls with increasing altitude

Atmospheric pressure at sea level is ~760 mmHg (101.3 kPa), and $O_2$ makes up 21% of the atmosphere; so, inspired $P_{O_2}$, is around 160 mmHg (21 kPa). The French physiologist Paul Bert first established that inspired $P_{O_2}$, rather than atmospheric pressure *per se* contributes to altitude sickness, by independently varying the percentage of inspired $O_2$ and air pressure in a chamber. He described this in his work *La Pression Barométrique* (1878).

Alveolar $P_{O_2}$ is around 100 mmHg (13 kPa), and lower than inspired $P_{O_2}$, because some of the $O_2$ has been extracted by the pulmonary blood. $P_{O_2}$ is only slightly lower than alveolar $P_{O_2}$ because $O_2$ equilibrates across the pulmonary capillary wall, and there is only a slight mismatch of ventilation with perfusion in the lung as a whole ($V_{\dot{A}/\dot{Q}} = 0.8$). There is usually an A–a gradient of no more than 15–30 mmHg (2–4 kPa) depending on age. Arterial haemoglobin saturation is 97% at sea level.

Atmospheric pressure, inspired $P_{O_2}$, alveolar $P_{O_2}$ and arterial $P_{O_2}$ all fall with increasing altitude. Atmospheric pressure and therefore inspired $P_{O_2}$ halve with roughly a 5500 m ascent. Arterial saturation shows little fall up to 2000 m, owing to the plateau on the oxyhaemoglobin dissociation curve (Figure 15.3). Saturation begins to fall significantly when arterial $P_{O_2}$ falls below 60 mmHg (8 kPa), at 3000 m – an altitude commonly experienced by skiers, tourists and climbers. On a major Alpine summit (~4000 m), arterial $P_{O_2}$ is less than half normal, ~45 mmHg (6 kPa). Even so, there is permanent human habitation up to 5000 m in the Andes and in Tibet, and acclimatized individuals have survived without supplementary $O_2$ above 8000 m on Himalayan peaks. While Sir Edmund Hillary and Tenzing Norgay were the first to summit Everest (at approximately 8848 m) using supplemental $O_2$ in 1953, Reinhold Messner and Peter Habeler were the first to summit without the use of supplemental $O_2$ in 1978.

Humans respond to acute arterial hypoxia with four primary compensatory changes: resting hyperventilation; increased cardiac output; pulmonary vasoconstriction and peripheral vasodilatation.

## Resting hyperventilation improves arterial $P_{O_2}$

The hypoxic stimulation of peripheral arterial chemoreceptors (Section 16.6) causes a reflex increase in resting alveolar ventilation. This raises alveolar $P_{O_2}$ closer to the inspired $P_{O_2}$, and thus raises arterial $P_{O_2}$. The hyperventilation also reduces alveolar and arterial partial pressure of $CO_2$ ($P_{CO_2}$; Figure 18.1). This shifts the haemoglobin dissociation curve to the left (reverse Bohr shift) and enables arterial blood to bind more $O_2$ at the prevailing arterial $P_{O_2}$. The hypocapnia also attenuates peripheral and central chemoreceptor activity, so it limits the ventilatory response. (By contrast, in **asphyxiation** the arterial $P_{CO_2}$ rises as arterial $P_{O_2}$ falls, thereby augmenting the chemoreceptor activity and ventilatory drive.)

## Resting heart rate and cardiac output increase

An increase in resting cardiac output is necessary to maintain $O_2$ delivery to the cells of the body. Since arterial $P_{O_2}$ is low, the blood-to-cell diffusion gradient for $O_2$ is reduced; so, less $O_2$ diffuses out of each millilitre of blood, and the $O_2$ **arteriovenous difference falls**. For example, at 7.5% inspired $O_2$ (Himalayan hypoxia), the arterial $O_2$ content is 120 mL $L^{-1}$ (normal 195 mL $L^{-1}$), mixed venous $O_2$ is 90 mL $L^{-1}$ (normal 145 mL $L^{-1}$) and the $(A – V)_{O_2}$ is 30 mL $L^{-1}$ (normal 50 mL $L^{-1}$). An increase in resting cardiac output compensates for the fall in $(A – V)_{O_2}$, as dictated by **Fick's principle** (Section 7.1), so that tissue $O_2$ consumption is not impaired. In our example, a rise in resting cardiac output to just over 8 L min$^{-1}$, when multiplied by the reduced $(A – V)_{O_2}$ of 30 mL $L^{-1}$, allows basal metabolism to proceed at its normal rate, of ~250 mL $O_2$min$^{-1}$.

The raised cardiac output is brought about by a **resting tachycardia** of up to 100 min$^{-1}$, due to the withdrawal of vagal inhibition of the pacemaker (Figure 18.1). What drives vagal withdrawal is not entirely clear, perhaps the cardiac vagal motor neurons are suppressed by the hyperactive inspiratory neurons (Figure 16.17).

## Peripheral vasodilatation increases tissue perfusion

Arterial hypoxia causes dilatation of the systemic resistance vessels, particularly in the human coronary and splanchnic circulations (Figure 18.1). The resulting fall in peripheral resistance prevents systemic hypertension as cardiac output rises, and facilitates the increased peripheral perfusion. The hypoxaemic vasodilatation is mediated by adenosine and adrenaline. Vasodilatation is restrained by an increase in sympathetic vasomotor activity due to the arterial chemoreflex, as proved by enhanced hypoxic vasodilatation after $\alpha$ adrenergic receptor blockade. By contrast, the $CO_2$-sensitive cerebral vessels show little vasodilatation at altitude because hyperventilation-induced hypocapnia has a counterbalancing vasoconstrictor effect (Figure 15.13).

## Systemic arterial pressure falls while pulmonary arterial pressure rises

The hypoxic reduction of peripheral resistance outweighs the rise in cardiac output, so systemic arterial pressure falls (Figure 18.1). In the lungs, by contrast, pulmonary hypertension develops, due to the raised cardiac output and hypoxic pulmonary vasoconstriction (Section 15.5). Mean pulmonary artery pressure can double to ~30 mmHg at rest; it trebled in one group of healthy mountaineers who climbed rapidly to 4560 m. Pulmonary hypertension confers certain advantages, in that it improves apical perfusion in the upright position (Figure 15.20) and reduces ventilation/perfusion ratio inequality; however, it is dangerous when prolonged, as in chronic emphysema or an extended stay at extreme altitude. The chronic increase in right ventricular workload, along with the negative inotropic effect of the hypoxaemia (Section 6.12), can lead to right ventricular failure.

## Hypoxaemic exercise requires exaggerated cardiac outputs

During submaximal hypoxaemic exercise, the cardiac output is higher than normal for a given work rate and $O_2$ consumption. Blood flow to the active muscle is likewise higher than normal. However, during maximal hypoxaemic effort the maximal heart rate and output are lower than at sea level, due to hypoxic depression of the pacemaker. Consequently, the maximum $O_2$ transport rate is reduced. This severely limits physical performance at high altitudes.

## High altitude can cause mountain sickness

Unacclimatized, individuals who ascend too rapidly to 2500–3000 m (8000–10 000 ft) often experience **acute mountain sickness** after 8–24 h. This is a cerebral disorder, comprising headache, dizziness, sweating, nausea, vomiting, sleeplessness and irritability. The symptoms are attributed to the effects of hypoxaemia and acute respiratory alkalosis (low arterial $P_{CO_2}$) on cerebral neurons. Treatment includes descent to a lower altitude, supplementary $O_2$ and acetazolamide (to stimulate the renal excretion of bicarbonate, to counter respiratory alkalosis). Severe cases receive the steroid dexamethasone to reduce cerebral oedema.

Acute mountain sickness can also progress into high-altitude pulmonary oedema. It can develop after a rapid ascent to high altitude, especially if the individual has a predisposing factor such as ischaemic heart disease. Pulmonary oedema is also common in climbers exposed to extreme altitude for too long. It is thought to arise from uneven hypoxic pulmonary vasoconstriction, which raises pulmonary artery pressure. This in turn raises pressure in patches of capillaries where the feeding vessels are relatively less vasoconstricted. This forces fluid from pulmonary capillaries into alveoli to cause patchy oedema. Some long-term high-altitude dwellers in South America can develop chronic mountain sickness (**Monge's disease**) due to excessive red cell production raising their haematocrit to pathological levels.

## Acclimatization to hypoxia follows chronic exposure

Slow, progressive exposure to moderately high altitudes over several days allows time for acclimatization and prevents acute mountain sickness. Acclimatization involves the following adaptations:

- There is a **further rise in resting alveolar ventilation**. This is traditionally attributed to correction of the respiratory alkalosis by the kidneys. However, this factor alone seems inadequate, because normalization of blood and cerebrospinal fluid pH lag behind the ventilatory response. Adaptation within both the peripheral and central chemoreceptors is thought to contribute. This shifts the control of breathing curves over time as shown in Figure 18.2. This shift can only be achieved through exposure to hypoxic hypocapnia. Normoxic hypocapnia and hypoxic normocapnia cannot fully produce this in isolation. These findings indicate that adaptation of both peripheral (sensing hypoxia) and central chemoreceptors (sensing mainly hypocapnia and alkalosis) is required.
- The **haemoglobin dissociation curve** shifts to the right (Bohr shift; Figure 15.3) at moderate to high altitudes (up to 6000 m), due to an increase in red cell 2,3-diphosphoglycerate. This improves $O_2$ unloading in the tissues. At extreme altitudes (8000 m), the curve shifts to the left because of severe alkalosis caused by

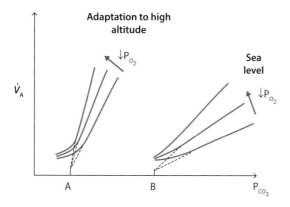

**Figure 18.2** Alveolar ventilation rate ($\dot{V}_a$) varies with rising arterial partial pressure of carbon dioxide ($P_{CO_2}$) at different fixed arterial partial pressures of $O_2$ ($P_{O_2}$). Note that following acclimatization to high altitude, the 'fans' of control curves shift to a lower overall $P_{CO_2}$ (B to A) and the gradient of the fans becomes steeper and closer together, reflecting an enhanced sensitivity to arterial $P_{CO_2}$.

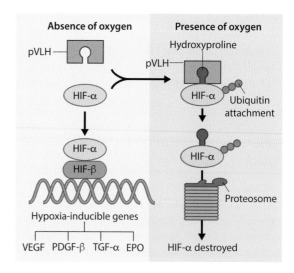

**Figure 18.3** The molecular basis of cellular $O_2$ sensing. Hypoxia inducible factor (HIF-1) is a heterodimer containing $\alpha$ and $\beta$ subunits, but in the presence of $O_2$ (as well as iron and 2-oxoglutarate) as shown on the right, HIF hydroxylases create a binding site for von Hippel–Lindau tumour suppressor (pVHL) on HIF-1-$\alpha$. This directs the polyubiquitination of HIF-1-$\alpha$ (ubiquitin represented by the green circle), ensuring that this protein will be degraded by the proteasome. In hypoxic conditions as shown on the left, HIF-1-$\alpha$ subunits accumulate and bind HIF-1-$\beta$. This heterodimer binds to HIF responsive elements (HREs) to increase the transcription of proteins such as vascular endothelial growth factor (VEGF), platelet derived growth factor subunit $\beta$ (PDGF-$\beta$), transforming growth factor $\beta$ (TGF-$\beta$) and erythropoietin (EPO).

excessive ventilation. This facilitates loading of $O_2$ into the lung.

- The **$O_2$-carrying capacity of blood** is increased by a rise in the haematocrit, which can reach 0.65 (i.e. 65% of blood volume is red cells). At a haematocrit above 0.65, chronic mountain sickness (or Monge's disease) can develop leading to reduced mental and physical capacity. The attendant high viscosity increases the risk of thromboembolic events such as a high-altitude stroke. The rise is due to increased bone marrow erythropoiesis, driven by renal erythropoietin release. The cellular mechanisms behind $O_2$ sensing in renal erythropoietin-producing cells have recently been elucidated. **Hypoxia-inducible factors (HIFs)** are transcriptional activators. HIF-1 is a heterodimer containing $\alpha$ and $\beta$ subunits; in the presence of $O_2$ (as well as iron and 2-oxoglutarate), HIF hydroxylases create a binding site for von Hippel–Lindau tumour suppressor protein on HIF-1-$\alpha$. This directs the polyubiquitination of HIF-1-$\alpha$, ensuring that this protein will be degraded by the proteasome. In hypoxic conditions, HIF-1-$\alpha$ subunits accumulate and bind HIF-1-$\beta$. This heterodimer binds to HIF responsive elements to increase the transcription of proteins such as erythropoietin and vascular endothelial growth factor (Figure 18.3).

## 18.2 SHOCK AND HAEMORRHAGE

### Clinical shock is acute circulatory failure

The term 'shock' is used by the medical profession and general public alike, but in very different senses. In general conversation, 'shock' means a psychological reaction to a traumatic experience, without organic pathology. Clinical shock, by contrast, is a **potentially fatal, pathophysiological disorder**

characterized by acute failure of the cardiovascular system to perfuse the tissues of the body adequately. This results in the following characteristic signs:

- the pulse is rapid and weak, due to tachycardia and a reduced stroke volume;
- mean arterial pressure may be reduced or normal, but pulse pressure is always reduced;
- breathing is rapid and shallow;
- urine output is reduced;
- there may be reduced mental awareness or confusion, muscular weakness and collapse.

### Causes of clinical shock

These can be divided into four categories:

1. **Hypovolaemic shock** is caused by a fall in circulating blood or plasma volume, following haemorrhage, diarrhoea and vomiting, dehydration, extensive burns, crush injuries or pancreatitis.
2. **Cardiogenic shock** is caused by the acute impairment of cardiac function by myocardial infarction, myocarditis, tachy- or bradyarrhythmia or acute valve rupture.
3. **Distributive shock** is caused by excessive vasodilatation. This occurs in septic shock due to endotoxins such as lipopolysaccharide from a bacterial infection. These trigger an immune response that causes the widespread

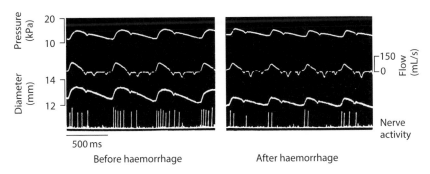

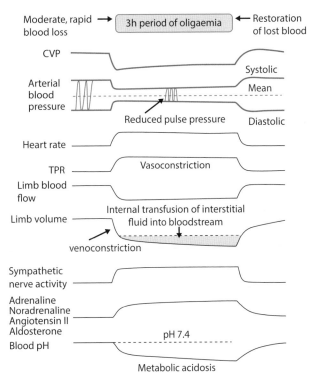

**Figure 18.4** Single aortic baroreceptor fibre activity and aortic parameters before (left) and after (right) a slow, 20% blood volume loss in a dog. Pulse pressure fell (because stroke volume fell), but mean pressure was unchanged (compensated haemorrhage). The reduced baroreceptor activity is caused by the reduced pulse pressure and reduced aortic diameter (caused probably by catecholamines). (After Hartikainen J, Ahonen E, Nevalainen T, et al. *Acta Physiologica Scandinavica* 1990; 140(2): 181–89, with permission from Wiley-Blackwell.)

release of vasodilatory substances (such as nitric oxide). Anaphylactic shock is caused by an intense allergic reaction to antigens to which the patient has become sensitized, such as foodstuffs, insect bites, antibiotics. It is usually a type 1 hypersensitivity reaction that involves immunoglobulin E and mast cell-dependent release of vasodilators (such as histamine).

4. **Obstructive shock** is caused by a large pulmonary embolus or cardiac tamponade.

Categories 1, 2 and 4 are associated with a compensatory peripheral vasoconstriction, but category 3 (distributive shock) shows a loss of peripheral vascular tone. Thus, the pathophysiology varies to some degree. We will concentrate here on one of the most common medical emergencies, namely acute haemorrhage leading to hypovolaemic shock.

## Haemorrhagic shock triggers compensatory reflexes

A 10%–15% blood loss (standard blood donation) is not a significant threat to the circulation. A rapid 15%–30% blood loss causes clinical shock, but, given prompt treatment, is not usually life-threatening. A 30%–40% blood loss reduces arterial pressure to 50–70 mmHg and causes severe, sometimes irreversible shock, with anuria and impaired cerebral and coronary perfusion.

The immediate effect of acute hypovolaemia is to reduce the central blood volume and thus the ventricular end-diastolic volume. This reduces the ventricular contractile energy through the **Frank–Starling mechanism**, so stroke volume and pulse pressure decline. Note that the fall in arterial pressure is mediated by the Frank–Starling mechanism; it is in no way analogous to the loss of pressure in a punctured tyre!

Following the onset of hypovolaemia, reflexes are activated to maintain mean arterial pressure, and thus cerebral and myocardial perfusion. **Cardiopulmonary stretch receptor** and **arterial baroreceptor activity** decline (Figure 18.4). **Arterial chemoreceptor activity** increases, partly because of the metabolic acidosis caused by tissue hypoperfusion (Figure 18.5) and partly because of reduced chemoreceptor perfusion (stagnant hypoxia). This drives the characteristic rapid breathing of shock.

**Figure 18.5** Compensated haemorrhage (blood loss <20%). Pulse pressure falls but mean blood pressure is preserved by tachycardia and peripheral vasoconstriction. The rapid, initial fall in limb volume is caused by venoconstriction; the slow fall (pink area) is caused by transcapillary absorption of interstitial fluid into circulation. A more severe blood loss reduces mean arterial pressure (decompensated phase). (Adapted from Chien S. *Physiological Reviews* 1967; 47(2): 214–88, with permission from the American Physiological Society; Jacobsen J, Søfelt S, Sheikh S, et al. *Acta Physiologica Scandinavica* 1990; 138(2): 167–73, with permission from Wiley-Blackwell; and Länne T, Lundvall J. *Acta Physiologica Scandinavica* 1992; 146(3): 299–306, with permission from Wiley-Blackwell.)

The changes in afferent input to the nucleus tractus solitarius evoke a reflex increase in **sympathetic outflow** and **circulating vasoactive hormones** (adrenaline, noradrenaline, angiotensin II, vasopressin). If the blood loss is <15%, the increased neuroendocrine outflow can maintain mean arterial pressure at a near-normal level (**compensated haemorrhage**). However, if the blood loss is ~30% a later phase of falling BP can supervene (**decompensated haemorrhage**).

During compensated, non-hypotensive hypovolaemia, the body's defences operate over three time scales: rapid reflexes that take effect within seconds; intermediate responses that act over 5–60 min; and slow responses that act over days to weeks, as follows.

## Rapid neurohumoral reflexes provide immediate support for the blood pressure

The reflex increase in sympathetic vasoconstrictor activity raises **vascular resistance** in the cutaneous, skeletal muscle, splanchnic and renal circulations. This provides immediate support to the arterial pressure. However, the **reduced tissue perfusion** also causes muscular weakness, lactic acidosis, oliguria (low urine flow) and skin pallor. Increased sympathetic cholinergic discharge to the skin causes sweating, hence the characteristic cold, clammy skin. In severe shock, white cell adhesion in microvessels contributes further to poor tissue perfusion.

Sympathetic-mediated **venoconstriction** in the splanchnic and cutaneous circulations partially restores the thoracic blood volume and cardiac filling pressure. It also increases the difficulty of cannulating a vein for intravenous fluid replacement. Filling pressure remains subnormal despite the venoconstriction, so stroke volume remains low. The effect of this on cardiac output is partly counteracted by a reflex, sympathetic-mediated **tachycardia**.

The sympathetic-mediated vasoconstriction is reinforced by increased levels of **circulating vasoconstrictor hormones** (adrenaline, noradrenaline, angiotensin II, vasopressin). Catecholamine and angiotensin II levels increase substantially during compensated, normotensive haemorrhage. **Angiotensin II** contributes to peripheral vasoconstriction by both peripheral and central actions (Section 14.8), and accounts for ~30% of the initial recovery of arterial pressure in venesected dogs. **Vasopressin** only reaches high enough levels to cause vasoconstriction during severe, hypotensive haemorrhage (Figure 14.11).

Due to increased peripheral resistance, reduced peripheral venous capacitance and increased cardiac performance, mean arterial pressure may be well maintained after a moderate haemorrhage. Consequently, **mean arterial pressure is not a reliable index of blood loss**.

## Absorption by capillaries causes a slow, internal fluid transfusion

The fall in venous pressure, coupled with the sympathetic-mediated rise in pre- to postcapillary resistance ratio $R_A/R_V$, lowers capillary BP (Figure 11.4). This enables plasma colloid osmotic pressure (COP) to establish a net absorption force across the capillary wall (Figure 11.11b). Consequently, there is a slow **absorption of interstitial fluid** into the depleted circulation, called the 'internal transfusion'. There is also increased lymphatic pumping. Up to 500 mL fluid can be transferred into the human circulation within an hour. This partially restores the depleted plasma volume and produces haemodilution. Consequently, haemorrhagic patients generally have a **reduced haematocrit** by the time they reach hospital. Although this reduces the $O_2$ carrying capacity of blood, it also reduces its viscosity, and thus improves tissue perfusion. The internal transfusion ceases within an hour because of the attendant fall in interstitial fluid pressure, rise in interstitial COP and fall in plasma COP (haemodilution) (Figure 11.11c).

The transfusion of interstitial fluid into the circulation is helped by fluid translocation from the much bigger **intracellular fluid compartment** into the interstitial compartment. Circulating adrenaline and glucagon stimulate hepatic glycogenolysis, which increases glucose concentration and extracellular fluid osmolarity by up to 20 mOsm. This draws fluid osmotically from the large intracellular compartment into the smaller interstitial compartment, allowing capillary absorption to continue for 30–60 min. It is estimated that about half of the internal transfusion comes, indirectly, from the intracellular compartment.

## Long-term renal and biosynthetic responses restore blood volume

The above responses preserve cardiac and cerebral perfusion over the short term in compensated shock. Over the following days to weeks the lost water, salts, plasma proteins and red cells are gradually made good. First, the water and salt deficits are corrected through increased fluid intake and reduced renal excretion. **Glomerular filtration rate** is reduced by a sympathetic-mediated contraction of the afferent arterioles. **Salt and water reabsorption** are stimulated by circulating aldosterone and vasopressin. Circulating angiotensin II stimulates not only aldosterone secretion but also **thirst**, by activating the subfornical organ of the brain. The increase in water intake, coupled with oliguria, quickly replenishes body water mass. The normal dietary intake of 2–10 g salt per day, along with renal salt retention, restores body salt mass in a few days.

**Albumin synthesis** by the liver gradually restores the plasma protein mass over a week or so. **Red cell production** by the bone marrow is stimulated by erythropoietin secreted by the kidney. Erythropoiesis restores the haematocrit to normal in a few weeks, given an adequate dietary iron intake.

## Decompensated (hypotensive) shock leads to organ failure

The account in the previous section describes reversible, compensated shock. If the blood loss is >30% and external fluid transfusion is delayed 3–4 h, shock enters a second, decompensated stage, which is often irreversible despite subsequent blood transfusion. In this phase, the arterial pressure falls, leading to myocardial underperfusion and possibly death (Figure 18.6). Thus, the 'golden hour' for transfusion is soon after the initial haemorrhage.

The collapse of BP in the decompensated phase is due primarily to a **fall in peripheral resistance** (except in skin), caused by reduced sympathetic vasoconstrictor outflow.

| | Stage 1 | Stage 2 | Stage 3 | Stage 4 |
|---|---|---|---|---|
| Blood loss (mL) | <750 <15% | 750–1500 15–30% | 1500–2000 30–40% | >2000 >40% |
| Heart rate (bpm) | <100 | >100 | >120 | >140 |
| Mean arterial pressure | Normal | Reduced | Reduced | Reduced |
| Respiratory rate (breaths/minute) | 14–20 | 20–30 | 30–40 | >35 |
| Urine output (mL/hour) | Normal >30 | Oliguria 20–30 | Oliguria 5–15 | Anuria |
| Neurological status | Normal | Agitated | Confused | Lethargic |
| ATP status | Supply = demand | Supply = demand | Supply < demand | Supply << demand |

$\dot{V}_{O_2}$

Blood flow redistributed to critical organs | Internal fluid transfusion | Anaerobic metabolism

$DO_2$crit

Cell death

$-DO_2$

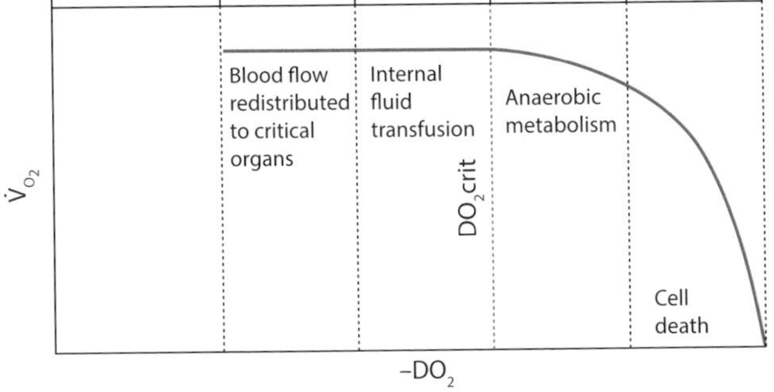

**Figure 18.6** A summary of the four stages of hypovolaemic shock as characterized by the physiological, neurological and cellular responses to worsening $O_2$ delivery ($-DO_2$) and metabolic rate ($\dot{V}_{O_2}$). Compensation occurs up to a critical point of $O_2$ delivery ($DO_2$crit) beyond which anaerobic metabolism and eventually cell death/ occurs. (Adapted from Kalla M, Herring N. *Surgery [Oxford]* 2013; 31(11): 545–51.)

The latter may be triggered by a central **depressor opioid pathway**. Endogenous opioids (enkephalins, β-endorphins) acting on δ and κ opiate receptors may depress the medullary vasopressor region. In support of this hypothesis, the administration of the opioid antagonist **naloxone** into the fourth ventricle of the brain helps to restore the sympathetic outflow and prevent decompensation.

As arterial pressure falls, the attendant fall in coronary perfusion and increasing metabolic acidosis impair myocardial contractility. This reduces cardiac output, which further reduces arterial pressure and coronary perfusion. Thus, **acute cardiac failure** sets in and establishes a deleterious **positive feedback loop**.

Decompensated shock can damage the kidneys, heart and other organs. Ischaemic damage to the renal tubules, called **acute tubular necrosis**, can cause acute renal failure, so urine output is monitored closely. In patients with pre-existing ischaemic heart disease, **myocardial infarction** can be precipitated by the reduced coronary pressure and **increased blood coagulability**. The latter can create numerous microthrombi in small vessels, which further impairs tissue perfusion. **Acute cardiac failure** may develop even without pre-existing coronary disease due to of the low perfusion pressure, microthrombi and white cell adhesion in microvessels. The condition can progress to **multiple organ failure** in severe cases.

## 18.3 TRANSIENT LOSS OF CONSCIOUSNESS (SYNCOPE)

Syncope is a sudden, transient loss of consciousness resulting from an abrupt fall in arterial pressure, sufficient to halve cerebral blood flow. The critical mean cerebral artery pressure is ~40 mmHg, which corresponds to ~70 mmHg at heart level during orthostasis. Syncope can be initiated by haemodynamic stresses, such as severe hypovolaemia, postural hypotension (Figure 18.7), vasovagal syndrome (inappropriate activation of the vagus nerve), paroxysmal coughing (impaired venous return to thorax), brady- or tachyarrhythmia, or exercise combined with severe aortic valve stenosis (Clinical Case 5). Vasovagal syncope can also be triggered by emotional stress, such as fear, pain or horror (Figure 18.8). The sight of blood, especially one's own, often induces emotional fainting in young adults. Vasovagal syncope occurs almost exclusively when upright because it requires a low central venous pressure (CVP) to inappropriately activate a vagal response. Consequently a person feeling faint should be advised to lie down.

Vasovagal syncope is usually preceded by the alerting response (tachycardia, muscle vasodilatation, cutaneous vasoconstriction, sweating). During this pre-faint period or 'prodrome', the individual looks pale and sweaty, hyperventilates and, characteristically, yawns. Then a sudden increase in vagal outflow causes **a profound bradycardia**; in the medical student of Figure 18.7, for example, there was no heartbeat for 8 s.

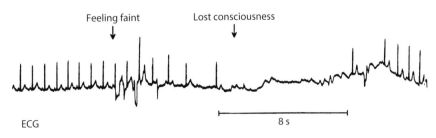

Feeling faint

Lost consciousness

ECG

8 s

**Figure 18.7** Electrocardiogram recorded during a transient loss of consciousness (vasovagal attack) in a healthy medical student. The student had received the vasodilator nitroglycerine and was then tilted from supine to upright. There was a period of 8 s asystole during the faint. The wobbly baseline is a movement artefact.

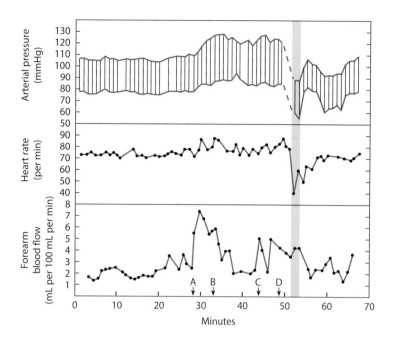

**Figure 18.8** Circulatory changes in a male student during an emotional transient loss of consciousness. The student showed forearm vasodilatation (alerting response) while watching the preparation for venepuncture (A) and the venepuncture of a colleague (B), but did not faint as the experimenter intended. Insertion of a needle into his arm (C) again produced vasodilatation, but no faint. Therefore, the student was asked to drink some of the blood taken from his colleague (D). He became pale, yawned, said 'I'm going' and fainted (tinted area). No heartbeat was detected by electrocardiogram for 11 s and his heart rate then averaged 37 min⁻¹. Forearm blood flow remained above resting level despite the slump in blood pressure, showing that vasodilatation had occurred. Consciousness was regained after 2 min. (From Greenfield ADM. *Lancet* 1951; 257(6668): 1302–3, with permission from Elsevier.)

The bradycardia is accompanied by a sudden **peripheral vasodilatation**, due to an abrupt fall in peripheral sympathetic vasoconstrictor activity. As a result, mean arterial pressure falls precipitously (Figure 18.8), cerebral perfusion falls below the autoregulation range, and loss of consciousness follows within seconds. This sequence can also be accompanied by nausea.

The pathways that cause the sudden changes in vasomotor and vagal activity are not clear, but the brainstem **depressor opioid pathway** may be involved (Section 18.2). Vasovagal syncope is thought to be related to the 'playing dead' response of small animals, which emanates from the cingulate gyrus (Section 16.8). Orthostatic and posthaemorrhagic syncope used to be attributed to a reflex from ventricular mechanoreceptors in a near-empty heart; however, echocardiography shows no presyncopal fall in cardiac volume; moreover, vasovagal syncope can occur in cardiac transplant patients with denervated ventricles.

## Recovery

The patient should not be propped up because the collapsed, supine position raises the intrathoracic blood volume and filling pressure, which increases the stroke volume by the Frank–Starling mechanism. First aid treatment is to raise the legs up from the supine position to further facilitate the venous return. Cerebral hypoperfusion in a propped up patient can cause them to fit. As the bradycardia fades and vascular tone returns, cardiac output and arterial pressure are restored. Consciousness is regained in ~2 min.

The best **treatment strategies** for vasovagal syncope include keeping well hydrated, adding salt to food and wearing compression stockings to help maintain CVP. Awareness and avoidance strategies, such as not standing for long periods of time and avoiding situations that may trigger the response are also important. As the vagal response includes both

bradycardic and vasodilatory elements, the implantation of a permanent pacemaker rarely helps. It is sometimes considered on specific occasions when there is repeated syncope secondary to prolonged periods of asystole, which cause serious injury and have no prodromal warning symptoms (**malignant vasovagal syncope**).

If a patient has clear prodromal symptoms and the episode occurs while standing, such that safety measures can be taken, then vasovagal syncope does not usually carry restrictions from driving a motor vehicle. However, if the episode occurs while sitting, or if no prodromal symptoms occur such as with malignant vasovagal syncope and cough syncope, then driving restrictions will apply.

## 18.4 HYPERTENSION

### What exactly is hypertension?

Clinical hypertension is the most common chronic disease, affecting an estimated billion individuals worldwide. It might be defined, simplistically, as a chronic, usually progressive, raised arterial BP. But this begs the following question: how high does the pressure have to be to be deemed 'raised'? This is a non-trivial problem, because arterial pressure is distributed in a negatively skewed, unimodal fashion across the population. Consequently, a clinically distinct group cannot be identified based on the population distribution alone. Moreover, hypertension is difficult to define on the basis of risk of sequelae, because the incidence of strokes, myocardial infarction, heart failure and renal failure increases linearly with increasing BP, rather than there being a clear inflection point. A pragmatic, partial solution is to adopt a clinical criterion, namely evidence of **substantial harm that we can afford to treat in an acceptable way**.

On this basis, stage 1 hypertension is diagnosed when repeated measurements of resting brachial artery pressure in clinic exceed 140/90 mmHg, and ambulatory BP exceeds 135/85 mmHg. In stage 2 hypertension, ambulatory BP exceeds 150/95 mmHg (according to the current National Institute for Health and Care Excellence guidelines in the UK). Hypertension thus defined is associated with ~7 million early deaths per year worldwide, from heart disease, stroke and renal failure. Humans with a systolic pressure of 130 mmHg, although not formally hypertensive, have a demonstrably higher risk of cardiovascular disease than humans with a systolic pressure of 120 mmHg. Therefore, with stage 1 hypertension, it is also recommended that the subsequent approach to treatment (lifestyle versus drugs) should depend on evidence of end organ damage (such as retinopathy, left ventricular hypertrophy or proteinuria) or the estimated 10-year cardiovascular risk being >20%.

## Classification of clinical hypertension

**Essential** or **primary hypertension** is hypertension without an obvious predisposing organic cause. It was called 'essential' because it was thought that the rise in pressure was essential to maintain tissue perfusion. Essential hypertension follows one of two courses. Hypertensive people are usually asymptomatic, so it usually comes to light though a routine check-up; or it may present much later through manifestations of end organ damage (coronary artery disease and myocardial infarction, left ventricular hypertrophy and heart failure, renal failure, or intracerebral haemorrhage and strokes). Aetiological factors include high dietary salt intake, genetic predisposition, obesity, excessive alcohol consumption, stress and lack of exercise. When hypertension develops acutely (>180/110 mmHg), it is termed **accelerated (previously 'malignant') hypertension**. In this rare condition, BP increases rapidly, leading to cardiac failure, peripheral oedema, renal damage with proteinuria, hypertensive encephalopathy (brain oedema, papilloedema) and accelerated hypertensive retinopathy.

**Secondary hypertension** has an identifiable pathological cause and is less common, but should especially be considered in young patients without obvious risk factors.

**Pre-eclamptic toxaemia** is defined as a brachial artery BP >140/90 mmHg during pregnancy, with proteinuria of >0.3 g/day, resolving post-partum. It occurs in the third trimester of 2%–6% of pregnancies. It is more common in those with a family history of the condition, the obese, older mothers and multiple (e.g. twin) pregnancies. It most commonly occurs in the first pregnancy (primiparous) and decreases with subsequent pregnancies with the same partner; however, the risk resets with a new partner. Failure of the placental spiral arteries to dilate normally results in placental ischaemia and the release of toxins into the maternal circulation. The toxins impair endothelial NO and prostacyclin production, and raise circulating endothelin, leading to peripheral vasoconstriction, reduced renal excretion and hypertension. Untreated, the hypertension may progress rapidly and cause cerebral oedema and seizures (termed 'eclampsia').

In **primary hyperaldosteronism** (Conn's syndrome), excessive secretion of aldosterone by an adrenal tumour stimulates renal salt and water retention, leading to hypertension (Figure 16.12). This condition is probably underdiagnosed. Excessive adrenal glucocorticoid secretion (Cushing's disease) can likewise cause hypertension.

**Aortic coarctation**, **renal artery stenosis** and certain other renal diseases which activate the renin–angiotensin–aldosterone system (RAAS), lead to hypertension (Figure 16.12).

A **phaeochromocytoma** is a rare, catecholamine-secreting tumour, usually in the adrenal medulla. The resulting activation of vascular α adrenergic receptors, and cardiac and renal β adrenergic receptors causes hypertension.

In >95% of non-pregnant hypertensives, no organic cause is found and the disorder is classed as essential hypertension. The overall condition is felt to be a disease of the vasculature, kidney and autonomic nervous system, reflecting the factors that contribute to the long-term control of BP (see Section 16.5).

## Altered renal pressure natriuresis and high vascular resistance

In established hypertension, vascular resistance increases in virtually every organ, including the kidney, due to a narrowing of the small resistance arteries and rarefaction. This shifts the renal pressure natriuresis curve to higher BPs as illustrated in Figure 18.9, and also produces a high total peripheral resistance against which the heart has to work.

A core feature of hypertension is a **narrowing of arterioles**. This is visible in retinal vessels as 'silver wiring'. In the early stages, the narrowing is caused by an increase in vascular tone, and may be reversible by vasodilator drugs. However, as time passes the structure of the tunica media changes. In mild hypertension, a rearrangement of the vascular myocytes, along with a modest increase in extracellular matrix, narrows the lumen by ~10%, with little change in wall area (**inward eutrophic remodelling**; little hypertrophy). The ratio of wall thickness to internal radius increases by around 30%. Even maximal vasodilatation now fails to rectify the abnormal resistance (Figure 18.10). In severe human hypertension (and hypertensive rats), there is also hypertrophy of the vascular myocytes, which increases the vascular wall area. The wall changes are thought to be triggered by increases in wall stress, high sympathetic drive, angiotensin II and plasma $Na^+$. Angiotensin II is not only a vasoconstrictor agent but also a growth factor, stimulating vascular hypertrophy (increased cell size) and hyperplasia (increased cell numbers). When the RAAS is stimulated by clipping a rat renal artery, the tunica media throughout the body remodels and hypertrophies in days to weeks.

**Rarefaction**, a reduction in the number of vessels per unit tissue volume, has also been demonstrated in the retina, skin and intestine. In the skin, the capillary density falls by ~21% in established hypertension.

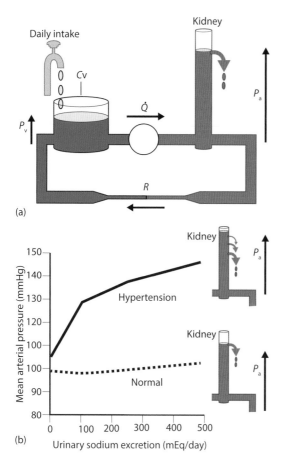

(a)

(b)

**Figure 18.9** Long-term control of blood volume in health and hypertension. **(a)** Representation of the open circulation model. In the chronic setting, arterial pressure (Pa) depends on daily water and $Na^+$ intake (dripping tap) and the renal pressure–natriuresis relationship (represented by the height of the holes in the arterial column) rather than cardiac output ($\dot{Q}$) and peripheral resistance (R). **(b)** Experimental models of hypertension (e.g. long-term angiotensin II infusion) with controlled $Na^+$ intake (and therefore excretion) demonstrate a reset pressure–natriuresis curve in hypertension. This may be represented by kidney holes positioned further up the arterial column. Natriuresis occurs to a degree similar to that in normotension, to maintain a stable body water volume, but requires a higher arterial pressure to do so. Pv, venous pressure. (a: Redrawn from Dorrington KL, Pandit JJ. The obligatory role of the kidney in long-term arterial blood pressure control: extending Guyton's model of the circulation. *Anaesthesia* 2009; 64(11): 1218–28; b: Data from Hall JE. The kidney, hypertension, and obesity. *Hypertension* 2003; 41(3 Pt 2): 625–33.)

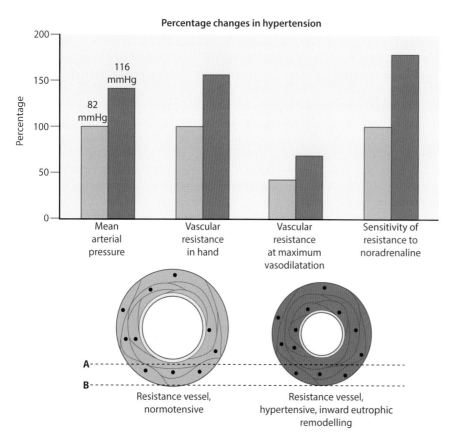

**Figure 18.10** Changes in resistance vessels of the hand in hypertensive patients (red) relative to normal individuals (grey). (Upper panel) In the hypertensive patients, vascular resistance is raised at rest and after maximum vasodilatation, and the vasoconstrictor response to noradrenaline is increased. (Results of Sivertsson R, Olander B. *Life Sciences* 1968; 7(23): 1291–7.) (Lower panel) Hypertension narrows the lumen and increases the wall thickness of human gluteal and subcutaneous small arteries. This is inward eutrophic remodelling; the total wall area is unchanged. The changes were reversed by angiotensin-converting enzyme inhibitors, but not by β blockers. (Results of Thybo NK, Stephens N, Cooper A, et al. *Hypertension* 1995; 25(4 Pt 1): 474–81.)

As the media of small vessels remodels and hypertension progresses, **endothelial dysfunction** can also develop, which may result in reduced endothelium-dependent vasodilatation and atherosclerosis. While this may be secondary to other cardiovascular risk factors such as smoking, obesity, dyslipidaemia and diabetes mellitus, it may also facilitate the maintenance of high vascular resistance later in the disease.

The **baroreflex** remains functional in hypertensive patients, but its sensitivity is reduced by the stiffening of the artery wall, and it operates around a higher set point due to peripheral resetting (Section 16.2). It is accepted that the baroreflex changes are a consequence of the hypertension, not a cause.

## Large artery stiffening exacerbates systolic hypertension

Although small artery narrowing is the primary pathology, secondary changes in the large, elastic arteries exacerbate the rise in systolic pressure and pulse pressure. This is important because morbidity and mortality correlate more closely with **systolic** than diastolic **hypertension**. The elastic arteries show elastin fragmentation, dilatation and increased wall stiffness (reduced compliance). The picture is, in effect, one of **accelerated ageing** (Section 17.7). The structural deterioration raises systolic pressure through two effects:

- **Arterial stiffness** (elastance) is increased; compliance is reduced. Since pulse pressure depends on stroke volume × elastance, a rise in elastance raises the pulse pressure (Figure 18.11). Consequently, systolic pressure increases much more than diastolic pressure.
- **Pulse wave velocity** increases due to the increased wall stiffness (Section 8.4). Consequently, the reflected wave arrives back in the ascending aorta at an earlier time. Moreover, the degree of reflection is enhanced by the raised peripheral resistance. The early return of a bigger reflected pressure wave greatly augments the original or 'incident' systolic pressure wave (Figure 18.12). This **systolic augmentation** can add as much as 50 mmHg to the systolic pressure in a hypertensive patient.

Aortic systolic hypertension is thus the product of three biophysical mechanisms, namely an increase in peripheral resistance, a fall in central artery compliance and the rapid return of a larger, reflected pressure wave. The first two mechanisms increase the incident wave (Figure 18.11) and the third increases the degree of systolic augmentation by wave reflection (Figure 18.12).

## The left ventricular wall hypertrophies and eventually fails

The high systolic pressure increases the work of the left ventricle, leading to **concentric hypertrophy** (as with strength

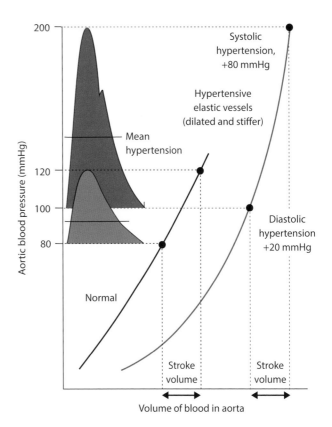

**Figure 18.11** Increased stiffness of elastic vessels contributes to systolic hypertension. The central elastic arteries are dilated because elastin fragments with ageing and hypertension. They are stiffer (steeper slope) due to collagen deposition and stress at the raised pressure. The same stroke volume causes a bigger pulse pressure and systolic pressure, due to the increased slope (elastance, 1/compliance). Diastolic pressure was raised 20 mmHg by increased peripheral resistance, but systolic pressure increased by 80 mmHg due to the reduced compliance, even neglecting augmentation by wave reflection. (Based on Nichols WW, O'Rourke MF. *McDonald's Blood Flow in Arteries*. London: Arnold, 2005.)

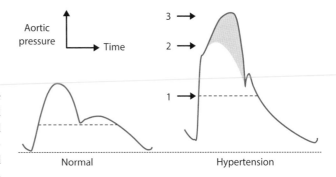

**Figure 18.12** Changes in the aortic pressure wave in hypertension. Arrow 1 and dashed lines show the increase in mean pressure, caused by the increased resistance of small arterial vessels. Arrow 2 highlights the effect of reduced aortic compliance, namely a disproportionate increase in the systolic incident wave (clear area). Arrow 3 shows the augmentation of pressure in late systole by the early return of a large reflected wave (pink area). Augmentation can account for as much as half the systolic hypertension. (Based on Nichols WW, O'Rourke MF. *McDonald's Blood Flow in Arteries*. London: Arnold, 2005.)

training; Section 17.4). The addition of sarcomeres in parallel within the cardiac myocytes can increase ventricular wall thickness ($w$) up to about threefold. This normalizes the stress $S$ on the individual cardiac myocyte, since according to Laplace's law, $S = (P/2w) \times$ radius (equation 6.2), where $P$ is systolic pressure (afterload). Thus, hypertrophy enables the ventricle to maintain a normal ejection fraction, despite the increased systolic pressure (afterload). The hypertrophy may be driven by wall stress, cardiac sympathetic stimulation, angiotensin II and possibly plasma $Na^+$ changes.

However, eventually the left ventricle begins to fail (**decompensated hypertrophy**). The cardiac myocytes begin to degenerate and die by necrosis and apoptosis, possibly because the increased diffusion distance into the thickened myocytes causes intracellular hypoxia. The loss of myocytes leads to a dilated cardiomyopathy. As ventricle radius increases and $w$ decreases, wall stress $S$ increases (Laplace's law), which exacerbates the myocyte death rate. This is one of several reasons for treating systolic hypertension. Angiotensin-converting enzyme (ACE) inhibitors and $Ca^{2+}$ channel blockers are particularly effective at reducing hypertensive left ventricle hypertrophy.

## What initiates the resistance vessel and renal pathology?

The answer to this key question remains incomplete, but both genetic and environmental factors are involved. Impaired renal salt handling (possibly genetic) and sympathetic hyperactivity coupled with a high dietary salt intake (environmental) are pivotal in many patients.

### Genetic factors

Genetic factors account for distinct familial and racial tendencies towards hypertension. For example, BP correlates better between monozygotic twins than adopted siblings; the response of BP to a standard intravenous or dietary salt load reveals salt-sensitive families; and hypertension is more common in blacks than caucasians. Only rarely is a single gene defect responsible, for example, the renal $Na^+$ channel gene in Liddle syndrome. Generally, multiple genes are implicated. Most of the hypertension-susceptibility genes identified to date, such as angiotensinogen and ACE gene variants, affect renal $Na^+$ handling. We may also have protective genes; a gain-of-function mutation in the human vascular smooth muscle $BK_{Ca}$ channel promotes hyperpolarization and vasorelaxation, and is associated with a reduced incidence of hypertension. About 30%–60% of BP variation is estimated to be genetic (cf. environmental).

### Environmental factors

Both epidemiological and direct, interventional studies show a link between hypertension and **high dietary $Na^+Cl^-$ intake**, **low dietary $K^+$**, **obesity**, **stress** and **alcohol consumption**. This has led to a number of causative theories, among which high dietary salt intake and impaired renal salt handling are pivotal.

## Salt imbalance renal hypothesis

### High salt intake

The natural diet of primates is low in salt ($Na^+Cl^-$) and rich in $K^+$, so the kidney has evolved powerful $Na^+$-retaining mechanisms. The salt hypothesis proposes that a small but sustained discrepancy between the high, modern dietary $Na^+$ intake and renal $Na^+$ excretion raises the body salt mass, which then causes hypertension through multiple mechanisms (see later in the chapter). Epidemiological studies and direct, interventional studies of humans, primates, dogs and rats show a strong association between a high salt diet (>10 g/day) and hypertension. Salt sensitivity evidently has a genetic component since it often runs in families; the salt-sensitive Dahl strain of rats develops hypertension on a salt intake that is harmless to ordinary rats.

### Low $K^+$ intake

Hypertension correlates even better with the dietary $Na^+$:$K^+$ ratio than with salt intake *per se*. The ratio is >2.5 for a typical Western diet. Given a fixed daily salt intake, $K^+$ supplementation by fruit and vegetables ($Na^+$:$K^+$ ~0) lowers BP. Conversely, reducing the $K^+$ intake raises BP, because it promotes renal tubular $Na^+$ reabsorption.

### How does salt overload cause hypertension?

Plasma [$Na^+$] increases by ~2 mM in hypertensive patients. The **cardiac hypothesis** proposes that an increase in salt mass, acting via the central osmoreceptor–antidiuretic hormone (ADH) pathway and thirst centre, raises the extracellular fluid volume at an early stage (Figure 16.12). The attendant rise in the plasma volume increases the cardiac filling pressure, stroke volume and arterial BP, which in turn provokes tunica media remodelling and a rise in peripheral resistance.

However, contrary to the cardiac hypothesis, extracellular fluid volume and plasma volume are not consistently raised in hypertensives, so researchers have sought additional mechanisms. There is some evidence that a small, chronic increase in plasma [$Na^+$] directly affects vascular tone and remodelling. Also, a high $Na^+$ intake stimulates the adrenal cortex and brain to release a steroidal, **endogenous digitalis-like factor** (ouabain, or its stereoisomer). Circulating digitalis-like factor is raised in 40%–50% of hypertensives, and its action is to inhibit the electrogenic $3Na^+$/$2K^+$ pump of vascular myocytes (Figure 12.5). The resulting partial depolarization increases the L-type $Ca^{2+}$ channel open probability; also, the rise in intracellular [$Na^+$] reduces $Ca^{2+}$ expulsion by the $3Na^+$/$Ca^{2+}$ exchanger. Consequently, intracellular $Ca^{2+}$ increases, raising vascular tone.

### What disturbs renal $Na^+$ regulation in hypertension?

Normally, a high $Na^+$ intake triggers a fall in circulating RAA (Figure 14.12). This reduces distal tubular $Na^+$ and water reabsorption, and thus maintains $Na^+$ balance. Therefore, the question arises as to what causes the kidneys to retain too much $Na^+$ in hypertensive patients.

A subgroup of hypertensives (particularly white patients <55 years old), the **high RAA subgroup**, have raised RAA levels. This may contribute to the renal salt retention in these individuals. Not all hypertensives have raised RAA levels and ~25%, the **renal defect subgroup**, have low renin levels. Excessive renal $Na^+$ reabsorption in such cases may be due to an acquired dysfunction or genes encoding renal ion channels and transporters. In keeping with the renal defect hypothesis, normal rats develop hypertension when transplanted with kidneys from spontaneously hypertensive rats with narrow afferent renal arterioles.

## The sympathetic nervous system and neurogenic hypothesis

The sympathetic nervous system plays an important role in regulating renal haemodynamics, influencing the release of renin and being able to shift the renal pressure natriuresis curve to higher BPs. Recordings of sympathetic activity in mixed peripheral nerves show elevated activity in many human hypertensives. There is also a wealth of evidence from animal models that increased sympathetic activity precedes the development of hypertension. Multiple abnormalities that increase neuronal excitability have been identified such as those related to inflammation, reactive $O_2$ species, abnormal mitochondrial function and $Ca^{2+}$ handling. These may arise in afferents, for example, arising from the kidney and carotid body, in brainstem nuclei controlling sympathetic outflow and in postganglionic sympathetic neurons. Neuronal dysfunction at any or all of these sites may increase resting sympathetic drive. In addition, cerebral hypoperfusion can cause a reflex increase in sympathetic activity and BP via the Cushing reflex. Therefore, it is possible that brainstem hypoperfusion could drive hypertension in what has become known as the **selfish brain hypothesis**. Remodelling of cerebral resistance vessels has been shown to occur before the onset of hypertension in some animal models and a large imaging study in humans has reported a higher prevalence of congenital cerebrovascular variants, along with increased cerebral vascular resistance, reduced cerebral blood flow and a higher incidence of small ('lacunar') infarcts in patients with hypertension. Cerebral vascular resistance was also observed to be elevated before the onset of hypertension along with elevated sympathetic nerve activity.

Prolonged sympathetic activation may not only reset the renal pressure natriuresis relationship, but can also promote the development of left ventricular hypertrophy and vascular remodelling. Therefore, it may represent a key link between the kidney, vasculature and heart, which may initiate, amplify or perpetuate the development of hypertension.

## The multifactorial hypothesis

The long-term regulation of BP involves complex interactions between dietary, neural, hormonal and renal mechanisms

(Section 16.5), and hypertension may only develop when one or more of the regulatory processes is disturbed in a genetically susceptible individual. Whatever the initial cause, the process is self-perpetuating once media remodelling develops; a rise in arterial pressure evokes media remodelling/hypertrophy, which normalizes the wall stress but raises the resistance and arterial pressure, which evokes further wall changes, and so on.

## Clinical sequelae and therapeutic strategies

Hypertension itself is virtually symptomless; contrary to popular belief, it rarely presents with nosebleeds or headaches. Untreated, however, hypertension (and especially systolic hypertension) damages the heart, brain, retina and kidneys, leading to:

- hypertensive heart failure;
- coronary artery atheroma and myocardial infarction;
- cerebrovascular accidents (strokes);
- hypertensive retinopathy;
- chronic renal failure.

Therefore, it is important to treat hypertension. The SPRINT (Systolic Blood Pressure Intervention Trial) trial showed that aggressive reduction of systolic BP (target <120 mmHg compared with <140 mmHg) gave a 25% reduction in cardiovascular morbidity and mortality. The trial was ended early due to the large differences between groups. Six types of lifestyle change have been shown to reduce BP: reduction of dietary salt to 5 g daily (~4 mmHg); increased fruit and vegetable intake (~5 mmHg at seven portions/day); reduction of obesity (~2 mmHg per kg lost); reduction of fat intake; limitation of alcohol consumption; and >30 min dynamic exercise three times per week. Further reduction is achieved through a graded pharmacological approach, the **ACD** regime:

- **'A': ACE inhibitors/angiotensin receptor blockers.** Captopril, enalapril and ramipril block ACE and therefore reduce levels of angiotensin II and aldosterone. This causes peripheral vasodilatation as well as dilating the glomerular afferent arteriole, and inhibiting tubular $Na^+$ reabsorption. They reduce the operating value of the renal pressure natriuresis curve to lower mean arterial pressures particularly at lower urinary $Na^+$ excretion rates; therefore, they may work best when combined with dietary salt restriction (see Figure 18.13). A common side effect is a dry cough, due to the concurrent inhibition of bradykinin breakdown (via kininase II). Losartan and valsartan block the $AT_1$ receptor and avoid this side effect. Aliskiren binds to and inhibits renin.
- **'C': $Ca^{2+}$ channel blockers** (nifedipine, amlodipine) are vasodilators that can act on the renal afferent arteriole to shift the pressure natriuresis curve to a lower mean arterial pressure, as shown in Figure 18.13. Alpha$_1$ adrenergic receptor inhibitors (prazosin, long-acting doxazosin) reduce sympathetic vasoconstrictor tone and may alter renal pressure natriuresis via a similar mechanism, but this often results in postural

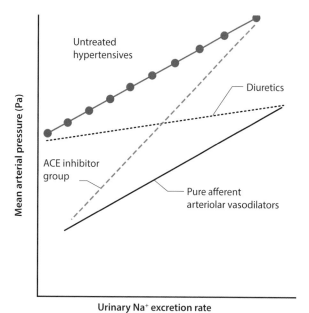

**Figure 18.13** Effects of antihypertensive agents on the pressure-natriuresis relationship for untreated hypertensives (red circles). See Figure 18.9 as a comparison. Pure vasodilators, such as $Ca^{2+}$ antagonists, tend to shift the pressure-natriuresis relationship towards the lower $Pa$ without a change of slope, by preferentially dilating the afferent renal arteriole; a similar effect is achieved by removal of a renal artery stenosis. Agents in the ACE-inhibitor group tend to shift the pressure-natriuresis curve to lower values of $Pa$ while also increasing its gradient. Drugs in this group would be expected also to include $\beta_1$ adrenergic receptor antagonists, centrally acting agents such as $\alpha_2$ adrenergic receptor agonists, and angiotensin II receptor antagonists because they all have renal actions predominantly via central or peripheral modulation of the renin–angiotensin system. The third group is that of diuretics, which shift the pressure-natriuresis line to lower values of $Pa$ while decreasing its gradient. (Adapted from Dorrington KL, Pandit JJ. *Anaesthesia* 2009; 64(11); 1218–28.)

hypotension from peripheral vasodilatation, so they are used less often.

- **'D': diuretics.** Thiazide diuretics (e.g. bendroflumethiazide, hydrochlorothiazide) inhibit $Na^+$ reabsorption (via inhibition of the $Na^+Cl^-$ cotransporter) at the distal convoluted tubule of the nephron. This reduces water reabsorption in the distal nephron and collecting duct to reduce the extracellular fluid volume. They also have a poorly explained vasodilator action. They tend to lower the gradient of the renal pressure natriuresis curve, as shown in Figure 18.13.

- **β adrenergic receptor blockers** (propranolol, atenolol, metoprolol) reduce cardiac output, so are not ideal in those over 55. They also reduce the sympathetic outflow and activation of the juxtaglomerular apparatus (renin secretion), leading to a gradual lowering of BP over several days. These have fallen out of favour as a treatment for hypertension, but are used where there is another indication for β blockade (e.g. angina, anxiety).

The current NICE guidelines and others are heavily influenced by two clinical trials that compare different antihypertensive medications. The ALLHAT (Antihypertensive and Lipid Lowering Treatment to Prevent Heart Attack Trial) trial

demonstrated relative clinic equivalence between several single first-line antihypertensives (including ACE inhibitors, β blockers, $Ca^{2+}$ channel blockers and thiazide diuretics) although $\alpha_1$ adrenergic receptor inhibitors performed less well. The ASCOT (Anglo-Scandinavian Cardiac Outcomes Trial) trial compared combinations of two antihypertensive medications (which the majority of patients require for adequate BP control). This found that a combination of ACE inhibitors and $Ca^{2+}$ channel blocker to be superior to a combination of a thiazide diuretic and β adrenergic receptor blocker. Therefore, the aim is to start patients on either 'A' or 'C' and then if a second-line agent is required, combine A with C. RAA inhibitors are the first-choice treatment for white patients under 55 because this subgroup often has high renin activity levels, although they tend to be poorly represented in clinic al trials. $Ca^{2+}$ blockers are recommended for white patients over 55 and black patients (who have lower plasma renin activity). If treatment A or C proves inadequate, the next stage is A + C + D, followed if necessary by the addition of further drug classes.

The central role of the kidney and the autonomic nervous system prompted investigation of renal denervation (an interventional procedure using catheters) for the treatment of drug-resistant hypertension. Early trials (SYMPLICITY HTN-1 and -2) showed promising results but were controversial because of lack of an adequate control group. SYMPLICITY HTN-3 was a large, sham-controlled randomized trial designed to address these concerns. It was negative, which has significantly reduced excitement about the renal denervation procedure. However, initial results from the SPYRAL HTN OFF-MED study (catheter-based renal denervation in patients with uncontrolled hypertension in the absence of antihypertensive medications), which uses a new spiral-shaped multi-electrode catheter to deliver the ablation treatment, look promising in patients with mild to moderate hypertension not taking antihypertensive medications. It may be that the denervation procedure can be improved further or that it might have a more specific role in certain patient subgroups with high sympathetic drive.

The overall aim of lifestyle intervention and treatment is to reduce systolic pressure to 135–145 mmHg or less, and diastolic pressure to 85 mmHg or less. This reduces the incidence of strokes by 38% and cardiovascular deaths by 21%. Untreated, ~50% of patients develop heart failure, 25% renal failure and 25% cerebral complications (retinopathy, encephalopathy, strokes).

## 18.5 CHRONIC HEART FAILURE

Chronic heart failure (or congestive cardiac failure) is a chronic inability of the heart to maintain adequate tissue perfusion at a normal filling pressure. Starling, working with the isolated heart-lung preparation, observed that when the heart begins to fail, it requires a higher filling pressure and higher end diastolic volume to maintain its stroke volume (Figure 18.14).

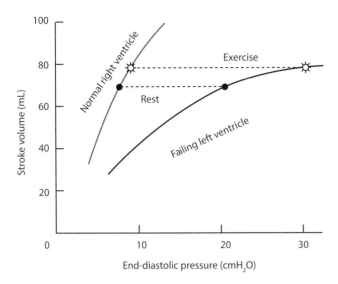

**Figure 18.14** Operation of the Frank–Starling mechanism in a patient with a failing left ventricle but still normal right ventricle. The left ventricle function curve is depressed. Under resting conditions (filled circles), the left ventricle requires an elevated filling pressure to match the right ventricle stroke volume. During exercise (open symbols), the disparity in filling pressure becomes extreme owing to the near-plateau on the function curve of the failing left ventricle. The attendant pulmonary congestion will cause severe exertional dyspnoea.

At a normal filling pressure, the stroke volume would decline. Thus, the immediate cause of cardiac failure is a fall in the energy of contraction at a given end diastolic volume (preload). This fall can arise from reduced myocardial contractility (systolic heart failure) or from impaired relaxation and filling (diastolic heart failure).

## Causes and clinical course

In many but not all patients, a recognizable pathology initiates heart failure. The most common **causes of chronic left ventricular failure** are: (1) diffuse coronary artery disease; (2) reduced myocardial mass due to an infarct (two-thirds of cases have a history of ischaemic heart disease); (3) excessive work (afterload) due to clinical hypertension or aortic valve disease; and (4) cardiomyopathy. Cardiac failure in older patients, not attributable to these causes, is thought to be an idiopathic myopathy, arising from myocyte senescence and death.

The most common **causes of chronic right ventricular failure** are (1) pulmonary hypertension due to chronic lung disease or high altitude and (2) left ventricular failure, which increases the pressure work of the right ventricle. Biventricular failure is therefore common.

The clinical features of left and right ventricular failure are summarized in Table 18.1. The most common presenting features are **exercise intolerance**, that is, excessive fatigue during moderate exercise; or **breathlessness (dyspnoea)**, especially on lying down (orthopnoea) and at night (nocturnal dyspnoea), due to left ventricular failure; or **ankle swelling** (peripheral oedema), due to right ventricular failure. Reduced systolic ('squeezing') function is most commonly diagnosed with echocardiography, and is manifest as a reduced left (LV) or right ventricle (RV) ejection fraction. The mortality rate is 50% over 5 years, and the cause of death is usually **pump failure** or **ventricular arrhythmia**. The cellular basis of pump failure and arrhythmia is described next, followed by the pathophysiological changes in the heart and circulation.

More recently, it has been recognized that up to 50% of cases of heart failure have normal or near-normal myocardial contractility. This condition is known as heart failure with preserved ejection fraction (HF-PEF) or 'diastolic heart failure', and is less well understood than heart failure with reduced ejection fraction (HF-REF). It appears that a majority of such cases involve an impairment of diastolic ('relaxing') function of the left ventricle. This initially may seem counterintuitive, but it is important to realize whilst relaxation is mainly a passive process in the normal heart (see Chapter 2.2), if the ventricle becomes stiff and loses its elastic recoil, then it becomes more reliant on active relaxation and atrial contraction in order to adequately fill. Conditions that affect the diastolic relaxation of heart muscle such as diabetes, or that stiffen the heart such as hypertension are risk factors for the development of HF-PEF. There is no proven treatment, although diuretics can be useful to reduce symptoms but have no prognostic benefit.

## Impaired excitation-contraction coupling reduces contractility

Cardiac myocytes from failing ventricles show multiple structural, transporter and channel abnormalities, namely:

- loss of T-tubules leading to inefficient excitation-contraction coupling;

**Table 18.1** Characteristic signs and symptoms of chronic left- or right-sided heart failure[a]

| Left ventricular failure | Right ventricular failure |
|---|---|
| Shortness of breath (dyspnoea) | Oedematous swelling of feet, ankles and legs (sacrum if bed-bound) |
| Orthopnoea (dyspnoea on lying down) | Hepatomegaly (enlarged, palpable, tender liver) |
| Paroxysmal nocturnal dyspnoea | Ascites (fluid in abdominal cavity) |
| Pulmonary congestion and oedema (crackles) | Excessive nocturnal urination (caused by oedema fluid excretion) |
| Exercise intolerance | Raised jugular venous pressure (JVP) |
|  | Exercise intolerance |

[a] It is common for both left and right ventricular failure to coexist. Additional diagnostic signs include a laterally displaced, weak apex beat, third heart sound and chest X-ray abnormalities, such as a cardiothoracic ratio of >0.5 in the postero-anterior projection or pulmonary oedema.

- reduced Ca$^{2+}$ pumping into the sarcoplasmic reticulum (SR) due to lower levels of sarcoplasmic/endoplasmic reticulum Ca$^{2+}$ ATPase 2a expression;
- impaired, leaky SR Ca$^{2+}$ release channels (ryanodine receptor 2) and increased phosphorylation by Ca$^{2+}$-calmodulin-dependent protein kinase II;
- reduced SR Ca$^{2+}$ content;
- upregulation of the sarcolemmal Na$^+$/Ca$^{2+}$ exchanger;
- downregulation of K$^+$ channels (inwardly rectifying, K$_{ir}$; transient outward current ($i_{to}$), K$_v$4.3).

Systolic contractile failure arises primarily from these cellular abnormalities, as follows.

The reduced contractility of failing myocytes is due primarily to a **reduced, slow systolic Ca$^{2+}$ transient**. This is caused by a fall in the size of the SR Ca$^{2+}$ store, and impaired Ca$^{2+}$ release (Figure 18.15). The fall in store size is the result of a reduced expression and activity of the SR Ca$^{2+}$ pumps (SERCA2a), exacerbated by a diastolic leak of Ca$^{2+}$ out of altered Ca$^{2+}$ release channels (RyR2). In addition, the loss of T-tubules leads to inefficient Ca$^{2+}$-induced Ca$^{2+}$ release and excitation-contraction coupling. The diastolic Ca$^{2+}$ leak, coupled with slow Ca$^{2+}$ reuptake in early diastole by the reduced SR pump, impairs diastolic relaxation. The failing ventricle thus displays diastolic dysfunction (stiffness), as well as systolic dysfunction. The slow diastolic relaxation impairs ventricular filling and is always present to some degree where there is systolic heart failure.

Several additional factors contribute to systolic dysfunction, namely a fall in the sensitivity of troponin to Ca$^{2+}$, wall fibrosis, dilatation (see later) and impaired energy use. One concept is that the failing heart is an 'engine out of fuel' and that this contributes to the pathophysiology. There is evidence for:

- impaired overall substrate use and a switch from fatty acids to glucose as the chief energy substrate;
- impaired oxidative phosphorylation with structural abnormalities observed in mitochondria and reduced adenosine triphosphate (ATP) synthase capacity;
- impaired ATP transfer and use. Creatine kinase, which transfers high energy phosphate from creatine phosphate to adenosine diphosphate (ADP) to maintain ATP availability, declines not only in the myocardium but also in skeletal muscles – a factor that may contribute to the characteristic exercise intolerance.

## Multiple electrophysiological abnormalities cause arrhythmia

Ventricular arrhythmia is a common cause of death in cardiac failure patients, especially when secondary to ischaemic heart disease. While the overall Ca$^{2+}$ transient is reduced and action potential duration prolonged in chronic heart failure, this does not occur homogeneously across the ventricle. The edge or 'borderzone' of myocardial infarction scars can remodel differently,

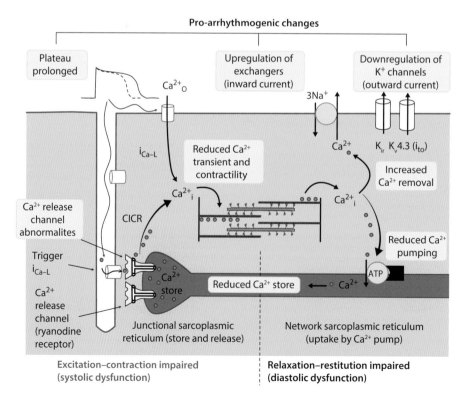

**Figure 18.15** Changes in cardiac myocyte Ca$^{2+}$ cycle, ionic currents and action potential in chronic heart failure. The dashed line is the normal action potential. ATP, adenosine triphosphate; CICR, Ca$^{2+}$-induced Ca$^{2+}$ release (Section 3.7). (Based on information in Sipido KR, Eisner D. *Cardiovascular Research* 2005; 68(2): 167–74; and Bers DM. *Physiology* 2006; 21: 380–7.)

and regional variation in the effects of high sympathetic drive can lead to some areas of the ventricle at times developing significant shortening of action potential duration and overload of intracellular $Ca^{2+}$ stores. Ventricular arrhythmia can therefore be triggered by a **delayed afterdepolarization** (DAD; Figure 3.16). DADs occur when the SR $Ca^{2+}$ store discharges spontaneously during diastole, stimulating the depolarizing $3Na^+/Ca^{2+}$ exchanger current, $i_{Na-Ca}$ (Section 3.10). Due to the **upregulation of the $Na^+/Ca^{2+}$ exchanger** (more inward, depolarizing current) and **downregulation of the inwardly rectifying $K^+$ channel** (less outward, polarizing current), a relatively modest SR $Ca^{2+}$ discharge can generate a DAD of sufficient size to trigger an extra-systole (or ectopic beat) which may have the required substrate to form a re-entrant circuit and ventricular arrhythmia. The SR discharge in diastole may be the result of $Ca^{2+}$ overload (driven by the raised **sympathetic activity** of heart failure) and leakiness of the $Ca^{2+}$ release channels due to channel phosphorylation, particularly by **$Ca^{2+}$-calmodulin-dependent protein kinase II (CaMKII)**. CaMKIIδ, the main cardiac isoform, appears to be an important nodal point integrating several cellular signalling pathways. Prolonged stimulation by $Ca^{2-}$/calmodulin as a result of β adrenergic stimulation, or modification by reactive $O_2$ species, can lead to autophosphorylation and $Ca^{2+}$-independent activation of the enzyme. CaMKIIδ can cause myocardial hypertrophy through altering transcriptional regulation, but also phosphorylates RyR2 and phospholamban. This increases SR $Ca^{2+}$ loading and diastolic SR $Ca^{2+}$ release, which may predispose to delayed afterdepolarizations. In addition, CaMKIIδ may have proarrhythmic actions on ventricular electrophysiology, including increasing L-type $Ca^{2+}$ current and late $Na^+$ current. Heart failure is also accompanied by upregulation of the $β_2$ receptor, which may increase conduction velocity, and increase action potential duration heterogeneity in failing hearts. Excessive sympathetic activity is a prominent feature of heart failure and predisposes to arrhythmia. Consequently, β blockers can reduce the risk of ventricular arrhythmia and mortality.

Another proarrhythmic change is that other areas of the ventricle develop **action potential prolongation**, therefore further increasing **heterogeneity** in severe failure (Figure 18.15). This is caused by the **downregulation of $K_v4.3$ channels**, which carry the early repolarizing current $i_{to}$. The delayed rectifier ($K_v$) is also often downregulated. Repolarization depends on the outward $K^+$ currents exceeding the (increased) inward current $i_{Na-Ca}$; so the plateau is prolonged. This is seen as an increased QT interval in the electrocardiogram (ECG). The lengthening of the plateau, and hence the refractory period, is greater in some myocytes than others. This heterogeneity in electrophysiology as well as patchy fibrosis throughout the ventricle increases the likelihood of **re-entry circuits** developing, and hence ventricular tachycardia or fibrillation (Figure 5.10).

To summarize, the upregulation of the $Na^+/Ca^{2+}$ exchanger, heterogeneous downregulation of $K^+$ channels and sympathetic activation contribute to the high incidence of arrhythmia in failing hearts because these changes facilitate (1) the development of the DADs that trigger arrhythmia and (2) the re-entry circuits that sustain arrhythmia.

## Resting cardiac output may/may not be reduced substantially: compensatory rise in filling pressure

A fall in myocardial contractility depresses the ventricular function curve (Figure 18.14) and pump function curve (stroke volume versus arterial pressure; Figure 6.15). However, in **moderate failure** there is surprisingly little reduction in the resting stroke volume, owing to a compensatory rise in ventricular filling pressure to >12 cmH$_2$O. This raises both EDV and end-systolic volume, so there is **ventricular dilatation** throughout the cardiac cycle (Figure 18.16). Consequently, the **cardiothoracic ratio** (cardiac shadow width/thoracic cavity width in postero-anterior projection chest radiogram) exceeds its normal value of 0.5 (Figure 18.17). The increase in the filling pressure and EDV shifts the ventricle up the depressed ventricular function curve, restoring contractile energy through the Frank–Starling mechanism (Figure 18.14). Due to this interaction, resting stroke volume and cardiac output can be almost normal in moderate failure (Figure 6.13). The ejection fraction, by contrast, is always reduced (Figure 18.16). In **severe failure**, the ventricular function curve is so depressed that the stroke volume falls despite the increased EDV. The **ejection fraction**, measured by echocardiography, falls from its normal resting value of 65% to as little as 10%–20%.

To summarize, the resting cardiac output can be within the normal range in **compensated failure** (Figure 18.16) or subnormal in **decompensated failure**. In either case, ventricular filling pressure is raised, and the heart is dilated throughout the cardiac cycle.

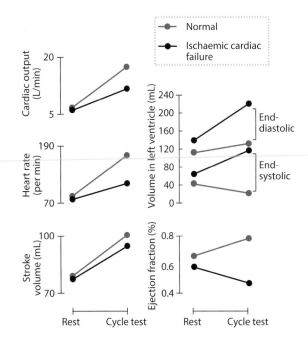

**Figure 18.16** Effect of chronic cardiac failure on cardiac performance at rest and during a standard exercise test, submaximal bicycle ergometry. Data from Table 17.2.

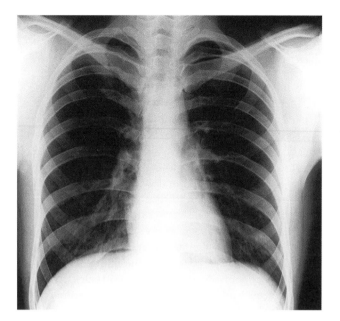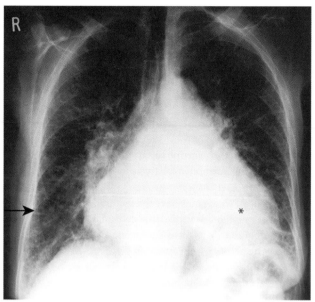

**Figure 18.17** Antero-posterior radiograph of chest. (Left) Normal individual; cardiothoracic ratio 0.45. (Right) Patient with left ventricular failure; cardiothoracic ratio 0.72. The asterisk marks a grossly dilated left ventricle. Arrow, septal line caused by interstitial oedema (Kerley B lines). Radiating opacities due to pulmonary interstitial oedema are present in the left lung field (Kerley A lines). Also note the 'air bronchogram' (the outlining of the major bronchi by surrounding oedema) and blunting of the costophrenic angle images by oedema. (Courtesy of Dr A Wilson, St George's Hospital, London.)

## How is the filling pressure raised in heart failure?

The compensatory increase in ventricular filling pressure is responsible for most of the clinical features of heart failure, including cardiac dilatation, pulmonary congestion (causing dyspnoea), jugular venous pressure elevation and ankle oedema (Table 18.1). But how does ventricular dysfunction raise the filling pressure? Multiple mechanisms are involved. The first is the **sump pump effect** (Figure 6.12). The cardiac pump removes blood from the feed line (the sump – central veins/pulmonary veins) and transfers it into the outflow line (pulmonary artery, aorta). If the pump becomes less effective, returning blood is removed less quickly from the feed line, so pressure builds up there. However, haemodynamic modelling indicates that the sump pump effect cannot account for the entire rise in filling pressure. A second factor is **increased sympathetic venomotor activity**, which causes marked peripheral venoconstriction and thereby shifts peripheral venous blood into the thorax. A third factor is **increased renal salt and water retention** (see later). This expands the extracellular fluid compartment by up to 30%, and the attendant increase in plasma volume helps raise the cardiac filling pressure.

## Cardiac output fails to increase normally during exercise

An **exercise test** reveals cardiac failure even when the output is compensated at rest. Figure 18.16 shows that a standard exercise test raised cardiac output in normal patients to 18 L/min, whereas in heart failure the output increased to only 11 L/min. The inadequate output during exercise is due to two factors: stroke volume impairment and, surprisingly, impaired tachycardia (Figure 18.16).

**Stroke volume** fails to increase adequately for several reasons: (1) stroke volume is less responsive than normal to the exercise-induced rise in the filling pressure (preload) because the slope of the ventricular function curve is reduced (Figure 18.14); (2) stroke volume is more susceptible to depression by the raised arterial pressure (afterload) of exercise because the pump function curve is depressed (Figure 6.15); (3) the $\beta_1$ adrenergic receptor pathway, which normally raises contractility and ejection fraction during exercise, is impaired in heart failure; (4) diastolic relaxation is impaired by the slow reuptake of $Ca^{2+}$ into the SR, so diastolic filling is impaired ('diastolic failure' or 'HF-PEF').

The **impaired heart rate response and contractile reserve** is due partly to a fall in tyrosine hydroxylase activity in cardiac sympathetic terminals, leading to NAd depletion. Also, $\beta_1$ adrenergic receptors are downregulated in failing cardiac myocytes, due to increased phosphorylation by $\beta$ adrenergic receptor kinase 1 ($\beta$-ARK1, otherwise known as G-protein-coupled receptor kinase 2). Binding of $\beta$-arrestin-1 then leads to desensitization of the receptor and its internalization via endocytosis. The activity of $\beta$-arrestin-1 and $\beta$-ARK1 are influenced by levels of cAMP, the second messenger of the $\beta$ adrenergic receptor itself.

## The puzzle of exercise intolerance

Excessive fatigue during moderate exercise is a common presenting symptom of cardiac failure. Surprisingly, patients often experience fatigue at low work levels, that call for little increase in cardiac output – so exercise intolerance is not fully explained by the limited rise in cardiac output or by the exertional dyspnoea. It appears that $Ca^{2+}$ handling is abnormal in the skeletal muscle fibres, as well as cardiac fibres. Slow skeletal muscle fibres and cardiac myocytes express the same isoform of SR $Ca^{2+}$ ATPase; in animal models of heart failure, skeletal muscle fibres show reduced $Ca^{2+}$ reuptake, slow relaxation and impaired fatigue resistance. There is also evidence of reduced mitochondrial function and creatine kinase levels. Changes in the skeletal muscle themselves thus contribute to exercise intolerance during heart failure.

## Compensatory mechanisms to support the failing heart cause many problems

Chronic cardiac failure evokes responses in other tissues/organs that can be a mix of helpful and harmful. The chief responses are:

- compensatory influences on the heart;
- sympathetic redistribution of the cardiac output among the peripheral tissues;
- renal retention of salt and water;
- pulmonary congestion and oedema;
- peripheral oedema.

This section deals with the first of these – compensatory influences on the heart. The output of the failing heart is supported by an increase in **filling pressure**, as described earlier, and also by an increase in **adrenergic stimulation** by circulating catecholamines and sympathetic activity. The resulting compensation is effective in mild failure at rest, but not during exercise or severe failure. Moreover, the compensatory mechanism can have harmful side effects, such as dyspnoea.

### Circulating catecholamine concentration rises but $\beta_1$ adrenergic receptors are downregulated

Plasma adrenaline and NAd concentration increases markedly in heart failure, though the cardiac sympathetic terminals become depleted of NAd in severe failure. During mild failure the inotropic action of the catecholamines helps to support the stroke volume. However, as the disease progresses the uncoupling and downregulation of myocardial $\beta_1$ adrenergic receptors vitiate the inotropic effect.

### Raised filling pressure: friend or foe?

In mild failure the rise in filling pressure and diastolic dilatation improves the contractile energy by the Frank–Starling mechanism, so resting stroke volume is almost normal (Figure 18.16). However, as failure worsens the ventricular function curve becomes flatter, so increases in filling pressure and cardiac dilatation achieve little increase in stroke volume; rather, they cause serious problems, as follows:

- Cardiac dilatation impairs the **mechanical efficiency** of systole, as dictated by **Laplace's law** (equation 6.1, Section 6.8). That is to say, the contractile force needed

to generate systolic pressure increases with ventricular radius (Figure 6.14). Cardiac dilatation thus increases the energy cost of systole.
- In a grossly dilated heart, **tricuspid/mitral valve leakage** may occur during systole due to the widened atrioventricular orifices and separation ('lateralization') of the papillary muscles, which pull on the free margins of the valve leaflets through the chordae tendineae. If the free margins cannot meet and seal properly, regurgitation reduces the effective stroke volume. Tricuspid regurgitation can also cause a palpable liver pulsation during systole.
- The high filling pressures associated with left ventricular failure causes **pulmonary vascular congestion** (Figure 18.17) and **extra-alveolar oedema**. The stiffened lungs require more effort to inflate, generating a sensation of difficulty in breathing called **dyspnoea**.
- The high CVP associated with right ventricular failure causes **peripheral oedema**, a visibly **raised jugular venous pressure** and **hepatomegaly**.

Thus, there are many reasons for reducing the cardiac filling pressure and dilatation therapeutically.

## Sympathetic-mediated peripheral vasoconstriction redistributes cardiac output and supports blood pressure

The limited cardiac output is preferentially distributed to the coronary, cerebral and skeletal muscle circulations through intense vasoconstriction of other tissues (Figure 18.18). In the cutaneous, renal and splanchnic vascular beds, resistance vessels and veins are constricted by **increased sympathetic vasomotor activity**, along with increased circulating **catecholamines**, **angiotensin II** and **endothelin-1**. Increased sympathetic activity is a pronounced feature of heart failure, driven perhaps by the hypothalamic paraventricular nucleus and baroreflex. Resistance vessel vasoconstriction maintains the arterial pressure, which would otherwise be threatened by a low cardiac output; venoconstriction contributes to the rise in cardiac filling pressure. In mild failure, these responses can be beneficial. However, in severe failure venoconstriction contributes to the excessive cardiac dilatation, and the afterload created by the maintained arterial pressure curtails the stroke volume of the enfeebled ventricle (Figure 6.15).

## Renal salt and water retention expands the extracellular fluid compartment, contributing to oedema

During cardiac failure, the kidneys retain salt and water. The resulting expansion of the extracellular fluid compartment, by up to 30%, contributes to cardiac dilatation and oedema formation. Salt and water retention is caused by the **increased renal sympathetic activity**, which causes **renal vasoconstriction** (Figure 18.18) and activates the **RAAS**. Circulating aldosterone

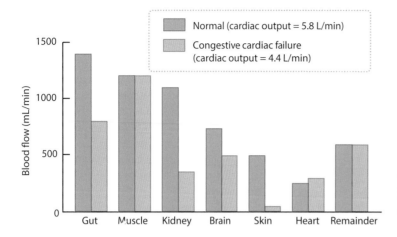

**Figure 18.18** Redistribution of cardiac output in a resting patient with chronic cardiac failure and an output of 4.4 L/min (grey columns). Note the reduced perfusion of the kidney, gut and skin, caused by a high sympathetic activity. (From Wade OL, Bishop JM. *Cardiac Output and Regional Flow*. Oxford: Blackwell, 1962, by permission.)

is raised further through reduced degradation in the congested, underperfused liver. Circulating **natriuretic factors** (NFs) are also raised, due to atrial NF secretion by the distended atria and a big increase in brain NF secretion by the distended ventricles. NFs may have a beneficial role in attenuating the excessive renal retention of salt and water. Raised plasma brain natriuretic peptide is used clinically as a marker of heart failure.

## Pulmonary congestion, pulmonary oedema and/or peripheral oedema occur in heart failure

### Pulmonary congestion, oedema and dyspnoea result from left ventricular failure

Ischaemic failure affects the LV primarily. If the LV transiently pumps out less blood than the right, blood accumulates in the lungs, raising pulmonary venous pressure ('sump pump' effect, see earlier) until the Frank–Starling mechanism restores left-right equality (Figure 18.14). The resulting pulmonary congestion (vascular distension) is obvious in chest radiographs (Figure 18.16). The congestion reduces lung compliance, making them stiffer and harder to inflate, thus **increasing the work of breathing**. The unpleasant sensation of having to work inappropriately hard to draw each breath is called **dyspnoea** (difficulty in breathing). Dyspnoea is a major symptom of left ventricular failure (Table 18.1).

Because capillary pressure is higher than venous pressure, the increased pulmonary venous pressure raises pulmonary capillary pressure, which increases transcapillary filtration. This leads to **pulmonary oedema**. In moderate pulmonary oedema, the excess fluid collects in the pulmonary interstitium and inside the bronchi, causing basal crackles (**crepitations**) during breathing, audible through a stethoscope. In severe pulmonary oedema, fluid also accumulates in the alveoli, impairing $O_2$ transport, with potentially fatal results.

Pulmonary vascular congestion and interstitial oedema become worse on lying down because of the shift of blood into the thorax. Consequently, cardiac dyspnoea becomes worse on lying down (**orthopnoea**). Pulmonary oedema gradually increases as the night wears on, awakening the patient with an

attack of **paroxysmal nocturnal dyspnoea.** Consequently, patients in failure tend to sleep propped up by several pillows.

### Peripheral oedema results from right ventricular failure

When the RV fails, CVP is raised by the sump pump effect, peripheral venoconstriction and renal salt and water retention. The rise in CVP raises venous pressures throughout the systemic circulation; for example, pressure in the venous limb of human skin capillaries at heart level rises to 20–40 mmHg (normal 12–15 mmHg). Also, the plasma COP falls by ~7 mmHg because of the increase in plasma volume caused by salt and water retention. The altered Starling forces increase the transcapillary filtration rate, leading to peripheral oedema (Section 11.10). Oedema is usually located in a dependent region (feet, ankles, leg; Figure 11.16), or over the sacrum in bedridden patients. The combination of **distended jugular veins** and **pitting peripheral oedema** points strongly to right ventricular failure.

Failure occurs not infrequently in both the right and left ventricles, so patients may have both peripheral and pulmonary oedema.

### Treatment is based on physiological principles

The treatment of cardiac failure is an exercise in applied physiology, aimed at relieving the symptoms and improving the condition of the heart. Specifically, the objectives are to:

1. reduce myocardial $O_2$ demand, by reducing cardiac work;
2. improve stroke volume, by reducing arterial BP (afterload);
3. improve mechanical efficiency, by reducing cardiac dilatation (Laplace's law);
4. reduce pulmonary congestion/oedema by reducing plasma volume and filling pressure;
5. prevent arrhythmias;
6. improve myocardial contractility.

These objectives are addressed as follows:

1. **Cardiac work** can be reduced by bed rest, afterload reduction and filling pressure (preload) reduction. **Afterload** can be reduced by peripheral vasodilators, such as ACE inhibitors (ramipril, lisinopril) or angiotensin receptor blockers (ARBs) such as candesartan and losartan. In those where ACE inhibitors or ARBs are contraindicated (pregnancy, renal failure), hydralazine can be used with a nitrate to produce vasodilatation. **Filling pressure** can be reduced by venodilators (intravenous nitroprusside or nitroglycerine in acute heart failure, or again ACE inhibitors). An **ACE inhibitor** is usually the drug of first choice because it has multiple actions, namely relaxation of resistance and capacitance vessels, reduction of sympathetic activity and reduction of renal fluid retention. **ARBs** (losartan, candesartan) are slightly more expensive alternatives, commonly used when ACE inhibitors cause persistent coughing (due to increased bradykinin from kininase II inhibition). **β adrenergic receptor blockers** (bisoprolol, carvedilol and metoprolol) oppose the increased sympathetic tone seen in chronic heart failure. Beta blockers slow the heart rate, which reduces cardiac work, increasing the diastolic interval for coronary perfusion (Figure 15.5) and helping compensate for slow relaxation (diastolic dysfunction). Beta blockers substantially reduce mortality in heart failure but must be used carefully. The patient must be euvolaemic when the medication is started, and the dose should be titrated up slowly, aiming for the highest tolerated dose over weeks and months. **Ivabradine** is a newer drug that acts on the pacemaker ('funny') current (hyperpolarization-activated cyclic nucleotide-gated channels) at the sino-atrial node to reduce heart rate and hence cardiac work. It is used where the patient cannot take a β blocker at all, or cannot tolerate an effective dose (resting heart rate >70 bpm). The patient must be in sinus rhythm because it has no effect in atrial fibrillation.

2. **Stroke volume** and ejection fraction can be markedly improved by reducing the pressure opposing ejection with the peripheral vasodilators discussed previously. Because of the steepness of the pump function curve, a small reduction in afterload can improve the stroke volume substantially; see Figure 6.15, point 4.

3 and 4. **Cardiac dilatation**, **pulmonary congestion** and **oedema** can be reduced by **diuretics**, such as furosemide (frusemide), which reduce extracellular fluid and plasma volume. **ACE inhibitors/ARBs** also help, by reducing aldosterone levels. If necessary, the aldosterone receptor antagonists **spironolactone** or eplerenone can also be added. These various pharmacological interventions reverse physiological compensations that have been overdone in cardiac failure. Neprilysin is an enzyme that breaks down natriuretic peptides; inhibition of this enzyme increases $Na^+$ loss and reduces plasma volume. However, neprilysin also breaks down angiotensin and endothelin, so **neprilysin inhibitors** are given in combination with an **ARB (sacubitril/valsartan)**.

5. **Arrhythmia**, an important cause of mortality in cardiac failure patients, is reduced by β **adrenergic receptor blockers**. ACE inhibitors also reduce the risk of sudden death through somewhat obscure mechanisms, probably relating to beneficial remodelling and reduction of sympathetic tone. The antiarrhythmic drug, amiodarone, is safe for use in structural heart disease but has only very modest effects on sudden death and its use is confined to patients who have already experienced ventricular arrhythmias. **Implantable cardioverter defibrillators** are far more effective and are increasingly widely used as a primary prevention measure when left ventricular systolic function is severely impaired.

6. **Myocardial contractility** could be improved acutely with emergency revascularization if acute myocardial infarction is the underlying cause of the heart failure. This approach was tested in the SHOCK trial, which demonstrated an improved mortality at 6 months after the event. Inotropic drugs, such as the $β_1$ agonists **dobutamine** and **dopamine,** the phosphodiesterase 3 inhibitor **milrinone** and the $Ca^{2+}$ sensitizer **levosimendan**, are used to provide short-term emergency support for the heart during acute failure. Milrinone increases mortality if used chronically. Temporary support can also be provided by mechanical means such as intra-aortic balloon counterpulsation or ventricular assist devices.

Otherwise, contractility can be partially restored by **digoxin**, which remains the only relatively safe inotropic drug for chronic oral use. The first published description of digoxin by William Withering in 1785 is a nice example of the roles of chance and a prepared mind in scientific discovery. Dr Withering was journeying through Shropshire when he was asked to see a woman suffering from severe dropsy (cardiac failure). He could do little for her; on his return journey, he was astonished to find her not only alive but much improved. On enquiring, he discovered that she had been taking a local folklore remedy, an infusion of the leaves of the foxglove, *Digitalis purpurea*. The efficacy of the digitalis infusion is illustrated in Figure 3.15. Digoxin boosts the intracellular $Ca^{2+}$ store (Section 3.8). Unfortunately, this can trigger afterdepolarizations and arrhythmia (coupled beats, called bigeminy; ventricular tachycardia; ventricular fibrillation), so plasma digoxin is usually monitored and maintained at 1–2.6 nM. However, digoxin toxicity can occur at 'safe' plasma levels and is increased by loop diuretics such as furosemide, which lower plasma [$K^+$]. $K^+$ and digoxin compete for the same $Na^+$–$K^+$–ATPase binding site. Because of these complications, and limited evidence of efficacy in heart failure, digoxin is not as widely prescribed as formerly. Digoxin is now used mainly when there is concomitant **atrial fibrillation**, because digoxin enhances parasympathetic activity through a central action, slowing atrioventricular (AV) node conduction and thus reducing ventricular rate (though generally not as effectively as β blockers).

Given this extensive pharmacological armoury, where does one start? Commonly used medications are summarized in Table 18.2, along with their evidence base, mechanism of action and common side effects. It is usual to commence therapy with

**Table 18.2** Medications used in chronic heart failure

| Drug class | Example (and trial)[a] | Mechanism of action | Side effects |
|---|---|---|---|
| ACE inhibitor | Enalapril (SOLVD), ramipril (AIRE) | Vasodilatation reduces afterload and cardiac work; opposes negative remodelling | Hypotension, hyperkalaemia, angio-oedema, cough (from kininase II inhibition and accumulation of bradykinin), renal impairment (especially in renal artery stenosis) |
| Angiotensin receptor blocker (ARB) | Losartan (ELITE II) | Vasodilatation reduces afterload and cardiac work; opposes negative remodelling | Hypotension, hyperkalaemia, renal impairment, angio-oedema |
| Combined neprilysin inhibitor and ARB | Sacubitril/valsartan (PARADIGM-HF) | Increases natriuretic peptides causing $Na^+$ loss and decreased plasma volume in addition to the action of valsartan | Hypotension, hyperkalaemia, renal impairment, angio-oedema (largely related to ARB) |
| β blocker | Metoprolol M/R (MERIT-HF), bisoprolol (CIBIS II), carvedilol (CAPRICORN) | Reduces cardiac work; oppose sympathetic overactivity | Bradycardia, hypotension, lethargy, impotence, nightmares |
| HCN channel blocker | Ivabradine (SHIFT trial in patients already on a β blocker with a resting pulse >70 bpm) | Reduces cardiac work by reducing heart rate | Visual disturbance |
| Aldosterone antagonist | Spironolactone (RALES), eplerenone (EPHESUS and EMPHASIS-HF) | Reduces plasma volume; opposes fibrosis and negative remodelling | Hyperkalaemia, renal impairment, hypotension, gynaecomastia (not eplerenone) |
| Hydralazine | Vascular smooth muscle vasodilatation and nitric oxide donor (useful in combination with isosorbide dinitrate in African-Americans: A-HeFT) | Vasodilatation reduces afterload and hence cardiac work | Hypotension, headache, reflex tachycardia, drug-induced lupus |
| Nitrate | Isosorbide dinitrate (A-HeFT) | Vaso- and venodilatation reduces preload and afterload and hence cardiac work | Hypotension, headache |
| Loop diuretic | Furosemide, bumetanide | Reduces plasma volume and filling pressure | Hypotension, hypokalaemia, hyponatraemia hypomagnesaemia, renal impairment, gout, ototoxicity |
| Thiazide diuretics | Metolazone | Reduces plasma volume and filling pressure | Hypotension, hypokalaemia, hyponatraemia, hyperglycaemia, gout, hypercalcaemia, metabolic alkalosis, agranulocytosis, thrombocytopenia, pancreatitis |
| $Na^+/K^+$ pump inhibitor | Digoxin (DIG) | Mild positive inotropy, reduces heart rate via atrioventricular (AV) node blockade | Hypokalaemia potentiates the effects of digoxin. AV block, ventricular tachycardia, gynaecomastia, xanthopsia, nausea, diarrhoea |

*Note:* ACE, angiotensin-converting enzyme; HCN, hyperpolarization-activated cyclic nucleotide-gated.

[a] A-HeFT, African-American Heart Failure; AIRE, Acute Infarction Ramipril Efficacy; CAPRICORN, Carvedilol Post-Infarct Survival Control in LV Dysfunction; CIBIS II, Cardiac Insufficiency Bisoprolol Study II; DIG, Digitalis Investigation Group; ELITE II, Losartan Heart Failure Survival Study; EMPHASIS-HF, Eplerenone in Mild Patients Hospitalization and Survival Study in Heart Failure; EPHESUS, Eplerenone Post-Acute Myocardial Infarction Heart Failure Efficacy and Survival Study; MERIT-HF, Metoprolol CR/XL Randomized Intervention Trial in Congestive Heart Failure; PARADIGM-HF, Prospective Comparison of ARNI with ACEI to Determine Impact on Global Mortality and Morbidity in Heart Failure; RALES, Randomized Aldactone Evaluation Study; SHIFT, Systolic Heart failure treatment with the If inhibitor Ivabradine Trial; SOLVD, Studies of Left Ventricular Dysfunction.

an ACE inhibitor where there is left ventricular systolic impairment, adding in spironolactone in symptomatic patients and then a loop diuretic (furosemide or bumetanide) if there is persisting pulmonary or peripheral oedema. Beta blockers are added in and titrated up slowly and carefully to the maximum tolerated dose, once the patient is euvolaemic. ACE inhibitors, aldosterone antagonists and β blockers have each been shown to prolong life; other treatments, such as furosemide and digoxin, can improve symptoms and quality of life, but do not significantly prolong it.

## Implantable cardiac devices in systolic heart failure

Devices aimed at rebalancing autonomic tone, improving cardiac contractility and treating ventricular arrhythmias have been developed for patients with systolic heart failure. Stimulating the cervical vagus nerve has been trialled as a way of improving cardiac function, patient symptoms and outcome, but to date results have been disappointing, (e.g. ANTHEM-HF, NECTAR-HF and INOVATE-HF). These trials have focused on cardiac function and heart failure symptoms, but not on the potential role in suppressing ventricular arrhythmia. Similar disappointment has been seen with spinal cord stimulation (e.g. the DEFEAT-HF trial). Spinal cord stimulation at the level of T1-3 may reduce cardiac sympathetic drive and target neural processing via intrathoracic extracardiac and intrinsic cardiac ganglia, as well as local circuit neurons. These approaches are still in their infancy.

Considerable success has been achieved with other device-based approaches targeting cardiac contractility and ventricular arrhythmias. In some cases, severely impaired left ventricular systolic function is exacerbated because of the presence of a broad left bundle branch block. This leads to uncoordinated, contraction between the left ventricular septum and lateral wall, known as 'dyssynchrony', that worsens the overall ejection fraction. Biventricular pacemakers, or **cardiac resynchronisation therapy pacemakers (CRTPs)**, pace the septum via a right ventricular lead and the left ventricular lateral wall via a left ventricular lead introduced via the coronary sinus into an epicardial posterolateral vein. Ventricular pacing can also be co-ordinated following atrial depolarization via sensing through an atrial lead to optimize ventricular filling. All three leads are introduced via the subclavian or axillary veins, usually on the patient's left (non-dominant) side, and attached to a programmable pulse generator placed in a prepectoral or

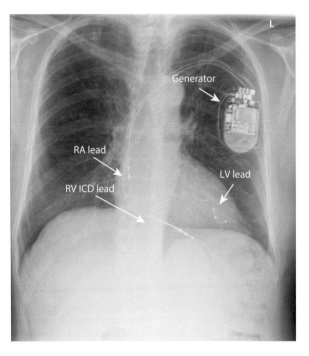

**Figure 18.19** Chest radiograph (postero-anterior projection) demonstrating a cardiac resynchronisation defibrillator. The generator is located on the patient's left-hand side (L) and is positioned subcutaneously in front of the pectoral muscle. This is connected to a right atrial (RA) lead, a right ventricular (RV) lead which contains a single defibrillating coil and a left ventricular (LV) lead.

subpectoral pocket. In a subset of patients, a remodelling process occurs in the months that follow leading to an improvement in left ventricular systolic function beyond just the electrical correction of the ventricular dyssynchrony and these patients are known as 'super-responders'. Overall, clinical trials have demonstrated an improvement in symptoms in up to two thirds of patients who are already on maximal medical therapy. However, as heart failure is a progressively deteriorating condition, it may be that cardiac resynchronization is simply slowing this progression in the other third of cases. Cardiac resynchronisation devices may also incorporate a cardioverter defibrillator function via a coil on the right ventricular lead with the generator also serving as a defibrillator electrode. These devices are known as **cardiac resynchronisation defibrillators (CRTDs)** and trials suggest that in appropriately selected patients, CRTPs and CRTDs improve mortality (Figure 18.19).

## SUMMARY

### SYSTEMIC HYPOXAEMIA

- Systemic hypoxaemia can be caused by a low inspired $P_{O_2}$ (at high altitude), a low alveolar $P_{O_2}$ (due to impaired alveolar ventilation), an increased A–a gradient (due to impaired diffusion of ventilation-perfusion mismatch) or reduced $O_2$ carrying capacity of the blood.
- In the case of high-altitude hypoxaemia, increased peripheral arterial chemoreceptor activity drives a reflex hyperventilation,

which improves arterial oxygenation, but causes hypocapnia and a reversed (left) Bohr shift.
- Tachycardia increases the resting cardiac output to maintain $O_2$ delivery in the face of reduced arterial $O_2$ saturation. Increased peripheral perfusion is also promoted by vasodilatation, except in the cerebral circulation, where the vasoconstrictor effect of hypocapnia offsets hypoxic vasodilatation.

- In the lungs, hypoxic pulmonary vasoconstriction causes pulmonary hypertension, which promotes apical perfusion, but can also lead to right ventricular failure.
- Maximum cardiac output and arterial $O_2$ saturation fall, so exercise performance is impaired.
- Acclimatization to altitude involves a correction of the respiratory alkalosis, a further increase in resting ventilation, increased haematocrit and a right Bohr shift that facilitates peripheral $O_2$ unloading.

## SHOCK AND HAEMORRHAGE

- Acute circulatory failure, or clinical shock, can be classified as obstructive (e.g. pulmonary embolism or cardiac tamponade), distributive (e.g. septicaemia, anaphylaxis) or caused by hypovolaemia (e.g. haemorrhage).
- Hypovolaemia reduces CVP, which reduces stroke volume and pulse pressure (Frank–Starling mechanism). Reduced cardiopulmonary and baroreceptor activity, along with increased arterial chemoreceptor activity, evoke a reflex increase in sympathetic outflow, circulating catecholamines, angiotensin II and, in severe cases, vasopressin.
- If the hypovolaemia is <15%, mean BP is maintained near normal (compensated, non-hypotensive phase), due to reflex tachycardia, increased cardiac contractility, increased peripheral resistance and venoconstriction. Pulse pressure is reduced. The skin is pale, cold and sweaty. Hyperventilation is driven by arterial chemoreceptors, stimulated by lactic acidosis.
- Over 30–60 min, the reduced capillary pressure allows plasma COP to draw ~500 mL interstitial fluid into the circulation. This 'internal transfusion' is facilitated by a shift of intracellular fluid into the interstitial compartment.
- The kidneys conserve salt and water, due to increases in renal sympathetic activity, aldosterone and vasopressin (ADH). Fluid intake is increased by angiotensin II-stimulated thirst. Extracellular fluid volume is thereby restored over a few days. Plasma proteins and red cells are resynthesized more slowly.
- In severe hypotensive haemorrhage, with delayed transfusion, an irreversible, decompensated phase sets in. Peripheral vessels relax, causing BP to collapse. Poor coronary perfusion sets up a negative feedback loop leading to acute cardiac failure. Poor renal perfusion leads to acute renal failure, signalled by anuria.

## TRANSIENT LOSS OF CONSCIOUSNESS (SYNCOPE)

- Emotional stress, hypovolaemia or prolonged orthostasis can cause an abrupt, profound vagally mediated bradycardia and peripheral vasodilatation (vasovagal attack).
- As mean arterial pressure falls below ~70 mmHg, a fall in cerebral perfusion causes a loss of consciousness. The collapsed, supine position raises stroke volume, and the heart rate soon picks up. Consciousness is regained in ~2 min.

## HYPERTENSION

- Resting BPs of >140/90 mmHg increase the incidence of myocardial infarction, heart failure, strokes, retinopathy and renal failure. Systolic hypertension in particular is harmful.
- Systolic pressure increases more than diastolic pressure with age. This is due to (1) reduced aortic compliance, which raises the pulse pressure; and (2) systolic augmentation by an early reflected wave, caused by the increased wave conduction velocity.
- Essential hypertension is a disease of the kidneys, vasculature and autonomic nervous system, due to an interaction between susceptibility genes (probably affecting aldosterone or endothelin secretion in some subgroups) and environmental factors, notably high salt intake, low $K^+$ intake, stress and obesity.
- Hypertension can be controlled with the 'ACD' regime: ACE inhibitors/ARBs, $Ca^{2+}$ channel blockers and diuretics. Beta adrenergic receptor blockers can be added, but are not considered first-line antihypertensive drugs.

## CHRONIC HEART FAILURE

- Chronic heart failure is an inability to maintain adequate tissue perfusion to meet the body's supply needs at a normal filling pressure. Systolic heart failure due to reduced ventricular contractility can be secondary to ischaemic heart disease, cardiomyopathy, or systemic hypertension. In some cases heart failure may be predominantly diastolic due to impaired elastic recoil, relaxation and ventricular filling. Heart failure results in exercise intolerance, dyspnoea and pulmonary/peripheral oedema. Death arises from pump failure or ventricular arrhythmia.
- Pump weakness is exacerbated by a small, sluggish systolic $Ca^{2+}$ transient, reduced $Ca^{2+}$ store, and inefficient excitation-contraction coupling. This is exacerbated by a fall in the sensitivity of troponin to $Ca^{2+}$, wall fibrosis, dilatation and impaired energy use.
- Fatal arrhythmia may be initiated by DADs, and re-entrant circuits sustained by heterogeneity of refractory period/action potential duration and interstitial fibrosis. Sympathetic stimulation of the heart can both initiate and sustain ventricular arrhythmias; consequently, $\beta$ blockers can reduce the risk of mortality.
- The ventricular function (Starling) curve, pump function curve and ejection fraction are depressed. The heart is enlarged (cardiothoracic ratio >0.5 or, more accurately, dilatation on echocardiography or cardiac MRI), due to a raised filling pressure. In mild, compensated failure, the stroke volume and output are almost normal at rest, due to the raised filling pressure (Frank–Starling mechanism) and raised plasma catecholamines. In severe failure, the output is low even at rest, due to further Starling curve depression, mechanical inefficiency caused by dilatation (Laplace's law; mitral/tricuspid regurgitation) and $\beta_1$ adrenergic receptor downregulation.
- During exercise, the heart rate and stroke volume both fail to increase adequately due to cardiac sympathetic NAd depletion, $\beta_1$ adrenergic receptor downregulation and the low slope

of the depressed Starling curve. Exercise intolerance is due to the poor cardiac output, dyspnoea and altered skeletal muscle $Ca^{2+}$ handling.

- In the cutaneous, splanchnic and renal circulations, constriction of resistance vessels supports the arterial BP. Venoconstriction elevates CVP. Constriction is driven by increased peripheral sympathetic activity and raised plasma angiotensin II, endothelin and catecholamines.
- The kidneys retain fluid because of high aldosterone levels and renal vasoconstriction. The plasma volume expansion, along with venoconstriction and the sump pump effect, raises ventricular filling pressure. In right ventricular failure, the increased CVP raises systemic capillary pressure, leading to oedema of the legs/sacrum. In left ventricular failure, the increased pulmonary venous pressure causes pulmonary congestion, pulmonary oedema and dyspnoea.

- ACE inhibitors and spironolactone, often supplemented by loop diuretics reduce afterload and cardiac work, promote renal fluid excretion, reduce cardiac dilatation and improve stroke volume. Hydralazine with nitrates is an alternative in certain circumstances. Beta adrenergic receptor blockers reduce cardiac work and the incidence of arrhythmia. They must be titrated up carefully when the patient is stable and euvolaemic.
- When severe left ventricular function is worsened by dyssynchronous contraction due to a left bundle branch block, this can be improved using a cardiac resynchronization therapy pacemaker (CRTP). Cardiac resynchronization devices, which may also incorporate a cardioverter defibrillator function (CRTDs), improve symptoms and mortality even when used as a primary prevention measure before the development of ventricular arrhythmias.

## FURTHER READING

### Hypoxaemia

Frise MC, Robbins PA. The pulmonary vasculature – lessons from Tibetans and from rare diseases of oxygen sensing. *Experimental Physiology* 2015; **100**(11): 1233–41.

West JB. High-altitude medicine. *Lancet. Respiratory Medicine* 2015; **3**(1): 12–13.

Wilkins MR, Ghofrani HA, Weissmann N, et al. Pathophysiology and treatment of high-altitude pulmonary vascular disease. *Circulation* 2015; **131**(6): 582–90.

West JB. Centenary of the Anglo-American high-altitude expedition to Pikes Peak. *Experimental Physiology* 2012; **97**(1): 1–9.

Wilkins BW, Pike TL, Marting EA, et al. Exercise intensity-dependent contribution of beta-adrenergic receptor-mediated vasodilatation in hypoxic humans. *The Journal of Physiology* 2008; **586**(4): 1195–205.

Longhurst J. Exercise in hypoxic environments: the mechanisms remain elusive. *The Journal of Physiology* 2003; **550**(Pt 2): 335.

Robbins PA. Is ventilatory acclimatization to hypoxia a phenomenon that arises through mechanisms that have an intrinsic role in the regulation of ventilation at sea level? *Advances in Experimental Medicine and Biology* 2001; **502**: 339–48.

### Shock and haemorrhage

Kalla M, Herring N. Physiology of shock and volume resuscitation. *Surgery (Oxford)* 2013; **34**(11): 543–9.

Angele MK, Schneider CP, Chaudhry IH. Bench to bedside review: latest results in haemorrhagic shock. *Critical Care* 2008; **12**(4): 218.

Frithiof R, Eriksson S, Rundgren M. Central inhibition of opioid receptor subtypes and its effect on haemorrhagic hypotension in conscious sheep. *Acta Physiologica* 2007; **191**(1): 25–34.

Länne T, Lundvall J. Mechanisms in man for rapid refill of the circulatory system in hypovolaemia. *Acta Physiologica Scandinavica* 1992; **146**(3): 299–306.

Schadt JC, Ludbrook J. Hemodynamic and neurohumoral responses to acute hypovolaemia in conscious mammals. *American Journal of Physiology* 1991; **260**(2 Pt 2): H305–18.

### Transient loss of consciousness (syncope)

Wieling W, Jardine DL, de Lange FJ, et al. Cardiac output and vasodilation in the vasovagal response: an analysis of the classic papers. *Heart Rhythm* 2016; **13**(3): 798–805.

Sheldon RS, Grubb BP 2nd, Olshansky B, et al. 2015 Heart Rhythm Society expert consensus statement on the diagnosis and treatment of postural tachycardia syndrome, inappropriate sinus tachycardia, and vasovagal syncope. *Heart Rhythm* 2015; **12**(6): e41–63.

Lambert E, Lambert GW. Sympathetic dysfunction in vasovagal syncope and the postural orthostatic tachycardia syndrome. *Frontiers in Physiology* 2014; **5**: 280.

Julu PO, Cooper VL, Hansen S, et al. Cardiovascular regulation in the period preceding vasovagal syncope in conscious humans. *The Journal of Physiology* 2003; **549**(Pt 1): 299–311.

Jardine DL, Melton IC, Crozier IG, et al. Decrease in cardiac output and muscle sympathetic activity during vasovagal syncope. *American Journal of Physiology. Heart and Circulatory Physiology* 2002; **282**(5): H1804–9.

### Hypertension

Digne-Malcolm H, Frise MC, Dorrington KL. How do antihypertensive drugs work? Insights from studies of the renal regulation of arterial blood pressure. *Frontiers in Physiology* 2016; **7**: 320.

Warnert EA, Rodrigues JC, Burchell AE, et al. Is high blood pressure self-protection for the brain? *Circulation Research* 2016; **119**(12): e140–51.

Bhatt DL, Kandzari DE, O'Neill WW, et al. A controlled trial of renal denervation for resistant hypertension. *New England Journal of Medicine* 2014; **370**(15): 1393–401.

Mancia G, Fagard R, Narkiewicz K, et al. 2013 ESH/ESC guidelines for the management of arterial hypertension: the task force for the management of arterial hypertension of the European Society of Hypertension (ESH) and of the European Society of Cardiology (ESC). *European Heart Journal* 2013; **34**(28): 2159–219.

Feihl F, Liaudet L, Levy BI, et al. Hypertension and micro-vascular remodelling. *Cardiovascular Research* 2008; **78**(2): 274–85.

Gilbert JS, Ryan MJ, LaMarca BB, et al. Pathophysiology of hypertension during preeclampsia: linking placental ischemia with endothelial dysfunction. *American Journal of Physiology. Heart and Circulatory Physiology* 2008; **294**: H541–50.

Adrogué HJ, Madias NE. Sodium and potassium in the patho-genesis of hypertension. *New England Journal of Medicine* 2007; **356**(19): 1966–78.

Binder A. A review of the genetics of essential hypertension. *Current Opinion in Cardiology* 2007; **22**(3): 176–84.

Diwan A, Dorn GW 2nd. Decompensation of cardiac hyper-trophy: cellular mechanisms and novel therapeutic targets. *Physiology* 2007; **22**: 56–64.

Dahlöf B, Sever PS, Poulter NR, et al. Prevention of cardio-vascular events with an antihypertensive regimen of amlodipine adding perindopril as required versus atenolol adding bendroflumethiazide as required, in the Anglo-Scandinavian Cardiac Outcomes Trial-Blood Pressure Lowering Arm (ASCOT-BPLA): a multicentre randomised controlled trial. *Lancet* 2005; **366**(9489): 895–906.

Meneton P, Jeunemaitre X, de Wardener HE, et al. Links between dietary salt intake, renal salt handling, blood pres-sure and cardiovascular diseases. *Physiological Reviews* 2005; **85**(2): 679–715.

ALLHAT Officers and Coordinators for the ALLHAT Collaborative Research Group. The Antihypertensive and Lipid-Lowering Treatment to Prevent Heart Attack Trial. Major outcomes in high-risk hypertensive patients randomized to angiotensin-converting enzyme inhibitor or calcium channel blocker vs diuretic: the Antihypertensive and Lipid-Lowering Treatment to Prevent Heart Attack Trial (ALLHAT). *JAMA* 2002; **288**(23): 2981–97.

## Chronic cardiac failure

Seidel T, Navankasattusas S, Ahmad A, et al. Sheet-like remodeling of the transverse tubular system in human heart failure impairs excitation-contraction coupling and functional recovery by mechanical unloading. *Circulation* 2017; **135**(17): 1632–45.

Greenberg B, Butler J, Felker GM, et al. Calcium upregulation by percutaneous administration of gene therapy in patients with cardiac disease (CUPID 2): a randomised, multina-tional, double-blind, placebo-controlled, phase 2b trial. *Lancet* 2016; **387**(10024): 1178–86.

Ponikowski P, Voors AA, Anker SD, et al. 2016 ESC Guidelines for the diagnosis and treatment of acute and chronic heart failure: The Task Force for the diagnosis and treatment of acute and chronic heart failure of the European Society of Cardiology (ESC). Developed with the special contribution of the Heart Failure Association (HFA) of the ESC. *European Heart Journal* 2016; **37**(27): 2129–200.

Lang D, Holzem K, Kang C, et al. Arrhythmogenic remodeling of β2 versus β1 adrenergic signaling in the human failing heart. *Circulation. Arrhythmia and electrophysiology* 2015; **8**(2): 409–19.

Sato PY, Chuprun JK, Schwartz M, et al. The evolving impact of G protein-coupled receptor kinases in cardiac health and disease. *Physiological Reviews* 2015; **95**(2): 377–404.

Eisner D, Caldwell J, Trafford A. Sarcoplasmic reticulum Ca-ATPase and heart failure 20 years later. *Circulation Research* 2013; **113**(8): 958–61.

Luo M, Anderson ME. Mechanisms of altered $Ca^{2+}$ handling in heart failure. *Circulation Research* 2013; **113**(6): 690–708.

Lompré AM, Hajjar RJ, Harding SE, et al. $Ca^{2+}$ cycling and new therapeutic approaches for heart failure. *Circulation* 2010; **121**(6): 822–30.

van Oort RJ, McCauley MD, Dixit SS, et al. Ryanodine receptor phosphorylation by calcium/calmodulin-dependent protein kinase II promotes life-threatening ventricular arrhyth-mias in mice with heart failure. *Circulation* 2010; **122**(25): 2669–79.

Lyon AR, MacLeod KT, Zhang Y, et al. Loss of T-tubules and other changes to surface topography in ventricular myo-cytes from failing human and rat heart. *Proceedings of the National Academy of Sciences of the United States of America* 2009; **106**(16): 6854–9.

Nattel S, Maguy A, Le Bouter S, et al. Arrhythmogenic ion-channel remodeling in the heart: heart failure, myocardial infarction, and atrial fibrillation. *Physiological Reviews* 2007; **87**(2): 425–56.

Neubauer S. The failing heart – an engine out of fuel. *New England Journal of Medicine* 2007; **356**(11): 1140–51.

Sipido KR, Eisner D. Something old, something new: changing views on the cellular mechanisms of heart failure. *Cardiovascular Research* 2005; **68**(2): 167–74.

# Experimental models and measurements to study cardiovascular physiology

**19**

## LEARNING OBJECTIVES

*After reading this chapter, you should be able to:*

- appreciate the influence that the 'observer effect', '*signal-to-noise ratio*', 'sampling rate' and 'dynamic range' have on experimental measurements (19.1);
- understand the need for appropriate 'positive and negative controls', 'randomization', 'blinding' and adequate 'statistical power' when it comes to experimental design (19.1);
- understand the basic principles behind common experimental models and measurement techniques used to study cardiovascular physiology (19.3–19.7);

- appreciate the advantages and limitations of these techniques (19.3–19.7);
- see how using a variety of experimental techniques across different spatial domains leads to a better approach to hypothesis-driven science (19.1);
- appreciate the use of computational modelling to facilitate the reassembly and understanding of complex systems (19.8).

## 19.1 THE EXPERIMENTAL APPROACH

The range of different experimental preparations and types of measurements that can be made is becoming increasingly varied and complex in physiological research. Research groups now often employ a range of measurements and interventions (aimed at genes, proteins, cells, organs and whole animals, as shown in Figure 19.1) to answer hypothesis-driven science, rather than being masters of a single technique as was the case several decades ago. Methods sections of original research papers increasingly quote previous papers rather than give detailed descriptions of all the techniques used. For the student starting to read papers or undertaking a research-based degree, this variety of approaches can be daunting. The aim of this chapter is to give a brief description of the methodology behind common techniques used in cardiovascular physiology; however, this is far from exhaustive.

Even the most modern and complex of experimental techniques have their advantages and limitations. In the physical sciences, it has long been appreciated that the act of observation can influence the phenomenon being observed. This is often the result of instruments that, by necessity, alter the state of what they measure, something known as the **observer effect**. All experimental techniques also have a **signal-to-noise ratio**, that is the ratio between the level of the desired signal and the background noise that is also detected during measurement. For a variable that changes over time, this can be influenced by the **sampling rate**, that is, the frequency at which observations are made, which is important in relation to the rate at which the variable is changing. The concepts of signal-to-noise ratio and **dynamic range** are also closely related. Dynamic range measures the ratio between the strongest undistorted signal that can be measured and the minimum discernible signal, that is, the background noise level. Attempts at measuring below or above this range produce unreliable data.

Experimental measurements should also have a **positive and negative control**, so that there is confidence that a detected change is real. A negative control is a measurement where no change is expected. This could be a sham procedure, a time control or administration of a placebo. The use

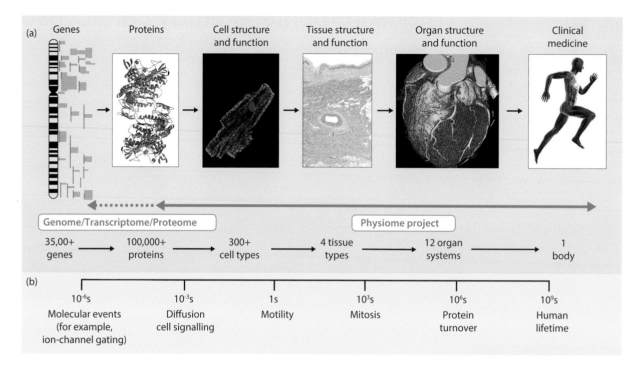

(a)

| Genes | Proteins | Cell structure and function | Tissue structure and function | Organ structure and function | Clinical medicine |

Genome/Transcriptome/Proteome          Physiome project

| 35,00+ genes | → | 100,000+ proteins | → | 300+ cell types | → | 4 tissue types | → | 12 organ systems | → | 1 body |

(b)

| $10^{-6}$s | $10^{-3}$s | 1s | $10^3$s | $10^6$s | $10^9$s |

| Molecular events (for example, ion-channel gating) | Diffusion cell signalling | Motility | Mitosis | Protein turnover | Human lifetime |

**Figure 19.1** Spatial domains and vertical integration. Studying the genome, transcriptome, metabolome and proteome, and integrating results at the cellular, multicellular, whole-organ and whole-organism level. (Adapted from Hunter PJ, Borg TK. *Nature Reviews Molecular Cell Biology* 2003; 4(3): 237–43.)

of multiple known positive controls at different levels of positivity may allow a standard curve to be produced and allow **calibration** of a measurement.

Where possible, measurements should be **randomized** to minimize systematic errors (e.g. due to imperfect calibration or the method of observation); the experimenter should be **blinded** to avoid confirmation bias. Sufficient experimental replicates or an adequate sample size are also needed to be confident of rejecting the null hypothesis ($H_0$) that an intervention produces no change and accept the alternative hypothesis ($H_1$) that it does. For this **statistical power**, calculations are often employed. For a particular level of statistical power (usually taken to be at least 80%), the sample size can be calculated given the estimated magnitude of the effect (although this may be completely unknown until one has done the study!), and the variability in the measurement (from the standard deviation). Ideally, a power calculation should be undertaken before embarking on a set of experiments so that an adequate sample size or number of replicates can be gathered. Importantly, these approaches are designed to increase the reliability of data, so they can be reproduced and stand the test of time.

In the subsequent sections, we describe a variety of experimental preparations across different spatial domains that are commonly used in cardiovascular physiology. For each preparation, we describe the kind of measurements that can be made. In Chapter 20, we go on to discuss the different types of perturbations (physical, chemical and genetic) that can be used to disrupt the system and thereby study function. While most of the experimental preparations can be obtained from humans, this is often both technically and ethically challenging! Experimental

perturbations in human patients are also limited to comparing patients with and without disease, or with and without a treatment. Therefore, most research in cardiovascular physiology is carried out on animal models ranging from rodents to large animal models (such as pigs or dogs). Thought needs to be given to the type of animal model used given what is known about how the physiology and gene expression differ from those of humans.

## 19.2 ISOLATED CELLS

One of the most reductionist approaches to studying physiology involves using an isolated cell preparation (or part thereof, such as an organelle). The advantage of isolating a cardiac myocyte allows measurements that are often difficult in multicellular preparations, such as patch clamping (especially voltage clamping) and high-resolution fluorescence imaging to measure local intracellular microdomains of ions or second messengers. However, isolated cells do not experience the same mechanical and biochemical environment that they experience *in vivo*. They are not electrically coupled to their neighbours via gap junctions, nor mechanically supported by the extracellular matrix. They do not experience the same movement of extracellular tissue fluid or receive communications via neurotransmitters released locally in a specific manner. They are also removed from the changing myriad of circulating hormones that influence their function. While these are certainly limitations, removing these factors from the cell of interest simplifies the experiment allowing confounding variables to be controlled and others to be manipulated.

## Freshly isolated cells

Circulating cell types can be easily purified from blood (although only white blood cells can subsequently be established in culture), but isolation of cells from intact tissue requires dissection, enzymatic digestion of the extracellular matrix (using enzymes such as trypsin and collagenase) and sometimes mechanical tissue trituration. For example, ventricular myocytes were first isolated and patch-clamped from the intact rat heart in 1976 by Powell and Twist; adaptions to this approach in a range of species (including humans) and cell types have revolutionized the study of cardiovascular physiology (for an example, see Figure 19.2). The process of isolation risks damaging the cell in question and the technique is sensitive to small changes in isolation conditions and procedure that greatly affect the health and survival of the cells. Therefore, there is often only a short period of time during which subsequent measurements can be reliably performed; time controls or reversal of effects are therefore very important. Sometimes, the membrane of the cell is deliberately removed (skinned or permeabilized). This allows a compound or substance to gain access to the cell interior, which might otherwise be impermeable, and allows the intracellular ion concentrations to be directly manipulated. This comes at the cost of losing localized membrane signalling via exchangers, ion channels and second messenger-producing receptors.

## Primary cell culture

One way to maintain cellular viability over a longer period of time is to establish isolated cells in culture. This involves maintaining cells in growth media at an appropriate temperature and gas mixture (usually 37°C with 5% $CO_2$) in a sterile incubator. The technique of tissue culture in warm saline solutions was pioneered at the end of the 19th century by Wilhelm Roux and Ross Granville Harrison. Cells can be grown in suspension or to an adherent plate containing components of the extracellular matrix, such as collagen or laminin. Culture conditions (especially the type of media, use of growth factors and plating density) can greatly influence the phenotype of the cells that over time change their protein expression profile compared to freshly isolated tissue. Furthermore, nutrient depletion, changes in media pH, accumulation of necrotic cells or contamination with other cell types or viruses can also influence cellular differentiation. These limitations should be considered when designing experiments and interpreting results. Cells can be plated to grow in isolation, in specific patterns or monolayers; more recent work has also used a variety of platforms to three-dimensional (3-D) cell culture including hydrogel scaffold systems to mimic the extracellular matrix.

## Established cell lines

Some cell lines are immortalized in that they have acquired the ability to proliferate indefinitely either through random mutation (such as some tumour cells) or artificial expression of particular proteins, such as telomerase. Numerous cell lines are well established as being representative of particular cell types. Examples include the HeLa cells obtained from human cervical cancer (the line having been obtained from cervical cancer cells taken from Henrietta Lacks who died of the disease in 1951), PC12 cells from rat phaeochromocytoma or human embryonic kidney cells 293. While cell lines can provide a human cell type that is easily obtainable and easy to work with, problems such as cell line misidentification, contamination with *Mycoplasma*, and genotypic and phenotypic instability can influence data quality and reliability.

## Induced pluripotent stem cells

Generating induced pluripotent stem cells (iPSCs) directly from adult fibroblasts, which can then be differentiated in a variety of different cell types, is a technology developed by Shinya Yamanaka. The introduction of four genes encoding transcription factors (octamer-binding protein 4, transcription factor SOX-2, proto-oncogene c-Myc and Krueppel-like factor 4 or related factors) can convert adult cells into pluripotent stem cells. Yamanaka was awarded the 2012 Nobel Prize in Physiology or Medicine for his work (together with Sir John Gurdon). iPSCs have been used in cardiovascular physiology to study human cell types that might be otherwise difficult to obtain, especially from patients with a genetic disease, and to study the actions of drugs on the cellular phenotypes from such patients. There is hope that the technology may in the future be useful for tissue repair and organ synthesis for transplantation, but safety concerns remain regarding their immunogenicity and teratogenicity; also, iPSC conversion efficiency is low.

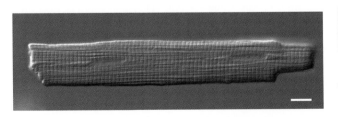

**Figure 19.2** Differential interference contrast (DIC)-image of a freshly isolated adult rat ventricular myocytes. Scale bar represents 10 μM. (Courtesy of Drs Andreas Koschinski, Nshunge Musheshe and Professor Manuela Zaccolo.)

## 19.3 MEASUREMENTS IN ISOLATED CELLS

### Protein expression at single time points

Protein localization in isolated cells can be determined using **immunohistochemistry**. Quantification of mRNA and protein expression in isolated cells is challenging given the very low quantities of mRNA or protein that can be extracted; therefore, this tends to be measured in multicellular preparations (see Section 19.5). Immunohistochemistry, developed by Albert Coons in 1941, can be performed on isolated cells or tissue sections that are fixed, for example, in paraformaldehyde. Multicellular preparations need to be embedded in a medium such as paraffin wax or cryomedia, and then thinly sliced with a microtome in a cryostat. Sections may then need to be permeabilized, dehydrated and mounted onto slides. Because some fixation methods can chemically modify and reduce the detectability of proteins, 'antigen retrieval' for example, by heating is sometimes required for formalin-fixed, paraffin-embedded tissues. The sections or isolated cells are then incubated with a primary antibody against the protein of interest, which can be directly conjugated to a fluorescent label, or incubated with a secondary antibody against the species of the primary antibody containing such a label. Nonspecific binding of the antibodies can be minimized by using blocking buffers and by optimizing the concentration of the antibodies used. Important control experiments include using a tissue known to express the antigen as a positive control, and a tissue known not to express the antigen as a negative control. It is also worth probing the tissue of interest with either omission of the primary antibody or absorption of the primary antibody by using high concentrations of exogenous antigen. Localization can also be assisted by co-staining for different structural components within the cell. In multicellular preparations, co-localization with markers of different cell types is also useful.

## Real-time spatial imaging of enzyme and ion activity

The imaging of cellular ion concentrations, membrane voltage and molecular interactions with high temporal and spatial resolution has been revolutionized by **fluorescence imaging**. The first fluorescent chemical indicators to be used in cardiovascular physiology were **$Ca^{2+}$-sensitive dyes** based on the highly specific small molecule $Ca^{2+}$-chelator BAPTA. Binding of $Ca^{2+}$ ions to a fluorescent indicator molecule leads to either an increase in fluorescence at a given wavelength (non-ratiometric dye, e.g. Rhod-2 or Fluo-4) or an emission/excitation wavelength shift (ratiometric dye, e.g. Fura-2). Ratiometric dyes have the advantage of producing a change in the ratios of emission at two wavelengths that is directly related to the amount of $Ca^{2+}$ bound. Therefore, they allow correction for uneven dye loading, photobleaching, changes in focus and variations in the intensity of the exciting LED light source. The first demonstration of real-time intracellular $Ca^{2+}$ fluxes in living cells was in cardiac myocytes by the Lederer group in the mid-1980s.

$Ca^{2+}$-sensitive dyes are often used as acetoxymethyl esters to render the molecule lipophilic and allow easy entrance into the cell. Once this form of the indicator is in the cell, cellular esterases free the carboxyl groups and the indicator can bind $Ca^{2+}$. However, esterase activity varies in different cellular compartments (such as the sarcoplasmic reticulum (SR) and mitochondria). The free acid form of the dyes can also

be directly injected into cells with a microelectrode to reduce uncertainty regarding intracellular localization. Genetically encoded ratiometric $Ca^{2+}$ indicators that use a variant of calmodulin and green fluorescent protein (GFP; cameleon) have also been developed by Roger Y Tsien and co-workers. He was awarded the 2008 Nobel Prize in Chemistry for the discovery and development of GFP from the jellyfish.

Different $Ca^{2+}$-sensitive dyes have different binding constants ($K_d$) and therefore measure $Ca^{2+}$ across different concentration ranges. This can be exploited to measure $Ca^{2+}$ concentrations in organelles where $Ca^{2+}$ concentrations are high (e.g. SR using low-affinity Mag-Fura-2 or Fluo-5N) when other dyes would be saturated. Fluorescent dyes also exist to measure intracellular $Na^+$ (e.g. SBFI), $K^+$ (e.g. PBFI), protons (e.g. SNARF), plasma membrane potential (e.g. RH237), mitochondrial membrane potential (e.g. tetramethylrhodamine ethyl ester) and nitric oxide (NO) concentration (e.g. diaminofluorescein).

When using fluorescent dyes, the type of dye (ratiometric versus non-ratiometric), the pattern of cellular loading, $K_d$, in relation to the variable being measured, and the ability to photobleach with repetitive excitation need to be considered. Molecules themselves act as buffers of the substance being measured; therefore, they can influence concentrations and subsequent cellular activity. The combination of these dyes with improved microscopy, particularly laser scanning and confocal fluorescence microscopy, has greatly improved our understanding of intracellular signalling. The Nobel Prize in Chemistry in 2014 was awarded to Betzig, Hell and Moerner for their work on the development of super-resolved fluorescence microscopy.

Improved imaging technology and exploitation of genetically encoded fluorescence technology have also been combined to measure subcellular microdomains of second messengers. Transfected proteins contain two different fluorescent molecules that come into close proximity to each other on binding of a second messenger. This produces a transfer of **fluorescence, or Förster resonance energy transfer (FRET)** between donor and acceptor chromophores such that the emission ratio between their two wavelengths changes as demonstrated in Figure 19.3. For example, cyclic adenosine monophosphate (cAMP) FRET sensors are structurally based on exchange protein directly activated by cAMP (Epac), protein kinase A, or cyclic nucleotide-gated channels and often use a cyan fluorescent protein donor and a yellow fluorescent protein acceptor to tag the regulatory and catalytic subunits, respectively. The FRET signal can be pH-sensitive; important control experiments involve demonstrating that the FRET signal is within the dynamic range and not saturated, and also transfecting a dead sensor control that contains the chromophores but has lost the ability to bind the second messenger.

## Electrophysiological measurements

The **patch clamp technique**, developed by Neher and Sakmann (1976) leading to the award of the Nobel Prize in

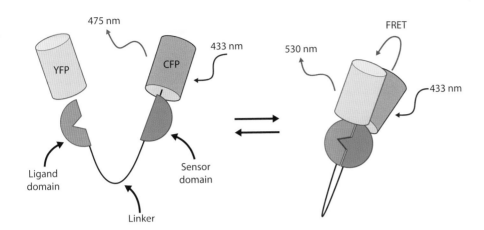

**Figure 19.3** A Förster resonance energy transfer (FRET) sensor containing a ligand and sensor domain that interact on binding of the ligand so that fluorescence resonance energy transfer can occur between the cyan fluorescent protein (CFP) donor and yellow fluorescent protein (YFP) acceptor chromophores. (Adapted from the PHOGEMON [**Pho**sphorylation and **G**uanine-nucleotide **E**xchange **Mon**itors] Project. Accessed 11 January 2018 from www.fret.lif.kyoto-u.ac.jp/e-phogemon/phomane.htm.)

Physiology or Medicine in 1991, allowed voltage and current clamping to be applied to isolated cells. The technique (introduced in Figure 4.3) involves using a polished microelectrode containing a similar ionic composition to the intracellular compartment, which is lowered onto the surface of a cell; suction is then applied to gain access to the cell interior via a giga-ohm seal. Electrical access to the cell interior can also be gained without rupturing the cell membrane (**whole-cell patch**), but instead antifungal agents (such as nystatin or amphotericin-B) to puncture holes in the cell membrane (**perforated patch**), thereby limiting the diffusion of intracellular contents into the patch. The electrode can then be used to record membrane current or voltage relative to an extracellular reference electrode; by using a feedback system, the current or voltage across the membrane can be clamped at a set level and 'stepped' to another level, and the response required to keep the new level constant is recorded. Before the invention of microelectrodes, the original voltage and current clamp set-up was used by Hodgkin and Huxley (1952) on the giant squid axon to uncover the ionic basis of the neuronal action potential. This was achieved using ion exchange to isolate the currents responsible, and by performing voltage clamp steps from a holding potential close to the resting membrane potential to look at the voltage- and time-dependent properties of the individual currents, which they then mathematically modelled. This led to them being awarded the Nobel Prize in Physiology or Medicine in 1963 with John Eccles.

The patch clamp technique can be used to **voltage, current or action potential clamp** (where the membrane voltage is varied in the same pattern as a recorded native action potential) the entire cell. It can also be used on a small patch of membrane to record the response of a single ion channel (cell-attached patch). If this small area of membrane is then separated from the rest of the cell, an **inside-out** or **outside-out** patch configuration can be formed and the ion channel interior or exterior exposed to different ionic concentrations or neurotransmitters (see Figure 19.4).

Electrophysiological techniques can also be used to detect neurotransmitter release. In cells with large enough vesicles, their incorporation into the cell membrane during exocytosis can be detected as an increase in cell capacitance as membrane

area increases. Alternatively, the release of neurotransmitters into the extracellular environment can be detected with a carbon fibre electrode very close to a release site, which is held at a particular potential at which the neurotransmitter may oxidize. Oxidation causes the transfer of electrons to the electrode, which can be detected as small currents via a process called **amperometry**. The size of the current spike can be used to estimate the number of vesicles released and the frequency of spikes gives an indication of release probability. The technique is challenging in single isolated neurons given the small amounts of vesicles being released at low probability; it works best with dense clusters of neurons, although it then becomes difficult to control because of the number of neurons contributing to the resultant release signal.

Another method for the electrical stimulation of isolated cells, or individual/groups of cells in multicellular preparations or *in vivo* is **optogenetics**. This technique, developed by the Miesenböck group in the early 2000s, involves expressing genetically modified, light-sensitive ion channels known as channelrhodopsins in a cell of interest. The expression of these ion channels can be linked to cell-specific promoters in multicellular tissue, and combined with a fibre-optic, solid state light source for illumination. This allows the stimulation of either an individual cell or groups of cells with millisecond temporal precision, without the need for microelectrodes. The technique has been widely used to study neurons and neuronal circuits *in vitro* and *in vivo* in the central nervous system, but is equally applicable to other excitable cells such as cardiac myocytes.

## Cell viability and proliferation

The health of isolated cells or their ability to maintain or recover viability can be assessed by a variety of viability assays. These are useful in assessing the toxicity of a substance or condition, or the ability to protect against such toxicity. Assays assess different aspects of cellular function, such as membrane integrity (e.g. staining with Trypan blue, or membrane leakage of lactate dehydrogenase), mitochondrial activity (e.g. staining with formazan (MTT/XTT) or resazurin dyes that are effectively reduced in the mitochondria and can therefore indicate apoptosis and cell death), signalling pathways that are activated

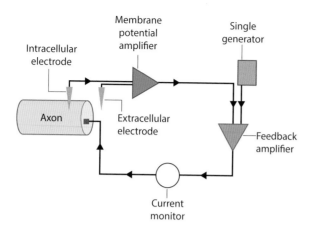

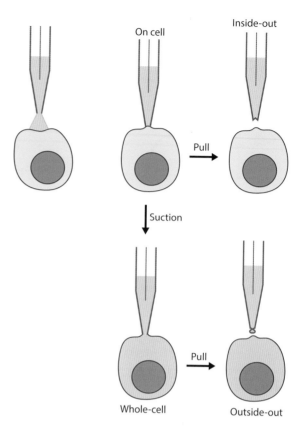

**Figure 19.4** A voltage clamp set-up (left) using an intracellular and extracellular (reference) electrode in a giant squid axon. Different patch clamp configurations (right) including whole-cell, and inside-out and outside-out. (Adapted from image of the four patch-clamp modes. Accessed 11 January 2018 from https://commons.wikimedia.org/wiki/File:Patchmodes.svg.)

by stress (e.g. via genomic and proteomic analysis) or directly assaying the behaviour of the cell. The latter will vary depending on the function of the type of cell being assayed but could, for example, include spontaneous beating of isolated sinoatrial (SA) node cells.

A variety of assays measure cellular proliferation, the simplest being counting cell number (e.g. with a haemocytometer microscope slide or flow cytometry). Other assays measure metabolic activity (with formazan or resazurin staining, or measuring adenosine triphosphate levels), cell surface antigens (such as Ki-67, type IIB topoisomerase, phospho-histone H3 and proliferating cell nuclear antigen) or directly measuring the rate of DNA replication. The latter makes use of measuring the incorporation of labelled nucleotide analogues, such as 3H-thymidine and the thymidine analogue bromodeoxyuridine into DNA during replication.

## 19.4 MULTICELLULAR PREPARATIONS

The ability to dissect multicellular preparations consisting of part of or an entire organ and maintain their viability was made possible by the introduction of artificial solutions resembling extracellular fluid by Sydney Ringer in the 1880s (Ringer, 1882). **Tyrode's solution** resembles Ringer's original solution, but contains bicarbonate and phosphate as a buffer (rather than lactate) and can be bubbled with 95% $O_2$ and 5% $CO_2$ to maintain a physiological pH. While isolated multicellular preparations allow more complex physiological

behaviours to be studied without the influence of changes in circulating hormones and haemodynamics experienced *in vivo*, they also have limitations. Tyrode's solution contains glucose rather than free fatty acids, the heart's main energy supply. It also lacks proteins. Therefore, during long experimental protocols, the lack of oncotic pressure can lead to tissue swelling. The lack of plasma proteins and haemoglobin also means that local signalling molecules which may bind to either of these may not behave in the same way as they do *in vivo*. In the following section we discuss some of the commonly used multicellular preparation used in cardiovascular physiology.

## Isolated vessels

Isolated vessels, from aortic rings down to small arterioles, can be dissected and perfused at physiological pressures so that they generate spontaneous tone. The response of the vessel in terms of vasoconstriction and vasodilatation to pharmacological agents or changes in flow can be measured through **wire myography** or video measurement of vessel diameter. Vessels can also be modified by removing the endothelium with strong detergents or through physical means. Branched vessels can also be studied with multiple cannulae, or a single cylindrical vessel can be cut open and pinned flat so that the endothelium can be studied with fluorescence imaging or electrophysiological techniques. Of note, perfusion systems generate a constant pressurized flow that is not pulsatile and may be unlike that experienced by larger arteries *in vivo*.

## Cardiac preparations

The heart can be dissected into individual components that may be suitable for measuring an aspect of the organ's function. For example, **SA node or atrial preparations** are useful in assessing local electrophysiology or even spontaneous beating rate without the added complication of atrioventricular node conduction or heart block. Atrial preparations, particularly with intact autonomic nerves, are also useful for measuring **radiolabelled neurotransmitter release** in response to stimulation of such nerves. This is because the neural innervation of the atria is particularly rich per unit volume of myocardial tissue. However, neuronal stimulation at particular frequencies, voltages and pulse widths may not reproduce the pattern seen *in vivo*. Moreover, direct stimulation of the cervical vagus nerve can stimulate efferent and afferent nerve fibres both anterogradely and retrogradely. This can activate reflexes and may produce different results if the nerve is severed compared to being intact.

The ventricular inotropic response can be conveniently assessed without the influence of vascular tone or neurohumoral activation using an **isolated papillary muscle preparation** (see Figure 6.2). These can be dissected without damaging the muscle and serve as excellent models for exploring the action of pharmacological agents or investigating transgenic animal models.

## Langendorff and working heart preparations

One method of studying the whole heart *in vitro* is through retrograde perfusion via the aorta, as first described by the German physiologist Oskar Langendorff (1895). This method closes the aortic valve and enables perfusion of the coronary arteries. The perfusate then passes into the coronary veins, coronary sinus and thebesian system and drains into the right atrium/ventricle. Using this system, the right ventricle remains relatively unloaded. The standard experimental set-up includes left ventricular pressure measurements by inserting a fluid-filled balloon via the left atrium (filled to a physiological end diastolic pressure), perfusion pressure measurements (if perfused in **constant flow mode**) or aortic flow measurements (if perfused in **constant pressure mode**), and electrocardiogram (ECG) monitoring (see Figure 19.5). It is an excellent system for assessing the actions of ischaemia/reperfusion, cardiac pacing, pharmacological agents and genetic manipulation independent of any haemodynamic or neurohumoral influences within the intact circulation.

Langendorff's perfusion in constant pressure mode allows autoregulation of coronary tone to remain intact and is particularly useful where there is ligation of a coronary artery to produce regional myocardial ischaemia. Constant flow preparations are of particular use when studying coronary vascular tone. Because perfusion pressure is measured at a known flow, coronary vascular resistance can be easily calculated. With constant flow perfusion, any intervention that causes coronary vasoconstriction does not reduce myocardial $O_2$ delivery because flow remains constant.

The Langendorff isolated heart method was modified by Neely and co-workers in 1967 to produce a model that allows

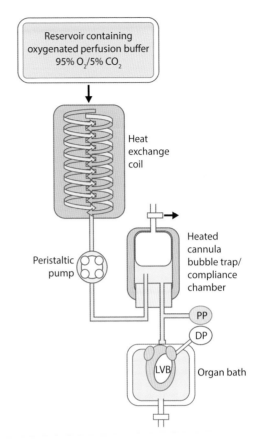

**Figure 19.5** A Langendorff heart set-up demonstrating perfusion of an isolated heart via the ascending aorta with measures of perfusion pressure (PP) and developed pressure (DP) via a left ventricular balloon (LVB).

the study of normal circulatory dynamics. In **the working heart model**, a second cannula perfuses the left atrium, which then pumps the fluid to the left ventricle and out of the aorta under experimentally controlled preload (atrial pressure) and afterload (aortic resistance). Flow in the atrial perfusion inflow cannula and aortic outflow cannula is measured to calculate cardiac output (aortic flow plus coronary flow) and coronary flow (atrial inflow minus aortic outflow). Other parameters that can be derived include stroke volume, stroke work and coronary vascular resistance. It should be noted that because these preparations are perfused with Tyrode's solution lacking haemoglobin, they rely on low levels of dissolved $O_2$ and high flow rates.

## Working heart-brainstem preparation

Langendorff and working heart preparations have become increasingly more complex, with microdissection techniques enabling removal of the heart with intact nerves, including the stellate ganglia and cervical vagi. Perhaps the most impressive preparation for studying central and reflex cardiac control is the working heart-brainstem preparation devised by Paton in the mid-1990s (see Figure 19.6). This set-up involves perfusion of the heart with Tyrode's solution via the descending aorta in constant flow mode. Perfusion pressure, left ventricular pressure and the ECG can be recorded as with a standard working

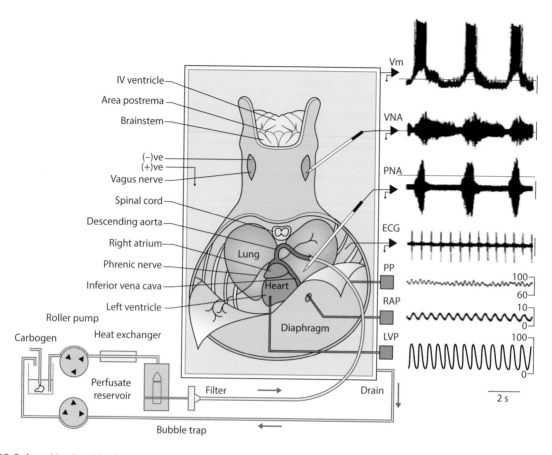

**Figure 19.6** A working heart-brainstem preparation in the mouse. Perfusion is via the descending aorta, while recordings are made of left ventricular pressure (LVP), right atrial pressure (RAP), perfusion pressure (PP), the electrocardiogram (ECG), phrenic nerve activity (PNA), vagus nerve activity (VNA) and intracellular recording of membrane potential are made from neurons of the medulla. (Adapted from Paton JF. *Journal of Neuroscience Methods* 1996; 65(1): 63–8.)

heart, but in addition a motor pattern can be recorded during spontaneous respiration from the phrenic and vagus nerves. Because the model incorporates non-pulsatile intra-arterial perfusion, there is minimal cardiac-related movement of the brainstem, which also enables simultaneous electrophysiological recording from medullary neurons (extracellular, intracellular and whole-cell recording).

## 19.5 MEASUREMENTS IN MULTICELLULAR PREPARATIONS

### RNA/Protein expression at single time points

Isolated tissue samples can be snap frozen (in liquid nitrogen) following an intervention, and the expression or activity of gene products of interest evaluated in several ways. It should be remembered that multicellular samples may contain a variety of cell types. The contribution of each cell type to the overall change in gene expression can sometimes be difficult to ascertain. Therefore, localization of the protein in conjunction with these measurements using immunohistochemistry as described in Section 19.3, is also important with co-staining for different cell types.

In terms of mRNA, the presence and level of expression can be evaluated using **reverse transcription** followed by **polymerase chain reaction** (PCR) with detection of the resulting complementary DNA (cDNA) products. The technique was developed by Mullis and Smith who received the Nobel Prize in Chemistry for their work in 1993. The first step requires the isolation of RNA from tissue (e.g. by homogenization and acid-guanidinium thiocyanate-phenol-chloroform extraction) and quantification of the amount of RNA extracted. A set amount of RNA is then reverse transcribed to cDNA. The cDNA is used as a template for exponential amplification with PCR guided by primers complementary to the three prime ends of the sense and antisense strands of the cDNA of interest. As well as primers, PCR requires a DNA polymerase with a temperature optimum at around 70°C, deoxynucleoside triphosphate nucleotides for cDNA synthesis and buffer solution with appropriate concentration of monovalent and bivalent cations. PCR then undergoes 20–40 amplification cycles, each with several temperature steps in a thermal cycling machine. First, there is a high temperature denaturation step (e.g. 94°C–98°C), followed by an annealing temperature for the primers to bind (e.g. 50°C–65°C), and then an extension stage at which DNA polymerase synthesizes the DNA product (around 70°C) as shown in Figure 19.7. This enables very small amounts of a specific mRNA to be detected. (Northern blotting requires a

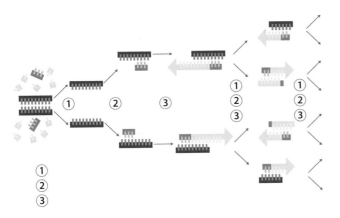

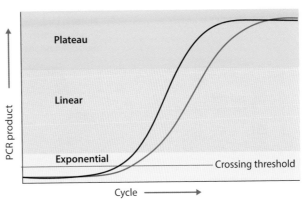

**Figure 19.7** Polymerase chain reaction (PCR) cycles demonstrating denaturation (1), annealing of primers (2) and elongation by synthesis of nucleotides (3). (Adapted from a schematic drawing of the PCR cycle. Accessed 11 January 2018 from https://commons.wikimedia.org/wiki/File:Polymerase_chain_reaction.svg.)

**Figure 19.8** The exponential increase in polymerase chain reduction product over increasing number of cycles. Measurements of products should be taken during the linear phase of amplification before a plateau is reached. PCR, polymerase chain reaction. (Adapted from VanGuilder HD, Vrana KE, Freeman WM. Twenty-five years of quantitative PCR for gene expression analysis. *Biotechniques* 2008; 44(5): 619–26.)

large amount of mRNA to start with.) Using real-time PCR with fluorescent DNA labelling techniques, the amount of cDNA over each amplification cycle can be measured, allowing a degree of indirect quantification of the differences in starting mRNA to be assessed as shown in Figure 19.8. The exponential amplification during the multiple cycles of PCR can produce inaccurate end-point quantification because of the difficulty in maintaining linearity through the cycles. Samples can also become contaminated or degraded due to the presence of RNases.

One way to analyse simultaneously the expression of many genes involves using a **microarray**. After mRNA has been isolated and reverse transcribed to cDNA, expression profiling then uses an **array plate** or **chip** containing many microscopic spots. Each spot consists of complementary nucleic acid sequences to the cDNA of the gene of interest. After washing off non-specific binding, fluorescently labelled target sequences bind to the probe sequence and generate a signal from a spot that depends on the amount of target sample binding. Microarrays use relative quantification in which the intensity of a spot is compared to the intensity of the same spot under a different condition and relies on the fact that no cross-hybridization between spots occurs. There should be sufficient technical and biological repeats so that appropriate statistical conclusions can be drawn from the large amount of data generated. Unfortunately, there is also a lack of standardization between different platforms and experimental conditions that makes inter-observer comparison of data difficult. Microarrays have to some extent been overtaken by **RNA sequencing** methods. This involves the creation of an mRNA library using poly (T) oligonucleotides covalently attached to magnetic beads to extract the mRNA (with its poly (A) tail). The mRNA library can then be analysed with direct RNA sequencing, or reverse transcribed to cDNA (which may introduce biases and artefacts), and analysed with high-throughput, next-generation sequencing. Differently expressed genes can be identified by using tools that count the sequencing reads per gene and compare them between samples.

mRNA localization can be assessed using *in situ* **hybridization**. Cells or tissue need to be fixed and membranes permeabilized before being incubated with a labelled complementary DNA or RNA probe that hybridizes to the sequence of interest. The probe can be labelled with either radio-, fluorescent- or antigen-labelled bases (e.g. digoxigenin) and then localized and quantified with either autoradiography, fluorescence microscopy or immunohistochemistry.

However, changes in the expression and localization of mRNA do not always translate into changes in the protein levels. **Western blotting** is perhaps the most commonly used method of quantitatively assessing protein expression (see Figure 19.9). Tissue samples are homogenized in lysis buffer with a mixture of protease inhibitors, and the protein is isolated and denatured. The amount of protein isolated is then quantified and equal amounts from different samples are loaded onto a sodium dodecyl sulphate polyacrylamide gel and separated according to their molecular weight. The protein is then transferred (or blotted) onto a nitrocellulose or polyvinylidene difluoride membrane that can be blocked (to prevent background antibody binding) and incubated with a primary antibody against the protein of interest. After washing to remove any unbound primary antibody, the membrane is incubated with a secondary antibody (raised against the species of the primary antibody), which is linked to an enzyme such as horseradish peroxidase (which can cleave a chemiluminescent agent and subsequently be detected), or with a fluorescence label (which can be excited at one wavelength and its emission recorded at a different wavelength), as shown in Figure 19.10. The resulting chemiluminescence or fluorescence signal can be detected with a camera or photographic film and analysed with densitometry. However, the use of film is less than ideal because of the non-linearity of the image, especially if under- or overexposed, leading to inaccurate quantification.

Membranes can be stripped of the bound antibodies and re-probed, and it is good practice to reprobe for a structural or

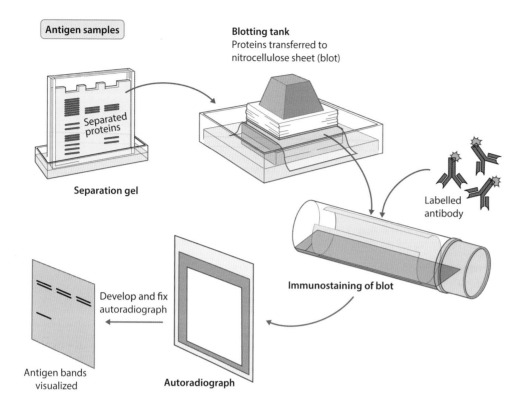

**Figure 19.9** The stages of Western blotting. Separation of proteins by electrophoresis followed by blotting and transfer of the proteins from the separation gel to a membrane. This is followed by incubation with labelled antibodies and analysis of the blot using autoradiography. (Adapted from *Virology Blog: About Viruses and Viral Disease.* Accessed 11 January 2018 from www.virology.ws/wp-content/uploads/2010/07/western_blot.jpg.)

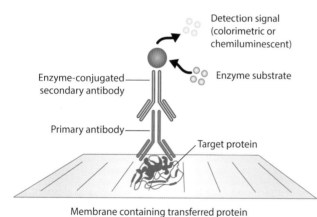

**Figure 19.10** Detection of transferred proteins in Western blotting using a primary, and enzyme-conjugated secondary antibody, followed by addition of substrate to detect a signal. (Adapted from Detection in Western Blots diagram, Leinco Technologies, Inc. Accessed 11 January 2018 from www.leinco.com/western-blotting-protocol.)

housekeeping protein, the expression of which would not be expected to be different between samples. Levels of expression of the protein of interest can then be normalized to this to account for any differences in gel protein loading or uneven transfer.

More recently protein chips/microarrays have been developed for **high-throughput screening** and measurement of multiple proteins simultaneously in small volumes of sample in a similar manner to DNA microarrays except using an antibody-based detection method.

Increased protein expression does not necessarily translate to increased protein activity, particularly if the protein is an enzyme. For example, this also depends on post-translational modifications, availability and localization of substrate and cofactors. **Enzyme activity assays** are therefore also important in assessing the effect of an experimental perturbation. All enzyme assays measure either the consumption of substrate or production of product over time for a given amount of enzyme protein. Many different methods of measuring the concentrations of substrates and products exist and many enzymes can be assayed in several different ways. Changes in substrate or product concentration can be measured with spectrophotometry, chemiluminescence or fluorescence, for example, and continuous assays are most convenient, with one assay then giving the rate of reaction. Such assays can be sensitive to the ionic concentrations, pH and high concentrations of substrate that eventually will become saturating.

Protein location can also be analysed with immunohistochemistry as detailed in Section 19.3. In multicellular preparations, tissue has to be fixed, sliced, permeabilized, dehydrated and mounted onto slides as previously described. Co-localization with antibody markers of different cell types is also useful. In neuroscience, tissue clearing techniques such as **CLARITY**, developed by the Deisseroth group, has allowed brain tissue to be made transparent so that gene-based labelling or fluorescently labelled antibodies can be used to visualize proteins in 3-D space within tissue. The approach is based on the removal of lipid from tissue and its replacement with acrylamide-based hydrogel monomers so that proteins and nucleic acids are held in place. A small amount of protein (up to 8%) can be lost during the lipid extraction, which takes several weeks. The immunostaining itself can take up to 6 weeks and stripping and reprobing with further antibodies can lead to further protein loss from the structure. This approach could theoretically be applied to other tissues, including the heart.

## Real-time spatial imaging of enzyme and ion activity

Fluorescence imaging as described in Section 19.3 with regard to single cells, can also be used in multicellular preparations using **optical mapping** techniques as pioneered by the Salama group. However, several limitations are particularly relevant to this approach in multicellular tissue. The first arises from the method of tissue perfusion, which may cause uneven loading of the dye throughout the tissue. The second arises in the mechanical restraint required to focus on a large area of curved tissue that may be spontaneously beating. This can be done via mechanical restraint for example, compressing a glass slide over a beating heart, or pharmacologically with a mechanical uncoupling agent such as blebbistatin, a small molecule inhibitor of myosin II. Blebbistatin will remove any mechano-electric feedback from the heart and may also directly interfere with cardiac electrophysiology, although this is controversial. Tissues, such as the epicardial surface of the heart, can also be loaded with more than one dye so that several parameters (membrane voltage, cytoplasmic calcium or SR $Ca^{2+}$) can be monitored with high temporal and spatial resolution across the tissue. This is particularly useful for the study of cardiac arrhythmias where intracellular $Ca^{2+}$ handling events can be related to the initiation and propagation of electrical waves of excitation.

## Electrophysiological measurements

While the voltage across regions of excitable tissue cannot be accurately clamped, electrical signals can be measured using unipolar or bipolar electrodes. In the heart, multi-electrode contact arrays can simultaneously measure electrical activation across the epicardial surface of the heart, for example, using a mapping sock in place of the pericardium (an example of this is shown in Figure 5.10, right). Activation on the endocardial surface of the heart can be mapped using non-contact basket catheters, or single or multiple contact electrodes. Multi-electrode mapping has a lower spatial resolution compared to voltage-sensitive dyes, but does not need to be used with a mechanical uncoupling agent. However, electrode positions may move as the heart contracts and the physical contact between the electrode and tissue may vary over time (as therefore will the signal magnitude). Long-term mapping may also cause localized pressure between the electrode and myocardium, which can lead to tissue necrosis. Electroanatomical mapping allows intracardiac electrical activation to be recorded in relation to anatomic location in a cardiac chamber of interest (e.g. using the EnSite™ NavX™ or Biosense CARTO® systems). They are also used *in vivo* for the mapping and ablation of cardiac arrhythmias in patients. These approaches allow spatial differences in activation recovery times, as well as patterns of activation and repolarization, and conduction velocity to be

determined. Pacing manoeuvres can also be used to measure the refractory period and how activation recovery times (a surrogate for action potential duration) vary with coupling interval (known as electrical restitution; see Chapter 5, Section 5.10).

## Real-time measurements of tissue mechanics

The tissue mechanics of multicellular preparations are relatively easily measured with force transducers, pressure catheters and flow (Doppler) catheters. Contraction rate can be calculated from these measurements along with the rate of change of pressure during contraction or relaxation ($dP/dt$). Volume changes can also be measured in the ventricle with multi-electrode impedance catheters.

## 19.6 ANIMAL STUDIES *IN VIVO*

Integrating results obtained from isolated cells, multicellular preparations and whole organs into observations in the whole organism is key to fully understanding physiological processes. However, the role and interactions of proteins and signalling pathways can become increasingly more complex and difficult to interpret moving from cell to organ to system, and when moving from *in vitro* (Latin *within the glass*) to the *in vivo* (Latin *within the living*) phenotype. Because of this, the mantra *in vivo veritas* ('in a living thing [there is] truth'), a corruption of the proverb *in vino veritas*, ('in wine [there is] truth'), is seen as important not just for understanding physiology, but also for trialling new therapies.

Animal studies *In vivo* have traditionally been conducted under **general anaesthesia**, allowing humane restraint and reducing the stress of complex instrumentation to measure simultaneously multiple physiological parameters. However, the general anaesthesia itself reduces sympathetic tone and lowers blood pressure (BP), and some anaesthetic agents also directly interact with cardiac ion channels. The use of miniaturized **radiotelemetry devices** has allowed many parameters (heart rate, ECG, BP, temperature and activity) to be recorded in awake, freely moving animals; their variability can also provide relevant information that cannot be obtained under general anaesthesia. However, ensuring full recovery from the surgical implantation of such telemetry devices and ensuring that implantation of the telemetry device itself does not influence the animal's physiology and well-being is critical.

## 19.7 MEASUREMENTS IN ANIMAL STUDIES *IN VIVO*

In the awake animal without telemetry, many non-invasive measures can be made including body weight, consumption of food and water, physical activity (e.g. voluntary wheel running), urine output and tail cuff measurements of BP (following a habituation period to the machine).

## Blood sampling

Blood samples can be taken either from peripheral veins, or (under general anaesthesia) from organ-specific arteries and veins (e.g. the left main coronary artery and coronary sinus) to measure arteriovenous difference. In smaller rodents with low blood volumes, the size and frequency of sampling that can be undertaken is limited. Blood samples should be immediately centrifuged to isolate plasma, then snap frozen and stored appropriately at −80°C. Blood can be analysed with **high-performance liquid chromatography** or if the analyte is a peptide, with an antibody-based **enzyme-linked immunosorbent assay (ELISA)** detection method against known calibration standards. With an ELISA, an antigen must be immobilized to a solid surface and then complexed with a highly specific antibody that is linked to an enzyme. Detection is accomplished by assessing the conjugated enzyme activity via incubation with a substrate to produce a measurable product. Measures should be made in duplicate, usually on 96-well plates, and the inter- and intra-plate variability measured for quality control. When there are only small volumes of sample from which multiple proteins need to be measured, **multiplex assays** can be used such as protein microarrays (see Section 19.5) and bead-based Luminex™ assays. The latter uses many colour-coded beads conjugated to analyte-specific capture antibodies. Biotinylated detection antibodies specific to the analyte together with phycoerythrin (PE)-conjugated streptavidin are then used for detection. The beads are read on a flow-based detection instrument, with one laser classifying the bead and analyte being detected, and a second laser determining the magnitude of the PE-derived signal and the amount of bound analyte.

## Haemodynamics

In animals, haemodynamic measurements can be made with pressure, flow (Doppler) and volume (multi-electrode impedance) catheters. Combining this with indicator or thermal dilution techniques, or measuring arteriovenous $O_2$ content can also allow the calculation of cardiac output as described in Chapter 7. The heart rate and BP responses to different manoeuvres aimed at activating the high (neck suction) or low pressure (lower body negative pressure) baroreflexes can also be measured. The use of vasoactive pharmacological agents to activate such reflexes should be used with care because many of these can directly interact with the reflex itself. For example, NO donors vasodilate but can also directly increase heart rate by stimulating the SA node as well as reducing the sympathetic and increasing the parasympathetic efferent response to the fall in arterial pressure.

Techniques for measuring transcapillary fluid movement and filtration rate in a limb (using plethysmography) and from a single capillary, as devised by researchers such as Krogh, Landis and Michel are described in Chapter 11 (see Figures 11.2 and 11.3). Interstitial fluid pressure and lymph flow can also be measured *in vivo* with a variety of methods as shown in Figures 11.10 and 11.20.

## Telemetry data

Analysis of heart rate and BP by telemetry can be used to give an indication of spontaneous baroreflex sensitivity (by examining the relationship between changes in systolic BP and pulse interval), or heart rate variability. Many measures of heart rate variability exist. Any signal that fluctuates can be analysed to see how often the signal occurs at different frequencies, something known as a power spectral analysis. The high and low frequency components of heart rate variability have often been taken to reflect the activity of the autonomic nervous system. Other measures, such as the standard deviation of the ECG RR (or NN) interval (SDNN), measure the overall heart rate variability that correlates with morbidity and mortality in human patients with heart failure. Heart rate variability is a controversial method of providing a quantitative measure of the contribution of the individual branches of the autonomic nervous system, particularly when the low frequency component or the LF/HF ratio are viewed in isolation; conclusion should be limited to the relative balance between the two.

## Electrophysiology

The most basic of electrophysiological measurements that can be undertaken *in vivo* is an ECG, although this can be made more complex by the addition of more leads to make up the 12-lead ECG (as described in Chapter 5) or even an ECG jacket containing many electrodes. This latter approach has been used to reconstruct potentials, electrograms and isochrones on the epicardial surface from body surface measurements through ECG imaging using algorithms that attempt to solve the **inverse problem** of electrocardiography (the **forward problem** being predicting the body surface measurements based on the epicardial potentials) as described in Chapter 5, Section 5.8 and Figure 5.10. Multi-electrode epicardial mapping can be undertaken following sternotomy, or using a single roaming percutaneous mapping electrode in the pericardial space with the chest unopened. As described in Section 19.5, endocardial electroanatomical mapping can also be undertaken *in vivo*.

## Imaging

Imaging is a key method of studying cardiovascular physiology and can make use of echocardiography, X-ray computed tomography (CT), magnetic resonance imaging (MRI), magnetic resonance spectroscopy (MRS) and single-photon emission CT (SPECT), as described in Chapter 2. A new molecular imaging technique enables the expression of tagged proteins to be imaged *in vivo*. **Bioluminescence** (or chemiluminescence) imaging makes use of luciferase, an enzyme that produces light emission from the conversion of D-luciferin to oxyluciferin. D-luciferin can be administered via an intravenous or intraperitoneal injection; then, the animal is anaesthetized to prevent movement artefact, and placed in a dark chamber before imaging with a charge-coupled device camera. The technique is cost-effective and has a high signal-to-noise ratio given the lack of background bioluminescence from mammalian cells. However, it requires genetically encoded luciferase, the injection of the substrate to enable light emission, and the resulting light signal will depend on the depth of tissue being imaged.

## 19.8 COMPUTER MODELLING

Computer modelling is a powerful tool that is becoming increasingly used in cardiovascular physiology. It was pioneered by among others Hodgkin and Huxley, who mathematically modelled the neuronal action potential based on experimental observations using the voltage clamp on the giant squid axon in 1952. The approach was taken further by Denis Noble (1960), who used a similar approach to model cardiac action potentials. Later, Noble together with others including Peter Hunter, modelled more complex electrophysiological, biochemical and mechanical properties of the heart. There is currently an international programme of research collaborations known as the **Physiome project**, the aim of which is to provide a comprehensive framework for modelling the human body using computational methods that can incorporate the biochemistry, biophysics and anatomy of cells, tissues and organs (Hunter and Borg, 2003).

The great power of computer modelling comes in its ability to integrate existing experimental data into a more complex system, which can then be used to run *in silico* experiments measuring variables or performing interventions that may not yet be possible *in vitro* or *in vivo*. Such models can be used to deepen our understanding of complex biological processes and also make predictions and generate hypotheses.

However, no matter how complex it may be, a computer model is only a simplified representation of reality based on our current understanding. A series of paintings by René Magritte in the 1920s make this point well, as shown in Figure 19.11. In *The Treachery of Images*, Magritte paints a very realistic picture of a pipe, yet the script below it reads *Ceci n'est pas une pipe* or This is not a pipe. In *The Two Mysteries*, he goes even further. The picture contains a pipe and a picture of a pipe and yet the pipe outside of the picture is still not a 'real' pipe.

We tend to learn most from computer models when their predictions prove to be wrong and it becomes apparent that the model, together with our understanding, needs to be revised.

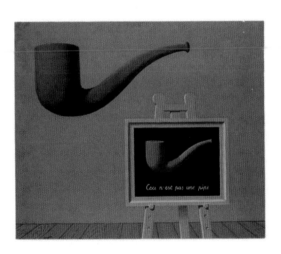
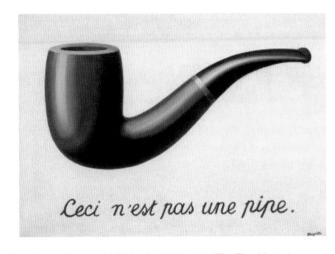

**Figure 19.11** *The Two Mysteries* (left) a painting of a painting of *The Treachery of Images* (right) by René Magritte. (*The Two Mysteries* painting is held by a private collector. *The Treachery of Images* painting is held by the Los Angeles County Museum of Art.)

## SUMMARY

- All experimental models and measurements have their advantages and limitations. Many measuring instruments by necessity, either directly or indirectly alter the state of what they measure, something known as the **observer effect**.
- The ratio between the level of the desired signal and the background noise is called the **signal-to-noise ratio**. All measurements have a degree of background noise and this should be factored into the experimental design.
- The frequency at which observations are made is called the **sampling rate**, and this is important in relation to the rate at which the variable being measured changes over time.

- Experiments should be designed with appropriate **positive and negative controls** and repeated to allow sufficient statistical power to draw conclusions.
- Where possible, measurements should be **randomized** and **blinded** to avoid confirmation bias.
- Single cells can be obtained by tissue digestion and cell isolation, primary cell culture, using established cell lines or induced pluripotent stem cells, which can then be differentiated in a variety of different cell types.
- Measurements on single cells include immunohistochemistry, real-time measurement of intracellular ion fluxes using

- fluorescent dyes, molecular interactions using FRET and electrophysiological stimulation and measurements through patch clamping and optogenetics. Cellular viability and proliferation can also be measured with a range of assays.
- Multicellular preparations include isolated vessels, atria, papillary muscle and also whole organs, such as the Langendorff and working heart preparations. Neural control can also be investigated *in vitro* using atria or Langendorff hearts with intact autonomic nerves or by using the working heart-brainstem preparation.
- Measurements in multicellular preparation include mRNA (quantitative PCR) and protein expression (Western blotting, microarrays) and localization (*in situ* hybridization, immunohistochemistry), real-time spatial imaging of enzyme and ion activity with one or more fluorescent dyes, electrophysiological measurements (using single electrodes or multi-electrode arrays and pacing) and tissue mechanics (by measuring force, pressure and volume).

- Animals can also be studied *in vivo* while awake (e.g. following instrumentation and radiotelemetry), or under general anaesthesia. While awake, body weight, urine output, activity, temperature, BP and heart rate can be measured. Under general anaesthesia, more invasive measures of haemodynamics, electrophysiology and blood sampling from anatomically privileged sites can be undertaken.
- Imaging is a key method of studying cardiovascular physiology and incorporates echocardiography, X-ray CT, MRI, MRS, SPECT and also bioluminescence imaging to track luciferase-tagged protein expression.
- Computer modelling allows the integration of experimental data into a more complex system, which can then be used to run *in silico* experiments measuring variables or performing interventions that may not yet be possible. Such models can be used to deepen our understanding of complex biological processes and generate hypotheses.

## FURTHER READING

### Isolated cells/measurements

Takahashi K, Tanabe K, Ohnuki M, et al. Induction of pluripotent stem cells from adult human fibroblasts by defined factors. *Cell* 2007; **131**(5): 861–72.

Zemelman BV, Lee GA, Ng M, et al. Selective photostimulation of genetically chARGed neurons. *Neuron* 2002; **33**(1): 15–22.

Klar TA, Jakobs S, Dyba M, et al. Fluorescence microscopy with diffraction resolution barrier broken by stimulated emission. *Proceedings of the National Academy of Sciences of the United States of America* 2000; **97**(15): 8206–10.

Zaccolo M, De Giorgi F, Cho CY, et al. A genetically encoded, fluorescent indicator for cyclic AMP in living cells. *Nature Cell Biology* 2000; **2**(1): 25–9.

Wier WG, Cannell MB, Berlin JR, et al. Cellular and subcellular heterogeneity of [Ca$^{2+}$]i in single heart cells revealed by fura-2. *Science* 1987; **235**(4786): 325–8.

Grynkiewicz G, Poenie M, Tsien RY. A new generation of Ca$^{2+}$ indicators with greatly improved fluorescence properties. *Journal of Biological Chemistry* 1985; **260**(6): 3440–50.

Neher E, Sakmann B. Single-channel currents recorded from membrane of denervated frog muscle fibres. *Nature* 1976; **260**(5554): 799–802.

Powell T, Twist VW. A rapid technique for the isolation and purification of adult cardiac muscle cells having respiratory control and a tolerance to calcium. *Biochemical and Biophysical Research Communications* 1976; **72**(1): 327–33.

Coons AH, Creech HJ, Jones RN. Immunological properties of an antibody containing a fluorescent group. *Experimental Biology and Medicine* 1941; **47**: 200–2.

### Multicellular preparation/measurements

Chung K, Wallace J, Kim SY, et al. Structural and molecular interrogation of intact biological systems. *Nature* 2013; **497**(7449): 332–7.

Paton JF. A working heart-brainstem preparation of the mouse. *Journal of Neuroscience Methods* 1996; **65**(1): 63–8.

Mullis K, Faloona F, Scharf S, et al. Specific enzymatic amplification of DNA in vitro: the polymerase chain reaction. *Cold Spring Harbor Symposia on Quantitative Biology* 1986; **51**(Pt 1): 263–73.

Burnette WN. "Western blotting": electrophoretic transfer of proteins from sodium dodecyl sulfate-polyacrylamide gels to unmodified nitrocellulose and radiographic detection with antibody and radioiodinated protein A. *Analytical Biochemistry* 1981; **112**(2): 195–203.

Salama G, Morad M. Merocyanine 540 as an optical probe of transmembrane electrical activity in the heart. *Science* 1976; **191**(4226): 485–7.

Gall JG, Pardue ML. Formation and detection of RNA-DNA hybrid molecules in cytological preparations. *Proceedings of the National Academy of Sciences of the United States of America* 1969; **63**(2): 378–83.

Neely JR, Liebermeister H, Battersby EJ, et al. Effect of pressure development on oxygen consumption by isolated rat heart. *American Journal of Physiology* 1967; **212**(4): 804–14.

Langendorff O. Untersuchungen am überlebenden Säugethierherzen. *Archiv für die gesamte Physiologie des Menschen und der Tier* 1895; **61**(6): 291–332.

Ringer S. Concerning the influence exerted by each of the constituents of the blood on the contraction of the ventricle. *The Journal of Physiology* 1882; **3**(5–6): 380–93.

## *In vivo* preparations/measurements

Parati G, Mancia G, Di Rienzo M, et al. Point: cardiovascular variability is/is not an index of autonomic control of circulation. *Journal of Applied Physiology* 2006; **101**(2): 676–8.

Taylor JA, Studinger P. Counterpoint: cardiovascular variability is not an index of autonomic control of the circulation. *Journal of Applied Physiology* 2006; **101**(2): 678–81.

Ramanathan C, Ghanem RN, Jia P, et al. Noninvasive electrocardiographic imaging for cardiac electrophysiology and arrhythmia. *Nature Medicine* 2004; **10**(4): 422–8.

McKay RG, Spears JR, Aroesty JM, et al. Instantaneous measurement of left and right ventricular stroke volume and pressure-volume relationships with an impedance catheter. *Circulation* 1984; **69**(4): 703–10.

Edler I. The use of ultrasound as a diagnostic aid, and its effects on biological tissues. Continuous recording of the movements of various heart-structures using an ultrasound echo-method. *Acta Medica Scandinavica. Supplementum* 1961; **370**: 7–65.

## Computer Modelling

Hunter PJ, Borg TK. Integration from proteins to organs: The Physiome Project. *Nature Reviews. Molecular Cell Biology* 2003; **4**(3): 237–43.

Noble D. Cardiac action and pacemaker potentials based on the Hodgkin–Huxley equations. *Nature* 1960; **188**: 495–7.

Hodgkin AL, Huxley AF. A quantitative description of membrane current and its application to conduction and excitation in nerve. *The Journal of Physiology* 1952; **117**(4): 500–44.

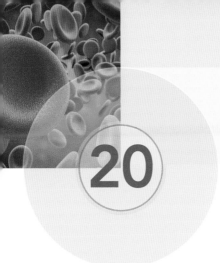

# Experimental perturbations to investigate cardiovascular physiology

**20**

## LEARNING OBJECTIVES

*After reading this chapter, you should be able to:*

- understand the basic principles behind the common experimental perturbations used to study cardiovascular physiology (20.1–20.4);

- appreciate their utility and the difficulties in interpreting the results of these perturbations (20.1–20.4);
- see the potential and limitations of undertaking measurements and experimental perturbations in human patients (20.1–20.4).

Chapter 19 describes a range of experimental models from single cells to whole-animal studies and some of the measurements that can be made on them. The aim of this chapter is to discuss some of the common experimental perturbations (physical, chemical and genetic) that can be used to investigate function, although the list is by no means exhaustive! Combinations of different manipulations can also be used in experimental design. For example, measurements can be made on isolated hearts (e.g. left ventricular developed pressure), the experimental perturbation could be knockout of a gene (compared with a wild-type animal) and the response of both groups to a physical manipulation, such as ischaemia/reperfusion or the addition of a drug evaluated.

When designing experiments, the way in which a perturbation can be induced and subsequently reversed needs to be considered. For interventions that can be reversed, paired statistical comparisons can be made within the same experimental individuals. If an intervention cannot be reversed, then two (or more) independent experimental groups are required and unpaired statistical comparisons are made. For a particular level of statistical power, more experimental replicates are required in each group when unpaired comparisons are made compared to paired comparisons within the same individual. This has implications for experimental design and the overall costs of the project. Importantly, before parametric statistics are used, the experimenter must make sure the data are normally distributed.

## 20.1 PHYSICAL MANIPULATION

### Isolated cells

Isolated cells are challenging to physically manipulate but this can be achieved directly, for example, using carbon fibres lowered onto each end of the cells. The spacing of these fibres can be set to investigate cellular behaviour at different preloads, or the response to an acute increase in **stretch**. The physical contact of the fibres pressing on localized regions of the cell membrane may influence cellular behaviour, and the fixed distance between the carbon fibres means that myocytes will contract in an isometric manner that is quite different to the situation in the whole organ. The physical forces experienced by cells in intact tissue include those related to the extracellular matrix, neighbouring electrically coupled myocytes, local capillary flow and the pressure of fluid in the contracting chamber itself. This is even more complex *in vivo* with pressure differentials inside and outside of the heart varying with respiration, movement and posture, which cannot be recreated *in vitro*.

Another way of physically manipulating an isolated cell without physical contact with the cell membrane, is through **osmotic stress**. This can cause the cell to swell or shrink and while this is useful for investigating the regulation of cell volume, it is not the same as manipulating the preload experienced by a myocyte in the intact organ. Changes in preload produce stretch between each end of the cell, together with a slight degree of curvature along its axis, rather than a change on whole-cell volume. Osmotic shock can also be used to produce detubulation in isolated myocytes, that is, loss of sarcolemma transverse tubule (T-tubule) invaginations, which is also observed in myocytes from failing hearts and may influence excitation-contraction coupling. This can be achieved by brief exposure to high concentrations of formamide (at 1800 mOsm/L), which produces a transient reduction in cell volume on perfusion. As formamide is membrane permeable, it then enters the cell dragging water, so the cell subsequently expands. During washout, the intracellular concentration of formamide is initially high so that water enters the cell, causing the rapid expansion that may cause the T-tubules to break from the surface membrane. While this is a useful model of manipulating the physical space between L-type $Ca^{2+}$ channels and ryanodine receptors, it is clearly different to the chronic structural remodelling that occurs in myocytes of the failing heart.

## Multicellular preparations

Physical stretch of multicellular preparations is considerably easier from a practical perspective than with isolated cells. With isolated papillary muscles, this can be applied between each end of the muscle, whereas in the isolated working heart, atrial filling pressure can be manipulated to vary preload and aortic pressure to vary afterload. The retrograde perfused Langendorff heart is an excellent model for studying the acute effects of **myocardial ischaemia**, for example, through ligation of a coronary artery and/or subsequent reperfusion. Regional ischaemia is generally carried out in constant perfusion pressure mode so that coronary autoregulation remains intact. While this is a convenient model, coronary artery occlusion in man is commonly via the rupture of an atherosclerotic plaque and subsequent activation of platelets and thrombus formation. Reperfusion through percutaneous coronary intervention, angioplasty and stenting results in distal embolization of thrombus and plaque. The influence of the autonomic nervous system *in vivo* on blood flow and the dynamic state of the heart is clearly missing in the Langendorff and working heart models as is normal $O_2$ delivery by haemoglobin at physiological flow rates.

Isolated resistance arteries/arterioles can also be cannulated, and their responses assessed through a video-monitored perfused system or via a myograph. Intraluminal pressure can be varied (via a servo-perfusion system) to measure the myogenic response, or flow-varied (via a peristaltic pump) to produce shear stress-mediated responses. The vessel itself can also be physically manipulated. **Endothelial denudation** was classically used in the Nobel Prize-winning work of Furchgott to suggest the existence of an endothelial-derived relaxing factor (subsequently identified as nitric oxide [NO]) released in response to acetylcholine.

## Manipulations *In vivo*

Physical manipulations *in vivo* can be used to investigate physiology, mimic a disease process or evaluate a potential surgical therapy. This requires intervention under general anaesthesia and may also require subsequent recovery to study the chronic effects of the intervention, and as such a **sham** group is important to control for the stress and inflammatory response of the surgery and anaesthesia itself.

### Investigating physiology

The simplest way of investigating the role of a tissue or nerve is through **surgical lesioning**. This has been used with varying success for specific brain regions, sectioning of nerves such as the vagus and carotid sinus nerves (see Figure 16.9), removal of the stellate ganglia and organ denervation including the kidneys and carotid body (see Chapter 18, Section 18.4). The results of such experiments are often more complex to interpret than they may first appear. Many nerves contain efferent and afferent fibres, and ganglia may also contain interneurons and are involved in complex reflex responses and neural integration. Sectioning or denervation may not be entirely complete or may recover following the intervention, and all interventions have the potential to damage neighbouring structures. Therefore, great care is needed to minimize heterogeneity within the experimental group, which will complicate the interpretation of results.

An alternative way of investigating physiology through physical means involves the activation of baroreceptors through **changes in posture**. This includes tilt-table testing or the application of negative pressure to the neck to activate the carotid sinus, or to the lower body to activate low pressure baroreceptors. In terms of practicality, these interventions are best suited to awake and compliant human patients rather than anaesthetized animal models.

### Mimicking disease

Physical intervention can be used *in vivo* to induce **acute ischaemia** with or without reperfusion, so that the local cellular response of the ischaemic tissue, or the systemic effects of the insult can be evaluated. In terms of the heart, acute reversible ischaemia can be induced by ligating a coronary artery around a small plastic tube, so that the ligature can subsequently be released for reperfusion. In larger animal models, balloon angioplasty can be performed (see Chapter 15, Section 15.1), and the balloon kept inflated until reperfusion is required. To produce a myocardial infarction without reperfusion in small rodent models, coronary artery clips, ligation or cryoinjury tend to be used. In larger animal models, percutaneous catheters can be used for coronary artery injection of alcohol, coil or microbead embolization. The chronic effects of myocardial infarction, remodelling or subsequent heart failure can also be evaluated with recovery anaesthesia.

Unlike humans, small rodent models never experience plaque rupture or myocardial infarction, even following

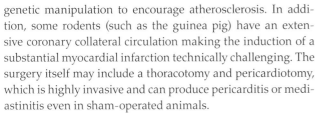

genetic manipulation to encourage atherosclerosis. In addition, some rodents (such as the guinea pig) have an extensive coronary collateral circulation making the induction of a substantial myocardial infarction technically challenging. The surgery itself may include a thoracotomy and pericardiotomy, which is highly invasive and can produce pericarditis or mediastinitis even in sham-operated animals.

The use of a **renal artery clip** to induce long-term hypertension was pioneered by the work of Goldblatt. This essentially mimics renal artery stenosis to produce renal hypoperfusion, and a rapid rise in plasma renin and activation of the angiotensin–aldosterone system. In the two-kidney, one-clip model, continuous activation of the renin–angiotensin–aldosterone system causes pressure diuresis of the contralateral normal kidney and prevents hypervolaemia. In contrast, in the one-kidney, one-clip model, volume retention by the single stenotic kidney eventually reduces renin secretion, providing a model of low-renin, volume-dependent hypertension. Both models develop cardiac hypertrophy and have been used as surrogates of hypertension and hypertensive diastolic and eventually systolic heart failure (see Chapter 18, Section 18.5). Most human hypertension is of unknown aetiology, with no clear structural, renal or endocrine abnormalities that can be identified as an underlying cause. Screening and aggressive treatment of hypertension in the Western world also now means that it rarely progresses to the development of systolic heart failure.

Heart failure can also be induced through **aortic banding**, mimicking severe coarctation to induce heart failure with pressure overload. Conversely, surgically induced **aortocaval fistulae** produce high-output volume overload heart failure. These models share many of the cardiac, renal and neurohumoral responses observed in human chronic heart failure. However, the most common cause of human heart failure in Western society is a cardiomyopathy, which is usually ischaemic or viral in origin.

## Testing surgical therapies

Surgical training often makes use of animal models as an educational tool, but the development of new techniques and the implantation of novel prostheses and devices often occurs in animal models before implementation in man. In terms of cardiovascular physiology, several recent developments stand out in this regard as being developed initially in animal models. This includes **renal sympathetic denervation** (see Chapter 18.4). However, with percutaneous radiofrequency ablation within the renal artery in man, there is no operative end point to establish that it has been successful. In rodent animal models, the approach to denervation is often via a flank incision and lesioning performed on the epivascular surface of the renal arteries where the neural plexus resides. Electrical stimulation of the vessel distal to the lesions failing to produce a rise in blood pressure (BP) is then used as an end point for the procedure to ensure successful denervation. Other examples include **stellectomy** as a treatment for ventricular arrhythmias (see Chapter 5, Section 5.11), and

**carotid body denervation** as a treatment for hypertension (see Chapter 18, Section 18.4). Implantation of a variety of **neural stimulators** targeting the cervical vagus nerve, thoracic spinal cord, dorsal root ganglia and deep brain nuclei has also been studied both in animal models and in man. How such stimulators interfere with reflex neural integration and how stimulators should be programmed in terms of frequency, intensity and pulse width to achieve therapeutic outcomes remains poorly understood.

## 20.2 CHEMICAL MANIPULATION

### Manipulation of ion concentrations/gas tensions

It is relatively simple to alter the composition of the perfusate when studying isolated cells or multicellular tissue in terms of the ion concentrations, blood gas tensions and pH to study their influence on cellular function. Multiple components can be changed simultaneously, for example, to mimic ischaemia. This is usually done with a perfusate containing high $K^+$, low pH and low $O_2$ tension. This does not mimic the tissue gradient of ion concentrations or temporal changes that occur *in vivo* during an ischaemic event. Many perfusate solutions contain glucose as the main metabolic substrate, but do not contain free fatty acids, ketone bodies or lactate. This is particularly relevant to the heart where under normal circumstances the main metabolic substrate for energy production are free fatty acids.

*In vivo*, blood gas tensions can be manipulated through **breathing circuits** which measure the concentrations of end-tidal gases and modify the fractions of inspired gases on a breath-by-breath basis using a feedback algorithm, such as those developed by Robbins and co-workers.

### Pharmacological agonists and antagonists

Drugs are used extensively in biomedical research to stimulate or inhibit an enzyme or receptor, and investigate the role of a signalling pathway in a physiological or pathophysiological process. Drugs are also tested as potential treatments in disease models. Chronic infusions of drugs can also be used to induce pathology. For example, prolonged infusions of angiotensin II produces hypertension and left ventricular hypertrophy.

Pharmacological agents can be used to activate reflexes, particularly the baroreflex in response to a vasodilator (e.g. an NO donor) or vasoconstrictor (e.g. an $\alpha 1$ adrenergic receptor agonist such as phenylephrine). Care must be taken with vasoactive compounds that may directly or indirectly interfere with the reflex response itself. An example of this is NO donors, which can influence the function of autonomic nerves as well as directly stimulate the sinoatrial node to increase heart rate in addition to causing vasodilatation.

When studying receptor **agonists**, ideally a full dose-response curve should be carried out, but this is often limited by the viability of experimental preparations over time. If a single dose or a few doses only are to be used, it is important to do preliminary experiments to establish that these are appropriate and not subthreshold or supramaximal. Also, when designing experimental protocols with agonists, it should be remembered that continual stimulation can lead to desensitization and eventually internalization of the receptors. An example of this is with the β adrenergic receptor, which after continued stimulation, becomes phosphorylated by a beta-adrenergic receptor kinase 1 (beta-ARK-1) or G-protein coupled receptor kinase 2. Binding of beta-arrestin-1 then leads to desensitization of the receptor and its internalization via endocytosis. The activity of beta-arrestin-1 and beta-ARK-1 are influenced by the levels of cyclic adenosine monophosphate, the second messenger of the β adrenergic receptor itself.

**Antagonists** bind to receptors; therefore, they have affinity but bring about no response in their own right, in other words, they have zero efficacy. Different types of antagonists or blockers are available, and their mechanism of action should be considered when planning experimental protocols. If an antagonist competes with the agonist for the same binding site and binds in a reversible manner, the result is a rightwards shift in the dose-response curve for the agonist as shown in Figure 20.1.

If an antagonist is competitive with the agonist but binds irreversibly, then at low doses the antagonist will shift the dose-response curve of the agonist to the right; at higher doses, it will start to reduce the maximal possible response to the agonist. This is because occupancy of only 30% of the total number of receptors is generally required for a maximal response to the agonist to be reached. Non-competitive antagonists bind to a region of the receptor other than the

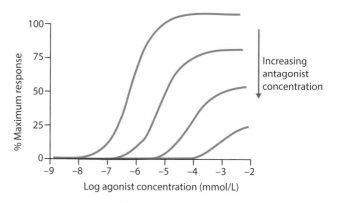

**Figure 20.2** Increasing concentrations of a non-competitive antagonist reduce the maximum response of the agonist dose-response curve. (Adapted from Wilkins R, Cross S, Megson I, et al., eds. *Oxford Handbook of Medical Sciences*, 2nd edn. Oxford: Oxford University Press; 2012. p. 83.)

agonist-binding site. These antagonists prevent activation of the transduction mechanism required to evoke a response; therefore, they reduce the maximum response of the agonist even at low concentrations as shown in Figure 20.2. Physiological antagonists act via a different receptor or second messenger system to reverse the effect of an agonist.

Many pharmacological antagonists and blockers also have non-specific, **off-target actions** on other receptors and signalling pathways; these need to be considered. Off-target effects are usually dose-related; therefore, a range of antagonist concentrations should be used. If this is not practical experimentally, then a suitable dose above the $K_i$ for the antagonist at the receptor of interest, but below that responsible for the off-target effects chosen. Some antagonists have structurally similar negative controls that can be used at the same concentration and produce similar off-target effects, but do not inhibit the receptor or enzyme of interest. When researching which pharmacological antagonists to use, it is worth remembering that the most recently discovered antagonists are always the most specific. This is not always because of refinement of their structure and better knowledge of drug-receptor interactions, but sometimes simply because their off-target effects have not yet been thoroughly studied!

## Pharmacokinetics

Even with isolated cells and multicellular preparations, pharmacokinetics is important to consider. With isolated cells, loading of a caged compound into a cell, which can be subsequently liberated through flash photolysis, is a useful technique to produce an abrupt rise in intracellular concentration. However, this is different from the microdomain signalling by which second messenger and intracellular ions communicate when signalling is through membrane receptors or liberated from intracellular organelles. Application of a neurotransmitter to tissue perfusate also does not mimic the highly localized release that is experienced through neural stimulation.

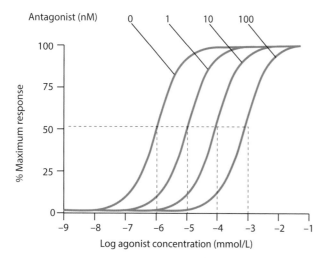

**Figure 20.1** Increasing concentrations of a competitive reversible antagonist shifts the dose-response curve of the agonist to the left. (Adapted from Wilkins R, Cross S, Megson I, et al., eds. *Oxford Handbook of Medical Sciences*, 2nd edn. Oxford: Oxford University Press; 2012. p. 83.)

Circulating levels of hormones and neurotransmitters measured *in vivo* are generally orders of magnitude lower than the concentrations of exogenous ligand that produce responses in isolated tissues. For example, circulating noradrenaline is in the low nanomolar range, whereas exogenous concentrations required for maximal stimulation of isolated cardiac tissue are in the micromolar range. Conversely, the concentration of a circulating drug is likely to be far higher than that which eventually diffuses to a tissue where its desired action is required. Tyrode's solution-based delivery of compounds is also different to that experienced *in vivo* because there are no plasma proteins or haemoglobin to which it may bind.

**Acute administration** of a compound under general anaesthesia via an intravenous, intraperitoneal, intramuscular or subcutaneous route is relatively straightforward; the pharmacokinetics that then result in a rise and fall in concentration at its desired site of action are not. The route of delivery, distribution, metabolism and excretion needs to be considered. **Chronic administration** of a compound *in vivo* in an animal model can be even more challenging. Approaches to this include **oral administration** via food or drinking water, although this may require the compound to be water-soluble and it will have to avoid being broken down by the liver once absorbed through the small intestine, otherwise known as first-pass metabolism. Reduced oral intake can also lead to dehydration and weight loss. Recurrent injections can be stressful for the animal and may require repeated anaesthesia. This also tends to produce peak and trough fluctuations in terms of drug delivery. **Osmotic minipumps** can be surgically implanted subcutaneously (usually on the dorsum, caudal to the scapulae); they allow a more constant delivery of drug over a longer period. Recovery surgery with appropriate post-operative analgesia is required for implantation and there is a risk of infection. Enough drug in an appropriate solvent also needs to be loaded into the pump and not result in excessive local irritation.

## 20.3 GENETIC MANIPULATION

The ability to **engineer** or manipulate gene expression has led to an explosion in the use of mouse models in biomedical research, although transgenic rat models are also now being developed. The ability to make animal models with a particularly gene **knocked out**, a variant of a gene **knocked in**, or with the expression of a gene upregulated, has allowed the role of such genes to be investigated *in vitro* and *in vivo* in a way that could never be achieved using a pharmacological approach. Genetic manipulation has also allowed animal models of human disease to be generated, and provided a method to track the localization and interaction of proteins using fluorescent tags; this has revolutionized biomedical research over the last 20–30 years. In this section, we describe the principles behind the commonly used methods of manipulating the genome that have become the cornerstone of biomedical research.

## Selective breeding

The generation of animal models of disease by selective inbreeding among those with the strongest phenotype has been very useful in cardiovascular research and has provided evidence that genetic factors are important in determining some of these disorders. Perhaps the most famous example is the **spontaneously hypertensive rat (SHR)**, which was developed by Okamoto and Aoki by selectively breeding littermates of Wistar-Kyoto rats with the highest BPs over multiple generations. After four generations, nearly all rats developed hypertension indicating that only a few genes may be involved in producing the phenotype. Other models of hypertension developed through selective breeding required many more generations of breeding (up to 20 for **New Zealand genetically hypertensive (NZGH) rats**) and may well be a result of many more genes, each influencing BP to a lesser degree. It is interesting to note that tail cuff BPs were used in the breeding of the SHR and NZGH rat; therefore, this may have specifically selected for stress-induced hypertension. The SHR model has also been used to study attention deficit hyperactivity disorder. The SHR is also a model of sympathetic hyperactivity that precedes the development of hypertension and can be observed before 4 weeks of age. By 6–8 weeks of age the animal has established hypertension with evidence of left ventricular hypertrophy by 12 weeks. By 9–10 months of age, impairment in left ventricular systolic function may start to develop before decompensated heart failure; premature death starts to occur around 16–20 months. The stroke-prone SHR is a substrain using the 24th generation of SHR with particularly severe hypertension and other genetic susceptibility to stroke compared to the SHR; they rarely survive beyond 12–15 months of age. Another example is the selective breeding for voluntary wheel-running behaviour in mice (based on the number of wheel revolutions per day) by the Garland group. This provides an interesting model for evaluating the heritability and neurobiology of locomotor behaviour and motivation, as well as the effects of exercise training on cardiovascular physiology.

## Gene knockout and knockin

The ability to modify genes in the mouse was first described by Thomas and Capecchi, and Smithies and co-workers. Capecchi and Smithies were awarded the Nobel Prize for Physiology or Medicine in 2007 with Martin Evans who pioneered the technique of isolating and culturing mouse embryonic stem cells (ESCs) and introducing a new gene (*hypoxanthine phosphoribosyltransferase 1*) using a retrovirus to make transgenic mice. The ability to modify or knockout endogenous genes in ESCs relies on the phenomenon of **homologous recombination**. This is a process by which nucleotide sequences are exchanged between identical or similar sections of DNA. It is the process by which genes are shuffled and genetic variation produced during meiosis, and the process by which double-stranded DNA breaks are repaired.

By transfecting a DNA construct that contains two homologous regions of DNA identical to sequences each side of the gene of interest into mouse ESCs, homologous recombination between these regions can result in a sequence of DNA from the construct being introduced into the host genome as demonstrated in Figure 20.3. The introduced sequence may contain a modified version of the gene or even encode an additional fluorescent tag that is **knocked in** or may contain no functioning gene at all resulting in **knockout**. Gain of function can also be achieved by introducing extra copies of a gene of interest or manipulating its promoter to upregulate gene expression. Introducing a sequence containing an antibiotic-resistant gene will help select for cells that have undergone successful recombination during subsequent culture. ESCs incorporating the alteration are then injected into blastocysts and implanted into surrogate mothers. Offspring are genotyped and interbred to identify homo- and heterozygotes for the manipulation, and control wild-type mice.

However, such technology is not without its limitations. It is worth bearing in mind that if a gene's function is critical in development, then knockout may well be embryonically lethal. The utility of a transgenic model also depends on the phenotype being measured. For example, if the protein product of a gene is being measured, then genetic knockout of the gene is likely to be an excellent experimental manipulation to achieve this. If the gene being manipulated is an enzyme, and the phenotype being measured is the conversion of a substrate to a product catalysed by the enzyme, other isoforms of the enzyme may also be upregulated. If the phenotype being measured is related to cellular, multicellular, whole-organ or even system-wide behaviour, then clearly the compensatory pathways become increasingly more complex. Experiments may be complicated by the result of gene knockout in different cell types and the response of the system to the change. For example, mice have been developed with genome deletion of endothelial NO synthase (eNOS). If the phenotype being studied is the role of

eNOS in ventricular myocyte function, then any changes observed compared with wild-type ventricular myocytes may be related directly to the knockout of eNOS. However, loss of eNOS-dependent vasodilatation in vascular smooth muscle also produces a model of hypertension and the differences in behaviour of ventricular myocytes may also be related to the development of left ventricular hypertrophy because of the hypertension. Moreover, while the mouse may be a suitable model for some aspects of human physiology, it is not a good model of all aspects of human health and disease. For example, the mouse has a high resting heart rate, very little resting vagal tone and very different cardiac electrophysiology in terms of the expression of voltage-gated ion channels. Mice also do not naturally develop atherosclerosis. Even following genetic manipulation (*low density lipoprotein receptor* $^{-/-}$ or *apolipoprotein E* $^{-/-}$) and a high fat diet, they develop stable plaque lesions at worse, which rarely rupture and result in infarction.

## Tissue- and time-specific knockout

Some of the issues with gene knockout models can be addressed with tissue- and time-specific knockouts. Tissue-specific knockout is achieved by incorporating locus of X-over P1 (loxP) sites either side of the gene of interest (**floxed gene**) using homologous recombination as described earlier. LoxP sites direct an enzyme called **Cre recombinase** that cuts and recombines sequences of DNA at these sites, thereby removing the sequence of DNA between them. The efficiency of the recombination tends to be lower the longer the length of DNA between the two loxP sites. The activity of Cre recombinase can then be controlled by crossing the mouse with the floxed gene with another mouse expressing Cre recombinase with a site- or cell-specific promoter as demonstrated in Figure 20.4. Examples of site/tissue-specific promoters with which Cre recombinase can be coupled include: synapsin (neuronal); PRSx8 (catecholaminergic neurons); alpha-myosin heavy chain (MHC; cardiac myocytes); smooth muscle MHC (smooth muscle); or tyrosine-protein kinase receptor Tie-2 (endothelial cells).

Time-specific gene knockout can also be achieved. This may be through the administration of doxycycline with the tetracycline **Tet-on** (where doxycycline activates expression) or **Tet-off** (where lack of doxycycline activates expression) system. Tetracycline transactivator (tTA) protein binds to sequences in the Tet response elements (TREs) to increase gene expression, but Tet binds to tTA and prevents TRE binding in the Tet-off system or encourages TRE binding in the Tet-on system. For temporally controlled, site-specific knockout, Cre recombinase can be fused with a mutated ligand-binding domain for the human oestrogen receptor. On the introduction of tamoxifen, the fusion protein can penetrate the nucleus and induce targeted recombination, whereas affinity for endogenous oestrogens is such that they are unable to achieve this. This gives irreversible knockout due to recombination unlike the Tet-on/Tet-off system.

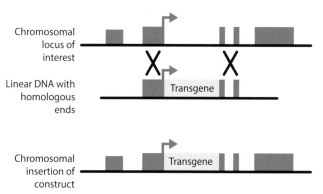

Chromosomal locus of interest

Linear DNA with homologous ends

Transgene

Chromosomal insertion of construct

Transgene

**Figure 20.3** Homologous recombination between a segment of linear DNA (or construct) and a chromosomal locus of interest occurs at regions of identical DNA sequences each side of a transgene, marked by the crosses on the diagram. This results in the incorporation of the transgene construct at a particular site in the chromosome.

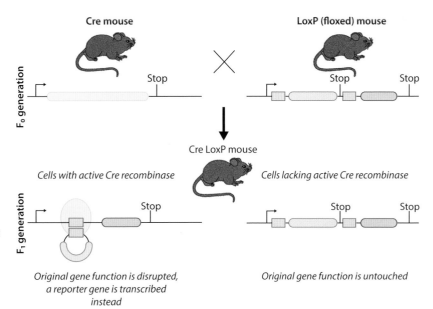

**Figure 20.4** Site-specific knockout is achieved by incorporating loxP sites either side of the gene of interest using homologous recombination to create a 'floxed' mouse. This mouse is crossed with a mouse expressing Cre recombinase under the control of a tissue-specific promoter. By using offspring that have both the floxed gene and Cre recombinase under the control of a tissue-specific promoter, the gene of interest will by excised in cells where only Cre recombinase is expressed.

Despite these innovations, often the resulting phenotype and the role played by the gene being manipulated can be difficult to interpret in experiments involving transgenic mice. For example, with site-specific knockout, low-level Cre recombinase expression in other tissues may succeed in producing additional gene knockout. Moreover, if the gene of interest being knocked out is an enzyme, cellular levels of the product of the reaction the enzyme catalyses may not be greatly influenced if the cell type where the gene is knocked out simply increases its extracellular uptake or synthesizes the product via an alternative pathway.

## Gene Knockdown

Another way of reducing gene expression without genomic knockout is through **interference RNA (RNAi)**. Small interfering RNA (siRNA) sequences or genomic non-coding microRNA can bind to specific mRNA molecules and prevent translation into protein. Endogenous double-stranded RNA (dsRNA) is cleaved into short interfering dsRNA (siRNA) by an endoribonuclease enzyme (endoribonuclease Dicer). siRNA can be unwound into a guide strand and a passenger strand with the guide strand targeting specific mRNA to the RNA-induced silencing complex (RISC), where the catalytic argonaute 2 cleaves the mRNA and prevents translation, as demonstrated in Figure 20.5. This pathway has been exploited by introducing dsRNA or siRNA to target specific mRNA. This was first achieved in *Caenorhabditis elegans* by feeding the worm with *Escherichia coli* carrying the required dsRNA; it led to the award of the 2006 Nobel Prize in Medicine or Physiology to Andrew Fire and Craig Mello. Introduction of RNAi can also be achieved with a viral vector delivery system. The challenge with RNAi is to find sequences that produce significant degrees of knockdown in protein expression without having off-target effects on other mRNAs. Scrambled sequences should also be used as a negative control.

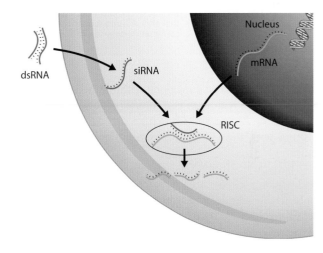

**Figure 20.5** The interference RNA pathway. Endogenous double-stranded RNA (dsRNA) is cleaved into short interfering dsRNA (siRNA) by an endoribonuclease enzyme (Dicer). siRNA can be unwound into a guide strand and a passenger strand with the guide strand targeting specific mRNA to the RNA-induced silencing complex (RISC), where the catalytic argonaute 2 will cleave the mRNA and prevent translation.

## Genome editing

Recently, a new technique to edit the genome has been adapted making use of the **clustered regularly interspaced short palindromic repeats (CRISPR)** system. In bacteria, this system allows short sequences of viral DNA known as spacer DNA to be inserted into the genome (between the short palindromic base sequences), recording over time which viruses the bacteria have been exposed to. The spacer sequences help the **CRISPR-associated system (Cas)** proteins identify and cut similar DNA from infecting viruses or plasmids, allowing a future adaptive immune response to be generated against them. In 2012, the Doudna and Charpentier groups described how a simple CRISPR/

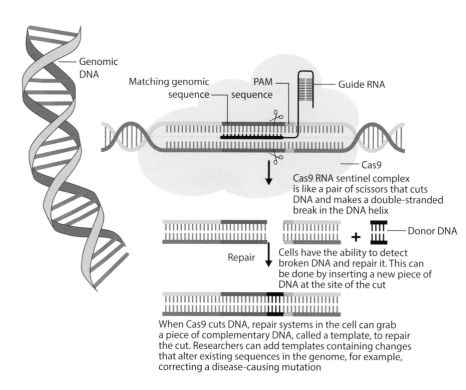

Genomic DNA

Matching genomic sequence — PAM sequence — Guide RNA

— Cas9

Cas9 RNA sentinel complex is like a pair of scissors that cuts DNA and makes a double-stranded break in the DNA helix

+ — Donor DNA

Repair

Cells have the ability to detect broken DNA and repair it. This can be done by inserting a new piece of DNA at the site of the cut

When Cas9 cuts DNA, repair systems in the cell can grab a piece of complementary DNA, called a template, to repair the cut. Researchers can add templates containing changes that alter existing sequences in the genome, for example, correcting a disease-causing mutation

**Figure 20.6** Genome editing using CRISPR/Cas9. The type II CRISPR/Cas9 system is carried by a plasmid and contains guide RNA (gDNA), a CRISPR RNA (crRNA) that binds only where editing is required, and transactivating RNA, which contains a hairpin loop and together with crRNA forms an active complex, as well as the Cas9 enzyme and a donor repair template. The synthetic gRNA along with a protospacer adjacent motif (PAM) sequence guide Cas9 to the appropriate section of DNA that is unwound and cleaved, allowing insertion of specific donor DNA sequence from the repair template up to 20 base pairs long.

Cas9 system could be used along with synthetic guide RNA (gRNA) to cut, remove or edit cellular genomic DNA. Then, in 2013, the Zhang and Church groups described genome editing with the CRISPR/Cas9 technique in human cell cultures.

The type II CRISPR/Cas9 system is carried by a plasmid and contains gRNA, a CRISPR RNA (crRNA), which binds only where editing is required, and transactivating RNA, which contains a hairpin loop and together with crRNA forms an active complex, as well as the Cas9 enzyme and a repair template. The synthetic gRNA, along with a protospacer adjacent motif sequence, guides Cas9 to the appropriate section of DNA which is unwound and cleaved, allowing insertion of specific DNA sequences from the repair template up to 20 base pairs long, as shown in Figure 20.6. The technique allows an accurate, cheap and rapid way of editing the genome that will have many uses in research.

## Viral vector delivery systems

Viral vector delivery systems offer a way of introducing genetic material into cells resulting in increased protein expression, or gene knockdown through the delivery of RNAi. This was first achieved by Paul Berg in 1976 using simian cultured kidney cells with a modified simian vacuolating virus 40 (SV40) containing bacteriophage λ DNA. This and other work on recombinant DNA led Berg being jointly awarded the Nobel Prize in Chemistry in 1980 with Gilbert and Sanger. A variety of different viral vectors have been used both for *in vitro* and *in vivo* gene delivery and each have their advantages and disadvantages. The most commonly used are adenoviruses (AVs), adeno-associated viruses (AAVs) and lentiviruses (LVs).

AVs are DNA viruses that do not integrate into the host genome. They produce short-lived gene expression over several days; this limits their use for long-term experiments or gene therapy. As they are common pathogens, hosts are likely to have already developed an immune response against them. However, they have a high transduction efficiency and have a large genome (~30 kb) compared to LVs (~8 kb) and AAVs (~5 kb). AAVs are less immunogenic and incorporate into the genome of dividing and non-dividing cells producing long-term gene expression. LVs are a class of retrovirus that integrate into the genome of non-dividing cells, and can be engineered so that they do not contain the machinery for replication. They also produce long-term, stable gene expression. For AAVs and lentiviruses, their site of integration into the host genome may disrupt normal cellular function and may potentially activate oncogenes. Gene expression from a viral vector may also not be under the same physiological control systems as the native gene, and large amounts of gene product may interfere with cellular function. Delivery of the genetic material in the viral vector to the site and cell type of interest and achieving high levels of transfection *in vivo* also remain major challenges. This can be helped through localized injections (e.g. into coronary arteries or into the pericardial space), using tissue-specific promoters (as described for the Cre/loxP system described earlier) and by encoding a fluorescent tag to the gene product of interest so that successfully transfected cells can be identified for further study (see Figure 20.7). Successful protein upregulation should also be confirmed through Western blotting.

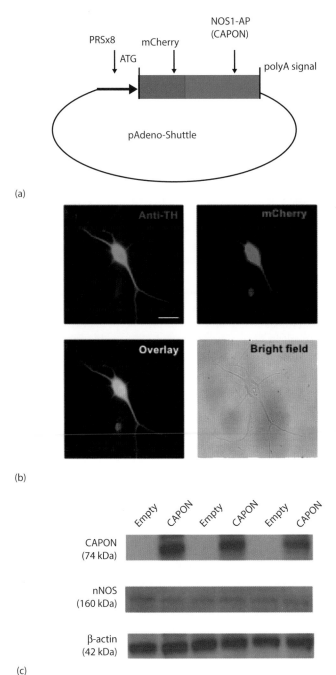

**Figure 20.7** (**a**) Map of adenoviral vector construct containing a noradrenergic neuron-specific promoter, PRSx8, neuronal nitric oxide synthase adaptor protein (NOS1-AP/CAPON) gene and red mCherry fluorescent protein (Ad.PRSx8-mCherry/CAPON). As a control, the same construct without NOS1-AP (CAPON) gene insert was used (Ad.PRSx8-mCherry). (**b**) Co-immunostaining of stellate neurons with anti-tyrosine hydroxylase (TH, green) and mCherry-tagged (red) viral construct showed viral transduction in sympathetic neurons. Nuclear staining with 4',6-diamidino-2-phenylindole (DAPI) is in blue. Scale bar, 25 μm. (**c**) Representative Western blot showing CAPON expression (74 kDa) and neuronal NOS expression in stellate ganglia from 4-week-old SHR 3 days after transduction with Ad.PRSx8-mCherry/CAPON and Ad.PRSx8-mCherry. (Adapted from Lu CJ, Hao G, Nikiforova N, et al. *Hypertension* 2015; 65(6): 1288–97.)

## 20.4 HUMAN CLINICAL STUDIES

While the measurements and perturbations discussed in Chapters 19 and 20 have focused mainly on animal research, translating the understanding gained from these experiments to human physiology and pathophysiology is key. Many modern research papers combine mechanistic studies in animal models with more observational human studies to demonstrate the potential applicability of their findings. Compared to animal research, human patients can have great diversity both in terms of genetics and environmental exposure, as well as multiple different underlying pathologies, which introduces a greater degree variability. Therefore, designing a study with the appropriate level of statistical power can be more challenging.

If appropriate legal and ethical permissions are in place, there are limited possibilities to obtain **tissue samples** from human patients, which can then undergo some of the single-cell and multicellular measurements, and physical and chemical perturbations we have described. For example, there are opportunities during cardiac bypass surgery to obtain tissue samples from the left atrial appendage, internal mammary artery and saphenous vein grafts; during right heart catheterization, right ventricular biopsies can be obtained that are sometimes taken by cardiologists to aid diagnosis. During bronchoscopy, biopsies can also be taken and bronchoalveolar lavage performed to sample the protein and cellular components of the epithelial fluid lining. **Fluid samples** from the pleural and pericardial space are also routinely obtained during certain pathological conditions for diagnostic and therapeutic purposes. More recently, **induced pluripotent stem cells** can be generated from fibroblasts in skin samples, which can then be differentiated into a variety of different cell types and studied either in isolation, cultured into layers or co-cultured with mixed cell types.

However, many of the measurements in animals *in-vivo* can also be undertaken in humans. This includes haemodynamic and electrophysiological measurements, imaging and holter monitoring. **Blood sampling** both peripherally and from anatomically privileged sites (such as the coronary sinus and coronary arteries) can also be obtained. The study of tissue and blood samples has been revolutionized recently with the advent of high-throughput screening techniques including functional genomics (e.g. with Illumina dye sequencing), RNA sequencing and mass spectrometry techniques to study metabolomics and proteomics. These approaches often generate a vast amount of information per sample. Adequate quality control, repeatability and appropriate statistical analysis of the resulting data are therefore key to interpreting the results. It is often best to have *a priori* hypotheses in mind when undertaking these analyses, rather than the approach simply being a 'fishing trip' to see what can be found. This is important given the statistical opportunity for findings to be related to random chance when so many variables are measured simultaneously.

Undertaking measurements in human research *in-vivo* is relatively straightforward; however, experimental perturbations are more difficult and confined to registered **clinical trials** of new therapies, interventions or treatment pathways. It is easier to make unpaired comparisons between diseased and normal individuals if the groups are otherwise well matched. While this only generates correlations, these can then be explored further with the aid of prospective studies where predictions are made on a different population of patients. Alternatively, more mechanistic studies can be carried out in animal models with more definitive experimental measurements and perturbations.

One area in which observational data between different human patients has been particularly useful is when the genetic basis of disease is being determined. This applies both to more conventional Mendelian inheritance through **genetic linkage studies**, but also for complex multigenic phenotypes. In conditions where there is some understanding of the underlying pathophysiology, case-controlled candidate gene studies can be undertaken to see if an allele of a candidate gene is observed more frequently in individuals with the conditions than those without. This approach is limited given the variance in penetrance and expressivity, and the ability of multiple genes to interact to give the same phenotype, and such studies have often been difficult to replicate in different populations. The ability to do whole-genome, single nucleotide polymorphism (SNP) genotyping cheaply on a large scale has allowed a non-candidate gene approach to complex phenotypes. In these studies, the association of SNPs related to genes with a phenotype can be assessed in what has become known as **genome-wide association studies**. Given the large number of SNPs in the human genome, only those with a very high probability of being linked with the phenotype (e.g. $p < 5 \times 10^{-8}$) in a large population of individuals should be considered. Such linkages should also then be explored in different populations to look for consistency. These studies work best when the phenotype is well defined and easily measured (e.g. QT interval on the electrocardiogram; see Chapter 5, Section 5.2). This phenotype-first approach can identify new genes that were not previously known, which only contribute a small amount to the overall complex phenotype. This has opened new avenues of research regarding the role of these genes and furthered our understanding of the physiology.

## SUMMARY

- For perturbations that can be reversed, paired statistical comparisons can be made within the same experimental patients. If a perturbation cannot be reversed, then two (or more) independent experimental groups are required and unpaired statistical comparisons are made.

- For a particular level of statistical power, more experimental replicates are required in each group when unpaired comparisons are made compared to paired comparisons within the same individual.

- Physical manipulations can be applied to isolated cells using carbon fibres to simulate axial stretch or through osmotic cell swelling. Osmotic shock can produce detubulation, a phenomenon also observed during congestive heart failure, and this approach has been used to assess the impact on excitation-contraction coupling.

- Physical manipulation of multicellular tissue can be used to assess the effect of pressure and flow, as well as regional ischaemia and subsequent reperfusion.

- Physical manipulations *in vivo* can be used to investigate physiology (by lesioning, denervation or by activating baroreflexes), mimic a disease process (by inducing ischaemia/infarction, clipping renal arteries or banding the aorta) or to evaluate potential surgical therapies.

- Chemical manipulation includes altering ion concentrations, pH and blood gas tensions, as well as pharmacological agents.

- Pharmacological agents can be used to inhibit or stimulate enzymes or receptors and with chronic administrations can also mimic disease phenotypes. The type of agonist (full versus partial) or antagonist (reversible versus irreversible, competitive versus non-competitive), the concentration used in relation to the drug selectivity and its pharmacokinetics must be taken into consideration when designing experiments.

- The ability to *engineer* or manipulate gene expression has revolutionized biomedical research over the last 20–30 years and has led to an explosion in the use of mouse models, although transgenic rat models are also now being developed.

- Genetic manipulation encompasses a range of approaches including selective breeding (such as with the SHR), as well as gene knockout, knockin or knockdown (using RNAi), which can be controlled to a certain degree in a tissue-specific (using the Cre-Lox system) or time-specific manner (using the Tet-on/Tet-off system). More recently, an accurate, cheap and rapid method of genome editing has been devised using the CRISPR/Cas9 system.

- The delivery of genetic material to a site and tissue of interest can also be achieved using viral vectors, which opens the possibility for gene therapy to non-germ line cells.

- There is huge potential for human research in cardiovascular physiology with appropriate ethical permissions. This encompasses a wide range of approaches from using tissue and blood samples to measurements *in-vivo*. Such research can be observational (comparing diseased and normal groups), but in the context of clinical trials can also evaluate pharmacological or surgical therapies, or different treatment pathways.

## FURTHER READING

### Physical

Esler M, Guo L. The future of renal denervation. *Autonomic Neuroscience* 2017; **204**: 131–8.

Ardell JL, Andresen MC, Armour JA, et al. Translational neuro-cardiology: preclinical models and cardioneural integrative aspects. *The Journal of Physiology* 2016; **594**(14): 3877–909.

Shivkumar K, Ajijola OA, Anand I, et al. Clinical neurocardiology defining the value of neuroscience-based cardiovascular thera-peutics. *The Journal of Physiology* 2016; **594**(14): 3911–54.

McBryde FD, Abdala AP, Hendy EB, et al. The carotid body as a putative therapeutic target for the treatment of neurogenic hypertension. *Nature Communications* 2013; **4**: 2395.

Green AL, Wang S, Owen SL, et al. Deep brain stimulation can regulate arterial blood pressure in awake humans. *Neuroreport* 2005; **16**(16): 1741–5.

White E, Le Guennec JY, Nigretto JM, et al. The effects of increasing cell length on auxotonic contractions; membrane potential and intracellular calcium transients in single guinea-pig ventricular myocytes. *Experimental Physiology* 1993; **78**(1): 65–78.

Furchgott RF, Zawadzki JV. The obligatory role of endothelial cells in the relaxation of arterial smooth muscle by acetyl-choline. *Nature* 1980; **288**(5789): 373–6.

Goldblatt H, Lynch J, Hanzal RF, et al. Studies on experimental hypertension: I. The production of persistent elevation of systolic blood pressure by means of renal ischemia. *Journal of Experimental Medicine* 1934; **59**(3): 347–79.

### Chemical

Smith JS, Rajagopal S. The β-arrestins: multifunctional regula-tors of G protein-coupled receptors. *Journal of Biological Chemistry* 2016; **291**(17): 8969–77.

Casadei B, Paterson DJ. Should we still use nitrovasodilators to test baroreflex sensitivity? *Journal of Hypertension* 2000; **18**(1): 3–6.

Kawai M, Hussain M, Orchard CH. Excitation-contraction coupling in rat ventricular myocytes after formamide-induced detubulation. *American Journal of Physiology* 1999; **277**(2 Pt 2): H603–9.

Robbins PA, Swanson GD, Micco AJ, et al. A fast gas-mixing system for breath-to-breath respiratory control studies. *Journal of Applied Physiology: Respiratory, Environmental and Exercise Physiology* 1982; **52**(5): 1358–62.

### Genetic

Rincon MY, VandenDriessche T, Chuah MK. Gene therapy for cardiovascular disease: advances in vector development, targeting, and delivery for clinical translation. *Cardiovascular Research* 2015; **108**(1): 4–20.

Cong L, Ran FA, Cox D, et al. Multiplex genome engineering using CRISPR/Cas systems. *Science* 2013; **339**(6121): 819–23.

Mali P, Yang L, Esvelt KM, et al. RNA-guided human genome engineering via Cas9. *Science* 2013; **339**(6121): 823–6.

Bush WS, Moore JH. Chapter 11: Genome-wide association studies. *PLoS Computational Biology* 2012; **8**(12): e1002822.

Jinek M, Chylinski K, Fonfara I, et al. A programmable dual-RNA-guided DNA endonuclease in adaptive bacterial immunity. *Science* 2012; **337**(6096): 816–21.

Risch NJ. Searching for genetic determinants in the new mil-lennium. *Nature* 2000; **405**(6788): 847–56.

Fire A, Xu S, Montgomery MK, et al. Potent and specific genetic interference by double-stranded RNA in *Caenorhabditis elegans. Nature* 1998; **391**(6669): 806–11.

Swallow JG, Carter PA, Garland T Jr. Artificial selection for increased wheel-running behavior in house mice. *Behavior Genetics* 1998; **28**(3): 227–37.

Gossen M, Freundlieb S, Bender G, et al. Transcriptional activation by tetracyclines in mammalian cells. *Science* 1995; **268**(5218): 1766–9.

Gu H, Marth JD, Orban PC, et al. Deletion of the DNA poly-merase beta gene in T cells using type-specific gene target-ing. *Science* 1994; **265**(5168): 103–6.

Thomas KR, Capecchi MR. Targeted disruption of the murine int-1 proto-oncogene resulting in severe abnormalities in midbrain and cerebellar development. *Nature* 1990; **346**(6287): 847–50.

Koller BH, Hagemann LJ, Doetschman T, et al. Germ-line transmission of a planned alteration made in a hypoxan-thine phosphoribosyltransferase gene by homologous recombination in embryonic stem cells. *Proceedings of the National Academy of Sciences of the United States of America* 1989; **86**(22): 8927–31.

Goff SP, Berg P. Construction of hybrid viruses containing SV40 and lambda phage DNA segments and their propaga-tion in cultured monkey cells. *Cell* 1976; **9**(4 Pt 2): 695–705.

Okamoto K, Aoki K. Development of a strain of spontaneously hypertensive rats. *Japanese Circulation Journal* 1963; **27**: 282–93.

## THE END BUT NOT THE END

'Begin at the beginning', said the King, very gravely, to the White Rabbit, 'and go on till you come to the end: then stop.' The scientific investigation of the circulation is far from at an end – too many mysteries remain unsolved. The discerning reader will have recognized the superabundance of unre-solved problems from the frequent use of 'may be', 'probably', 'is thought to' and so on. Our subject began essentially with the work of William Harvey over three centuries ago, yet a comment by Harvey is just as relevant today as it was then:

*I see a field of such vast extent that my whole life perchance would not suffice for its completion.*

(Mallock A. *William Harvey.* New York: Hoeber; 1929.)

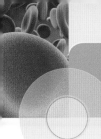

# CLINICAL CASES FOR PROBLEM-BASED LEARNING

## CASE 1: ELDERLY MAN WITH A MURMUR

*A 70-year-old man, keen on keeping fit, visited his doctor because he experienced a tight, constricting band across his chest during exercise, relieved by rest. He also complained of excessive breathlessness and dizziness during exercise, and had recently fainted while exercising.*

*On examination, his pulse was regular but slow-rising and of small amplitude. His brachial blood pressure (BP), 115/80 mmHg, confirmed a low pulse amplitude for his age. On palpation, the apex beat was in the fifth intercostal space, mid-clavicular line; however, a 'thrill' (vibration) was palpable during systole. Auscultation revealed a systolic crescendo–decrescendo murmur (diamond-shaped murmur, Figure 2.8), loudest over the aortic area. The second heart sound was soft, with reversed (or 'paradoxical') splitting, that is, splitting on expiration.*

*A chest X-ray showed a normal cardiothoracic ratio, but dilated ascending aorta. An electrocardiogram (ECG) showed left axis deviation, large QRS complex amplitudes in the chest leads, and lateral ST segment depression and T-wave inversion. An echocardiogram showed left ventricular concentric hypertrophy and poorly mobile, calcified aortic valve cusps. It was difficult to estimate the velocity across the aortic valve, and hence the gradient because of poor ultrasound windows. Cardiac catheterization subsequently revealed a left ventricular systolic pressure of 180 mmHg, but 115 mmHg in the aorta. The patient was referred for replacement of the stenosed aortic valve. In the meantime, he was advised against overexertion and given a β blocker, bisoprolol fumarate, to prevent angina.*

## QUESTIONS

1. Which valves create the second heart sound and why was it soft here?
2. What is the structure of the aortic valve and what orifices lie just behind the cusps?
3. Explain the reversed splitting of the second heart sound.
4. Does inspiration/expiration affect stroke volume and/or heart rate?
5. How big is the pressure gradient across the normal aortic valve during (1) ejection and (2) diastole? Why was the systolic gradient increased here?
6. What is a typical arterial pressure for a healthy 70-year-old?
7. How does the coronary circulation normally respond during exercise?
8. How is systolic coronary blood flow affected by a rise in ventricular systolic pressure?
9. Can exercise induce angina in the absence of coronary artery stenosis?
10. How does left ventricular hypertrophy affect pulmonary venous pressure, and could this contribute to exercise dyspnoea?
11. How might aortic valve stenosis lead to dizziness and fainting during exercise?
12. How does aortic valve stenosis cause a murmur and thrill?
13. Does a systolic murmur always indicate a valve lesion?
14. In electrocardiography, why is the ST segment normally isoelectric, and why is the T-wave normally upright?
15. What does 'electrical axis' mean, and how does left ventricular hypertrophy affect it?
16. How does myocardial ischaemia depress the ST segment?
17. How does a β blocker help to relieve exercise-induced angina?

## ANSWERS

1. The second heart sound is caused by the vibration of the aortic and pulmonary valve cusps on closing. When cusp mobility is impaired by calcification, as here, they have less far to travel, there is less vibration and therefore a softer sound.

2. A normal aortic valve has three cusps, but aortic stenosis also often develops in a congenitally bicuspid valve (present in 1%–2% of the population). Each cusp is a thin sheet of fibrous tissue covered by the endothelium. The openings of the right and left coronary arteries lie immediately behind the valve cusps, in the sinuses of Valsalva (Figure 1.4).

3. Normally, the aortic component of the second sound precedes the pulmonary component (Figure 2.4). The 'splitting' normally increases during inspiration because a transient increase in systemic venous return raises right ventricular filling, which prolongs right ventricular ejection (Figure 8.27); at the same time, pulmonary vascular expansion reduces flow into the left ventricle, shortening left ventricular ejection. In severe aortic stenosis, the aortic component comes second because of the increased resistance to left ventricular ejection, which is therefore prolonged. Inspiration again prolongs right ventricular ejection, this time bringing the two sounds together – 'reversed splitting'.

4. Expiration slows the heart rate by increased vagal inhibition (sinus arrhythmia; Figure 16.17). Expiration also reduces right ventricular stroke volume and increases left ventricular stroke volume – see (3).

5. The systolic pressure gradient across the aortic valve is normally only a few mmHg because the wide aperture offers little resistance to flow (Figure 2.4). The large systolic pressure gradient in the patient, 65 mmHg, is caused by the high resistance of the narrowed valve (Figure 2.8). In diastole, the gradient across the closed valve is large, namely diastolic aortic pressure (80 mmHg) minus diastolic left ventricular pressure (5–10 mmHg).

6. Ageing raises BP to ~140/75 mmHg for a 70-year-old white man (Figure 17.10). The exaggerated rise in pulse pressure and systolic pressure is due to arteriosclerosis, which reduces arterial compliance (Figure 18.7) and increased systolic augmentation by wave reflection (Figure 18.8).

7. During exercise, coronary blood flow normally increases in proportion to increased myocardial $O_2$ consumption, due to metabolic vasodilatation (Figure 15.4).

8. Coronary blood flow normally declines sharply in systole because the tense myocardium compresses the intramural coronary vessels (Figure 15.5). An exaggerated increase in ventricular systolic pressure, 170 mmHg here, further curtails systolic perfusion.

9. Yes. Ischaemic myocardial pain occurs whenever myocardial $O_2$ supply fails to meet demand. In this patient, myocardial $O_2$ demand is excessive (because the ventricle is pumping through a narrowed outlet) and

10. Because the ventricle wall is hypertrophied, it is stiffer than normal, so filling requires a higher diastolic pressure. The attendant increased left atrial pressure raises pulmonary venous pressure, which congests the lungs and makes them stiffer. Lung stiffness causes dyspnoea, as in Clinical Case 5.

11. During exercise, arterial pressure is normally maintained by the increased cardiac output, despite the fall in peripheral resistance caused by the muscle metabolic vasodilatation (Figure 17.5); mean arterial pressure = cardiac output × peripheral resistance. Severe aortic stenosis prevents an adequate increase in cardiac output, so arterial pressure falls during exercise. If pressure falls below the limit of cerebral autoregulation (Figure 15.13), cerebral hypoperfusion leads to dizziness or even fainting on exercise.

12. Aortic valve stenosis creates turbulent flow, which sets up the vibrations heard as a crescendo–decrescendo murmur (Figure 2.8) or felt as a thrill. Turbulence is favoured by the abrupt change in diameter at the stenosed valve exit, and by the high Reynolds number (fluid velocity × diameter × density/viscosity) generated by the high velocity of blood in the narrowed valve.

13. No. If the aortic Reynolds number exceeds ~2000 during peak systolic flow, turbulence can develop, creating a benign systolic murmur. This is particularly common in pregnancy, owing to the increased cardiac output and moderate anaemia (low viscosity).

14. The ST segment corresponds to the plateau of the ventricular myocyte action potential. Since all the ventricle myocytes are at approximately the same potential, no current flows between them and the ECG is isoelectric (baseline). The T-wave is upright because subepicardial myocytes have shorter plateaux than subendocardial myocytes (Figure 5.3), and therefore repolarize first (Figure 5.8).

15. The electrical axis is the direction of the largest dipole during ventricular depolarization (Figure 5.6). The axis depends on the physical angle of the heart and on left ventricular muscle mass relative to right ventricular mass. Left ventricular hypertrophy increases the magnitude of left-sided current, shifting the electrical axis to the left.

16. Ischaemia is most severe in the subendocardium of the hypertrophied ventricle, where compressive stress is highest. This reduces the size of the subendocardial resting and action potentials. The potential difference between the ischaemic and non-ischaemic regions generates an injury current, which displaces the ST segment (Figure 5.11).

17. Blockage of cardiac $\beta_1$ adrenergic receptors reduces the tonic effect of the cardiac sympathetic nerves on rate and contractility, lowering cardiac output. This reduces myocardial work and $O_2$ demand, and increases the diastolic period, during which coronary perfusion is highest. These changes help prevent angina.

## CASE 2: MAN WITH A CHEST PAIN

*A collapsed 60-year-old bus driver was brought into Accident & Emergency complaining of a severe, sustained crushing pain in a band across the chest, spreading into the arms. Previously, he had been well, but smoked 10 cigarettes a day.*

*On examination, he was pale, with cold, sweaty skin. His pulse was weak, with occasional extra systoles (ventricular ectopic beats). His arterial blood pressure (BP) was 95/70 mmHg. Heart sounds were normal. An electrocardiogram (ECG) revealed large*

*Q waves and ST segment elevation. He was admitted with a provisional diagnosis of myocardial infarction. Point of care blood testing showed raised high-sensitivity troponin T and laboratory testing later revealed a raised total cholesterol.*

*He was given aspirin, ticagrelor and morphine and was transferred immediately to the catheter laboratory for coronary angiography and primary percutaneous coronary intervention.*

## QUESTIONS

1. Name the major coronary arteries and their territories; define 'functional end artery'.
2. What is the likely coronary artery pathology here and how does endothelial dysfunction contribute to it?
3. Which afferents mediate ischaemic cardiac pain?
4. Since the left ventricle contains oxygenated blood, why is the left ventricle wall ischaemic?
5. If the patient's arterial blood contained 190 mL $O_2$ per L, mixed venous blood 90 mL $O_2$ per L and his $O_2$ consumption was 300 mL/min, what was the cardiac output? Name the principle involved.
6. How do you account for the low BP?
7. What makes the skin pale, cold and sweaty (clammy)? Of what general response is this a characteristic?

8. Draw a normal lead II ECG and show how it aligns with a ventricular action potential. What feature corresponds with the ST segment?
9. What causes ST segment displacement in myocardial ischaemia?
10. How does dual antiplatelet therapy (aspirin and ticagrelor) improve the prognosis?
11. What is the source of the raised troponin T?
12. What are the dangers of abruptly restoring blood flow to a tissue after prolonged ischaemia?
13. What is a ventricular ectopic beat, how does it affect stroke volume and what might cause it?

## ANSWERS

1. The left main coronary artery usually supplies the anterior and lateral parts of the left ventricle and the anterior two thirds of the septum. It divides into the left anterior descending and circumflex arteries. The right coronary artery supplies the inferior surface of the left ventricle, the inferior septum and the right ventricle. A functional end artery is one with insufficient arterial anastomoses to maintain tissue viability if the main vessel is obstructed (Figure 15.6).

2. A thrombus (organized blood clot) forms on an atheromatous plaque. Atheroma originates with the transendothelial passage of lipoproteins, fibrinogen and monocytes (Section 9.9). Endothelial nitric oxide, an inhibitor of platelet aggregation, is low in atheromatous regions, enabling platelets to aggregate and initiate thrombosis (Chapter 9, Sections 9.10 and 9.11).

3. Chemosensitive sympathetic afferents in the myocardium mediate cardiac ischaemic pain (Figure 16.10). Convergence with pathways from the arms in the spinal column may explain the 'referred pain'.

4. The left ventricle wall is ~1 cm thick. The time needed for $O_2$ diffusion increases as distance squared, so diffusion is too slow to support myocyte metabolism beyond ~100 μm from the chamber lumen (Table 1.1).

5. For an $(A - V)_{O2}$ of 100 mL/L (i.e. 190 − 90) and an $O_2$ uptake of 300 mL/min, the cardiac output must be 3 L/min (i.e. 300/100). This is Fick's principle (Section 6.1). Cardiac output is depressed.

6. Ischaemia impairs contractility (Figures 6.22 and 6.23). This reduces the stroke volume and BP.

7. The skin is pale and cold due to sympathetic-mediated veno- and vasoconstriction, respectively (Section 15.3). The 'clamminess' (cold sweat) is due to sympathetic sudomotor activity. The patient is in cardiogenic shock (Section 18.2).

8. See Figure 5.3. The ST segment corresponds to the plateau of the action potential.

9. The ST segment is displaced by injury currents (Figure 5.11b). Injury currents develop because the action potential of ischaemic myocytes is less positive than that of the neighbouring normal myocytes and the resting potential is less negative than normal.

10. The primary event of thrombosis is platelet activation and aggregation (see Chapter 9, Section 9.11). This is promoted by platelet thromboxane, which is synthesized through cyclooxygenase (Section 13.5). Aspirin inhibits platelet cyclooxygenase, helping prevent further platelet aggregation. Other antiplatelets (e.g. ticagrelor, cangrelor, clopidogrel, prasugrel) inhibit a platelet receptor, $P2Y_{12}$, preventing a different aggregation signal. The combination of aspirin and a further antiplatelet improves outcomes over aspirin alone.

11. Troponin T and I are components of the cardiac sarcomere. They are released into the blood when cardiomyocytes are damaged and are excreted through the kidneys, so exaggerated rises are seen in those with poor renal function.

12. There is reperfusion injury due to contracture (caused by cytosolic $Ca^{2+}$ overload), white cell activation and free $O_2$ radical generation (Sections 6.12 and 13.9). Reperfusion arrhythmias (such as ventricular tachycardia and fibrillation; see Chapter 5, Section 5.10) are common in the immediate phase after opening an occluded coronary artery, and are largely caused by cytosolic $Ca^{2+}$ overload.

13. A ventricular ectopic beat is a premature systole triggered from within the ventricle (Figure 5.13). The trigger is often a delayed afterdepolarization (Figure 3.16). Excitation does not follow the normal route, so the contraction is ill co-ordinated and generates little output. The pulse appears to miss a beat.

## CASE 3: THE HAEMORRHAGIC HEAVY DRINKER

*A 60-year-old civil servant, known to be a regular, heavy drinker, with a deteriorating work performance, collapsed after vomiting copious fresh blood (massive haematemesis). When examined in the Accident & Emergency Department, he was confused, with a pale, clammy skin. His pulse was regular, but weak and rapid (120 min⁻¹). Recumbent blood pressure (BP) was 100/75 mmHg. When the patient was sat up, he felt faint and pressure dropped to 80/65 mmHg. His history of alcoholism, coupled with a firm, palpably enlarged liver and characteristic skin changes, indicated hepatic cirrhosis. Rectal examination revealed black 'tarry' stools characteristic of melaena (old, partly digested blood from a bleed high in the gastrointestinal tract). Endoscopy revealed bleeding oesophageal varices (distended veins in the lower oesophagus), the result of portal vein hypertension caused by alcoholic cirrhosis.*

*A cannula was inserted into the small, constricted dorsal vein of the hand (with difficulty), to infuse a crystalloid fluid (Hartmann's solution) while awaiting type-specific blood. Large-bore venous access was difficult, so a central venous catheter was inserted into the internal jugular vein, which recorded a central venous pressure (CVP) of <4 cmH$_2$O (subatmospheric). This line was used to infuse vasopressin. Haematocrit was 0.36 on admission, and haemoglobin 11.8 g/dL. Urine output was 20 mL/hour, and the patient complained of thirst.*

*Rehydration and blood transfusion was followed by emergency endoscopy and the injection of a sclerosant solution into the gastro-oesophageal varices to induce local thrombosis. On discharge, the patient was prescribed daily propranolol.*

## QUESTIONS

1. What is a 'portal circulation'? Sketch the blood supply to the liver.
2. Why does hepatic cirrhosis cause oesophageal bleeding?
3. Was the CVP normal? Was stroke volume affected? (Hint: consider the pulse pressure.)
4. What was the recumbent patient's mean BP? Was he severely hypotensive when supine?
5. Why was the arterial pressure also measured in orthostasis and why did the pressure fall?
6. Which class of blood vessel regulates mean BP? Did the skin provide any evidence of vascular regulation?
7. Is the peripheral venoconstriction (obvious when venipuncture was attempted) likely to be of benefit?
8. What cardiac responses helped to maintain mean arterial pressure, and what induced them?
9. Identify three types of afferent receptor that drive the cardiovascular responses to hypovolaemia.
10. What accounts for the low haematocrit and haemoglobin concentration on admission, if the values were normal previously?
11. Why was the urine output monitored?
12. What mechanism might account for the patient's thirst?
13. How might the vasopressin infusion be of benefit?
14. What is propranolol and how might it help?

## ANSWERS

1. A portal circulation is one downstream of, and in series with, another circulation; the tissue receives venous blood from the upstream organ (Section 1.8). The liver has a dual blood supply: a small arterial supply from the hepatic artery and a much larger portal supply, namely intestine-derived venous blood in the portal vein (Figure 1.5). The hepatic vein drains the liver.

2. Hepatic cirrhosis distorts the liver and raises its vascular resistance. This raises portal vein pressure (normally 5–6 mmHg). The portal vein is linked to the lower oesophageal veins by venous collaterals, so swollen oesophageal veins (varices) develop. Being very superficial, they bleed readily.

3. The patient's CVP, <4 cmH$_2$O, was low (normal ~4 cmH$_2$O), due to hypovolaemia. The low CVP reduced stroke volume (Frank–Starling mechanism), as shown by the low pulse pressure, 25 mmHg (i.e. systolic minus diastolic blood pressure = 100 – 75 mmHg). Pulse pressure depends on stroke volume (Figure 7.4) and on arterial compliance.

4. Mean brachial artery BP is diastolic pressure plus one third of the pulse pressure (equation 8.4). The recumbent mean was 83 mmHg, that is, normotensive. The patient was therefore in compensated haemorrhagic shock (Figure 18.3).

5. The doctor was assessing the severity of the hypovolaemia, which is not apparent from the compensated supine value. Orthostasis causes peripheral venous blood pooling, lowering CVP and stroke volume further, so the pulse pressure fell to 15 mmHg (80 – 65 mmHg).

6. Resistance vessels (arterioles, terminal arteries) regulate mean BP (Section 1.6). The low skin temperature and pallor indicated cutaneous vaso- and venoconstriction, respectively, caused by increased sympathetic activity, circulating catecholamines, angiotensin II and vasopressin.

7. Peripheral venoconstriction displaces blood into the thorax and thus limits the fall in CVP and stroke volume.

8. Sympathetic-mediated tachycardia (120 min$^{-1}$) and increased contractility helped to maintain cardiac output and therefore arterial pressure. The tachycardia is also aided by reduced vagal parasympathetic activity.

9. (1) The activity of carotid sinus and aortic arch baroreceptors is reduced by the fall in pulse pressure (Figure 18.2). (2) Cardiopulmonary receptor input is reduced by the reduced CVP. (3) Peripheral arterial chemoreceptor activity is increased by hypoperfusion and metabolic acidosis (Figure 18.3). The altered input into the nucleus tractus solitarius triggers a reflex increase in sympathetic activity (Figure 16.18).

10. The patient's haemodilution is caused by an 'internal transfusion' of interstitial fluid into capillary and venular blood (Figure 18.3). Capillary pressure is reduced by the venous hypotension and precapillary resistance vessel contraction (Figure 11.4). This allows plasma colloid osmotic pressure to predominate and draw water into the circulation (Starling's principle of fluid exchange). The interstitium is topped up with water drawn osmotically from the intracellular compartment by extracellular fluid hyperglycaemia (Section 18.2).

11. Urine output was monitored because acute renal failure, caused by acute tubular necrosis, is a potentially fatal complication of severe hypotension.

12. Thirst is stimulated by the action of angiotensin II on the subfornical organ near the hypothalamus. Angiotensin levels are high due to the renal secretion of renin in response to the increased sympathetic activity, low perfusion pressure and low tubular salt load (Figure 14.12).

13. Vasopressin contracts the splanchnic resistance vessels feeding the portal vein. This temporarily reduces portal vein pressure.

14. Propranolol is a non-selective $\beta$ adrenergic receptor blocker. It reduces heart rate and cardiac output by blocking cardiac $\beta_1$ receptors, and it raises splanchnic vascular resistance by blocking vascular $\beta_2$ receptors. Together, these effects reduce portal vein pressure.

## CASE 4: THE HYPERTENSIVE FAINTER

A 45-year-old travelling salesman, attending a local Accident & Emergency Department after a minor accident, was told his blood pressure (BP) was 180/110 mmHg. His general practitioner subsequently recorded supine brachial artery pressures of 185/110 and 165/105 mmHg on 2 visits. On the last visit, the pressure during standing was 155/110 mmHg and his heart rate increased from 75 (supine) to 85 bpm (standing). The patient was obese and admitted to a regular, moderately heavy alcohol intake. Cardiac signs were normal. After checking the retina, the doctor made a provisional diagnosis of essential hypertension. He started the patient on doxazosin (an unusual first choice in the absence of benign prostatic hyperplasia) and advised the patient to lose weight, avoid added salt and salty processed foods and reduce his alcohol intake.

After a few days on doxazosin, the patient returned because he felt faint and dizzy on standing up, and on one occasion had collapsed for a few minutes. Exercise also made him feel faint and dizzy. The doctor recorded a supine pressure of 145/95 mmHg, falling to 90/65 mmHg on standing, with faintness and fading vision that made the patient lie down again. The doctor stopped the doxazosin and started the patient on ramipril, which resolved the problem.

## QUESTIONS

1. How is brachial arterial BP measured in humans?
2. What were the mean pressure and pulse pressure on the first visit to the GP? Why did the GP insist on a second visit?
3. At what systolic/diastolic pressure is hypertension usually diagnosed?
4. What two parameters determine mean BP? Which one is responsible for established hypertension?
5. Why should the patient reduce his salt intake?
6. What structural changes occur in peripheral resistance vessels in hypertension?
7. What are the principal factors regulating vascular tone?
8. What changes occur in elastic arteries in hypertension? Which aspects of arterial BP does this affect?
9. How might mental stress contribute to hypertension?
10. What are the long-term effects of systemic hypertension on the heart?
11. Since most drugs have side effects, why treat symptomless hypertension?
12. Doxazosin is an $\alpha_1$ adrenergic receptor antagonist. What is the role of $\alpha_1$ adrenergic receptors in vascular control?
13. Explain how doxazosin caused dizziness (1) on standing and (2) during exercise.
14. How does ramipril act?
15. Name three other classes of drug used to treat essential hypertension, and state their modes of action.

## ANSWERS

1. Brachial BP is traditionally measured by sphygmomanometry, with auscultation of the Korotkoff sounds (Figure 8.12). Automatic cuff devices are commonly used instead, but they are less accurate.

2. The pulse pressure was 75 mmHg (185 − 110). The mean pressure was 135 mmHg (diastolic plus one third pulse pressure). The alerting response (Section 16.8) often raises pressure during the initial visit to the doctor (white coat hypertension), hence the repeat visit.

3. Brachial artery pressure in normal 45-year-old white men averages 130/78 mmHg (Figure 17.10) and is a little higher in people of Afro-Caribbean origin. Systolic pressures >140 mmHg and diastolic pressures >90 mmHg in young to middle-aged patients substantially increase the risk of strokes, ischaemic heart disease, cardiac failure and renal failure, so 140/90 is considered the diagnostic level.

4. Mean BP = cardiac output × total peripheral resistance. In established hypertension, cardiac output is normal. One might expect that hypertension is solely due to increased vascular resistance; however, long-term blood pressure regulation is closely linked with control of circulating blood volume by the kidneys. (Compare the closed vs open model of the circulation in Figure 16.12.) The pathology of hypertension may involve the kidneys, vasculature and autonomic nervous system and is discussed in detail in Chapter 18, Section 18.4.

5. In some patients, hypertension correlates strongly with salt intake. Hypertension may be due to an imbalance between salt intake and defective renal salt excretion.

6. The media thickens and the lumen narrows (eutrophic inward remodelling, later hypertrophy; Figure 18.6). Resistance is inversely proportional to the fourth power of the lumen radius (Poiseuille's law), so a 10% narrowing raises resistance by 46%.

7. *Intrinsic factors* include the myogenic response (Section 13.2), shear stress-mediated vasodilatation by endothelial nitric oxide (Section 13.3), other endothelial products (prostacyclin, endothelium-derived hyperpolarizing factor, endothelin), tissue products mediating metabolic vasodilatation (Section 13.4) and autacoids. *Extrinsic factors* are the ubiquitous sympathetic noradrenergic vasoconstrictor fibres (Section 14.1), and circulating vasoactive hormones, notably adrenaline, angiotensin II and vasopressin.

8. Hypertension ages the elastic vessels prematurely, causing elastin fragmentation, dilatation and increased stiffness. The reduced compliance raises pulse pressure and systolic pressure (Figure 18.7). The rapid return of the reflected wave adds further to the systolic hypertension (Figure 18.8).

9. Stress evokes the alerting response, which comprises tachycardia, muscle vasodilatation, vasoconstriction in the renal, splanchnic and cutaneous circulations, and increased BP (Section 16.8). An exaggerated alerting response and the attendant repeated episodes of transient hypertension may contribute to resistance vessel remodelling.

10. Systemic hypertension increases left ventricular work (Section 7.5), the tension-time index (Section 7.14) and $O_2$ demand. The left ventricle myocytes hypertrophy, thickening the wall (concentric hypertrophy). Eventually, left ventricular failure may develop.

11. Treatment is justified by the increased morbidity and mortality from strokes, ischaemic heart disease, cardiac failure and renal failure.

12. Alpha$_1$ adrenergic receptors mediate the vasoconstriction evoked by sympathetic activity and circulating catecholamines (Sections 12.5 and 12.6). Consequently, $\alpha_1$ blockers reduce BP.

13. (1) On standing, BP falls initially because venous pooling in the legs reduces cardiac filling pressure and therefore stroke volume (Frank–Starling mechanism). The resulting postural hypotension reduces cerebral blood flow, leading to dizziness. Doxazosin (which should not have been the drug of first choice) blocks the compensatory, sympathetic-mediated contraction of resistance vessel. (2) During exercise, metabolic vasodilatation in the active muscles lowers total peripheral resistance, but BP is maintained by sympathetic vasoconstriction in inactive tissues, along with increased cardiac output. Also, increased sympathetic drive to the active muscle prevents excessive metabolic dilatation. When these effects are blocked by doxazosin, exercise can cause hypotension, cerebral hypoperfusion and giddiness.

14. The ACD therapeutic regime is considered best practice. 'A' is for angiotensin-converting enzyme inhibitors, such as ramipril, which reduce angiotensin II formation, or angiotensin receptor blockers (ARBs), such as losartan. Angiotensin II raises BP by direct vasoconstriction, peripheral neuromodulation, central presympathetic stimulation, thirst and aldosterone secretion. If side effects (cough) are a problem, ARBs are used instead.

15. (1) The 'C' of ACD refers to Ca$^{2+}$-channel blockers, for example, amlodipine. This reduces Ca$^{2+}$ entry into vascular myocytes and thus relaxes the resistance vessels, lowering BP. Sympathetic neurotransmission is not impaired, so postural hypotension is not a problem. (2) The 'D' of ACD refers to diuretics, such as the thiazide bendroflumethiazide. These cause salt and water excretion, and dilate resistance vessels (perhaps by opening $K_{ATP}$ channels), lowering BP. (3) β adrenergic receptor blockers, such as propranolol, reduce cardiac output and hence BP. They also reduce the sympathetic stimulation of the renin–angiotensin–aldosterone system and act centrally to reduce sympathetic outflow.

## CASE 5: THE BREATHLESS WOMAN

*A 70-year-old woman complains that she can no longer do her housework or climb the stairs without frequent rests; she also gets very breathless. At night she wakes up struggling to breathe, and finds that sleeping propped up by several pillows helps. Her ankles swell as the day progresses, but improve after a night's rest.*

*On examination the doctor notes that her breathing is rapid. Chest auscultation reveals fine, basal crackles (crepitations). The pulse is regular and arterial BP is within the normal range, but the neck veins are distended even in the upright position. The doctor estimates the central venous pressure (CVP) to be about 18 cmH$_2$O. The apex beat is palpable faintly in the anterior axillary line of the fifth intercostal space. Examining the puffy ankles, he presses on the skin over the tibia for a minute and observes that a deep pit forms.*

*A chest X-ray shows a cardiothoracic ratio of 0.69, congested pulmonary vessels and the thin horizontal lines of interseptal oedema. The electrocardiogram shows left bundle branch block and echocardiography reveals severe biventricular dysfunction with a dilated left ventricle. A diagnosis of biventricular cardiac failure is made. She is treated initially with ramipril, spironolactone and furosemide, with monitoring of her renal function and electrolytes. When central venous pressure reduces to normal by this treatment, she is started on bisoprolol and the dose slowly titrated up.*

## QUESTIONS

1. How is CVP estimated, using inspection of the jugular veins?
2. What is the relation between CVP and stroke volume?
3. What are the chief roles of the Frank–Starling mechanism in humans?
4. Which factors govern the size of CVP?
5. Can cardiac distension be disadvantageous?
6. Might lowering the arterial pressure help the failing heart?
7. What key intracellular parameter triggers cardiac contraction and how is it changed in cardiac failure?
8. Draw a pair of ventricular function curves to illustrate the meaning of 'impaired contractility'.
9. What factors can raise contractile energy besides the Frank–Starling mechanism?
10. How can cardiac contractility be assessed in humans?
11. What is the link between pulmonary vessel distension and dyspnoea?
12. What causes crepitations (crackles) in the lungs?
13. Why was the dyspnoea worse at night (paroxysmal nocturnal dyspnoea), and why did sleeping propped up help?
14. Why is the pitting test negative in normal tissues?
15. What factors govern the distribution of fluid between the vascular and interstitial compartment and how are they changed in cardiac oedema?
16. Why did the ankle swelling get worse during the day?
17. What might account for the patient's poor exercise tolerance?

# ANSWERS

1. The jugular vein is as a valveless tube connected to the right atrium (Figure 8.23). A vein collapses when its luminal pressure is below atmospheric pressure. If the point of jugular vein collapse (pressure equal to atmosphere) is, say, 18 cm vertically above the right atrium, atrial pressure (CVP) must be atmospheric pressure plus 18 cm of fluid.

2. CVP determines right ventricle diastolic distension, which governs the energy of contraction and stroke volume (Section 6.4, Figures 6.10 and 6.19).

3. (1) The Frank–Starling mechanism equalizes the outputs of the right and left ventricles. (2) It helps raise stroke volume during exercise. (3) It can cause postural hypotension (Section 17.1). (4) It mediates the arterial hypotension of hypovolaemia (Section 18.2).

4. CVP depends on blood volume and distribution. Blood distribution between the thoracic and peripheral veins depends on posture (effect of gravity), movement (muscle pump) and peripheral sympathetic venous tone.

5. As the ventricular function curve flattens, distension no longer raises contractile energy significantly, but it impairs the conversion of wall tension into luminal pressure (Laplace's law; Figure 6.14), and may cause functional incompetence of the atrioventricular valves.

6. If arterial pressure is lowered, less energy is used in raising ventricular pressure. This leaves more energy to eject the stroke volume; see the 'pump function curve' (Figure 6.15).

7. Release of the sarcoplasmic reticulum $Ca^{2+}$ store generates a systolic $Ca^{2+}$ transient that, via the troponin-tropomyosin complex, triggers myosin head-actin interaction and the sliding filament process (Sections 3.2 and 3.5). In heart failure, the $Ca^{2+}$ transient is small and sluggish.

8. See Figure 18.9. Impaired contractility is a reduced force of contraction for a given filling pressure or cardiac distension.

9. Sympathetic noradrenaline activates $\beta_1$ adrenergic receptors which, via the adenylate cyclase–cyclic adenosine monophosphate–protein kinase A pathway, increase the plateau $Ca^{2+}$ current, $Ca^{2+}$ store and systolic $Ca^{2+}$ transient, raising contractility (Section 6.10). Downregulation of $\beta_1$ adrenergic receptors weakens this mechanism in advanced cardiac failure (Section 18.5).

10. Human ventricular contractility is assessed by (1) the ejection fraction measured by echocardiography, cardiac magnetic resonance imaging or, less commonly, radionuclide angiography (normally > approximately 55%, depending on modality) and (2) ventricular $dP/dt_{max}$ measured through an intracardiac catheter (Figure 2.5).

11. The pulmonary vessels are distended because left atrial pressure is raised by left ventricular failure, renal salt and water retention and peripheral venoconstriction. Congestion and oedema stiffen the lungs, increasing the work of breathing.

12. Crepitations indicate oedema of the conducting airways, caused by increased pulmonary capillary pressure, secondary to the raised left atrial pressure.

13. The supine position redistributes peripheral venous blood into the thorax (Figure 8.24). This exacerbates pulmonary congestion and oedema. Movement of oedema fluid from the legs into the circulation overnight exacerbates the problem. Sleeping propped up helps prevent these gravity-based problems.

14. Normal interstitial fluid does not pit readily because the glycosaminoglycan (GAG) matrix offers a high resistance to flow (Figure 11.9). In oedema, GAGs are diluted, so fluid is easily displaced.

15. The Starling principle of fluid exchange describes the factors (Section 11.1). Capillary pressure is increased by the raised venous pressure (Figure 11.5). Also, dilution of plasma proteins by renal salt and water retention lowers plasma colloid osmotic pressure moderately.

16. Gravity raises leg capillary pressure (Figure 11.5). Oedema improves overnight because lower-limb capillary pressure falls in the supine position, allowing lymphatic drainage to outpace fluid filtration.

17. The exercise intolerance is caused by the impaired responses of heart rate and stroke volume to exercise (Figure 18.11), dyspnoea and increased skeletal muscle fatigability.

## FURTHER READING

Kumar PJ, Clark ML. *Clinical Medicine*, 9th edn. Edinburgh: Elsevier, 2017.

Lilly LS, ed. *Pathophysiology of Heart Disease: a Collaborative Project of Medical Students and Faculty*, 6th edn. Baltimore, MD: Williams and Wilkins, 2015.

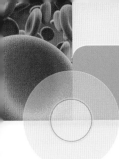

# Appendix 1: Human cardiovascular parameters

Values refer to a young, resting human adult at heart level unless specified otherwise.

## AORTIC PARAMETERS

| | |
|---|---|
| Cross-sectional area at root | 4–5 cm$^2$ |
| Reynolds number at peak flow | ~4600 |
| Stroke distance | 15–20 cm |
| Stroke volume, rest | 70–80 cm$^3$ |
| Stroke volume, exercise | 110–120 cm$^3$ |
| Velocity of blood, peak ejection | 70 cm s$^{-1}$ |
| Velocity, mean during ejection | 50 cm s$^{-1}$ |
| Velocity, mean over whole cycle | 20 cm s$^{-1}$ |
| Velocity, mean during ejection in heavy exercise | 250 cm s$^{-1}$ |

## AREA

| | |
|---|---|
| Body surface, 70-kg adult | 1.8 m$^2$ |
| Capillary endothelium of lungs (combined) | 90 m$^2$ |
| Capillary endothelium, all skeletal muscles | 280 m$^2$ |

## ARTERIAL PARAMETERS (SYSTEMIC AND PULMONARY)

| | |
|---|---|
| Brachial artery pressure at age 30 years | 125/70 mmHg |
| Foot artery, standing, mean | 183 mmHg |
| Compliance, elastic arteries at 30 years | 1.5 mL mmHg$^{-1}$ |
| Pulse velocity, young | 4–5 m s$^{-1}$ |
| Pulse velocity, old | 10–15 m s$^{-1}$ |
| Pulmonary artery pressure, supine | 25/12 mmHg |
| Pulmonary artery pressure, standing | 22/9 mmHg |
| Pulmonary artery pressure, heavy exercise | 40/24 mmHg |

## BLOOD BIOPHYSICAL PARAMETERS

| | |
|---|---|
| Blood volume, total | 5 L |
| Blood volume, venous | ~3 L |
| Blood volume, pulmonary | 0.6 L |
| Density, $\rho$ | 1.06 g cm$^{-3}$ |
| Haematocrit, female | 0.40 |
| Haematocrit, male | 0.45 |
| Oxygen content, see *Oxygen* | |
| Relative viscosity, blood/water | ~4 |
| Relative viscosity, plasma/water | 1.7 |
| Viscosity, water at 37 °C | 0.69 mPa s |

## BLOOD FLOW AND VELOCITY

| | |
|---|---|
| Cerebral, grey matter | 100 mL min$^{-1}$ 100 g$^{-1}$ |
| Coronary, resting individual | 70–80 mL min$^{-1}$ 100 g$^{-1}$ |
| Coronary, maximum | 300–400 mL min$^{-1}$ 100 g$^{-1}$ |
| Skeletal muscle, rest (phasic) | 3–5 mL min$^{-1}$ 100 g$^{-1}$ |
| Skeletal muscle, rest (postural) | 15 mL min$^{-1}$ 100 g$^{-1}$ |
| Skeletal muscle, maximum | 100–200 mL min$^{-1}$ 100 g$^{-1}$ |
| Skin, thermoneutral | 10–20 mL min$^{-1}$ 100 g$^{-1}$ |
| Skin, maximum | 150–200 mL min$^{-1}$ 100 g$^{-1}$ |
| Transit time, coronary circulation | 15 s |
| Transit time, systemic capillary bed | 0.5–2.0 s |
| Transit time, left ventricle to left ventricle | 1 min |
| Velocity, aortic, peak | 70 cm s$^{-1}$ |
| Velocity, capillary | 0.05–0.1 cm s$^{-1}$ |

## CARDIAC PARAMETERS

| | |
|---|---|
| Cardiac index | 3 L min$^{-1}$ m$^{-2}$ |
| Cardiac output, rest | 4–7 L min$^{-1}$ |
| Cardiac output, maximum | 20–35 L min$^{-1}$ |
| Electrical axis | −30 ° to +110 ° |
| Weight of heart | 300–350 g |

## TIMING

| | |
|---|---|
| Cardiac cycle, typical, rest | 0.9 s |
| ECG, P wave duration | 0.08 s |
| ECG, PR interval | <0.2 s |
| ECG, QRS wave | <0.1 s |
| ECG, ST segment | 0.2–0.4 s |

| | |
|---|---|
| Heart rate, rest | 50–100 min⁻¹ |
| Heart rate, maximum | 180–200 min⁻¹ |
| Intrinsic pacemaker rate | 105 min⁻¹ |
| Isovolumetric contraction | 0.05 s |
| Isovolumetric relaxation | 0.08 s |
| Ventricular filling | 0.5 s |
| Ventricular systole | 0.35 s |
| Ventricular ejection | 0.30 s |

## PRESSURE, RELATIVE TO ATMOSPHERIC (760 mmHg)

| | |
|---|---|
| Central venous pressure | 0–10 mmHg |
| Left ventricle, end-diastole, supine | 9 mmHg |
| Left ventricle, end-diastole, standing | 4–5 mmHg |
| Left ventricle, peak systolic | ~125 mmHg |
| Right ventricle, end-diastole, supine | 4 mmHg |
| Right ventricle, end-diastole, standing | 0 mmHg (atmospheric) |
| Right ventricle, peak systolic, supine | 25 mmHg |
| Right ventricle, peak systolic, standing | 22 mmHg |

## VOLUME

| | |
|---|---|
| End-diastolic volume, ventricle | 120 mL |
| End-systolic volume | 40–50 mL |
| Ejection fraction | 67% |
| Stroke volume (at rest) | 70–80 mL |
| Stroke volume (during exercise) | 110–120 mL |
| Stroke work (at rest) | 1 Joule |

## CELLULAR/SUBCELLULAR DIMENSIONS

| | |
|---|---|
| Contractile filament, myocardial actin (thin) | 6 nm diameter, 1.05 μm long |
| Contractile filament, myosin (thick) | 11 nm diameter, 1.6 μm long |
| Desmosome gap (cadherin) | 25 nm |
| Gap junction (nexus, connexon) | 2–4 nm |
| Muscle, cardiac myocyte | 10–20 μm diameter, 50–100 μm long |
| Muscle, cardiac Purkinje fibre | 40–80 μm diameter |
| Muscle, skeletal fibre (typically) | 50 μm diameter |
| Muscle, vascular myocytes | 4 μm diameter, 20–60 μm long |
| Red cell | 8 μm diameter |
| Sarcomere length, normal diastole | 1.8–2.0 μm |
| Sarcomere, maximum stretch | 2.2–2.3 μm |

## DENSITY AT 20 °C

| | |
|---|---|
| Blood | 1.06 g mL⁻¹ |
| Mercury | 13.55 g mL⁻¹ |
| Water | 1.00 g mL⁻¹ |

## DIAMETER

| | |
|---|---|
| Aortic root | 2.5 cm |
| Arteriole | 10–100 μm |
| Arteriovenous anastomosis | 20–130 μm |
| Artery, large named (e.g. iliac) | 1–2 cm |
| Artery, medium to small named (e.g. radial, cerebral, coronary) | 0.2–0.5 cm |
| Artery, resistance vessel | 100–500 μm |
| Capillary | 4–8 μm |
| Postcapillary (pericytic) venule | 15–40 μm |
| Venule | 50–200 μm |

## DISTANCE AND THICKNESS

| | |
|---|---|
| Aortic valve to iliac bifurcation | 0.5 m |
| Capillary to parenchymal cell | 10–20 μm |
| Capillary wall | 0.2–0.3 μm |
| Sympathetic neuromuscular gap | 0.1 μm |
| Wall of left ventricle | 1.0 cm |
| Wall of right ventricle | 0.5 cm |

## ELECTROPHYSIOLOGY

| | |
|---|---|
| Cardiac resting potential | −80 to −90 mV |
| Cardiac action potential | +20 to +30 mV |
| Cardiac pacemaker potential | −50 to −70 mV |
| Cardiac plateau potential | 0 to −20 mV |
| Cardiac action potential duration | 200–400 ms |
| Conduction velocity, atrial | 1 m s⁻¹ |
| Conduction velocity, atrioventricular node | 0.05 m s⁻¹ |
| Conduction velocity, Purkinje | 3–5 m s⁻¹ |
| Conduction velocity, ventricle wall | 0.5–1.0 m s⁻¹ |
| Equilibrium potential, $Ca^{2+}$ | +124 mV |
| Equilibrium potential, $Cl^-$ (vascular) | −23 mV |
| Equilibrium potential, $K^+$ | −94 mV |
| Equilibrium potential, $Na^+$ | +70 mV |
| Vascular myocyte, basal | −50 to −60 mV |

# IONIC AND OTHER CONCENTRATIONS

| | |
|---|---|
| ATP, intracellular | ~5 mM |
| $Ca^{2+}$, free ions, extracellular | 1.2 mM |
| $Ca^{2+}$, cardiac cytosol, diastole | 0.1 µM |
| $Ca^{2+}$, cardiac cytosol, systole | 2 µM |
| $Cl^-$, extracellular | 120–134 mM |
| $Cl^-$, intracellular (vascular muscle) | 54 mM |
| $HCO_3^-$, extracellular | 27 mM |
| $HCO_3^-$, intracellular | 10 mM |
| $K^+$, extracellular | 3.5–5.5 mM |
| $K^+$, intracellular | 140 mM |
| Myoglobin, cardiac | $3.4\ g\ L^{-1}$ |
| $Na^+$, extracellular | 135–145 mM |
| $Na^+$, intracellular | 10 mM |
| pH, extracellular | 7.4 |
| pH, intracellular | 7.0–7.1 |

# MASS OF SOFT TISSUE IN A 70-KG HUMAN

| | |
|---|---|
| Blood | 5 kg |
| Brain | 1.5 kg |
| Gastrointestinal tract and liver | 4 kg |
| Heart | 0.35 kg |
| Kidneys | 0.3 kg |
| Lungs | 1 kg |
| Skeletal muscle | 40 kg |
| Skin | 2–3 kg |

# OXYGEN (REST)

| | |
|---|---|
| Blood content, arterial | $195\ mL\ O_2\ L^{-1}$ |
| Blood content, mixed venous | $150\ mL\ O_2\ L^{-1}$ |
| Extraction, whole body | 25% |
| Extraction from coronary blood | 65%–75% |
| Consumption, basal, 70-kg adult | $250\ mL\ min^{-1}$ |
| Consumption, maximal ($V_{O_2max}$) | $\sim3000\ mL\ min^{-1}$ |
| Partial pressure, inspired | 160 mmHg (21 kPa) |
| Partial pressure, arterial | 100 mmHg (13 kPa) |
| Partial pressure, mixed venous | 40 mmHg |
| Partial pressure, cardiac myocyte | 5–20 mmHg |
| Saturation, arterial | 97% |
| Saturation, mixed venous | 72% |

# PRESSURE

See also *Arterial parameters*, *Venous pressure*, *Cardiac parameters* and Table 15.1 (*Pulmonary circulation*)

| | |
|---|---|
| Capillary, arterial limb, heart level | 32–36 mmHg |
| Capillary, venous limb, heart level | 12–25 mmHg |
| Capillary, foot during standing | 95 mmHg |
| Pulmonary capillary, supine | 13 mmHg |
| Pulmonary capillary, upright | 9 mmHg |
| Mean circulatory pressure (arrested) | 7 mmHg |
| Pressure drop across capillary bed | 20–30 mmHg |
| Pressure drop across resistance vessels | 40–50 mmHg |

# RESISTANCE

| | |
|---|---|
| Pulmonary circulation | $0.003\ mmHg\ min\ mL^{-1}$ |
| Systemic circulation, rest | $0.02\ mmHg\ min\ mL^{-1}$ |

# VENOUS PRESSURE

| | |
|---|---|
| Antecubital or femoral vein, heart level | 8–10 mmHg |
| Foot vein, standing | 90 mmHg |
| Pulmonary vein, supine | 9 mmHg |
| Pulmonary vein, standing | 5 mmHg |
| Systemic venule, heart level | 12–20 mmHg |
| Venoatrial junction | 0–10 mmHg |

# VOLUME

| | |
|---|---|
| Water as % body weight (male, female) | 60% (m), 55% (f) |
| Total water, 70-kg male, 55-kg female | 42 L (m), 30 L (f) |
| Intracellular water, (two thirds) | 28 L (m), 20 L (f) |
| Extracellular water, (one third) | 14 L (m), 10 L (f) |
| Interstitial water | 11 L (m), 8 L (f) |
| Plasma volume | 3 L (m), 2 L (f) |
| Blood volume | 5 L (m), 3.5 L (f) |

Note: page numbers in *italics* refer to figures and tables.

Index